CONTACT LENS PRACTICE AND PATIENT MANAGEMENT

CONTACT LENS PRACTICE AND PATIENT MANAGEMENT

by

IRVING P. FILDERMAN

and

PAUL F. WHITE

CHILTON BOOK COMPANY *PHILADELPHIA NEW YORK LONDON*

FIRST EDITION

PUBLISHED IN PHILADELPHIA BY CHILTON BOOK COMPANY
AND SIMULTANEOUSLY IN ONTARIO, CANADA,
BY THOMAS NELSON & SONS LTD.
LIBRARY OF CONGRESS CATALOG CARD NUMBER 68-23518
DESIGNED BY HARRY BRODSKY
MANUFACTURED IN THE UNITED STATES OF AMERICA

DEDICATED TO

THE BLESSED MEMORY

OF

JOHN W. WHITE, MOLLIE FILDERMAN, AND EDGAR C. HAAS, SR.

PREFACE

The primary purpose of this book is to prepare beginners and assist experienced practitioners in contact lens practice and patient management. A secondary purpose is to provide a foundation so that subsequent developments in contact lenses can be understood, evaluated, and integrated.

There is a large quantity of contact lens literature, which contains a mass of details. Most of these details are not complex in themselves; complexity comes from the amount of material. We have tried to select all the important principles from this mass, to integrate them with our own concepts, to organize them to fulfill the aforementioned purposes, and to present them clearly.

As private practitioners, we are acutely aware that the value of this book will be measured by its ability to give clinical assistance. As authors, we are equally aware that it is difficult to write so that theory is transferred easily to practice. Such awareness guides the style of presentation and the organization of the material.

Language is meant to communicate thoughts, not to cloud them. Because scientific facts are communicated more clearly by simplicity of expression, we have written this book using a simple, direct style.

We have tried to organize the material into a logical, comprehensive system of contact lens practice and patient care. There are two general sections in this book: Part I, Clinical Practice; and Part II, Clinical Reference.

Subject matter most often used in daily practice is presented in Part I in the sequence of stages used clinically.

When a patient seeks contact lenses, the advisability of application must be evaluated. The first stage of contact lens practice and patient management involves the selection of patients for whom contact lens application probably will be successful.

After a patient is accepted for contact lens fitting, the most logical lenses for this individual must be selected. The second stage of clinical practice involves the selection of lens designs and specifications that probably will achieve the best results.

Once such lenses are selected, they must be ordered, verified, and perhaps modified. The third stage of clinical practice involves the laboratory procedures used to prepare the lenses for dispensing.

After the lenses are ready for dispensing, the patient must be prepared to assume certain responsibilities. Thus, the fourth stage of clinical practice involves education directed toward establishment of proper patient techniques of lens handling and care, and the establishment of guides for wear and use.

Once the patient starts to use lenses, proper serial examination must be used to produce desired adaptation, and early detection and remediation of undesired responses. The fifth stage of clinical practice involves the control and management of adaptation for the duration of contact lens wear.

Knowledge of the technical aspects of contact lens application may not be adequate to produce the desired results for patient and practitioner. The sixth stage of contact lens practice and patient management involves practice management procedures. In effect, all six stages combine to form a system of contact lens practice and patient management.

Subject matter that supplements daily practice has been placed in Part II—the Clinical Reference section. It is presented separately to allow a relatively full development without obscuring the other material. When it is needed, the supplementary material can be consulted.

The last part of the clinical reference section is devoted to recent developments. This material is presented to make the book complete and to indicate that much clinical and laboratory research is needed. Although many people can be fitted successfully now, a great many problems remain. The ultimate will be attained when and if contact lenses are prescribed and used with the same degree of success, ease, and safety as spectacles.

Contemporary contact lens practice is demanding, frustrating, challenging, and rewarding. We hope that this book helps the reader meet the demands so that patient and practitioner have fewer frustrations and more rewards. We also hope that it produces an awareness of current problems and a desire to accept the challenge to eliminate the problems. The public's welfare will be served best if all segments of the ophthalmic field cooperate to meet this challenge.

ACKNOWLEDGMENTS

To present a comprehensive book, authors must synthesize and organize both their own ideas and those of others. Plan of organization, style of presentation, and inclusion of material depend on the author's judgment and philosophy of teaching. We have tried to evaluate all available information about contact lenses, and to the best of our ability, select with wisdom or discard with care. We are indebted to all who have contributed to the development of contact lenses. Many of their names are in the bibliography. There is special pleasure in acknowledging the important contributions made to this book by the following.

The authors gratefully acknowledge the technical assistance and advice of Nodema, Inc., and the support of the American Vision Research Foundation. Without their aid, this book could never have been completed.

Only the authors can fully appreciate the value of the counsel of Fernando A. Coletta on laboratory procedures. Many of the procedures discussed were developed or refined by him.

The invaluable contributions of Edward G. Eckstein, our illustrator, and Ken Ross, our photographer, are obvious.

Neal J. Bailey, O.D., Ph.D., The Ohio State University School of Optometry; Charles Chandler, B.S., Memphis, Tennessee; W. Jerome Heather, O.D., Keauu, Hawaii; Milton M. Kaplan, O.D., Eye-Bank for Sight Restoration, Inc.; Bascom H. Story, Ed.D., Director, Educational Section, Agency for International Development, United States Government; Phineas J. Sparer, M.D., University of Tennessee School of Medicine; and Paul G. Walcott, O.D., Boston, Massachusetts, all have been very helpful in reading and commenting on sections of the book.

Ralph W. Kalish, LL.B., St. Louis, Missouri, has been helpful in locating patents. Jayne Griffey has provided sustained assistance in typing the manuscript.

The knowledge, advice, and cooperation of the staff at Chilton Book

Company—especially Franklin H. Calsmer and Stephen B. Decker, editors, and Nic Groenevelt, General Manager and Editor-in-Chief—have contributed significantly to the quality of the book.

The most important acknowledgment is reserved for our families. We cannot adequately express our gratitude for their constant understanding and encouragement.

CONTENTS

PART TWO CLINICAL REFERENCE

APPENDICES

PART ONE

Clinical Practice

1

STAGE ONE

Patient Selection

Contact lenses are visual, protective, and cosmetic aids. Placing a lens in contact with the eye was originally considered advisable only in cases of certain relatively rare ocular abnormalities. In some such cases, contact lenses afford significant visual advantages. A prime example of this is replacing the highly irregular anterior surface of a keratoconic person with a regular contact lens surface (Fig. 1–1). In other such cases, contact lenses afford significant protective advantages. A prime example of this is protection of corneal integrity from disturbance by the scarred inner surface of a lid (Fig. 1–2).

Contact lens application is no longer reserved for such relatively rare cases. Contemporary art and science are sufficiently developed so that many people without unusual ocular abnormalities can successfully wear them.

Contact lens fitting involves understanding and clinically applying a great deal of theory. The transfer of theory to clinical application must be accomplished in a systematic, organized manner so that nothing of importance is omitted. This is best done by using a proper record form, which acts as a guide and outline for the clinical procedure. Form 1 (Appendix X) is designed for this purpose, and it is correlated with the presentation of material in this text.

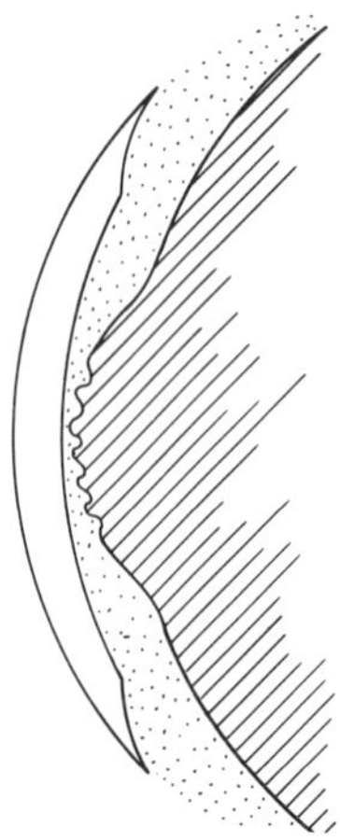

Figure 1–1. Regular surfaces of a contact lens replace the irregular anterior corneal surface of a keratoconic eye.

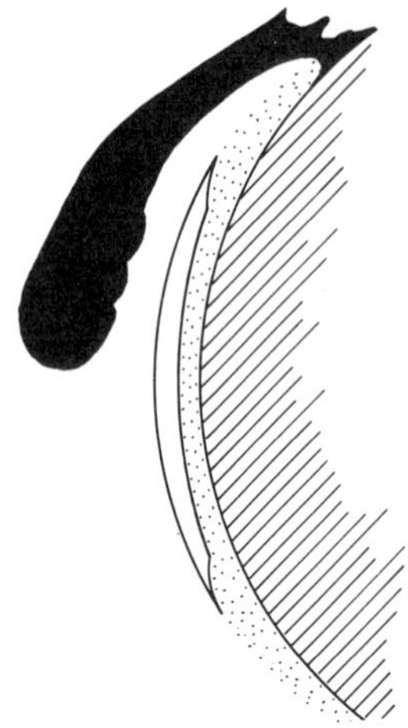

Figure 1–2. A contact lens protects the cornea from the scarred inner surface of a lid.

The first stage of contact lens fitting involves evaluating the advisability of application and the probability of success with each patient. This evaluation considers three goals, which constitute an operational definition of successful contact lens application. These goals are: objective evaluation showing that there is not and probably will not be significant ocular tissue disturbance; subjective evaluation showing that there is satisfactory visual performance, comfort, and daily wearing time; and cosmetic evaluation showing that the patient looks good while wearing the lenses.

Two related questions must be answered to determine whether these goals can probably be attained: can the patient be prepared to fulfill the goals, and can the practitioner design lenses to fulfill the goals?

PSYCHOLOGICAL FACTORS

There is almost unanimous agreement that psychological factors are extremely important in contact lens application.[1] Athough contact lens fitters are neither psychologists nor psychiatrists, they must understand psychological factors relevant to their work.[2] Such understanding assists them in evaluating a prospective wearer and managing an accepted wearer.[3]

Patients who seek contact lenses generally have conflicting feelings. They may be concerned about experiencing ocular discomfort or irritation, and at the same time they may be concerned about their inability to wear contact lenses.

The decision to be fitted with contact lenses by a particular practitioner implies that the patient has some confidence in both contact lenses and the practitioner. Such confidence must be reinforced during all relationships between patient and practitioner. Reinforcement of confidence is aided by a positive approach, a confident attitude, realistic encouragement, friendliness, patience, and empathy on the part of the practitioner.

In evaluating a prospective wearer, the practitioner must judge whether the patient is sufficiently motivated to overcome fear and discomfort related to initial contact lens wear. He must also judge whether the patient is sufficiently mature and cooperative to follow instructions concerning the use of contact lenses. Finally, he must deal satisfactorily with the patient's anxieties and misconceptions about contact lenses. Discussing these anxieties and misconceptions with the practitioner may help the patient understand them more clearly and help to suggest ways of overcoming them. The practitioner must also try to reassure the patient that the contact lens program will be managed properly.

Motivation

Motivation is directly related to the patient's true need to replace spectacles with contact lenses.[4] As need and motivation increase, advisability of contact lens application increases. Three needs may motivate a person to acquire contact lenses: visual enhancement, protection, and cosmetic and ego enhancement.

Vision is man's most important sense for orientation to his environment. If vision is unsatisfactory, the ability to function in our complex modern environment diminishes. The poorer an individual's uncorrected vision is, the greater his need for proper correction is. Generally, the greater this need is, the more advisable contact lens application is.

Contact lens application becomes more advisable for people whose visual needs cannot be satisfied as well with spectacles. Prime examples of this are the keratoconic, aphakic, or highly myopic individual. These people are frequently motivated to acquire contact lenses for the considerably better visual performance that can be obtained. Often such motivation results from the practitioner's suggestion that contact lenses are preferable to spectacles. The motivation of the relatively small group that acquires contact lenses because of a need for protection usually results from the practitioner's suggestion.

Spectacles or visual training can satisfy the visual and protective needs of most people. What then motivates them to acquire contact lenses?

Most Americans generally believe that spectacles detract from physical appearance. Some people also believe that spectacles are an undesirable sign of aging or weakness. Most contact lens patients are motivated by a desire for cosmetic and ego enhancement. They assume that physical appearance will be improved by replacing spectacles with contact lenses. They also assume that improved appearance will result in better acceptance by and better relationships with others, thus resulting in greater self-acceptance and self-satisfaction.

Motivation in young people at times is initiated by the parents' disapproval of the youngster's appearance with spectacles. When the patient is young, it is advisable to understand the desires of both the patient and the parents and their opinions of contact lenses.

Maturity

To produce the desired result, contact lenses must be used properly. The general emotional maturity of the patient and his ability to assume responsibility for obeying instructions, handling, and maintaining the lenses properly must be evaluated.

In the taking of the case history, certain factors about the patient's emotional makeup may be revealed. During the examination, a patient's reaction to the discussion of advantages and disadvantages of contact lenses, his initial ability to follow instructions and handle lenses, and his reaction to lenses placed on his eyes yield important information.

Conceptions

Every patient who comes to be fitted has certain conceptions about contact lenses. These are related to his reasons for wanting to be fitted and to assumed advantages and disadvantages of contact lenses. Often the reasons are inaccurate. To a great extent, this is due to inaccurate or insufficient information.[5] It is the practitioner's responsibility to provide accurate and complete information in each case concerning advantages and disadvantages of contact lenses.

Both practitioner and patient must make decisions concerning the advisability of contact lens application.[6] The practitioner must decide if the patient should be fitted and if there is a satisfactory probability of success. The patient must decide if he wishes to be fitted after being properly informed of the advantages, disadvantages, and probability of success in his case. The decisions by both the practitioner and patient are related to fulfillment of the three goals previously mentioned. Four key topics should be discussed with each patient: safety, visual performance, annoyance and discomfort, and cosmetic and ego enhancement.

Safety. Man has learned and unlearned protective responses that aid in keeping things out of his eyes.[7] Most patients who desire contact lenses also have some fear of them based on their learning and experiences. They come to be fitted when their motivation is temporarily strong enough to overrule their fear.

Patients usually ask four general types of questions related to fear of danger to physical well-being: First, can contact lenses become lost "behind the eye"? The patient should be told that the anatomic structure makes it impossible for loss "behind the eye." An illustrative diagram or picture is

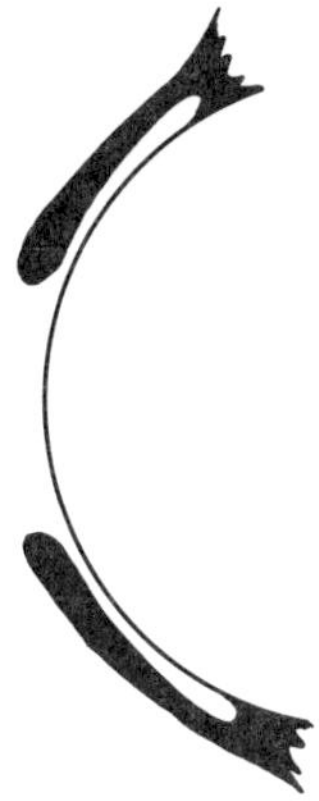

Figure 1–3. This illustration may be used for patient education to show why a contact lens cannot become lost "behind the eye."

often effective (Fig. 1–3). Practitioners should not assume that this fact, although apparent to them, is apparent to the patient.

Second, can contact lenses be broken on the eye? It is possible for a contact lens to be broken on the eye. However, because of the resiliency of contact lens materials, and the elasticity and protective mechanisms of the eye, this rarely happens. The eye is protected by the orbital bones, the eyelids, and the eyelashes. A contact lens on the eye is also protected by these anatomical structures. A spectacle lens is located in front of these protective mechanisms and has a greater tendency to break, although shattering can be reduced by using safety lenses. In some cases, a contact lens has protected the eye from flying objects that might otherwise have entered behind a spectacle lens and caused damage.

Third, can contact lenses damage the eye? There has been relatively little significant permanent damage caused by properly fitted and used contact lenses. Both the practitioner and the patient must try to eliminate any potential cause of damage. If probability of damage is considered to be high in a specific patient, contact lenses should not be applied (see p. 378).

Fourth, how can the eyes adapt to contact lenses? Patients know that a small particle on the eye causes considerable discomfort until the particle is removed. Many wonder why a contact lens will not produce similar continuous discomfort. They should be told that, although there is an adaptation period, which varies in duration and degree among patients, the front of the eye and the lids *usually* adapt to contact lenses. They may be told that this is due to the conformation of the lens to the eye and due to the smooth surfaces of the lens.

Visual Performance. Most patients assume that visual performance with contact lenses is the same as or better than with spectacle lenses. This is not always true. After the examination, probable visual performance should be evaluated for each patient and discussed with him. There are certain general considerations involved.

Visual performance with contact lens correction as compared to spectacle correction is aided by a slight increase in light transmission (assuming tinted contact lenses are not used), a slight increase in usable field, and a better quality of retinal image.[8] The quality of the retinal image is improved by reduction of aberrations and more consistent fixation through the optical center.[9] With high refractive powers, such as needed in aphakia or high myopia, all these benefits are increased. The high myope also obtains a considerably larger retinal image.

In other specific cases, the visual advantages are also considerable. Replacing an irregular corneal surface with a regular contact lens surface, such as in keratoconus, produces marked visual improvement. The amount of aniseikonia with a *refractive* anisometrope is considerably reduced. Because a contact lens follows eye movements, there is less vertical prismatic effect for any anisometrope. In a monocular aphakic, these factors often allow single binocular vision, whereas spectacles would produce diplopia or suppression. Cosmetic contact lenses that provide an artificial aperture may help vision in cases of aniridia or coloboma of the iris (see p. 110).

Patients who need constant correction and who do not wear spectacles while engaging in certain sports obviously derive considerable visual benefits from contact lenses. There is less fogging of contact lenses from perspiration in sports in which spectacles are worn. This is also true for people whose occupation involves frequent temperature changes.

Some patients dislike the cosmetic effect of spectacles so much that they use them only when it is absolutely essential. In such cases, vision with contact lens correction should not be compared to vision with spectacle correction. Rather, the comparison should be between vision with contact lens correction and vision with limited or no use of spectacles.

There are three relatively common visual disadvantages arising from the use of contact lenses. First, an astigmatic error may be left uncorrected or residual. Residual astigmatism is discussed on page 350. Second, contact lenses are generally made of hydrophobic plastic, which can become coated by transfer of materials from the fingers or precorneal fluid. Such a coating blurs vision, just as a coated spectacle lens blurs vision (see p. 358 for further discussion). Third, improper contact lens positioning may produce flare (see p. 228 for further discussion).

If these visual disadvantages are not present, general visual performance for most patients is slightly better with contact lenses than with spectacle lenses. Vision may be poorer when the above problems are present, and it is significantly better in special cases.

ANNOYANCE AND DISCOMFORT. Patients should not be misled into believing that there will be no annoyance or discomfort during or after adaptation. After adaptation, many patients are unaware of the lenses, aside from the occasional instances when dust or wind causes brief discomfort. Many other patients are slightly aware of but not annoyed by the presence of the lens. A few patients are annoyed by seemingly well fitted lenses to a degree that wear is discontinued or continued on a part-time basis.

Spectacles also cause discomfort and annoyance for some people. Such discomfort is greater for patients whose skin tonicity is reduced or for patients who have a strong correction, which causes use of a heavy lens.

Cosmetic Enhancement. Because cosmetic enhancement is usually the prime motivating factor, the patient assumes his appearance will be better with contact lenses than with spectacles. Properly fitted contact lenses can usually fulfill this need. Corneal lenses generally do this more adequately than scleral lenses.

When cosmetic need is great enough and is fulfilled, patients usually are satisfied with contact lenses in spite of some other disadvantages. When cosmetic need is slight or other disadvantages are great, patients may be dissatisfied.

Cosmetic need is especially great in the patient having strong corrections for myopia, keratoconus, hyperopia, aphakia, or astigmatism. Such strong spectacle corrections distort and change the size of underlying features. Rings and reflections are apparent in spectacle lenses. Contact lenses eliminate these problems. The advantages of cosmetic contact lenses for specific disfiguring conditions are apparent (see p. 298).

Some structural or positional anomalies of the anterior segment of the eye are more apparent with contact lenses than with spectacles because of the masking effect of spectacles. Strabismus, ptosis, coloboma of the lids, and pinguecula are examples. In such cases, the patient may mistakenly assume the condition will be no more or even less apparent with contact lenses. To avoid subsequent disappointment in such cases, the patient should be properly informed.

Economic factors should also be discussed with each patient. These are considered on page 254.

GENERAL PATHOLOGIC FACTORS

Persons with neither present nor past ocular pathologic conditions can usually wear safely contact lenses that are properly fitted, used and cared for. This fact is substantiated by the relatively few significant tissue disturbances compared to the relatively large number of wearers.

Research is being done to design tests that can predetermine the ability of an eye to adapt to contact lenses. These auxiliary tests are discussed on page 408.

In some cases, contact lenses cannot safely be used in persons with present or past ocular pathologic conditions. A thorough case history and examination must be used with every prospective contact lens patient to determine his pathologic status.[10] Case history is directed toward obtaining information about past ocular pathologic conditions and symptoms suggesting current ones. Examination is directed toward detecting signs of past or present ocular pathologic conditions. The case history is obtained and the examination is done in the usual manner, and the significance of any pathologic condition is evaluated in terms of the advisability of contact lens application.

Each present or past ocular pathologic condition has a specific relationship to the advisability of contact lens application, and each case must be considered on its individual merits. The more common and important ocular pathologic conditions in relation to contact lens application are discussed in Chapter 10 (p. 378). Each reader should familiarize himself with this material. The following is a general guide.

Present Ocular Pathologic Conditions

Any inflammatory and most degenerative ocular conditions should generally be cured before contact lenses are considered. Because degenerative conditions usually do not respond to treatment, the use of contact lenses usually is contraindicated. Keratoconic and postsurgical cataractous patients are exceptions. Any injury should be cured and the tissues allowed to develop adequate strength before contact lenses are considered.

There are two basic reasons for these generalizations: The contact lens may aggravate the pathologic condition or may cause misleading signs and symptoms that complicate diagnosis and treatment; and the pathologic condition may cause misleading signs and symptoms that complicate contact lens fitting.

Past (Cured) Ocular Pathologic Conditions

Once a pathologic condition is cured, the advisability of contact lens application depends to a large degree on the integration of five factors: (1) the seriousness of the pathologic condition, (2) the possibility of spontaneous recurrence or the chronicity of the pathologic condition, (3) the possibility that the contact lens may cause activation of the pathologic condition, (4) the fitting complication from residual structural changes caused by the pathologic condition, and (5) the ability of spectacle lenses to correct the visual anomaly. The more significant any one of these factors becomes, the less advisable is the application of contact lenses.

Consider the last factor in more detail. Even though the visual needs of many patients can be satisfied by spectacle lens correction, such patients may desire contact lenses to satisfy psychological needs related to cosmetic enhancement. When such patients have a significant history of ocular disease based on the first four factors, it is often best to be more conservative with contact lens application. On the other hand, some patients with a significant history of ocular disease are visually handicapped when corrected by spectacle lenses, but not when corrected by contact lenses. Better fulfillment of visual needs may warrant a more liberal application of contact lenses for these patients.

EXAMINATION FOR VISUAL NEED AND TENTATIVE LENS DESIGN

The case history and certain tests provide information that helps establish the patient's visual need and dependency on correction. These same tests also place each patient in a tentative lens design category. With determination of the visual need and the tentative lens design category, much valuable information about probability of success and complexity of fit is obtained.

Case History and Tests

The case history is taken and the visual acuity determined. Then, central ophthalmometry, static retinoscopy, and subjective lens acceptance tests are performed.

Case History. It should be determined if spectacles are worn constantly or just for specific tasks. Generally, the more constant the use, the greater the visual need is and the more advisable contact lens application is. The exception is in patients whose visual need is great enough to warrant constant use, but who refuse to wear spectacles because of dislike of their appearance.

Visual Acuity. It is always important to record acuities, and this factor becomes more important when contact lens application is considered.[11] If it is not recorded, subnormal acuity subsequently may mistakenly be considered a result of contact lens wear.

Uncorrected acuity is determined at distance and near. As uncorrected distant acuity decreases, the visual need for constant correction increases, which increases the advisability of contact lens application.

If uncorrected near acuity is poor as a result of presbyopia, the advisability of application of contact lenses may not be as great. Application of contact lenses for a presbyope is discussed on page 125. The approximate date of the last spectacle power change and corrected acuities with the patient's current spectacles are determined. This test helps to ascertain the rate of progression of the ametropia. The better the corrected acuities are, the less the ametropic change.

Best corrected spectacle acuities are also recorded, for legal reasons and to provide a basis of comparison with best corrected contact lens acuities.

Central Ophthalmometry (Keratometry). The Ophthalmometer (Keratometer) and its use are discussed on page 323. Central ophthalmometric readings give reasonably practical determinations of the central anterior corneal radii. The difference between the two principal meridians indicates the amount of astigmatism at the interface between air and the precorneal fluid. Regularity of the miral images gives an indication of the regularity of the anterior corneal surface.

STATIC RETINOSCOPY. The refractive error of the eye is determined objectively.

SUBJECTIVE LENS ACCEPTANCE. The refractive error of the eye is determined subjectively in the practitioner's usual manner. Best corrected acuity is recorded.

TENTATIVE LENS DESIGN CATEGORIZATION

On the basis of central ophthalmometry, static retinoscopy, and subjective lens acceptance, each patient can be categorized tentatively in terms of lens design requirements. The various lens design categories are related to general degrees of complexity and probability of success. Each category is discussed in detail in Chapter 2. A general overview is presented here.

SPHERICAL SINGLE VISION. Most patients can be fitted with nonprismatic, single vision lenses having single spherical central anterior and posterior curvatures. Generally it is easiest to attain the basic goals for patients in this category.

POSTERIOR TORIC CENTRAL CURVATURE. If central ophthalmometric astigmatism is more than 2.0 D, it may be impossible to produce an adequate relationship between a contact lens with a single spherical posterior central curvature and the toric corneal curvature. In such cases, the need for a contact lens with a toric posterior central curvature must be considered. This factor complicates contact lens application.

ANTERIOR TORIC CENTRAL CURVATURE. A contact lens with single spherical posterior central curvature eliminates astigmatism from the interface between air and the precorneal fluid. This amount of astigmatism is represented by the ophthalmometric astigmatism (AO). Total astigmatism (AT) of the eye at the corneal plane is represented by full spectacle power referred to the corneal plane.

Total astigmatism is composed of two elements. First is ophthalmometric astigmatism (AO); second is astigmatism from the eye internal to the interface between air and the precorneal fluid (AI) (see p. 350).

This internal astigmatism is not neutralized when a contact lens with a single spherical central curvature is placed on the eye.[12] The astigmatism remains uncorrected or is residual. When it is of sufficient degree, it affects visual acuity or comfort.

The amount of residual internal astigmatism is predicted with reasonable accuracy by the formula $AI = AT - AO$. When predicted residual internal astigmatism is 0.75 D or more, it often must be corrected or visual acuity and efficiency may suffer. It is most fully corrected by a lens with an anterior toric central surface. Application of an anterior toric surface to correct residual astigmatism complicates contact lens fitting.

Bifocal Lenses. It is quite difficult successfully to fit contemporary bifocal contact lenses. The need for bifocal or multifocal correction complicates contact lens application.

Subnormal Vision. The cause of partial sight must be considered. If the purpose is to increase retinal image size by microscopic or telescopic aids, contact lenses are often not the best means of correction. If the purpose is to supply a regular surface in place of an irregular cornea or to provide an artificial aperture, contact lenses are often the best means of correction.

The fitting of a keratoconic patient is complicated because of abnormal and irregular corneal topography, loss of corneal sensitivity, and structural weakness of corneal tissue. These factors are often more than offset by the vastly improved visual performance and possible retardation of the progression of cone formation.

Aphakia. To fit an aphakic is complicated because of the high refractive power needed and the resultant relatively thick lens, the residual scar tissue, possible corneal irregularity, loss of corneal sensitivity, possible abnormality of pupil shape, and the age of most aphakics. These factors are often more than offset by the vastly improved visual performance afforded by contact lenses.

Anisometropia. Overall or meridional anisometropia is determined by analyzing the needed spectacle correction. Aniseikonia related to refractive anisometropia is best corrected by contact lenses. Aniseikonia related to axial anisometropia is best corrected by spectacles.[13]

Clinical data help differentiate between axial and refractive anisometropia. If a patient with binocularity has worn spectacles and not experienced discomfort, the anisometropia is probably axial. If the ophthalmometric readings of the flattest principal meridian are similar, and also if the refractive error is high, the anisometropia is probably axial. This, of course, is not true in a monocular aphakic. If anisometropia is meridional, it is probably refractive.

COMPLICATING FACTORS

Certain factors that may complicate contact lens application in any tentative lens design category must be evaluated.

Anterior Segment Factors

Position of Lids. Typically, with primary fixation, the lower lid is approximately coincident with the lower limbus, and the upper lid covers one fifth of the superior cornea. Marked departure from these conditions may complicate contact lens fitting (see p. 31).

Vertical Palpebral Aperture Size. The average median vertical palpebral aperture size is between 9 and 10 mm.[14] Marked departure from this condition may complicate contact lens fitting (see p. 53).

Pupil Size. The average pupil size under ordinary illumination is 3 to 5 mm. Marked departure from this condition may complicate contact lens fitting (see p. 32).

Horizontal Visible Iris Diameter. The average size of the horizontal visible iris diameter is about 11.5 mm. Marked departure from this condition may complicate contact lens fitting (see p. 53).

Blink Rate and Amount. The average blink rate in women is 14 per minute. Average blink rate in men is 19 per minute. It is usual to have a full blink. Departure from this condition may complicate contact lens fitting (see p. 31 and 215). *Proper blink is essential.*

Position of Globe in Orbit. Marked exophthalmos or marked enophthalmos may complicate contact lens fitting (see p. 53).[15]

All these anatomical factors are more significant with corneal than with scleral contact lenses.

Physiologic Factors

The physiologic performance of a patient's eyes may be different when he uses contact lenses from when he uses spectacles.[16] The practitioner must judge whether problems will occur or can be corrected if contact lenses are applied.[17] If problems cannot be corrected, contact lens application is less advisable.

Case History. The case history is taken in the usual manner, and the information gathered is related to the advisability of contact lens application.

Spectacle Elements. If prisms are a part of the patient's spectacle correction, the prescription of contact lenses may be less advisable. Corneal contact lenses can have only a vertical prismatic effect, because gravity orients the base of the prism inferiorly. Use of a prism of more than 2 to 3^{Δ} in a corneal contact lens results in a thick lens that is difficult to fit. Scleral contact lenses may have either a vertical or a lateral prismatic effect on the eye.

Visual Training. If visual training has been used successfully by a patient, contact lens application is generally not contraindicated. If visual training has been unsuccessful, contact lens application may be complicated. The patient may feel that the use of contact lenses should relieve his asthenopia. In most cases it does not. In some cases, reduced aberrations, increased visual field, and changes of accommodation and convergence enhance binocularity and reduce asthenopia (see p. 15). If asthenopia is due to psychological resistance to wearing spectacles, contact lenses may be helpful.

Strabismus. The residual effects of strabismus surgery on contact lens application is discussed on page 384; the cosmetic aspect is discussed on page 9.

Examination. Examination is performed in the usual manner, and the information gathered is related to the advisability of contact lens application.

Tests. Among these tests should be chair skills, such as the cover test, determination of the near point of convergence, and version and rotation tests. Also, there should be phorometric tests to determine various factors in relation to accommodation and convergence. Phoria and duction tests should be done at distance and near. Crossed cylinder, relative accommodation, and amplitude of accommodation tests should be done at near. Gradient, fusion, and cyclophoria testing may also be done.

Accommodation and Convergence. When a patient changes from spectacle to contact lens correction, various changes related to accommodation, convergence, and fusion may occur (see p. 355). A myope must accommodate more for a given distance when corrected with contact lenses than when corrected with spectacle lenses. The opposite holds for a hyperope. This phenomenon has clinical significance for two reasons. First, a myopic incipient presbyope may function reasonably well with single-vision spectacle lenses, but he may need an addition for near work with contact lenses. The functional onset of presbyopia for a hyperope is slightly retarded for the same reason by contact lens application.

Second, more accommodative convergence is produced in a myope corrected by contact lenses and less in a hyperope corrected by contact lenses. These phenomena may cause problems of binocular coordination and result in excessive demands on fusional reserves.

A spectacle-corrected myope has base-in prism when fixating at near. A contact lens-corrected myope does not and must converge more for a given distance. A spectacle-corrected hyperope has base-out prism when fixating at near. A contact lens-corrected hyperope does not and must converge less for a given distance.

Image Size. Image size is greater for a myope and less for a hyperope corrected with contact lenses instead of with spectacle lenses (see p. 354). Clinically, this is most significant in high myopes, who appreciate the large image size, and in aphakics, who have better binocularity and spatial orientation.

Usable Field. The usable field of vision is greater with contact lenses than with spectacles, partly because of the rim of the frame, which limits the usable field of fixation. With plus corrections, the increase of prism with its base opposite to the direction of fixation toward the edge of the lens further reduces the usable field (see p. 121). A larger usable field may aid fusion because of greater supportive aid from peripheral fusion.

Aberrations. When contact lenses are worn, they usually have a reasonably consistent centration of the optic zone of the lens and the pupil. Most aberrations are less with contact lenses than with spectacle lenses. Coma, oblique astigmatism, distortion, and curvature of field are generally considerably less with contact lenses. Chromatic aberration is about the same with contact lens or spectacle lens correction. Spherical aberration in air is usually greater with contact lenses, but the eye eliminates most of it.

Environmental Factors

The patient's residential, vocational, and avocational physical environments may affect the advisability of contact lens application.

Residential Factors. The patient's residential environment may affect contact lens fitting owing to altitude, humidity, temperature, and wind. One of the requirements for comfort and tissue maintenance is a proper precorneal fluid evaporation rate. Evaporation has a concurrent cooling effect. If the evaporation of precorneal fluid is too slow, corneal temperature is elevated. This condition can cause burning and itching, and it can cause minor temporary tissue changes. If the evaporation rate is too fast, the protective, lubricating, and nutritional functions of the precorneal fluid may be altered. The eyes may feel dry, and excess lacrimation may be produced to relieve this condition.

Rate of evaporation is related to atmospheric pressure, humidity, temperature, and surface area. As atmospheric pressure, humidity, or surface area is increased, rate of evaporation is decreased. As temperature is increased, rate of evaporation is increased.

The effect of atmospheric pressure, humidity, and temperature on contact lens wear is most important when there are appreciable changes in these factors. All contact lens patients experience this effect when going from a hot, humid outdoor environment to a cooler, less humid indoor environment; when the seasons change; or when moving from one geographical location to another. Contact lens application may be less advisable for persons whose environment changes frequently or severely.

Other residential factors are wind and dust. Wind can increase lens movement and the evaporation rate of precorneal fluid, thus drying the lens and increasing mechanical irritation. To obtain a balance and to wash away the foreign body, hyperlacrimation often results. Wind may also introduce dust particles. Frequently, hyperlacrimation is produced to wash these particles away. Any windy or dusty location may make corneal contact lens application less advisable. Scleral lenses may be preferable.

Vocational and Avocational Factors. Some vocational or avocational environments are favorable, and some are unfavorable to contact lens application.

Favorable Factors. Contact lenses are often advantageous in sports.[18,19] Although corneal lenses can be used, scleral lenses are preferable for contact and water sports because they are retained better. When corneal lenses are used, it is advisable to have a spare pair in case of loss. Scleral lenses may also be preferable when a sporting event is played in a windy or dusty environment.

Airline stewardesses are usually not allowed to wear spectacles while on duty. Contact lenses are allowed when they can be worn for a sufficient number of daily hours and when uncorrected acuity is not too poor. Requirements vary among airlines, but usually eight to ten hours of daily wear and uncorrected acuity of about 20/100 or better are accepted. This standard of uncorrected acuity is required so that a stewardess can function adequately if her contact lenses are lost or removed.

Surgeons and dentists may find that there is less fogging of contact lenses than of spectacle lenses from perspiration. There is also less fogging in occupations that require frequent movement from hot to cold areas.

People in the performing arts may be highly motivated for cosmetic reasons to be fitted with contact lenses. Also, a cosmetic contact lens may be needed to change iris color.

Unfavorable Factors. An environment containing fumes may cause ocular irritation or corneal edema. An environment containing dust or small particles may necessitate the use of scleral lenses or corneal lenses and protective goggles with side shields.

2

STAGE TWO

Initial Design Selection

After the initial evaluation, two determinations must be made. Can lenses be processed that will probably fulfill the basic goals, and what are the most logical initial designs and specifications? There is no easy or simple way to make these determinations. It is important to understand the theory and limitations of contemporary procedures so that initial lens designs that will probably provide a satisfactory environment for adaptation are selected. *Pages 216 and 217 should be read now.*

PHYSICAL, ANATOMICAL, AND PHYSIOLOGIC FACTORS

Physical Structure and Terminology of Single-Vision Corneal Contact Lenses

For communication and prescription purposes, it is necessary to understand the physical structure and terminology of contact lenses. Single-vision corneal contact lenses with circular curvatures are considered here. Other types of lenses are considered subsequently. There are four categories of physical structure: curvature and refractive power, diameter or width, thickness, and auxiliary features.

Curvature and Refractive Power

Short radii produce steep curvatures, and long radii produce flat curvatures. Contact lens curvatures are described either in diopters of refractive power or by radii. The refractive power of a given curvature depends on the indicial difference between the lens and the surrounding media. Because indicial difference can vary, there can be many powers for any curvature.

Most lenses are made of polymethyl methacrylate (P.M.M.A.), which has an index of refraction of about 1.49 (see p. 400). Lenses are surrounded either by air or by precorneal fluid. The index of refraction of air is taken as 1.00; the index of precorneal fluid is usually taken as between 1.33 and 1.34. Because of indicial factors, communication errors may be produced in the description of contact lens curvatures by diopters of refractive power (see p. 326).

It is preferable to describe contact lens curvatures by radii, which are constant linear measurements designated in millimeters or inches. The relationship between millimeters and inches is 0.1 mm. = 0.004 inch. Because all other linear values of a contact lens are designated in millimeters, it is logical to describe radii in millimeters.

Refractive Power. A contact lens is physically thin, but it must be considered as a thick lens for optical purposes. The power of light entering the anterior convex surface and emerging from the posterior concave surface of an optically thick lens is not the same as the power of light entering the posterior surface and emerging from the anterior surface. When light enters the anterior and emerges from the posterior surface, the focal length is determined by measurement from the vertex of the posterior surface to the focal point. This measurement is termed the *posterior,* or *back, focal length.* The reciprocal of this measurement is the *posterior,* or *back, vertex power.* When a contact lens is worn, light enters the anterior surface and emerges from the posterior surface. It is this posterior vertex power (DP) that must be determined (see p. 340).

Optic-zone Curvatures. Figure 2–1 shows a single-vision, nonprismatic corneal contact lens. The posterior surface is divided into two general areas. The central zone is usually circular and is surrounded by a peripheral zone, which is usually annular and concentric.

The posterior curvature in the central zone is the primary, or basic curve. It is termed the *base curve* (*B.C.*), and its radius is termed the *base curve radius* (*B.C.R.*). This zone contains the refractive power, or optics, to correct the patient's ametropia, and it is termed the *optic zone* (*O.Z.*).

Anterior and posterior optic zone curves may be *spherical* or *toroidal.* Spherical surfaces have the same radius in each meridian. Toroidal surfaces have different radii in each meridian of any quadrant. On a toroidal surface, there is a progressive change in each quadrant from longest to shortest radii. The meridians of minimum (shortest) and maximum (longest) radii are termed the *principal meridians* (*P.M.*), and they differ by 90°.

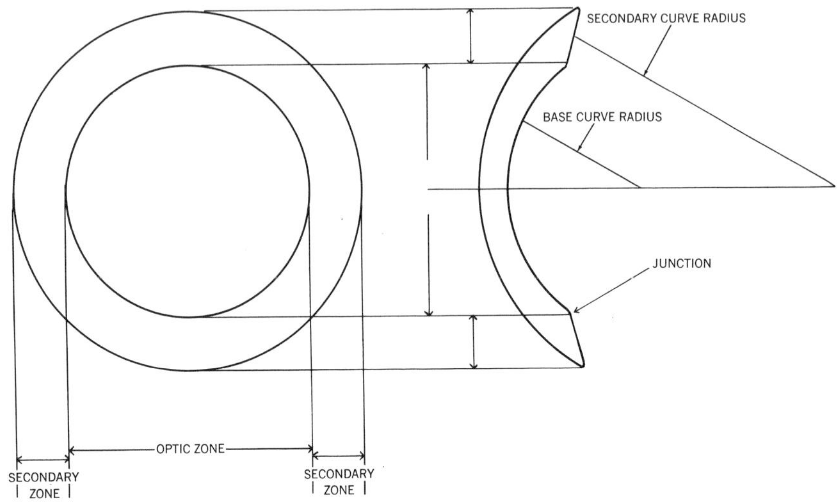

Figure 2–1. A bicurve contact lens with a central (optic) zone surrounded by a peripheral (secondary) zone.

On the basis of optic-zone curvature, single-vision contact lenses may be placed in four categories. When the anterior and posterior surfaces are spherical, the lens is termed a *spherical lens.* When the anterior surface is toroidal and the posterior surface is spherical, the lens is termed an *anterior, front,* or *outside surface toric lens.* When the posterior surface is toroidal and the anterior surface is spherical, the lens is termed a *posterior, back,* or *inside surface toric lens.* When both the anterior and posterior surfaces are toroidal, the lens is termed a *bitoric* lens. The axes of the toroidal anterior and posterior surfaces may coincide or be oblique to one another. Usually they coincide.

SECONDARY-ZONE CURVATURES. The curves in the peripheral zone are always longer in radius, or flatter, than the base curve(s). They are fabricated after, or secondary to, the fabrication of the base curve. These curvatures are termed the *secondary curve(s) (S.C.).*

When there are two curves of differing radii in this zone, the one closest to the edge is termed the peripheral secondary curve, or the *peripheral curve (P.C.).* If the width of this curve is 0.4 mm. or less, it is often termed a *peripheral bevel.* This term is used especially when the radius of this curve is considerably longer than that of the adjacent curve. The curve between the peripheral and base curves is termed the intermediate secondary curve, or *intermediate curve (I.C.)* (Fig. 2–2).

The radius of the peripheral curve is always the longest on the posterior surface, and the radius of the base curve is always the shortest on the posterior surface. The radius of the intermediate curve is always between these

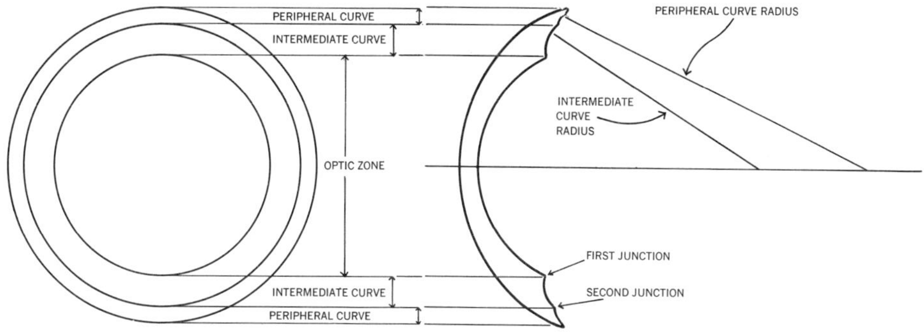

Figure 2–2. A tricurve contact lens with an optic zone surrounded by intermediate and peripheral secondary zones.

two. Secondary curves are usually spherical, but they may be toric. It is also possible to have aspherical secondary curves (see p. 390).

A lens may have more than two secondary curves. In this case, the curves are numbered in the same order in which they are fabricated. Fabrication is done by starting with the steepest secondary curvature and progressing to the flattest. As a result, the secondary curve adjacent to the optic zone is termed the *first secondary curve* (S_1). The next adjacent curve is termed the *second secondary curve* (S_2), and so on (Fig. 2–3).

On the basis of the number of secondary curves, single-vision contact lenses may be placed in three categories. When the lens has a base curve and one secondary curve, it is termed a *bicurve lens.* When the lens has a base curve and two secondary curves, it is termed a *tricurve lens.* When the lens has a base curve and three or more secondary curves, it is termed a *multicurve lens* (Figs. 2–1, 2–2, and 2–3).

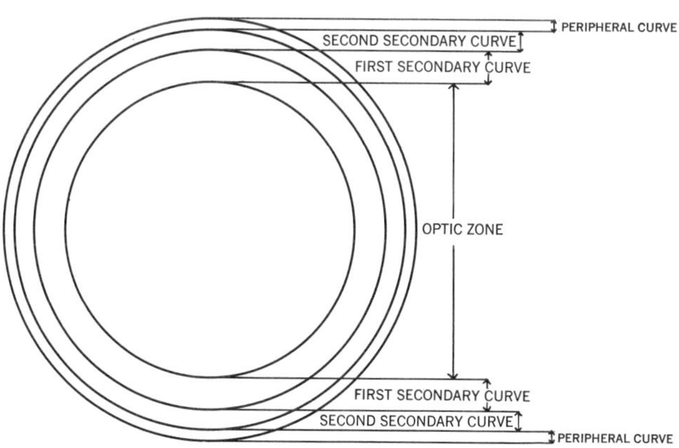

Figure 2–3. A multicurve contact lens with an optic zone surrounded by three secondary zones.

Blends. When there is a considerable difference in the radii of two adjacent curves, the point of transition from one curve to another is a sharp juncture. Such a sharp juncture may cause problems, and it is often necessary to remove it. This is done by fabricating a curve with a radius value between the values of the two adjacent curves. As a result, the curvatures will *blend* (*BL*) more smoothly into one another.[20]

On the basis of blends, single-vision contact lenses may be placed in three categories. When the transition between two adjacent curves is readily apparent, the juncture is *not blended* or *lightly blended*. A light blend is often called a *touch* or an *A blend*. When the transition between two adjacent curves is difficult or impossible to determine, the juncture is *heavily blended*. A heavy blend is often called a *complete* or a *C blend*. The degrees of blend between these extremes are called *medium* or *B blends*.

Blends are not considered true secondary curves, and they are not considered in the categorization of a lens according to its number of secondary curves.

Diameter or Width

There are three basic diameters or widths.

Total Lens Diameter (Overall Diameter, Lens Size). The chord value from one edge of the lens to the other is termed the *lens diameter* (*L.D.*). Lens diameter is usually the same in all meridians.

On the basis of lens diameter, contact lenses arbitrarily may be placed in three categories. When lens diameter is greater than 9.5 mm., the lens is termed *relatively large;* when between 9.5 and 8.6 mm., it is termed *medium;* and when 8.5 mm. or less, it is termed *relatively small.* It is important to realize that diameter is a relative concept. In this instance, it is related to the corneal and palpebral aperture sizes of each patient. A diameter that is large for one patient may be small for another.

Occasionally, a portion of the lens periphery is removed, producing different diameters in various meridians. Such a procedure is termed *truncation* (*Trunc.*). For practical purposes, two meridians are used to describe the lens diameters of a truncated lens. These are meridians of maximum and minimum diameter, which are usually horizontal and vertical (Fig. 2–4).

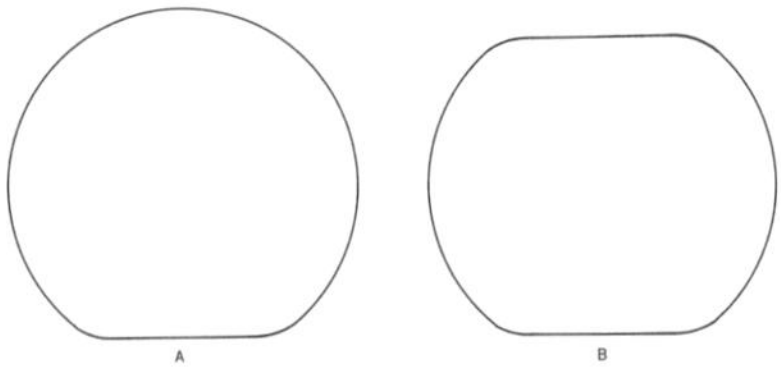

Figure 2–4. A, *Contact lens truncated on one side—a single truncation.* B, *Contact lens truncated on two sides—a double truncation.*

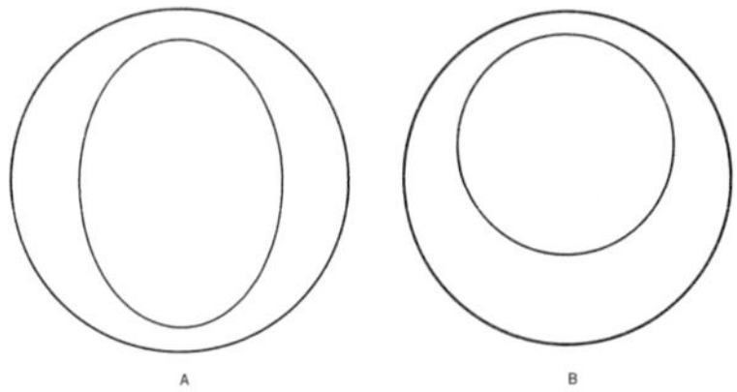

Figure 2–5. A, *Circular contact lens with oval optic zone.* B, *Circular contact lens with decentered circular optic zone.*

Optic-zone Diameter (Optic-zone Width). The chord value in a given meridian from one edge of the optic zone to the other is termed the *optic-zone diameter* (*O.Z.D.*) or *optic-zone width* (*O.Z.W.*).

On the basis of optic-zone diameter, contact lenses arbitrarily may be placed in three categories. When the optic zone is 7.5 mm. or more, it is termed *large;* when between 6.8 and 7.4 mm., it is termed *medium;* and when it is 6.7 mm. or less, it is termed *small.*

The optic-zone diameter is usually the same in all meridians, and the optic zone is round or circular. Occasionally, the diameter is different in various meridians, and the optic zone is oval. For practical purposes, the maximum and minimum diameters are used to describe an oval optic zone (Fig. 2–5).

Optic zones are usually centered in the lens. They may also be decentered vertically or horizontally (Fig. 2–5).

Secondary Curvature Width (Secondary Curvature Diameter). The chord value from one edge of a secondary curve to the other is termed the *secondary curve width* (*S.C.W.*) or *secondary curve diameter* (*S.C.D.*). This is the width on *each* side of the optic zone.

With a bicurve lens, secondary curve width is equal to half the difference between circular lens diameter and optic-zone diameter. In the tricurve or multicurve lens, the *sum* of the secondary curve widths is equal to half the difference between circular lens diameter and circular optic-zone diameter (Fig. 2–3).

On the basis of total secondary curve width, contact lenses arbitrarily may be placed in two categories. When the total width on each side of the optic zone is more than 0.7 mm., it is termed *wide;* when the total width on each side of the optic zone is 0.7 mm. or less, it is termed *narrow.*

Thickness

There are three basic aspects of lens thickness: center thickness, minus and plus thickness, and edge thickness.

Center Thickness. The separation between the anterior and posterior sur-

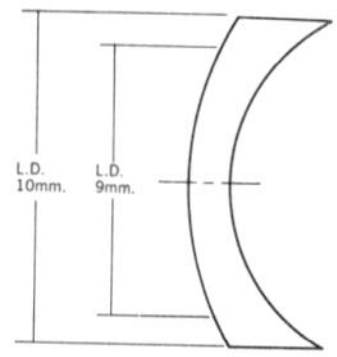

Figure 2–6. Thickness increases progressively from center to edge of a diverging (minus, negative) lens. (L.D., lens diameter.)

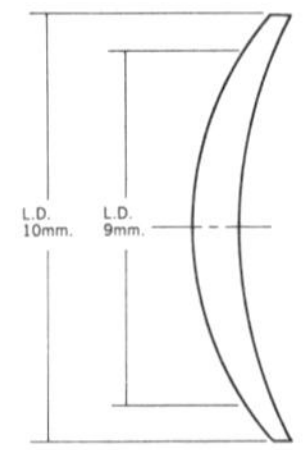

Figure 2–7. Thickness decreases progressively from center to edge of a converging (plus, positive) lens. (L.D., lens diameter.)

faces at the geometric center of the lens is termed the *center thickness* (*C.T.*). Center thickness for minus lenses usually ranges from 0.15 to 0.22 mm. Lenses with smaller center thickness are termed *thin lenses;* lenses with greater center thickness are termed *thick lenses.*

MINUS AND PLUS LENS THICKNESS. A lens with a single anterior and a single posterior curve may cause parallel rays of light to diverge or converge. A lens that causes light to diverge is termed a *minus* or *negative* lens. A lens that causes light to converge is termed a *plus* or *positive* lens.

Disregarding the effects of thickness on refraction, assume that the anterior and posterior surfaces of the lens are surrounded by the same medium. To produce diverging posterior vertex power, the anterior radius must be longer than the posterior radius. If these radii are fabricated with their centers of curvature on the same axis, there is a progressive increase of thickness from center to edge (Fig. 2–6). To produce converging posterior vertex power, the anterior radius must be shorter than the posterior radius. If these radii are fabricated with their centers of curvature on the same axis, there is a progressive decrease of thickness from center to edge (Fig. 2–7).

EDGE THICKNESS. The separation between anterior and posterior surfaces at the edge of the lens is termed *edge thickness* (*E.T.*). Edge thickness of a minus lens increases as diameter or power increases. Edge thickness of a plus lens of a given center thickness decreases as diameter or power increases.

Secondary curves are typically applied with their centers of curvature on the same axis as that of the base curve. Because secondary radii are always longer than base radii, application of secondary curves always decreases edge thickness. Edge thickness decreases more as secondary curve radius or width increases (Fig. 2–8).

Edge thickness before the application of secondary curves and edge finishing is termed *uncut* edge thickness. Edge thickness after application of secondary curves and edge finish is termed *finished edge thickness* (Fig. 2–9).

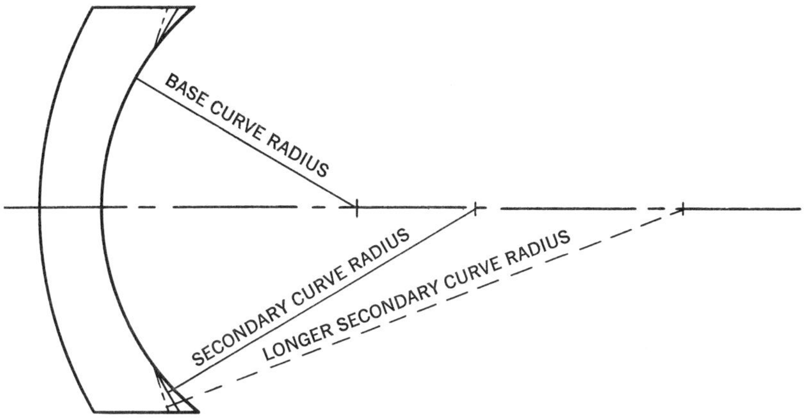

Figure 2–8. Application of secondary curvatures decreases edge thickness. Longer secondary radii produce a greater decrease.

AUXILIARY FEATURES

There are five common auxiliary features: tint; ballast; lenticular form; fenestrations, chamfers, and grooves; and lens material.

TINT. Contact lenses are clear, or they have through-and-through tints. Common tints are blue, brown, gray, green, and pink. Lavender, yellow, and smoky gray (black) are also available. Tints usually come in three shades: No. 1, lightest; No. 2, medium; and No. 3, darkest. It is also possible to obtain a No. 1½ shade in some tints. Tinted contact lenses are discussed on page 298.

BALLAST. Contact lenses rotate on the eye (see p. 32). They may have ballast incorporated to neutralize rotation. Ballast is usually provided by prism, the heavier base of which is oriented inferiorly on the eye by gravity. Normal terminology is used. The ability of the lens to displace rays of light

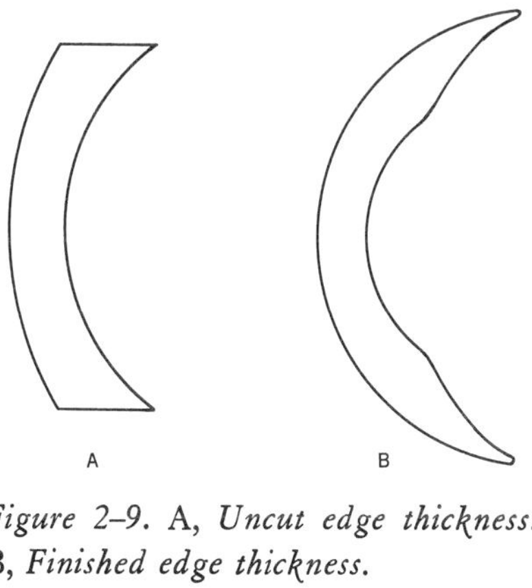

Figure 2–9. A, *Uncut edge thickness.* B, *Finished edge thickness.*

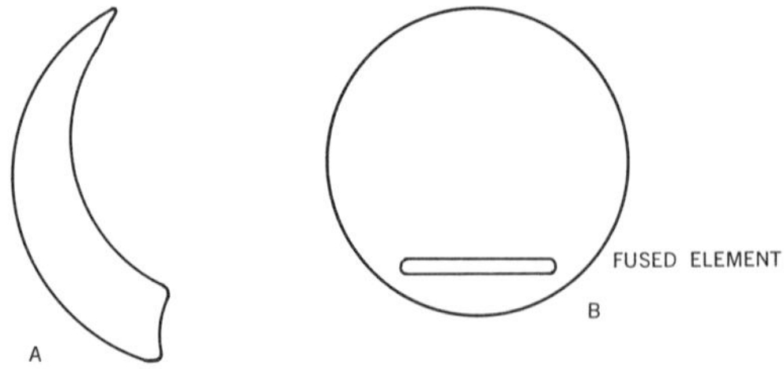

Figure 2–10. A, *Prism ballast contact lens, sectional view.* B, *Metallic ballast contact lens, front view.*

is expressed in prism diopters ($^{\Delta}$). The thickest part of the prism is the base, and the thinnest part is the apex. Ballast may also be in the form of a fused metallic element (Fig. 2–10).

Lenticular Form. A contact lens may be made in *anterior lenticular* (*Lent.*) form. Lenticular form produces an *anterior optic zone* (*bowl*) and an annular peripheral *carrier* section. Lenticular construction is used with a *high* minus lens to decrease the thickness of the peripheral portions of the lens (Fig. 2–11). Lenticular construction is used with a *high* plus lens to restrict or reduce the optics to the central portion of the lens. As a result, center thickness and lens weight are reduced (Fig. 2–12). Lenticular constructions may have any of the three forms shown in Figs. 2–11 and 2–12.

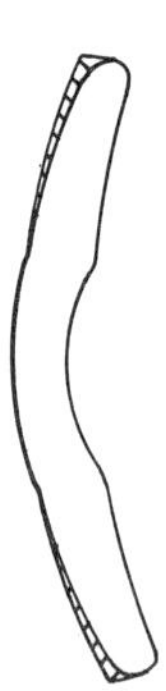

Figure 2–11. A minus lens with a lenticular construction to decrease edge thickness. The lined area indicates the plastic that was removed.

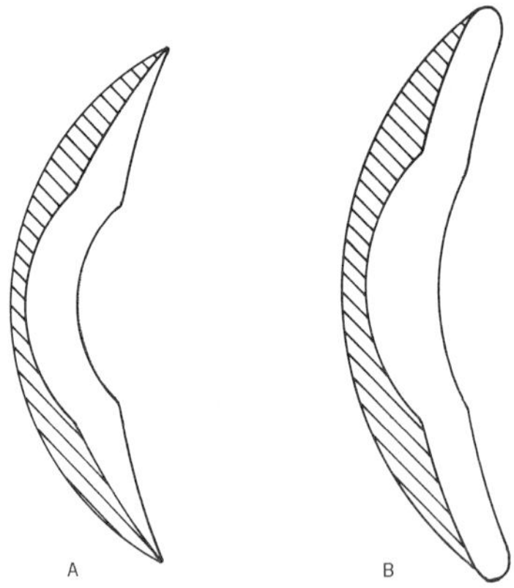

Figure 2–12. Plus lenses with lenticulars to reduce optic portion, center thickness, and lens weight. The lined area indicates the additional thickness needed if not made in lenticular form. A, *Plus-carrier lenticular.* B, *Minus-carrier lenticular.*

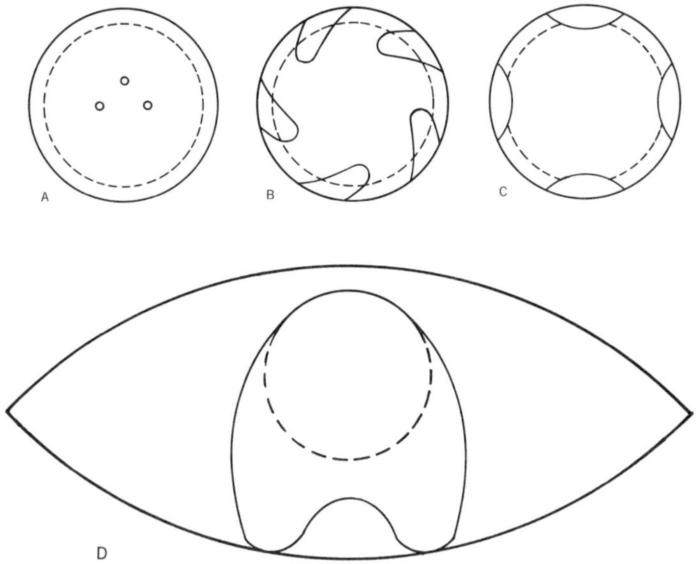

Figure 2–13. A, *Contact lens with apertures or fenestrations.* B, *Contact lens with Spiro-Vent grooves.* C, *Contact lens with Vent-Air grooves.* D, *Contact lens with Bi-Ped™ grooves.*

The anterior optic zone is usually about 0.5 mm. larger than the posterior optic zone. Lenticular form may alter lens position (see p. 44).

FENESTRATIONS, CHAMFERS, AND GROOVES. Fenestrations, chamfers, or grooves may be placed in the lens (see p. 139).[21–23] These are shown in Fig. 2–13.

LENS MATERIAL. Materials other than polymethyl methacrylate (P.M.M.A.) can be used or the surfaces can be treated to improve wetting (p. 401).[24–27]

SYNOPSIS OF CORNEAL TOPOGRAPHY RELATED TO CONTACT LENS APPLICATION

Posterior contact lens and anterior corneal curvatures have relationships that are important in establishing the physical fit of the lens (see also p. 35). To appreciate this fact better, certain aspects of corneal topography should be considered (see also p. 401).

Classically, the cornea has been considered to consist of two zones. First, there is a central zone, 4 to 6 mm. wide, over which the curvature in any meridian is relatively constant. This is termed the *corneal, optic,* or *apical cap.* The curvature of the corneal cap has been considered spherical or toric. Second, there is an area surrounding the corneal cap and extending to the limbus over which the curvature is flatter than the central curvature. It is termed the *peripheral,* or *basilar, zone.* It has been felt that the curvature of the peripheral zone progressively flattens from the transition of the corneal cap to the limbus. The transition from corneal cap to peripheral zone traditionally has been taken as that point in any meridian where the curvature is 0.25 D flatter than the central curvature (Fig. 2–14).

Currently, it is thought that most corneas do not have corneal caps as classically defined. The amount of flattening over a 4 to 6 mm. central diameter is probably 1 to 2 D. It is also believed that the curvatures of the cornea are aspheric and that flattening therefore is a continuous process from center to periphery. Flattening of the peripheral cornea is generally asymmetrical—that is, there is a variance in the rate and amount of flattening in the different quadrants. The only factual generalization that can currently be made about anterior corneal topography is that it is smooth, convex, asymmetrical, and aspheric, with a flattening from the central area to the limbus. This last factor has considerable clinical significance.

In terms of posterior curvatures, the simplest contact lens has a monocurve spherical surface. In the early days of corneal contact lens fitting, micro lenses with such spherical monocurve posterior surfaces and lens diameters of about 9.5 mm. were used. Because of the aspherical corneal topography, such surfaces do not produce satisfactory relationships with the anterior corneal surface, even if the cornea is neither toric nor asymmetrical. When the base curve radius equals the central corneal radius, as measured by ophthalmometry, the lens rests peripherally and clears centrally. When the base curve radius is lengthened to reduce central clearance and edge bearing, a

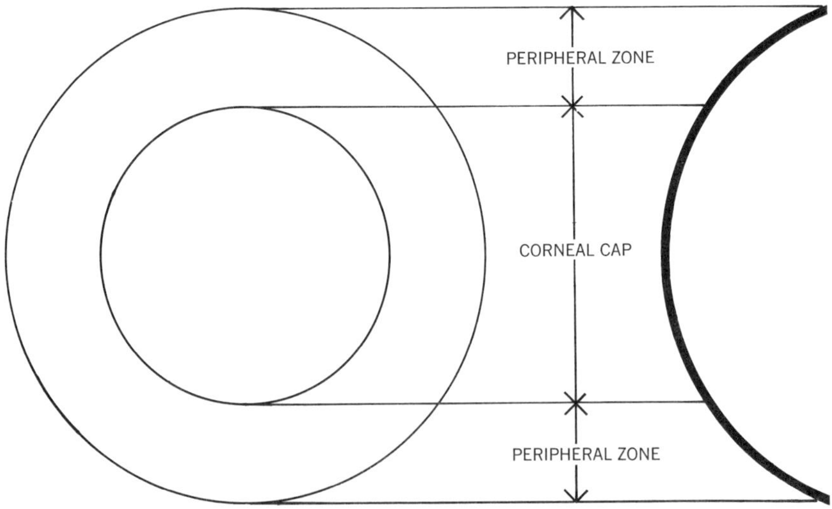

Figure 2–14. Front and sectional schematic representations of a two-zone cornea with a corneal cap of 4 to 6 mm. surrounded by a flatter peripheral zone.

small central bearing area surrounded by annular peripheral clearance results. These are poor relationships (see p. 39). When the base curve is kept equal to the ophthalmometric radius, and the lens diameter is reduced, precorneal fluid depth between lens and cornea decreases. When the lens diameter is 6.5 mm., there is often an apparent alignment between the posterior lens and anterior corneal curves. This is a good relationship (see p. 39); however, the overall performance of monocurve lenses with small diameters is usually poor.

Because lenses with monocurve spherical posterior surfaces do not usually perform satisfactorily, other options are used. These involve making the posterior surface aspherical to produce satisfactory lens-cornea relationships and overall performance. The most commonly used procedure involves the application of spherical secondary curves with longer radii than that of the base curve (p. 39). See page 390 for a discussion of aspheric curvatures.

When a two-zone lens with spherical curves is used, the base curve is restricted to a zone of 6.5 to 7.5 mm., which enables clinically satisfactory matching with the underlying cornea. The longer secondary radii produce progressively increasing linear depth from the optic zone–secondary zone transition to the edge of the lens. Introduction of an optic zone and a transition presents problems. First, power and prism variance between optic and secondary zones may produce visual problems (see p. 228). Second, when the rate of change between base and secondary curves is considerable, the transition juncture may be sharp.

The complexity of corneal topography related to contact lens fitting is increased by the fact that corneal topography may be altered by external pressure. Contact lenses apply external pressure to the cornea and usually alter corneal topography.[28]

Synopsis of Relationships Between Corneal Anatomy and Physiology and Contact Lens Application

The physical fit of the lens affects the ability of the cornea to maintain a desirable function. There is, therefore, a physicophysiologic fit. To appreciate this idea better, consider certain aspects of corneal anatomy and physiology. A more comprehensive discussion of corneal anatomy and physiology may be found on page 368.

There are five classically accepted layers in the cornea. From anterior to posterior, they are stratified epithelium, Bowman's membrane, stroma (substantia propria), Descemet's membrane, and endothelium (Fig. 2–15). The cornea is constantly bathed on its anterior surface by the precorneal fluid, whose three layers are the oily film, lacrimal layer, and mucoid layer. *Normal precorneal film is essential for successful contact lens wear.*

Because the cornea is avascular, the nutritional and oxygen supply and the removal of metabolic waste products are indirect. Nutritional supply to the

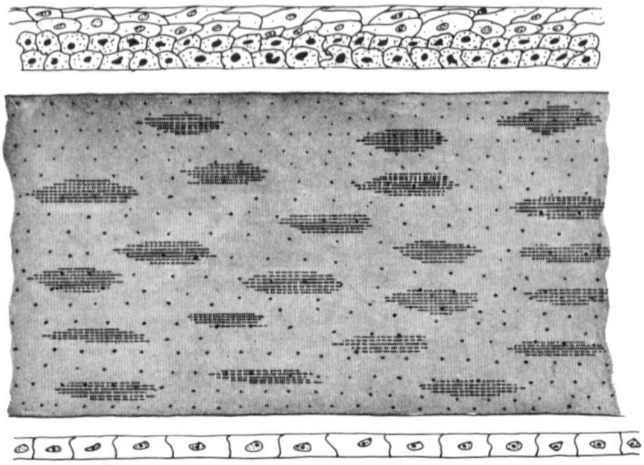

Figure 2–15. Sectional, schematic representation of corneal layers.

cornea is from lacrimal secretion, the fluid of the anterior chamber, and the capillary network surrounding the limbus. Oxygen supply to the cornea is from the limbal capillaries, the aqueous, and the atmosphere. Waste removal is through the precorneal fluid, exposure to the atmosphere, and the limbal capillaries.

The primary requirement of a useful cornea is to maintain transparency. Transparency is attained and maintained by a unique anatomic structure of the tissues, the unique functioning of these tissues, and an absence of blood vessels. Proper metabolism is necessary for maintenance of transparency.

To maintain transparency, the fluid level of the corneal tissue must be controlled. The cornea is relatively deturgescent, containing less water than it is capable of accepting from distilled water or salt solutions. When the fluid level of the cornea is increased—that is, becomes turgescent or swollen—the cornea starts to lose its transparency. Clinically, this turgescence is termed *edema*. Because the cornea has an affinity for absorbing fluid, some mechanism must neutralize this affinity and keep the cornea relatively deturgescent. The exact mechanism is unknown.

It is known that the cornea functions normally in an environment with four basic characteristics:

1. There is a relatively constant exposure to the atmosphere during all hours of wakefulness. This exposure allows atmospheric oxygen to become mixed with the precorneal fluid and produces a satisfactory evaporation rate of this fluid.

2. There is a constant coverage of the cornea by normal precorneal fluid. The action of the eyelids *spreads* the thin precorneal film over the cornea. This flow makes available nutrients and oxygen mixed in the precorneal fluid for corneal metabolism, and it aids in removal of metabolic waste products.

3. There is only *diffuse* external pressure from the lid against the cornea and limbus during the blink cycle. This type of pressure allows maintenance of the unique corneal anatomic structure. It also allows proper blood flow

through the limbal vessels, providing availability of nutrients and oxygen, and removal of metabolic waste products.

4. There is no excessive mechanical stimulation to tissues and nerve endings. This condition allows maintenance of a proper metabolic cycle. Because the nerve supply is richest at the apex of the cornea and gradually decreases toward the limbus, it is critical that the apex does not receive excessive mechanical stimulation.

The presence of a contact lens on the cornea changes this basic environment. There are four possible environmental changes: (1) The contact lens covers a certain portion of the cornea, thus reducing the exposure of the cornea to the atmosphere. (2) The contact lens may impede the flow of precorneal fluid over the corneal surface. (3) The pressure from the upper lid during the blink cycle is transmitted to the contact lens and then to the cornea. When this pressure is not disbursed over a large enough area or when it is disbursed to the limbal capillaries, anatomic structure or blood flow may be affected. (4) The movement and pressure of the contact lens may interfere with nerve impulses by causing excess peripheral stimulation.

The cornea can adapt to some environmental changes caused by the presence of a contact lens. Although the exact mechanism is not understood, it is known that adaptation is best when the environment is changed least. A contact lens should be fitted so that it causes minimal environmental changes.

Synopsis of the Relationship Between Eyelid and Pupil, and Contact Lens Application

Eyelids

The physicophysiologic fit is affected by the action of the eyelids, and the action of the eyelids is affected by the contact lens construction and fit.* As the upper eyelid blinks across the cornea, it spreads fresh precorneal fluid from the lid margin reservoirs. The upper and lower lids must meet and must remain in close apposition to the cornea to wet it properly. Incomplete or infrequent blinkers are poorer contact lens candidates (see p. 215), as are persons whose corneas wet improperly or abrade from normal lid pressure. Assuming a proper blink and proper corneal reaction, lenses must be fitted to maintain this. Lens thickness must not be so great that it lifts the lid away from, or bridges, corneal areas; edge configuration and thickness must permit normal blink action; lens movement must be slight so that blink action is not increased or decreased to reduce movement; and lens position must allow normal blink action.

When a contact lens is on the eye, the upper lid transmits its pressure to the lens and causes a movement and rocking of the lens. These pressures are then transmitted to the cornea and disbursed according to the relationship of the posterior surface of the lens and anterior corneal curves.

* Drs. Donald R. Korb and Charles R. Stewart have made significant contributions in this area of contact lens fitting.

Pressure is exerted on the lens during the closing phase of blinking and released during the opening phase of blinking. This lid pressure activates a pump system that causes the interchange of precorneal fluid between the lens and cornea. This interchange is aided by the movement of the lens in both superoinferior and anteroposterior directions. Anteroposterior movement is possible because of the elastic nature of the precorneal fluid. When the posterior surface of the lens and anterior corneal curvatures are relatively aligned over too great an area, precorneal fluid interchange may be impeded. *Full blink is essential to proper interchange.*

The upper lid also exerts a major influence on the positioning of the lens. The underside of the lid is lined with conjunctiva. This and the lid's tonicity may be sufficient to cause adherence and to position the lens superiorly. When the lens diameter is relatively large, the upper lid has a large lens area to adhere to. As a result, a lens of large diameter *tends* to position superiorly. When the lens diameter is relatively small, the opposite is true. A small lens does not provide a large area for the upper lid to adhere to, and the small lens does not adhere as readily to the cornea. As a result, a lens of small diameter *tends* to position in the palpebral aperture (see p. 45).

As lid tonicity or blink rate decreases, three concurrent results are produced: there is less pressure transmitted to the cornea, the pump mechanism and lens movement are less effective, and adherence of the lid to the lens is reduced.

The action of the lids, especially the upper lid, tends to rotate a contact lens. Rotation is usually up nasal and down temporal—that is, counterclockwise on the right eye and clockwise on the left eye.[29] In some cases, it is necessary to use ballast in the lens to maintain meridional stability.

The transitional epithelium of the lid margins is richly supplied with free sensory nerve endings, and it is quite sensitive to direct stimulation.

The lids, especially the upper lid, play one of the most important roles in corneal contact lens performance.

Pupil

The pupil acts as the entrance for light in the optical system of the eye. The range of pupil size in individuals is about 1.5 mm. to 8 mm. Fluctuation of the pupil size in an individual depends on the amount of illumination, degree of accommodation and convergence, and his emotional status.

The fluctuation of this entrance complicates contact lens fitting, because the optic zone is relatively small and the lens moves. A contact lens must be designed so that the optic zone adequately covers the pupil for all tasks under all levels of illumination. Fortunately, there is some flexibility in the amount of the pupil that must be covered by the optic zone. As a rule, if one eighth to one quarter or less of the pupil is covered by the secondary zone of the lens, visual performance is still satisfactory. The best theoretical explanation for this phenomenon is the Stiles-Crawford effect, which postulates that light passing through a unit area near the center of the pupil evokes a much greater sensation than light passing through a unit area near the periphery of the pupil.

PRECEPTS AND RELATIONSHIPS

Precepts

Contact lens application is most successful when certain precepts related to the physical, anatomical, and physiological factors are followed. These precepts can be grouped into four categories—bearing, venting, stability, and physical structure of the lens.

Bearing

Bearing refers to the areas of the cornea (also to the limbus or sclera in some lenses) on which the lens rests (bears).[30] During the blink cycle, pressures from the upper lid, and the weight and movement of the lens are transmitted to these bearing areas.

Five factors are essential for satisfactory bearing: (1) Posterior lens and anterior corneal curves must be relatively coincident over a fairly large area. This arrangement distributes the pressure throughout the area, and there is no great pressure on any small area. (2) Lens movement must be great enough to shift the bearing area *slightly* with blinking and eye movements, but not so great that pressure is increased significantly. (3) The limbus should be relatively free of bearing, so that there is no impairment of limbal circulation. The corneal apex should be relatively free of bearing, so that there is no excessive stimulation of the rich sensory nerve endings. (4) The periphery and edge of the lens should be close enough to the cornea so that the lid does not bear on it too abruptly. (5) Blink rate should not be excessive.

Venting

Venting is defined as exposure of the cornea to its normal environment.[31] Proper venting involves adequate flow of precorneal fluid over the cornea and adequate exposure to the air, which permit satisfactory nutrient and oxygen supply, metabolic waste removal, and normal precorneal fluid evaporation. Four factors are essential for satisfactory venting: (1) The posterior surface of the lens and anterior corneal curves must be noncoincident in some areas. The reservoirs and channels thus formed help promote good fluid interchange.[32] (2) Lens movement must be great enough in both a superoinferior and an anteroposterior direction to aid precorneal fluid interchange. (3) Lens diameter must be small enough to allow exposure of the cornea to the air.[33] (4) Blink rate and amount must not be insufficient.

A successful fit balances bearing and venting. In general, anything that improves one renders the other less effective. Thus, maximum bearing is attained when there is exact coincidence of lens and corneal curves over the entire posterior surface of the lens. In such a relationship, there are no fluid reservoirs or channels, and there is usually little or no lens movement. Fluid interchange is extremely poor. Maximum fluid interchange is attained when only a small central area is coincident with the cornea and the rest of the lens is removed from it. In such a relationship, pressures are restricted to a small area, and there is usually considerable lens movement. Bearing is extremely poor.

Stability

Stability of movement has been discussed in terms of bearing and venting. Movement must also allow satisfactory constant pupil coverage by the optic zone, and *movement should not be so great that blink action is radically increased or decreased in an attempt to maintain proper lens position.* This condition produces bearing, venting, and cosmetic problems, and the lids receive excessive mechanical stimulation. *Slight* movement is desired.

Stability of corneal topography is important; change of corneal topography from contact lens wear should be minimal. This stability provides a more consistent relationship between the posterior surface of the lens and anterior corneal curves. It decreases the amount of blurred vision when contact lenses are removed, and it permits an easier interchange of contact lenses and spectacles. If corneal topography remains stable, the patient is not forced to rely solely on contact lenses, and the possibility of problems from overwear is decreased.

Physical Structure of the Lens

The lens must be physically sound. Surfaces and edges must have proper configuration and smoothness. The proper refractive correction must be incorporated. The lens should be thin enough so that excessive lens weight is avoided. The lens should be thick enough so that there is no excessive change of curvature, no excessive adherence between lens and cornea, and no excessively thin edge (see p. 42).

Relationships

To fulfill the basic precepts, certain hypotheses based on theory and clinical experience are established as guidelines. These hypotheses are considered in terms of the physical characteristics of the lens and the relationships produced between it and the eye. The three general categories of physical characteristics are lens and corneal curvatures, thickness of the lens, and diameters or widths of the lens.

Lens and Corneal Curvatures

Specifically, this aspect involves the relationships between the posterior surface of the lens and the anterior corneal curves. As discussed here, these relationships are important in producing desirable bearing, venting, and movement.

General Curvature Relationships. When two structures having single spherical curvatures are placed in apposition without any tilt, there are three possible general curvature relationships. The rear curvature of the anterior structure may be the same as, steeper (having a shorter radius) than, or flatter (having a longer radius) than the front curvature of the posterior structure (Fig. 2–16).

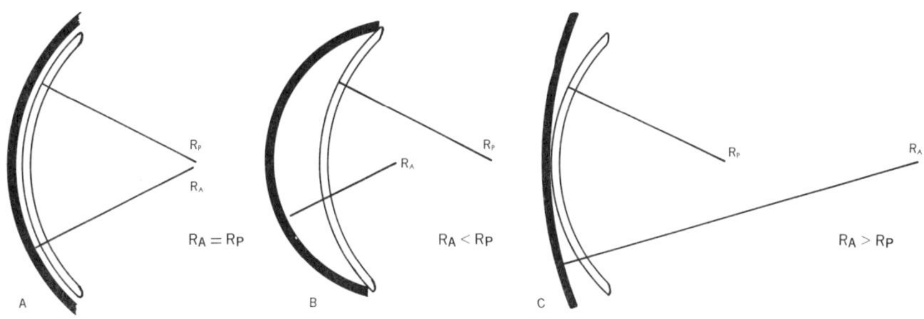

Figure 2–16. Relationships of two apposed spherical curvatures. A, *Curvatures are the same.* B, *Anterior curvature is steeper.* C, *Anterior curvature is flatter.* (*B and C are greatly accentuated for illustration.*)

When the curvature is the same, there is a *parallelism* or *alignment* of the two structures. When the curvature of the anterior structure is steeper than that of the posterior structure, there is a touch area around the periphery and *central clearance*. When the curvature of the anterior structure is flatter than that of the posterior structure, there is *central touch* and peripheral clearance.

In considering these relationships in terms of the posterior lens and anterior corneal curvatures, we will make four initial assumptions for ease of explanation: (1) The cornea has a centered, spherical corneal cap 6.5 mm. wide. (2) The peripheral cornea is spherical and flattens in a symmetrical manner. There is, therefore, a two-zone cornea. (3) The contact lens has an optic zone 6.5 mm. wide and an annular secondary zone of flatter curvature surrounding it. There is, therefore, a two-zone contact lens. (4) The 6.5 mm. optic zone is completely centered with the 6.5 mm. corneal cap, and there is no tilt of the contact lens. The two-zone lens can now be related to the two-zone cornea.

Optic-zone Relationships. Figure 2–17 shows the three possible relationships between the optic zone of the contact lens and the corneal cap. Figure

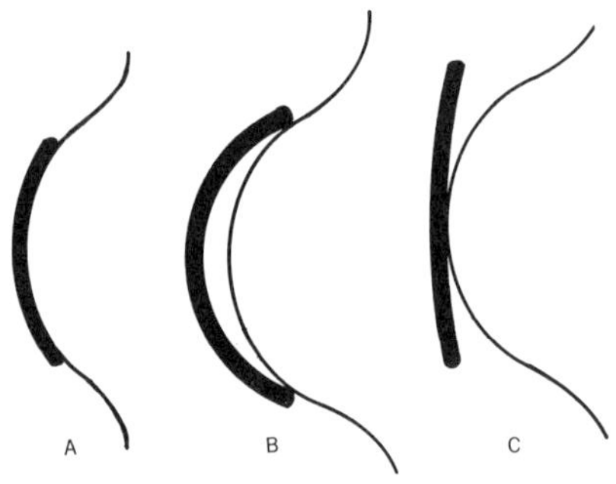

Figure 2–17. Relationships between the optic zone and corneal cap. A, *Apical (central) alignment with a parallel or maximum bearing relationship.* B, *Apical (central) clearance with a steep relationship.* C, *Apical (central) touch with a flat relationship. (B and C are greatly accentuated for illustration.)*

2–17A shows the relationship when the curvatures are the same. This is called an *apical* or *central alignment*—a *parallel,* or a *maximum bearing area* relationship. Figure 2–17B shows the relationship when the curvature of the optic zone is steeper than that of the corneal cap. This is called an *apical* or *central clearance*—a *steep* relationship. Figure 2–17C shows the relationship when the curvature of the optic zone is flatter than that of the corneal cap. This is called an *apical* or *central touch*—a *flat* relationship.

Even if there were a true corneal cap, the optic-zone diameter is almost always larger than that of the corneal cap. The cornea as classically defined flattens from corneal cap to limbus. As a result, the transition between optic and secondary zones of the contact lens rests on the flat peripheral cornea. This arrangement tends to push the optic zone away from the cornea (Fig. 2–18).

A 6.5 mm. optic zone with base curve radius equal to a central *spherical* ophthalmometric reading often produces apparent relative alignment. When optic-zone diameter is increased and this base curve is used, central clearance is often produced. This effect is due to two factors. First, the optic-zone transition is on a relatively flatter corneal area, which causes a greater lift effect. Second, as the chord length of two dissimilar superimposed curvatures is increased, the apparent sagittal depth between them is increased (Fig. 2–19).

As a clinical guideline, to compensate for alteration of fitting relationships produced by a change in optic-zone diameter, the base curve radius

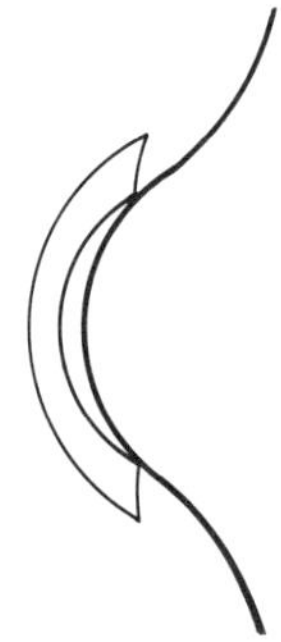

Figure 2–18. When an optic zone has the same radius but a greater diameter than the corneal cap, the transition between optic and secondary zones rests on the flatter peripheral cornea. This produces central clearance.

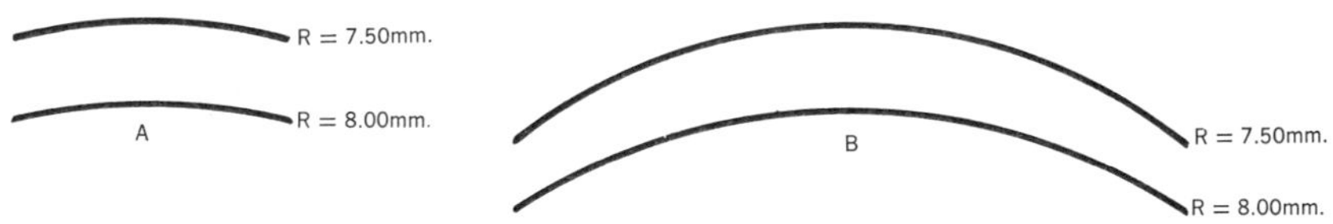

Figure 2–19. Because of a greater chord length, it is easier to appreciate sagittal differences between the curves on B.

must be lengthened by 0.01 mm. for every 0.1 mm. of increase of optic-zone diameter over 6.5 mm. to maintain the same relative central relationship. The opposite is true when optic-zone diameter is decreased. For example, assume that a desired relationship is obtained with a 7.5 mm. optic-zone diameter, but that a 7.0 mm. optic-zone diameter is to be used. The base curve radius must be shortened by 0.01 mm. for every 0.1 mm. decrease of optic-zone diameter to maintain the same relative central relationship.

Secondary-zone Relationships. Figure 2–20 shows the three possible relationships between the secondary zone of the contact lens and the peripheral cornea. Figure 2–20A shows the relationship when the curvatures are the same. This is called a *secondary-alignment relationship.* Figure 2–20B shows the relationship when the curvature of the secondary zone is steeper than that of the peripheral cornea. This is called a *secondary-touch relationship.* Figure 2–20C shows the relationship when the curvature of the secondary zone is flatter than that of the peripheral cornea. This is called a *secondary-clearance relationship.* Note that apical and secondary touch are produced by opposite types of curvature relationships. The same is true for apical and secondary clearance.

Figure 2–21 shows a lens with a secondary curve of a given radius. The depth of the plastic removed depends on the width of the secondary curvature. With a given secondary radius, the depth of the plastic removed at the edge of the lens is increased as the width of the secondary curve is increased.[34–35]

This is an important concept. In fabrication, *radii* are used to signify the secondary curve. This is done only for purposes of communication; it is the

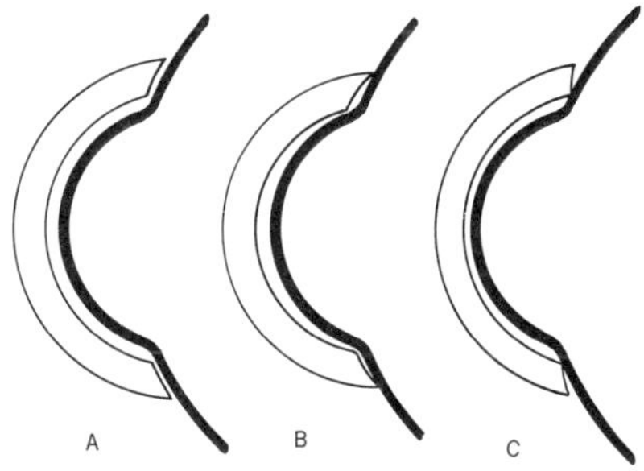

Figure 2–20. Secondary zone and peripheral corneal relationships. A, *Secondary alignment.* B, *Secondary touch.* C, *Secondary clearance. For diagrammatic purposes, the corneal flattening is accentuated.*

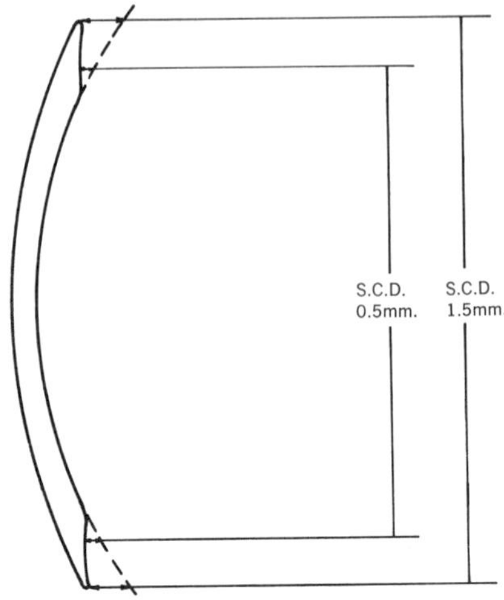

Figure 2–21. As the width of a secondary curve increases, the depth of plastic removed at the edge increases.

depth of the plastic removed that is important in establishing the relationship between the lens and the corneal curves. To a great extent, this is because the centers of curvature of a contact lens lie on the same axis, but the centers of curvature of the various areas of the cornea do not (Fig. 2–22). In contact lens fitting, linear-depth relationships are established between posterior lens and anterior corneal curves.

In addition, even if a single secondary curvature is used, there is a change of depth of plastic removed from the optic zone to edge (Fig. 2–21). This arrangement is advantageous because there is also progressive flattening of the cornea toward its periphery. As a result, a single secondary curvature may provide satisfactory relationships throughout its width with the underlying cornea.[36]

Another important related factor is that, for a given secondary width, the rate of change increases as the radius increases (Fig. 2–8), for there is

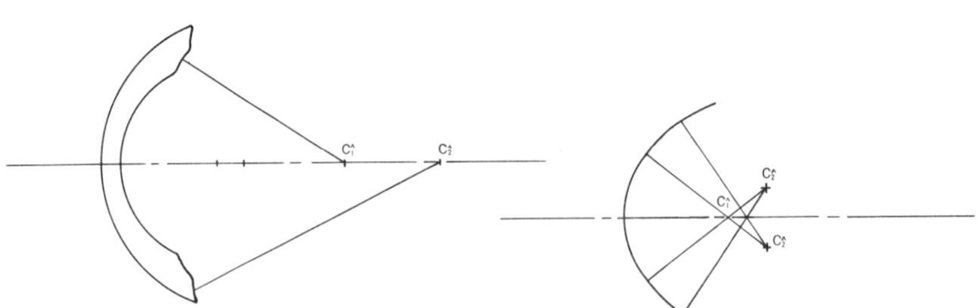

Figure 2–22. A, *The centers of various contact lens curvatures lying on a common axis.* B, *The centers of various corneal curvatures not lying on a common axis.*

a progression from maximum depth at the edge to no depth at the transition between optic and secondary zones.

Four concepts are important relative to secondary-zone fluid reservoirs: (1) For a given width, the depth of plastic removed is increased as the radius is increased. (2) For any secondary curve, there is a progressive increase in the depth of plastic removed, going from the transition between base and secondary curves to the edge of the lens. (3) For a given secondary radius, the depth of plastic removed is increased as the secondary-zone width is increased. (4) For a given secondary width and a given amount of difference between base and secondary curvatures, the depth of plastic removed and the resultant linear clearance between secondary curve and cornea is less for flatter bases.[35] To obtain a similar linear clearance, the secondary curve radius must vary directly with base curve radius, because of the *geometry of the lens* and not because of any correlation between central corneal curvature and rate of peripheral corneal flattening.

COMBINED OPTIC AND SECONDARY RELATIONSHIPS. Clinical application of contact lenses has shown that apical touch is generally not an acceptable relationship, because bearing is on a small area, producing a relatively great pressure on each area. Furthermore, this area is usually at or near the highly sensitive central cornea. Because of the small area of coincidence between lens and corneal curves, there is relatively poor adherence and often excessive movement. Precorneal fluid interchange is usually good, but the bearing is poor.

Clinical application of contact lenses has also shown that secondary edge touch is generally not an acceptable relationship. The touch at the edge of the lens pushes the center of the lens away from the cornea. At the same time, it produces a binding, or damlike, effect at the edge of the lens. Precorneal fluid interchange is usually poor because of the binding, and the bearing is usually poor because of its restriction to a narrow area.

Practically, this leaves two optic-zone relationships that may be combined with two secondary-zone relationships, resulting in four combinations: a combination of apical alignment and secondary clearance or secondary alignment; and a combination of apical clearance and secondary clearance or secondary alignment.

APICAL ALIGNMENT. *Apical Alignment and Secondary Clearance.* The optic zone is aligned with, and the secondary zone is clear of, the underlying corneal area (Fig. 2–23). As long as the optic zone is not too small, the pressures of the lens are spread over a relatively wide area and bearing is fairly good. The clearance of the secondary curves allows precorneal fluid to enter between them and the cornea, producing a reservoir. The pumping action of the lid, and lens movement and rocking move fluid from the reservoir over the optic-zone area and irrigates it. Secondary clearance should not be excessive, so that there is some auxiliary bearing support in this area. This arrangement still is one of the most widely used relationships.

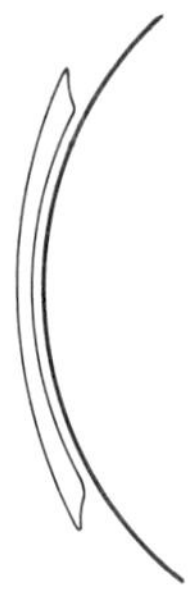

Figure 2–23. Apical alignment and secondary clearance.

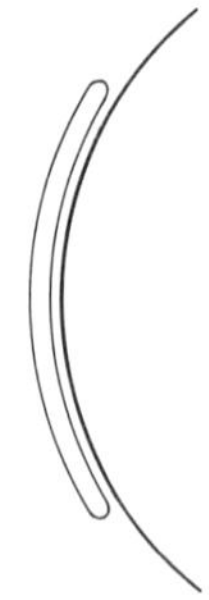

Figure 2–24. Apical alignment and secondary alignment.

Apical Alignment and Secondary Alignment. Both optic and secondary zones are aligned with the underlying cornea (Fig. 2–24). Bearing is good because the pressures are disbursed over a wide area. Interchange of precorneal fluid is usually poor because of the close curvature coincidence and the poor lens movement and rocking. If a material is developed that allows adequate fluid and gas interchange *through* the contact lens, this relationship may be acceptable.

Apical Clearance. *Apical Clearance and Secondary Clearance.* Both the optic and secondary areas of the lens are clear of the underlying corneal areas. Bearing is on the annular transition between optic and secondary areas (Fig. 2–25). When there is considerable apical clearance, bearing on the annular transition area is harsh. The transition bearing may produce a binding effect around the optic zone, which inhibits precorneal fluid interchange. However, there is less inhibition with *small* steep lenses than with larger steep lenses.

When there is minimum apical clearance and no excessive secondary clearance, these problems are reduced. Transition bearing is usually not so great that inhibition of fluid interchange and binding are caused. This fit is similar to the apical alignment–secondary clearance fit. It differs mainly in its attempt to ensure a very slight clearance from the highly sensitive cen-

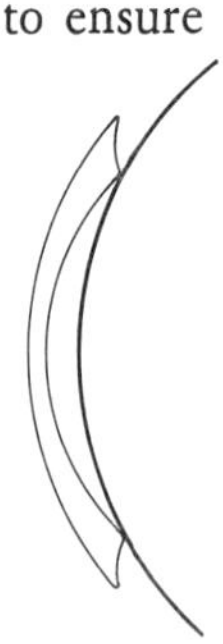

Figure 2–25. Apical clearance and secondary clearance.

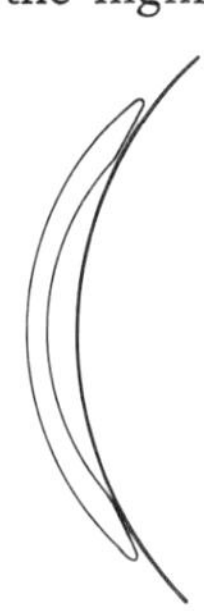

Figure 2–26. Apical clearance and secondary alignment.

tral cornea. Minimum apical clearance and moderate secondary clearance is the relationship preferred by the authors.

Apical Clearance and Secondary Alignment. The secondary area of the lens is aligned with, and the optic area is clear of, underlying corneal areas (Fig. 2–26). If the secondary zone of the lens is wide enough, bearing may be satisfactory. True secondary alignment may impede precorneal fluid interchange. This disadvantage can be overcome to a degree by the use of a relatively small lens diameter and a small optic-zone diameter. The small lens diameter aids venting by increasing corneal exposure. The small optic-zone diameter aids venting by decreasing the area needing irrigation. The combination of a small lens diameter and a small optic-zone diameter may also aid venting by increasing lens movement.

The basic relationships between corneal curves and the optic zone and the secondary-zone curves are not so clear-cut as presented, because most corneas are aspherical, toric, asymmetrical, and do not have corneal caps as classically described. In addition, the lens moves and tilts over different areas of the cornea.

Toric Corneas. A single spherical base curve cannot have the same relationship with the various meridians of a toric central cornea, and spherical secondary curves cannot have the same relationship with the various meridians of a toric peripheral cornea. When there is relative alignment across the flatter meridians, there is clearance along the steeper meridians.

It is important to remember that a toric surface does not have only the meridians of minimum and maximum curvature—that is, the two principal meridians. There is a gradual, progressive change of curvature from one meridian to another in any quadrant between the two principal meridians. As a result, spherical base or secondary curves can have relatively the same type of relationship with a considerable area of a not too highly toric cornea. The variance of linear depth between the lens and the cornea is extremely small over this area.

When corneal toricity is less than 0.4 mm. (about 2 D of astigmatism), it is often possible to obtain satisfactory relationships with spherical lens curves. At times, the best overall optic-zone relationship is obtained with a base curve slightly steeper than that needed for relative alignment across the flatter corneal meridians. This steepness produces a slight clearance over these meridians, but at the same time reduces the clearance over the steeper meridians. This procedure of *splitting "K"* is most often used when central corneal toricity is between 0.2 to 0.4 mm.—that is, 1 to 2 D. The relationships for appreciable with-the-rule and against-the-rule toricity are shown in Fig. 2–27.

When central corneal toricity is greater than 2 D, this procedure of splitting "K" may be used in some cases. In other cases, a toric base curve must be used to obtain satisfactory bearing (see p. 86).

Corneal Asymmetry. Not only are most corneas toric, but also they are

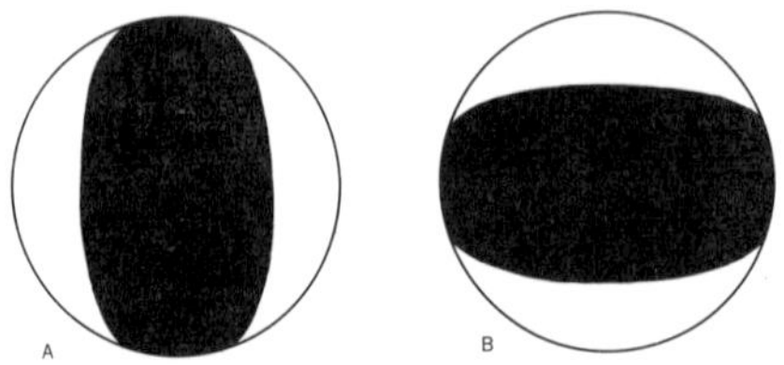

Figure 2–27. Schematic representation of relationship produced by use of a spherical base steeper than that needed for relative alignment with flatter meridians of a cornea that is considerably toric. White indicates relative alignment, and black indicates clearance. A, *With-the-rule corneal toricity.* B, *Against-the-rule corneal toricity.*

usually asymmetrical—that is, the rate and amount of curvature change in the various quadrants are unequal. Neither spherical nor toric-lens curvatures can have the same relationship to the corneal curvatures in all quadrants. If, for example, the nasal side of the cornea is flatter than the temporal, a secondary curvature that is aligned nasally will have clearance temporally.

It is felt that corneal asymmetry is greater peripherally than centrally. As a result, the problem in providing a desirable relationship in all quadrants of the secondary area is greater than in the optic area. When the secondary area is not too wide, however, satisfactory relationships are often obtained.

Lens Tilt. Up to this point, it has been assumed that the lens does not tilt on the eye. In practice, almost all lenses tilt to varying degrees when on the eye. This tilt changes the relationships between lens and corneal curves.

The upper lid often tilts the top of a superior-positioned lens toward, and the bottom away from, the cornea. Inferior-positioned lenses may be tilted this way if the lower lid pushes the bottom of the lens away from the cornea. Inferior-positioned lenses may also be tilted in the opposite direction. This tilt usually occurs when the lower lid does not support the lens. Generally, there is less tilt with inferior-positioned than with superior-positioned lenses.

Thickness of Lens

The three general aspects of contact lens thickness are center thickness, edge thickness, and anterior surface configuration.

To arrive at a logical center thickness, what happens when thickness is decreased or increased must be considered.[37,38] When center thickness is decreased, the weight of the lens, and pressure on the cornea is decreased. At the same time, the center of gravity moves toward or behind the rear surface (Fig. 2–28A), which increases adherence between the lens and the cornea and decreases movement. Structural stability of the lens is decreased as center thickness is decreased. When center thickness is increased, the weight of the lens is increased, thus increasing pressure on the cornea. At

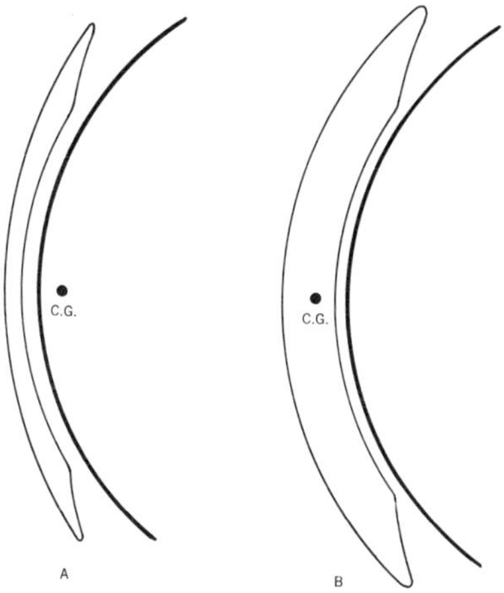

Figure 2–28. Position of center of gravity (C.G.) *related to lens thickness.* A, *Thin lens.* B, *Thick lens.*

the same time, the center of gravity moves toward the front surface (Fig. 2–28B), which decreases adherence between the lens and the cornea and increases movement. Structural stability of the lens is increased as center thickness is increased. A balance must be obtained between the relatively good bearing, good adherence, and poor structural stability of a thin lens and the relatively poor bearing, poor adherence, and good structural stability of a thick lens. *Thickness must not push the lid far from the cornea.*

Our conception of balanced center thicknesses is shown in Table 2–11 (see p. 63). With present manufacturing techniques of polymethyl methacrylate, lenses with center thicknesses less than 0.13 mm. frequently have poor structural stability. Hydration and lid pressures often flatten or warp the curvatures significantly, lens breakage is not uncommon, and surfaces cannot be readily polished to remove scratches or to alter refractive power. Different materials or annealing processes may minimize some of these problems and permit more liberal use of lenses with center thicknesses less than 0.13 mm.

Our conception of appropriate edge thickness is 0.13 ± 0.02 mm. on a *finished but unedged lens.* Edging procedure reduces this thickness somewhat and produces a proper edge contour. Edge contour should be such that the rounded apex is one-third closer to the posterior surface of the lens (see Figures 3–38, page 175). There should be no "lips," or sharp transition junctures, between the edge and the surfaces. When the upper lid tries to blink over an edge thicker than 0.15 mm., discomfort or displacement of the lens may occur, especially with small lenses that position in the palpebral aperture. *To reduce discomfort or lens movement, the patient may inhibit blinking, which results in poor venting.* When the edge is too thin it may be difficult to contour properly, and the residual sharpness may produce discomfort. There is also a greater probability that the edge will be chipped by handling, and there is insufficient stock for subsequent modification of secondary curves.

Because of the complex relationships of refractive power, lens diameter, optic-zone diameter, and secondary curvatures, our suggested center thicknesses may produce *finished but unedged* edge thicknesses outside of the range from 0.13 ± 0.02 mm. Table 2–11 should be used as a guide and thickness should be computed by the practitioner or manufacturer for each lens (App. VIII, p. 473). When undesired edge thickness is produced, center thickness can be increased or decreased slightly, or the original center thickness can be maintained and an anterior lenticular form can be used. Plus carrier lenticular form decreases edge thickness, and minus carrier lenticular form (myoflange) increases edge thickness.

Manufacture of an anterior lenticular form must be precise. The anterior optic-zone, or the bowl, should be about 0.30 to 0.50 mm. larger than the posterior optic-zone. The transition between the carrier and the bowl should be smooth. This smoothness should be produced without marring the optic quality of the periphery of the bowl area. Juncture thickness of a lens with positive refractive power should be about 0.13 to 0.15 mm. to reduce thickness and weight. Thinner junctures decrease stability, and may produce disengagement of the carrier from the bowl.

As the anterior surface curvature of a contact lens becomes flatter, there is an increase of base away from center prism, and the ability of the upper lid to grasp the lens increases. This anterior surface configuration is one reason that minus lenses usually position higher than plus lenses. A minus carrier lenticular form flattens the anterior surface curvature toward the periphery of the lens, and it can be used to raise a corneal contact lens.* Diagnostic lenses with various minus carriers can be used to control position. A minus carrier can either be ordered by power; such as −6 D carrier, or it can be ordered to produce a desired edge thickness, such as minus carrier to produce a 0.13 mm. edge thickness. A plus carrier lenticular steepens the anterior curvature near the periphery of the lens, and it can be used to lower a corneal contact lens, especially one with high minus power.

Diameters or Widths

Three categories of importance are lens diameter, optic-zone diameter, and secondary-zone width.

Lens Diameter. There are two important considerations related to lens diameter. First, the minimal functional lens diameter possible should be used in each fitting technique. This procedure allows for the maximum exposure of the cornea to its normal environment. Second, at the same time, the lens diameter used should allow for proper movement and position. Movement should be neither excessive nor insufficient, and the optic zone

* Drs. C. Edward Williams and Irvin M. Borish have made significant contributions in this area of contact lens fitting.

should adequately cover the pupil at all times. A balance must be obtained between these two considerations.

The lens diameter that produces the best balance is related to the corneal size, palpebral aperture size, lid position, lid tonicity, blink rate and amount, lens thickness, lens weight, optic-zone and secondary-zone diameters, the relationship between posterior surface of the lens and anterior corneal curves, and the viscosity of the precorneal fluid. Because of these many factors, lens diameter cannot be related accurately to lens position and movement. However, certain general guidelines may be used.[39]

As lens diameter is decreased, adherence of the lens to the cornea and the surface area of the lens that can be held by the upper lid are decreased. As a result, there are three general categories of lens diameter.

1. When the lens diameter is 9.5 mm. or larger, adherence of the lens to the cornea and of the lid to the lens tends to maintain the lens in a superior position. The geometric center of the lens is superior to the center of the cornea. About 20 to 25 per cent of a minus lens is covered by the upper lid in primary fixation. Plus lenses position somewhat lower.

2. When the lens diameter is 9.4 to 8.6 mm., adherence of the lens to the cornea and of the lid to the lens is such that there may be superior positioning, considerable lens movement, centered positioning, or positioning in the palpebral aperture.

3. When lens diameter is 8.5 mm. or less, and when it is at least 0.5 to 1.0 mm. less than median vertical palpebral aperture size, adherence of the lens to the cornea and of the lid to the lens is such that the lens tends to remain in an inferior position. The geometric center of the lens is inferior to the center of the cornea. Usually, none of the upper lid covers the lens in primary fixation, and the lens positions within the palpebral aperture. Small lenses that are thin, steep, or have minus carriers may go up.

Optic-zone Diameter. There are two important considerations related to optic-zone diameter with apical alignment or minimum apical clearance relationships. First, the optic zone should be large enough so that bearing is spread over a relatively large area, so that adherence is great enough to prohibit excessive movement, and so that the optic zone covers a sufficient amount of the pupil at all times. Second, the optic zone should be small enough so that a desired relationship can be obtained, so that the optic zone can be readily irrigated, and so that movement is not retarded too greatly.

Clinically, the range of optic-zone diameters that best balances bearing, venting, and movement with apical alignment or minimum apical clearance relationships is 6.5 to 7.5 mm. In terms of bearing, when the optic zone is larger than 7.5 mm., it is often difficult to obtain a desired central relationship because of the asymmetry and flattening of the peripheral cornea. When the optic zone is less than 6.5 mm., a desired central relationship can usually be obtained, but the area over which the pressures are disbursed is relatively small. As a result, the pressure on this smaller area is increased, assuming that there is a constant total force being exerted. However, the total force typically is increased because the smaller optic zone decreases adherence and increases movement. Because of this excess movement, as well as the basically small optic-zone diameter, it is more likely that inadequate pupil coverage will result.

In terms of venting, when the optic zone is larger than 7.5 mm., it is often difficult to obtain proper central irrigation because of the size of the zone and the reduced lens movement. When the optic zone is less than 6.5 mm., venting is good, but bearing is often poor.

In an apical clearance and secondary bearing technique, the most logical optic-zone diameter is 6.6 mm. or less. There are two reasons for this. First, this diameter provides a relatively small central area requiring irrigation. Second, for a given base curvature, clearance is inversely related to the optic-zone diameter (see p. 36).

Secondary-zone Width. Total secondary-zone width on each side of the optic zone is simply half the difference between lens diameter and optic-zone diameter. When a secondary clearance relationship is used, total secondary width of small contact lenses is usually 0.50 to 0.75 mm. and total secondary width of medium or large contact lenses is usually 1.00 to 1.25 mm. These widths provide a satisfactory volume of fluid in the secondary reservoir while maintaining a satisfactory optic-zone diameter. When a secondary alignment relationship is used, total secondary width is 0.70 to 1.00 mm., which distributes the pressures over a satisfactory bearing area.

Any contemporary corneal contact lens can be evaluated in terms of its curvature relationships, center thickness, and diameters and widths. The combination of these values establishes a lens design that tends to assume a certain position on the eye.

CONTEMPORARY LENSES IN TERMS OF RELATIONSHIPS AND POSITIONING

Superior Positioning Lenses

On the basis of lens diameter and secondary width, there are three frequently used types of lens construction that *tend* to position superiorly.

Contour (Large Lens Diameter and Wide Secondary)

A popular contemporary lens design is the contour or modified contour.[40–44] It is based on apical alignment or minimum apical clearance and moderate secondary clearance relationships. The lens diameter is usually 9.0 to 10.2 mm., and the optic-zone diameter is usually 6.5 to 7.5 mm. Use of these diameters usually results in a secondary width of approximately 1.0 to 1.5 mm.

When a bicurve construction is used, the secondary radius is usually 0.7

to 1.3 mm. longer than the base curve. When a tricurve construction is used, the intermediate curve radius is usually 0.7 to 1.3 mm. longer than the base curve. The peripheral curve is usually 0.2 to 0.4 mm. wide, and its radius is usually 1.5 to 4 mm. longer than the base curve. There is often a blend between the peripheral and intermediate curves. A tricurve construction is used more frequently when the lens diameter is greater than 9.8 mm. It is possible to use a multicurve construction, but it is rarely necessary. Center thickness is computed to produce an edge thickness of 0.15 mm. on a finished but unedged lens. About 20 to 25 per cent of a minus lens is covered by the upper lid with primary fixation. Because of its greater weight and the position of its center of gravity, the plus lens usually positions lower. This lens design is discussed in more detail on page 55.

Spherocon® (Medium Lens Diameter and Narrow Secondary)

This configuration is also a popular contemporary lens design.[45] A basic reason for its popularity is that most of the specifications are standardized, making it easier to design. However, because of the wide variability among patients, excess standardization presents many problems.

This lens design is based on an apical alignment or minimum apical clearance, and secondary clearance relationships. Lens diameters usually range from 8.9 to 9.4 mm. When a relatively flat cornea, a relatively large cornea, a low lower lid, a wide palpebral aperture, or a strong refractive power is encountered, larger diameters in the range (9.3 or 9.4 mm.) are recommended. When a relatively steep cornea, a relatively small cornea, a high lower lid, or a narrow palpebral aperture is encountered, smaller diameters in the range (8.9 or 9.0 mm.) are recommended.

The secondary curve is usually about 0.4 mm. wide, and its radius is usually standardized at 12.25 mm. Subtraction of the secondary curve width from the lens diameter gives an optic zone of 8.0 to 8.6 mm. To obtain approximate apical alignment with such large optic zones, it is often necessary to use a base curve radius 0.10 to 0.15 mm. longer than the central spherical ophthalmometric reading.

Often a series of blends is placed between the secondary curve and the optic zone. This procedure decreases the sharp juncture between the grossly dissimilar base and secondary radii. At the same time, it decreases the optic-zone diameter. When this procedure is used, the base curve radius need not be lengthened as much. These blending curves usually have radii of 11.50, 10.50, and 9.50 mm.

Lenses of this design usually position superiorly or move from superior to central positioning.

Ultrathin (Medium Lens Diameter and Wide Secondary)

This lens design has lens diameters about 8.6 to 9.4 mm. and secondary curve widths about 0.8 to 0.9 mm. Optic zones of 7.0 to 7.6 mm. result.

A bicurve construction usually is used, and secondary curve radii are usually 1.0 to 1.5 mm. longer than the base curve. These medium lens diameters are used to increase corneal exposure.[46]

Because aperture positioning or excessive movement often results from such diameters, compensations are made in an attempt to center the lens or reduce movement. These compensations usually involve the use of a thin center thickness and mild apical clearance. Such a lens design is termed a *thin lens* or *thin, steep lens design.*

Reduction of thickness decreases lens inertia, moves the center of gravity toward the cornea, and reduces the holding ability of the upper lid. These factors increase adherence of the lens to the cornea and reduce movement. Steepening the base curve further increases adherence. In a thin lens, the proximity of the lens to the cornea is such that the depth of the fluid between them is not altered greatly by shortening of the base curve radius by 0.05 to 0.10 mm.

This lens design is more applicable in minus lenses from −2.00 D to about −6.00 D than in plus and in low or very high minus lenses. Plus and low or very high minus lenses in small diameters usually have too much weight per unit area, and a relatively large amount of inertia, resulting in excessive movement.

Thickness is determined by *computation* of the center thickness that produces a 0.10 mm. edge thickness on a finished but unedged lens. Computation at times produces a center thickness of less than 0.10 mm. The minimum center thickness for a thin lens, however, should be 0.10 mm. Thicknesses are often about one-quarter less than standard (Table 2–1). Positioning may be superior, central, or inferior. At times, there is considerable movement.

TABLE 2–1

CENTER THICKNESS GUIDE FOR SMALL, ULTRATHIN MINUS LENSES

Power	Center Thickness
−2.00 D	0.15 mm.
−2.75 D	0.14 mm.
−3.50 D	0.13 mm.
−4.25 D	0.12 mm.
−5.00 D	0.11 mm.
−5.75 D	0.10 mm.

Palpebral Aperture Positioning Lenses (Intrapalpebral Lenses)

When the lens diameter is 8.5 mm. or less, the lens tends to position in the palpebral aperture. Lenses that position in the palpebral aperture are termed *aperture lenses, palpebral aperture lenses,* or *intrapalpebral lenses.* The diameter that will result in this positioning in a given individual depends to a large degree on the vertical median palpebral aperture size.

The minimum diameter in an intrapalpebral lens without infringement of the edge onto the pupil is equal to the distance from the lower lid to the top of the pupil. This determination assumes that the lower lid is at or above the lower limbus. The maximum diameter for a completely aperture-contained lens is equal to the vertical median palpebral aperture size. Any lens meant to position in the palpebral aperture has an overall diameter less than palpebral aperture size. The closer the lens diameter is to the minimum, the greater the probability is that it will position in the aperture. There are four frequently used types of lens constructions that *tend* to position in the aperture.

Ultrathin (Small Lens Diameter and Narrow Secondary)

This lens design is based on apical alignment or slight apical clearance and secondary clearance relationships. The lens diameter is usually 7.3 to 8.8 mm. The secondary curve width on each side is usually 0.5 to 0.6 mm. Optic-zone diameter is usually 6.3 to 7.8 mm. Thin center thickness, such as that just discussed, is often used. A bicurve or a blended bicurve construction usually is used. Secondary radii are usually 2 to 8 mm. longer than the base curve.[47–48] One such lens (L.D. +2 or O.C. +2) is designed by a Topogometer attachment on a Keratometer or Ophthalmometer (see p. 334).

Bayshore Technique (Small Lens Diameter and Wide Secondary)

This design is based on apical clearance and secondary alignment. The lens diameter is 0.2 mm. less than the vertical median aperture size, but not less than 7.0 mm. or more than 8.8 mm. It is of tricurve construction.[49–51]

The intermediate curve width on each side is 0.8 mm. when the lens diameter is 7.0 to 8.0 mm., 0.85 mm. when the lens diameter is 8.0 to 8.5 mm., and 0.90 mm. when the lens diameter is 8.5 to 8.8 mm. Intermediate radii are often 0.9 to 1.6 mm. longer than the base. The intermediate radius *must* be chosen by use of diagnostic lens procedures (see p. 81). The peripheral curve width is 0.10 mm. when the lens diameter is 7.0 to 8.0 mm., 0.15 mm. when the lens diameter is 8.0 to 8.5 mm., and 0.20 mm. when the lens diameter is 8.5 to 8.8 mm. The peripheral curve radius is usually standardized at 17.0 mm. The optic-zone diameter is simply the difference between the lens diameter and twice the secondary-curvature width.

The base curve is chosen with an allowance to the flatter ophthalmometric reading plus one third of the corneal astigmatism. The base curve radius is *steepened* by subtraction of the allowance factors in Table 2–2.

TABLE 2–2

B.T. BASE CURVE ALLOWANCE

Optic Zone	Subtract Base Curve Allowance
5.6 mm.	0.65 mm.
5.8 mm.	0.50 mm.
6.0 mm.	0.40 mm.
6.2 mm.	0.35 mm.
6.4 mm.	0.30 mm.
6.5 mm.	0.30 mm.
6.6 mm.	0.25 mm.

Edge thickness usually is slightly larger than standard, or about 0.22 mm.

Nodema® Contact Lens (Small Lens Diameter and Variable Secondary)

This lens design is based on apical alignment or minimum apical clearance and moderate secondary clearance relationships. The lens diameter is between the minimum and maximum aperture positioning lens diameters, and usually ranges from 7.5 to 8.8 mm., with an average of 8.3 mm. (Fig. 2–29).

The secondary curve width on each side of the optic zone is usually 0.5 to 0.75 mm. A bicurve or tricurve construction is usually used. Secondary curve radius for a bicurve lens and intermediate curve radius for a tricurve lens is usually 1.0 to 1.6 mm. longer than base curve radius. Peripheral curve width is 0.30 mm. for a tricurve lens. The center thickness is computed to produce edge thicknesses as discussed on p. 43. This lens design is discussed in more detail on page 55.

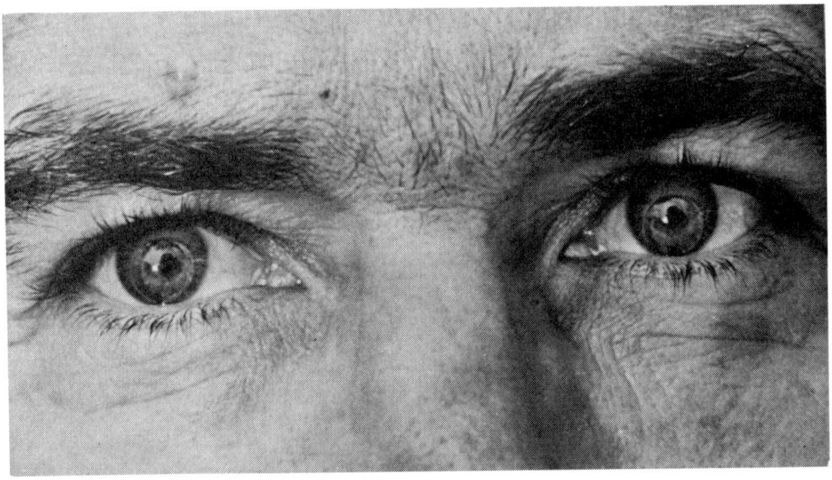

Figure 2–29. Nodema® contact lenses.

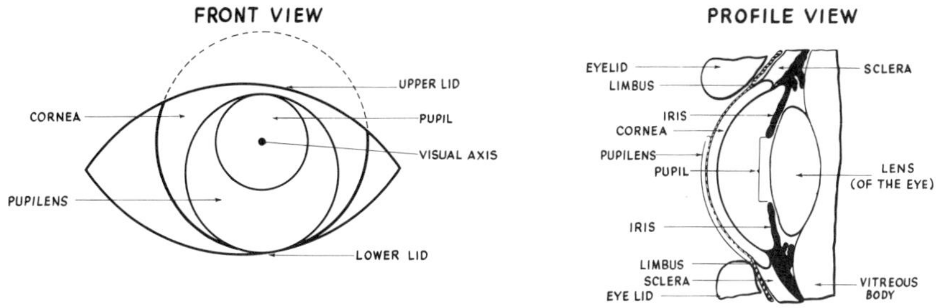

Figure 2–30. "F" Pupilens® contact lenses.

"F" Pupilens® (Lower Lid-Bearing Lenses)

Many aperture-positioning lenses rest, or bear, on the lower lid. This is especially true in the lens design ("F" Pupilens) described here (Fig. 2–30).[52–55]

The lens diameter is equal to the distance from the lower lid to the superior pupillary margin. Apical alignment or minimum apical clearance and moderate secondary clearance relationships are used.

The secondary curve width on each side is equal to about three sixteenths of the pupil size under ordinary room illumination (Table 2–3).

TABLE 2–3

SECONDARY CURVE WIDTHS FOR "F" PUPILENS® CONTACT LENSES

Pupil Size	Secondary Curve Width
3 mm.	0.55 mm.
4 mm.	0.75 mm.
5 mm.	0.90 mm.
6 mm.	1.10 mm.
7 mm.	1.30 mm.

A bicurve construction is generally used. The secondary radius is similar to that in the Nodema® contact lens. Computation of the center thickness is discussed on page 43.

BASIC CLINICAL PROCEDURE FOR GENERAL SPHERICAL SINGLE-VISION LENSES

Selection of a tentative lens design category for a given patient is discussed starting on page 12. Most patients are best fitted with nonprismatic, single-vision lenses having single spherical central anterior and posterior curvatures. The clinical procedure used with this group is considered here. Clinical procedures used with patients requiring "special design lenses" because of special topographical, structural, or visual needs are considered starting on page 86.

The practitioner must make two important initial decisions when fitting general spherical single-vision lenses.[56] The *lens design* that will probably best fulfill the precepts and attain the basic goals for each patient must be selected. Then the *lens specifications* of this design must be determined.

Selection of Lens Design

Many patients can be successfully fitted with any one of several of the contemporary designs discussed here. Others are best fitted using a particular design. Maximum overall success is attained by determination of which lens design probably will be most successful for the patient. Clinically, the most logical lens design for a patient is determined by the practitioner's knowledge and experience, the lid positioning and palpebral aperture size, the refractive power and corneal topography, and the patient's reaction to, and the performance of, lenses placed on the eye.

Experience and knowledge direct the authors' thinking in making certain judgments. The first is that certain superior (large) or intrapalpebral aperture (small) lens designs are preferable; the second is that some patients are better fitted by superior-positioning lenses and others by aperture-positioning lenses.

For a superior-positioning lens design, the preference of the authors is to use a modified contour with a minimum apical clearance and moderate secondary clearance. When necessary, it is usually possible to produce apical alignment with this same lens by reducing the optic-zone diameter 0.3 to 0.4 mm.

The Sphercon is used as an auxiliary superior-positioning design when aperture size is small, corneal size is small, and the pupil is large. This lens design provides a relatively smaller lens diameter, indicated by corneal diameter and aperture size, while providing a large optic zone, indicated by the pupil size.

In aperture-positioning, the preferred basic design is the Nodema contact lens. Minimum apical clearance and moderate secondary clearance relationships are preferable. Ultrathin lenses or the Bayshore technique are used as auxiliary designs.

The authors prefer to use relatively small contact lenses, which usually position in the palpebral aperture, for all patients. Relatively larger lenses, which usually position superiorly, are used only when the performance of and reaction to small diagnostic contact lenses is unfavorable or when the patient cannot adapt to small intrapalpebral lenses. This judgment is based upon the following general bearing, venting, vision, and comfort characteristics of these two lens types.

Bearing. (1) Aperture-positioning lenses are usually covered by the upper eyelid only during the closure phase of blinking, but superior-positioning lenses are almost always partially covered by the upper eyelid. The contact lens and the cornea receive more pressure with superior-positioning lenses. (2) Aperture-positioning lenses often move less than superior-positioning lenses. (3) Aperture-positioning lenses are usually smaller and lighter than superior-positioning lenses. (4) The upper edges of superior-positioning lenses are usually tucked underneath the upper eyelid and the bearing of the eyelid against the edge is less abrupt.

VENTING. (1) The relatively smaller diameters of aperture-positioning lenses cover less of the cornea. (2) Because the upper eyelid almost always covers part of superior-positioning lenses, the pump action of the upper eyelid is usually more effective. This pump action becomes extremely bad with aperture-positioning lenses when the patient inhibits blinking in an attempt to reduce the bearing of the upper eyelid against the edge of the lens. (3) Aperture-positioning lenses often move less than superior-positioning lenses.

COMFORT. (1) Initial comfort is often better with superior-positioning lenses because their edges are tucked underneath the upper eyelid. (2) Adaptation and long-term comfort are often better with aperture-positioning lenses because they move less, because they follow the eye during fixation changes, and because they produce fewer physical and physiological changes of the anterior segment tissues. The relative ease of adaptation to aperture-positioning lenses often reinforces the patient's motivation.

VISION. (1) Because of their small size, aperture-positioning lenses may produce more visual problems from flare (see p. 228). Even those practitioners who prefer to use relatively large lenses for most patients should consider fitting small lenses to patients with certain anatomical, topographical, or refractive characteristics.

First, when the palpebral aperture is less than 8.5 mm., the upper lid is low, the patient is enophthalmic, or the cornea is more than 45 diopters, small lenses are highly desirable. When these anatomical characteristics are associated with one another, and intrapalpebral contact lenses are contraindicated, small lenses may be fitted so that their upper edge is underneath the upper eyelid with primary fixation. This positioning may tend to allow more corneal exposure to the atmosphere, fewer problems of flare, less abrupt bearing of the upper eyelid against the edge of the lens, and a better bearing relationship of lens to the lower lid or limbus.

When small lenses are fitted to a person with a palpebral aperture more than 10.5 mm., with a lower lid that is below the inferior limbus, an upper lid that is high, or with exophthalmia, superior positioning may again be desired. This positioning may enhance the pumping action of the upper eyelid and may lessen an abrupt bearing of the lens on the lower limbus or lid.

Second, when the central corneal toricity is less than 0.2 mm.—or about 1 D of astigmatism—a good central bearing relationship may be obtained with a single spherical base curve. When the corneal toricity is greater than this value, it is more difficult to obtain desirable bearing with a single spherical base curve. In such cases, an intrapalpebral lens is preferred. In this position, the upper lid exerts less pressure on the lens. Lens weight is usually reduced as smaller diameters are used. These factors aid bearing. Venting is usually satisfactory owing to lack of coincidence between the lens and corneal curves and the relatively greater corneal exposure.

Third, small lenses are indicated for single cut low minus and low or medium plus lenses. Basic ophthalmic optics shows that the center thickness necessary to achieve a desired plus correction and a satisfactory edge thickness is directly proportional to the lens diameter, assuming that all other factors are constant. A relatively thinner lens with more desirable position and movement often results. Minus carrier lenticular forms often produce better position and movement with low minus or any plus lens.

Selection of Lens Specifications

Once the most logical lens design is selected, the specifications that will provide the desired relationships must be determined from data from properly applied tests and measurements. *Understanding of theory and limitations of contemporary procedures allows a logical selection of lens specifications* (see p. 216).

There are three general methods for determining specifications: those employing measurements and standards, diagnostic lens procedure, and a combination of both.

Measurements and Standards

In this method of selection of lens specifications, measurements of various factors are taken. They are then related to standards or norms for a given lens design, and the specifications are determined. The most common means for measuring corneal topography is by ophthalmometry or keratometry (p. 323). This method is neither entirely accurate nor valid for determining the posterior curvatures of a contact lens, which are needed to establish desired lens-cornea relationships.[57–59] It is possible, however, to make empirical average allowances in ophthalmometric findings that will result in satisfactory relationships in some cases. Because these are average allowances and there are many deviations from average, satisfactory relationships are not produced in some cases.

Measurement of anterior segment anatomy by a ruler or gross inspection as an aid for determining lens diameters and widths is not very accurate. Furthermore, there is no refined accurate or valid way to correlate these findings as an aid to selecting lens characteristics. Again, it is possible to correlate these findings empirically and to determine grossly specifications that are satisfactory in some cases.

Diameters and Widths. Tables 2–4 and 2–5 have the suggested initial lens diameters, optic-zone diameters, and secondary curve widths for aperture-positioning small Nodema contact lenses and superior-positioning contour (large) contact lenses.

TABLE 2–4

DIAMETERS AND WIDTHS FOR NODEMA™ CONTACT LENSES

Flat "K"	H.I.D.	V.P.A.	L.D.	O.Z.D.	S.C.W.
Less than 42.00 D	12.5 mm. or more	10.5 mm. or more	8.8 mm.	7.5 mm.	0.65 mm.
42.00 to 42.75 D	12.0 mm.	10.0 mm.	8.5 mm.	7.2 mm.	0.65 mm.
43.00 to 43.75 D	11.5 mm.	9.5 mm.	8.3 mm.	7.0 mm.	0.65 mm.
44.00 to 44.75 D	11.0 mm.	9.0 mm.	8.0 mm.	6.7 mm.	0.65 mm.
45.00 to 46.00 D	10.5 mm.	8.5 mm.	7.8 mm.	6.5 mm.	0.65 mm.
More than 46.00 D	10.0 mm. or less	8.0 mm. or less	7.5 mm.	6.2 mm.	0.65 mm.

H.I.D. = Horizontal iris diameter
V.P.A. = Vertical palpebral aperture
L.D. = Lens diameter
O.Z.D. = Optic-zone diameter
S.C.W. = Secondary curve width
Flat "K" = Ophthalmometric or keratometric power of the flatter principal meridian

TABLE 2–5

DIAMETERS AND WIDTHS FOR CONTOUR LENSES

Flat "K"	H.I.D.	V.P.A.	L.D.	O.Z.D.	S.C.W.
Less than 42.00 D	12.5 mm. or more	10.5 mm. or more	9.8 mm.	7.8 mm.	1.00 mm.
42.00 to 42.75 D	12.0 mm.	10.0 mm.	9.5 mm.	7.5 mm.	1.00 mm.
43.00 to 43.75 D	11.5 mm.	9.5 mm.	9.3 mm.	7.3 mm.	1.00 mm.
44.00 to 44.75 D	11.0 mm.	9.0 mm.	9.0 mm.	7.0 mm.	1.00 mm.
45.00 to 46.00 D	10.5 mm.	8.5 mm.	8.8 mm.	6.8 mm.	1.00 mm.
More than 46.00 D	10.0 mm. or less	8.0 mm. or less	8.5 mm.	6.5 mm.	1.00 mm.

H.I.D. = Horizontal iris diameter
V.P.A. = Vertical palpebral aperture
L.D. = Lens diameter
O.Z.D. = Optic-zone diameter
S.C.W. = Secondary curve width
Flat "K" = Ophthalmometric or keratometric power of the flatter principal meridian

Lens Diameter. With a Nodema contact lens design, the average or standard lens diameter is taken as 8.3 mm. This value then may be modified with consideration of other factors. The three important measurements related to lens diameter modification are a vertical measurement, a horizontal measurement, and a keratometric or ophthalmometric measurement.

The vertical measurement is from the lower lid or inferior limbus, whichever is higher, to the upper lid or superior limbus, whichever is lower. This

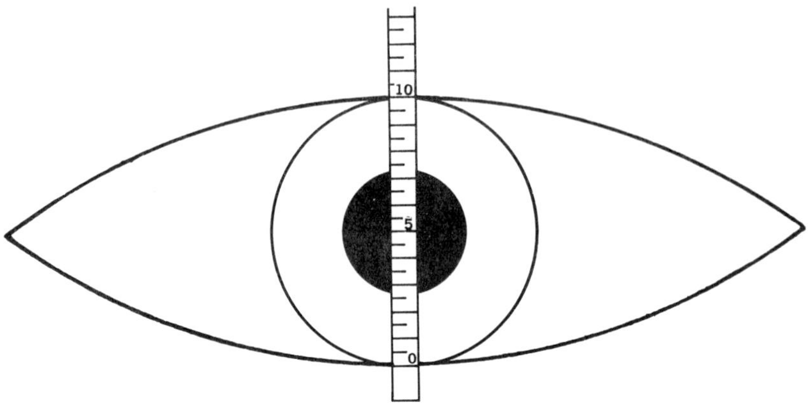

Figure 2–31. Measurement of median vertical palpebral aperture size with a millimeter rule.

measurement is made in the median vertical plane, and it is usually equal to median vertical palpebral aperture (V.P.A.) size. To determine median vertical aperture size, the patient is instructed to fixate a distant eye-level target. A millimeter rule is placed as shown in Fig. 2–31. Estimation to the nearest 0.5 mm. is made. This measurement is relatively gross. When patients narrow the aperture in a defense reaction as the ruler is positioned, the measurement is not as valid. Under such circumstances, visual estimation without the use of a ruler may be more accurate. The measurement is related to Table 2–4.

The horizontal measurement is from the nasal limbus to the temporal limbus in the median horizontal plane. Clinically, this is a measurement of visible horizontal iris diameter (H.I.D.), and it is somewhat more accurate than the preceding measurement. It is taken as shown in Fig. 2–32. Estimation to the nearest 0.5 mm. is made. The measurement is related to Table 2–4.

Some practitioners recommend that lens diameter should be altered in relation to the ophthalmometric reading. Smaller diameters are used with steeper corneas, and larger diameters are used with flatter corneas. This practice is based on the assumption that steep corneas are small and flat corneas are large and on the assumption that steep corneas have small corneal caps and large corneas have large corneal caps. The measurement is related to Table 2–4.

For a contour lens design, the average or standard lens diameter is 9.3 mm. This value may be modified in consideration of the three important measurements related to lens diameter modification—that is, vertical palpebral aperture, horizontal iris diameter, and keratometric or ophthalmometric

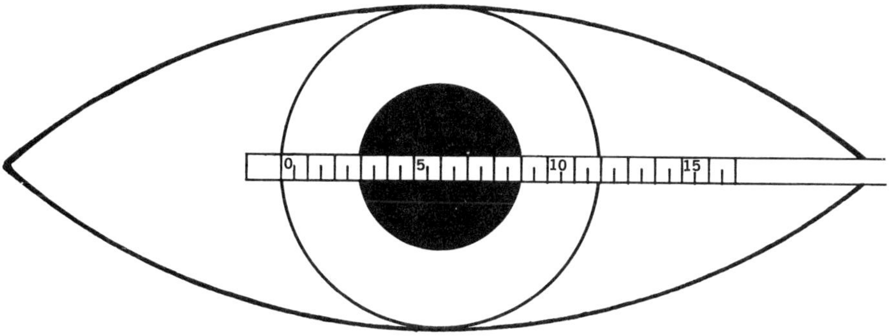

Figure 2–32. Measurement of visible horizontal iris diameter with a millimeter rule.

measurement. These measurements are related to Table 2–5. Note that the lens diameter of a contour contact lens is about 1 mm. more than that of a Nodema contact lens for a given eye.

In some cases, the measurements of vertical palpebral aperture, horizontal iris diameter, and keratometric or ophthalmometric reading will produce different diameters when related either to Table 2–4 or to Table 2–5. If two of the three measurements produce the same lens diameter, the third measurement is disregarded. If none of the three measurements produces the same lens diameter, the middle lens diameter value is used.

Optic-Zone Diameter. The range of optic-zone diameters used is 6.5 to 7.5 mm. This range balances bearing and venting (see p. 45).

Secondary Curve Width and Number. Total secondary curve width on each side of the optic zone is simply half the difference between lens and optic-zone diameters. Total average secondary curve width of Nodema contact lenses is 0.65 mm. (Table 2–4). Total average secondary curve width of contour lenses is 1.00 mm. (Table 2–5).

The authors prefer to order bicurve lenses rather than tricurve lenses. When problems from improper precorneal fluid interchange occur, the bicurve lens can be made into a tricurve lens by the addition of a peripheral curve. This peripheral curve increases the volume of the secondary reservoir of precorneal fluid and helps to shear the precorneal fluid toward the edge of the lens. The secondary curve of the bicurve lens should be ground on and then polished with a hard pad. A 0.10 mm. wide touch blend with a radius 0.60 flatter than the base curve radius should then be applied with a soft pad (Table 2–6). Practitioners who prefer to order tricurve lenses can use the secondary curve tables on pages 67 and 68.

TABLE 2–6

SECONDARY CURVE WIDTHS

T.S.C.W.	BL. W.	S.C.W.
0.50 mm.	0.10 mm.	0.40 mm.
0.65 mm.	0.10 mm.	0.55 mm.
0.75 mm.	0.10 mm.	0.65 mm.
1.00 mm.	0.10 mm.	0.90 mm.
1.25 mm.	0.10 mm.	1.15 mm.

T.S.C.W. = Total Secondary Curve Width
S.C.W. = Secondary Curve Width
BL. W. = Blend Width

CURVATURES. Tables 2–7, 2–8, and 2–10 show the suggested base and secondary radii.

TABLE 2–7

B.C.R. WHEN L.D. IS LESS THAN 8.8 MM. AND O.Z.D. IS 6.7 TO 7.2 MM.*

Amount of Ophthalmometric or Keratometric—"K"— Astigmatism	B.C.R.
0.00 to 0.37 D	Flat "K"
0.50 to 1.00 D	Flat "K" +0.25 D
1.12 to 1.50 D	Flat "K" +0.37 D
1.62 to 2.00 D	Flat "K" +0.50 D
2.00 D and over	$\text{Flat "K"} + \left(\frac{\text{Steep "K"} - \text{Flat "K"}}{3}\right)$ A toric base curve should also be considered

* When O.Z.D. is 6.2 to 6.6 mm., steepen B.C.R. found in this table by 0.25 D. When O.Z.D. is 7.3 to 7.8 mm., flatten B.C.R. found in this table by 0.25 D. To compensate for lengthening of B.C.R. from hydration, shorten B.C.R. found in this table an empirical average of 0.03 mm. for *all* plus and minus less than 6 D and 0.05 mm. for over minus 6 D.

B.C.R. = Base curve radius
L.D. = Lens diameter
O.Z.D. = Optic-zone diameter

Flat "K" = Power of flatter ophthalmometric or keratometric principal meridian

Base Curve. Determination of base curve radius is by average allowances made in central ophthalmometric (or keratometric) readings. To obtain the most accurate readings, the instrument must be focused, calibrated, and used properly (p. 328).

Three readings are taken on each eye, and the mean values for the flatter ophthalmometric principal meridian—that is, flat "K"—and the oph-

TABLE 2–8

B.C.R. WHEN L.D. IS MORE THAN 8.9 MM. AND O.Z.D. IS 6.7 TO 7.2 MM.*

Amount of Ophthalmometric or Keratometric—"K"— Astigmatism	B.C.R.
0.00 to 0.37 D	Flat "K" −0.25 D
0.50 to 1.00 D	Flat "K"
1.12 to 1.50 D	Flat "K" +0.12 D
1.62 to 2.00 D	Flat "K" +0.25 D
2.00 D and over	Flat "K" + $\left(\frac{\text{Steep "K"} - \text{Flat "K"}}{3}\right)$ A toric base curve should also be considered

* When O.Z.D. is 6.2 to 6.6 mm., steepen B.C.R. found in this table by 0.25 D. When O.Z.D. is 7.3 to 7.8 mm., flatten B.C.R. found in this table by 0.25 D. To compensate for lengthening of B.C.R. from hydration, shorten B.C.R. found in this table an empirical average of 0.03 mm. for *all* plus and minus less than 6 D and 0.05 mm. for over minus 6 D.

B.C.R. = Base curve radius
L.D. = Lens diameter
O.Z.D. = Optic-zone diameter
Flat "K" = Power of flatter ophthalmometric or keratometric principal meridian

thalmometric astigmatism are determined. These values are then related to Table 2–7 when the lens diameter is less than 8.8 mm., as is common with Nodema intrapalpebral contact lenses. This table lists average allowances and can be used when minimal apical clearance relationships are desired.

As shown in Table 2–8, it is recommended that, for lens diameters more than 8.8 mm., as are common in superior-positioning lenses, base curve radius be 0.25 D flatter than that used for small diameters, as are common with aperture positioning lenses.

When Table 2–7 or Table 2–8 is used with optic zones larger than 7.2 mm. the base curve radius is lengthened. When Table 2–7 or 2–8 is used with optic zones smaller than 6.7 mm., the base curve radius is shortened (see p. 36).

The need to change the allowance factor as central corneal toricity increases is discussed on page 41. Base curves should be ordered slightly steeper than optimum because lenses typically flatten after they are hydrated.[60–62] Although the amount of flattening is not constant in all lenses, 0.03 mm. is used as an average amount for plus or low minus lenses.

Because the drum readings of the Ophthalmometer or Keratometer are in diopters, they must be converted to radii (Table 2–9). A more extensive surface power table is given in Appendix VI.

TABLE 2–9

CONVERSION TABLE FROM DIOPTERS ($\nabla N = 1.3375 - 1.0000$) TO RADII*

D	R	D	R	D	R	D	R
50.87	6.63	47.87	7.05	44.87	7.52	41.87	8.06
50.75	6.65	47.75	7.07	44.75	7.54	41.75	8.08
50.62	6.67	47.62	7.09	44.62	7.56	41.62	8.11
50.50	6.68	47.50	7.11	44.50	7.58	41.50	8.13
50.37	6.70	47.37	7.12	44.37	7.61	41.37	8.16
50.25	6.72	47.25	7.14	44.25	7.63	41.25	8.18
50.12	6.73	47.12	7.16	44.12	7.65	41.12	8.21
50.00	6.75	47.00	7.18	44.00	7.67	41.00	8.23
49.87	6.77	46.87	7.20	43.87	7.69	40.87	8.26
49.75	6.78	46.75	7.22	43.75	7.72	40.75	8.28
49.62	6.80	46.62	7.24	43.62	7.74	40.62	8.31
49.50	6.82	46.50	7.26	43.50	7.76	40.50	8.33
49.37	6.84	46.37	7.28	43.37	7.78	40.37	8.36
49.25	6.85	46.25	7.30	43.25	7.80	40.25	8.39
49.12	6.87	46.12	7.32	43.12	7.83	40.12	8.41
49.00	6.89	46.00	7.34	43.00	7.85	40.00	8.44
48.87	6.91	45.87	7.36	42.87	7.87	39.87	8.46
48.75	6.92	45.75	7.38	42.75	7.90	39.75	8.49
48.62	6.95	45.62	7.40	42.62	7.92	39.62	8.52
48.50	6.96	45.50	7.42	42.50	7.94	39.50	8.55
48.37	6.98	45.37	7.44	42.37	7.97	39.37	8.57
48.25	7.00	45.25	7.46	42.25	7.99	39.25	8.60
48.12	7.01	45.12	7.48	42.12	8.01	39.12	8.63
48.00	7.03	45.00	7.50	42.00	8.04	39.00	8.65

* This table is accurate to the nearest 0.12 D. It is valid for measuring *convex* surfaces with a Bausch & Lomb Keratometer. For measuring convex surfaces with an American Optical Co. Ophthalmometer, 0.03 mm. is subtracted from the radius determined. For measuring concave surfaces, the following allowances are added to the convex radius:

Radius 7.10 or less	add 0.02 mm.
Radius 7.10 to 8.30	add 0.03 mm.
Radius 8.30 or more	add 0.04 mm.

Secondary Curve Radii. Secondary curve radius is determined by addition of a given amount to base curve radius. Table 2–10 can be used with blended or unblended bicurve lenses, and it was computed to maintain mild to moderate secondary clearance and a satisfactory secondary reservoir of precorneal fluid as secondary curve width is varied.

The depth of the plastic removed and the resultant lacrimal reservoir depth and volume for a given secondary radius are directly related to secondary curve width. To maintain satisfactory fluid reservoirs, secondary

TABLE 2–10

SECONDARY CURVE RADII

S.C.W.	BL. R.	S.C.R.
0.50 mm.	0.60 mm.	1.6 mm.
0.65 mm.	0.60 mm.	1.4 mm.
0.75 mm.	0.60 mm.	1.2 mm.
1.00 mm.	0.60 mm.	1.0 mm.
1.25 mm.	0.60 mm.	0.8 mm.

S.C.W. = Secondary Curve Width on each side of the optic zone
S.C.R. = Secondary Curve Radius. Add this value to B.C.R. and order to nearest 0.1 mm.
BL. R. = Blend Radius. Add this value to B.C.R. and order to nearest 0.10 mm.

curve radii must be inversely related to secondary curve width. Blend curve radius is also found from Table 2–10.

Because it is difficult to verify the zone diameters of a heavily blended lens, and because the practitioner can better manage performance of lenses with modifications following clinical observations of lenses ordered for the patient, the authors usually prefer to order touch blended lenses. When it is necessary, heavier blends are placed between adjacent curves. Blend radius is about halfway between the radii of adjacent curves. Blend width is about 0.20 mm. If the practitioner does not do his own modifications, lenses may be ordered from the manufacturer with the heavy blends. If such lenses are ordered, the secondary curve width should be reduced by the amount of the blend width to maintain the optic-zone diameter. Blends should be fabricated with a soft pad, such as velveteen.

Secondary curve radii also have been determined by peripheral ophthalmometric measurements (see p. 322). We do not believe that they give sufficiently valuable information as they are generally done now. However, it is conceivable that a satisfactory system for taking and translating such measurements into the selection of secondary radii can be developed. If such a system is developed, it will be preferable to use this system rather than to use arbitrary allowances. Base and secondary radii have also been determined by photokeratoscopic readings (see p. 369).

Examples

Take an example of a touch blended Nodema aperture-positioning lens and a touch blended superior-positioning (contour) lens fitted by use of these tables. The following measurements are found: horizontal iris diameter (H.I.D.) = 11.5 mm., vertical palpebral aperture (V.P.A.) = 9.5 mm., and central keratometric readings = 43.75/44.50 @ 90 or 7.72 mm./7.58 mm. (Table 2–9).

Nodema Aperture Positioning. Using H.I.D., V.P.A., and Flat "K" in Table 2–4, we find the following diameters and widths: L.D. = 8.3 mm., O.Z.D. = 7.0 mm., and S.C.W. = 0.65 mm. Using S.C.W. of 0.65 in Table 2–6, we find BL. W. = 0.10 mm. and S.C.W. = 0.55 mm.

Using a Flat "K" reading of 7.72 and a "K" astigmatism of 0.75 D in Table 2–7, the B.C.R. is desired 0.25 steeper than the flatter keratometric principal meridian—44.00 D or 7.67 mm., it should be ordered 0.03 mm. shorter than desired—7.64 mm.—to compensate for flattening from hydration. An S.C.R. with an S.C.W. of 0.65 mm. is 1.4 mm. longer than the B.C.R., or 9.04 mm. (Table 2–10). For practical purposes, it may be ordered to the nearest 0.10 mm., or 9.00 mm. BL. R. is 8.20 mm.

Superior-Positioning Lens. Using H.I.D., V.P.A., and Flat "K" in Table 2–5, we find the following diameters and width: L.D. = 9.3 mm., O.Z.D. = 7.3 mm., and S.C.W. = 1.00 mm. Using S.C.W. of 1.00 in Table 2–6, we find S.C.W. is 0.90 mm., and BL. W. = 0.10 mm.

With a keratometric astigmatism of 0.75 D in Table 2–8, the base curve radius (B.C.R.) desired is "on K,"—that is 43.75 D or 7.72 mm. It should be ordered 0.03 mm. shorter than desired—7.69 mm.—to compensate for flattening from hydration. A secondary curve radius (S.C.R.) with an S.C.W. of 1.00 mm. is 1.00 mm. longer than the B.C.R., or 8.69 mm. (Table 2–10). For practical purposes, it may be ordered to the nearest 0.10 mm. or 8.70 mm. BL. R. is 8.30 mm. (Table 2–10).

Lens Thickness. The authors' concept of an appropriately balanced thickness is discussed on page 42. Tables 2–11 and 2–12 may be used as general guides for center thickness.

Refractive Power. A full discussion is presented on page 338. Clinically, the following procedure is used to compute refractive power to fit a contact lens with central spherical anterior and posterior curvatures:

1. The needed spectacle plane refractive power is written in minus cylinder form.
2. It is placed on an optical cross.
3. The vertex distance of the spectacle correction is determined.
4. The spectacle plane refractive power in each meridian is converted to equivalent corneal plane refractive power. Assuming a 12 mm. vertex distance, this conversion is done by finding the spectacle plane refractive power in the left hand column of the vertex distance table and going across to the right for each meridian (Table 2–13). For other vertex distances, the formula below the table is used or the more comprehensive vertex table is used (p. 454).
5. The values are taken from the optical cross and made into a spherocylindrical prescription.
6. The formula $AI = AT - AO$ is used,

where: AI = Residual internal astigmatism
AT = Total spectacle astigmatism at the corneal plane
AO = Ophthalmometric astigmatism

TABLE 2–11

APPROXIMATE STANDARD CENTER THICKNESS FOR MINUS LENSES*

Refractive Power	7.5 to 8.0 mm. L.D.	8.1 to 8.5 mm. L.D.	8.6 to 9.0 mm. L.D.	9.1 to 9.5 mm. L.D.	9.6 to 10.00 mm. L.D.
−1.00 to −1.87 D	0.16 mm.	0.17 mm.	0.18 mm.	0.20 mm.	0.22 mm.
−2.00 to −2.87 D	0.15 mm.	0.16 mm.	0.17 mm.	0.18 mm.	0.19 mm.
−3.00 to −3.87 D	0.14 mm.	0.15 mm.	0.16 mm.	0.16 mm.	0.17 mm.
−4.00 to −4.87 D	0.13 mm.	0.14 mm.	0.15 mm.	0.15 mm.	0.16 mm.
−5.00 to −5.87 D	0.13 mm.	0.13 mm.	0.14 mm.	0.14 mm.	0.15 mm.
−6.00 to −6.87 D	0.12 mm.	0.12 mm.	0.13 mm.	0.13 mm.	0.14 mm.
−7.00 and over	0.11 mm.	0.11 mm.	0.12 mm.	0.12 mm.	0.13 mm.

* If computed center thickness for a standard thickness minus lens is less than 0.13 mm., an anterior lenticular construction with a 0.13 mm. center thickness may be considered. The anterior optic zone is 0.5 mm. larger than the posterior optic zone. If ultrathin lenses are desired, 0.03 mm. is subtracted from the value in the table.

TABLE 2–12

APPROXIMATE STANDARD CENTER THICKNESS FOR PLUS LENSES

Refractive Power	7.5 to 8.0 mm. L.D.	8.1 to 8.5 mm. L.D.	8.6 to 9.0 mm. L.D.	9.1 to 9.5 mm. L.D.	9.6 to 10.00 mm. L.D.
+1.00 to +1.87 D	0.19 mm.	0.20 mm.	0.22 mm.	0.23 mm.	0.25 mm.
+2.00 to +2.87 D	0.21 mm.	0.22 mm.	0.24 mm.	0.26 mm.	0.28 mm.
+3.00 to +3.87 D	0.22 mm.	0.24 mm.	0.26 mm.	0.28 mm.	0.31 mm.

7. Half of any *AI* is then added to the spherical component of corneal plane refractive power. This procedure compensates for vertex distance factors and produces the spherical equivalent power needed to place the circle of least confusion on the retina. This procedure should be followed in all cases to form the proper habit for determining refractive power.

8. Finally, the relationship of the base curve to the flatter central ophthalmometric reading must be considered (see p. 349). When the base curve and the flatter ophthalmometric reading have the same radius, no compensation is made. When the radius of the base curve is longer than that of the flatter ophthalmometric reading, +0.25 D is added to the value found in Step 7 for each 0.04 or 0.05 mm., or 0.25 D difference. When the radius of the base curve is shorter than the flatter ophthalmometric reading, −0.25 D is added to the value found in Step 7 for each 0.04 or 0.05 mm., or 0.25 D (Table 2–9).

Auxiliary Features. Aside from tint and anterior lenticular construction, auxiliary features are usually not indicated at this point.

Effect of Modification on Determining Lens Specifications. As has been implied, certain aspects of a finished contact lens can be modified;

TABLE 2–13

VERTEX DISTANCE COMPENSATION FOR 12 MM.
(accurate to nearest 0.12 D)

Spectacle Plane Power	Corneal Plane Power Minus	Corneal Plane Power Plus	Spectacle Plane Power	Corneal Plane Power Minus	Corneal Plane Power Plus
3.00	2.87	3.12	9.00	8.12	10.12
3.25	3.12	3.37	9.25	8.37	10.37
3.50	3.37	3.62	9.50	8.50	10.75
3.75	3.62	3.87	9.75	8.75	11.00
4.00	3.87	4.25	10.00	8.87	11.37
4.25	4.00	4.50	10.25	9.12	11.62
4.50	4.25	4.75	10.50	9.37	12.00
4.75	4.50	5.00	10.75	9.50	12.37
5.00	4.75	5.37	11.00	9.75	12.62
5.25	5.00	5.62	11.25	9.87	13.00
5.50	5.12	5.87	11.50	10.12	13.37
5.75	5.37	6.12	11.75	10.25	13.75
6.00	5.62	6.50	12.00	10.50	14.12
6.25	5.87	6.75	12.25	10.62	14.25
6.50	6.00	7.00	12.50	10.87	14.75
6.75	6.25	7.37	12.75	11.12	15.12
7.00	6.50	7.62	13.00	11.25	15.37
7.25	6.62	8.00	13.25	11.50	15.87
7.50	6.87	8.25	13.50	11.62	16.12
7.75	7.12	8.50	13.75	11.75	16.37
8.00	7.25	8.87	14.00	12.00	17.00
8.25	7.50	9.12	14.25	12.25	17.25
8.50	7.75	9.50	14.50	12.37	17.50
8.75	8.00	9.75	14.75	12.50	17.87

$$D_c = \frac{D_1}{1 - sD_1}$$

D_c = Power need at corneal apex
D_1 = Lensometer or phoropter value of spectacle lens
s = Vertex distance in meters

other aspects can be altered only by processing a new lens. The following are among the modifications that can be made to a finished lens: lens diameter can be reduced; secondary curves can be flattened, added or widened, and optic-zone diameter can be decreased.

When the practitioner is doubtful of the specifications to order, he should tend to use slightly larger lens diameters, slightly larger optic-zone diameters, and slightly steeper secondary curves. If necessary, these characteristics can be appropriately modified on the initial lenses.

The practitioner should know the *minimum* changes of lens parameters that may alter lens performance. Changes of lens diameter or optic-zone diameter less than 0.3 mm., changes of intermediate curve radius less than

0.2 mm., changes of peripheral curve radius less than 0.5 mm., changes of center thickness less than 0.02 mm., and changes of base curve radius less than 0.04 mm. generally are clinically insignificant in altering lens performance. Note that both lens diameter and optic-zone diameter are often changed simultaneously by the same amount. If this is not done, total secondary curve width will also be changed. The authors almost never use lenses with total secondary curve width less than 0.5 mm.

Diagnostic Lens Procedure

In this method of selection of lens specifications, lenses with known characteristics are systematically observed and tested on the patient's eyes. The results are related to standards or norms for a given lens design, and the specifications are determined.

This method has been called diagnostic, fitting, control, or trial lens procedure. With the use of all four of these designations, the procedure is best defined.

One definition of diagnosis is a critical scrutiny and resultant judgment. On this basis, the diagnostic lens procedure may be defined as a method for determining the characteristics of a contact lens based on critical scrutiny and resulting judgment from the systematic trial of lenses with controlled specifications (diagnostic lenses).

The diagnostic lenses are placed on an eye the characteristics of which are not completely known. Various tests, measurements, and observations are used to determine the relationship of lens to eye. The results are related to the desired, or standard, findings for a given lens design. When results are unsatisfactory, another diagnostic lens that will theoretically improve the results is selected, placed on the eye, and evaluated. By systematic continuation of this procedure, the specifications of the lenses to be ordered are determined.

The diagnostic lens procedure is also used with lenses processed for the patient to evaluate resulting performance from initial specifications. When undesired performance results, lens specifications may be modified or new lenses processed. *Determination of modifications or specifications of new lenses is based on both the diagnostic lens evaluation of patient's lenses and evaluation of the lenses from the diagnostic sets.* Because of this factor, even practitioners who order all their initial designs by means of measurements and standards must understand diagnostic lens procedure.

Need. The method of measurements and standards is not entirely accurate and valid for determination of initial contact lens specifications. The most valid and accurate determination of lens specifications is made with a lens having all desired specifications on an adapted eye. This determination cannot be done for two reasons:

First, to have lenses with all possible combinations of lens variables constitutes an additional economic investment; and second, it is not usual for the amount of lacrimal fluid and the blink action to remain completely unaltered when contact lenses are initially worn. On initial insertion of a contact lens, many patients react with the defense mechanisms that protect the eye from a foreign body. Excessive lacrimal fluid is produced in an effort to wash out the "foreign body." Excessive winking or blinking (blepharospasm) may be produced in an effort physically to expel the "foreign body." If these reactions are severe and prolonged, the practitioner must judge whether contact lenses are contra-indicated, whether lens specifications should be determined by the measurements and standards procedure, or whether the patient should be seen again before a decision is made.

However, use of the diagnostic lens procedure employing a properly designed and used set can often approximate the ideal situation well enough so that a valid and accurate selection of initial lens specifications and designs results. In keratoconus and irregular cornea, refraction over diagnostic lenses is the only way to determine proper power. With aphakia, refraction over diagnostic lenses allows more accurate power determination, because it eliminates vertex distance errors.

Design. A diagnostic lens unit should be designed to obtain the maximum accurate information about all lens designs from a minimum number of lenses.[63] The *first* consideration in designing a diagnostic lens unit relates to refractive power. Records indicate that, excluding aphakics, well over 90 per cent of contact lens patients are myopes. More than 75 per cent of these need a spherical refractive element ranging between −1.75 and −5.00 D. It is logical to select a power that will give maximum information for this large group. A median power, about −3.25 D, produces relatively small differences between the diagnostic lens and needed power in a large number of cases, and the majority of diagnostic lenses should have this power. Supplementary diagnostic lenses with −1.25 D and +2.50 D are also desirable.

The *second* consideration in designing the diagnostic lens unit relates to diameters, thickness, and anterior surface configuration. The range of diagnostic lens diameters used most often by the authors is 7.5 to 9.0 mm. Secondary curve width on each side of the optic zone is either 0.50 or 0.75 mm. Some −3.25 D diagnostic lenses have a standard center thickness (about 0.15 to 0.16 mm.) and some have an ultrathin center thickness (about 0.10 mm.). Ultrathin center thicknesses are also used with the −1.25 D (about 0.15 mm.) and the +2.50 D (about 0.21 mm.) diagnostic lenses. All ultrathin lenses are made to produce a 0.10 mm. edge thickness on a finished but unedged lens. Minus six diopter carriers are frequently used with the ultrathin −3.25 D diagnostic lenses.

The *third* consideration in designing the diagnostic lens unit relates to base and secondary curves. Base curves usually range from 7.10 to 8.40 mm.[64]

The *fourth* consideration in designing the diagnostic lens unit relates to secondary curves. In accordance with his fitting philosophy, the practitioner can use the following outline to develop diagnostic lens sets of *bicurve, unblended tricurve,* or *blended tricurve* lenses. Lens diameters, optic-zone diameters, refractive powers, and thicknesses are the same for any of these three lens constructions. Base curves range from 7.10 to 8.40 mm. in 0.10 mm. increments. Secondary curve widths and radii are determined from the following tables. All blends should be fabricated with a soft pad, such as velveteen. The secondary curves of all bicurve lenses and the intermediate and peripheral curves of all tricurve lenses should be ground on and then polished with a hard pad. However, all tricurve lenses with secondary curve widths of 0.50 mm. should have their intermediate curves fabricated with a soft pad, to act as a blend.

SECONDARY CURVES FOR DIAGNOSTIC LENSES

Bicurve Lenses

S.C.W.	S.C.R.
0.50 mm.	1.6 mm.
0.65 mm.	1.4 mm.
0.75 mm.	1.2 mm.
1.00 mm.	1.0 mm.
1.25 mm.	0.8 mm.

S.C.W. = Secondary Curve Width
S.C.R. = Secondary Curve Radius. Add this value to the base curve radius and order to the nearest 0.10 mm.

Unblended Tricurve Lenses

S.C.W.	I.C.W.	P.C.W.
0.50 mm.	0.20 mm.	0.30 mm.
0.65 mm.	0.35 mm.	0.30 mm.
0.75 mm.	0.45 mm.	0.30 mm.
1.00 mm.	0.70 mm.	0.30 mm.
1.25 mm.	0.95 mm.	0.30 mm.

S.C.W.	I.C.R.	P.C.R.
0.50 mm.	1.6 mm.	12.50 mm.
0.65 mm.	1.4 mm.	12.00 mm.
0.75 mm.	1.2 mm.	11.00 mm.
1.00 mm.	1.0 mm.	10.50 mm.
1.25 mm.	0.8 mm.	10.50 mm.

S.C.W. = Secondary Curve Width
I.C.W. = Intermediate Curve Width
P.C.W. = Peripheral Curve Width
I.C.R. = Intermediate Curve Radius. Add this value to the base curve radius and order to the nearest 0.10 mm.
P.C.R. = Peripheral Curve Radius. Order as shown in table.

Blended Tricurve Lenses

S.C.W.	B.L.W.	I.C.W.	P.C.W.
0.50 mm.	0.10 mm.	0.10 mm.	0.30 mm.
0.65 mm.	0.15 mm.	0.20 mm.	0.30 mm.
0.75 mm.	0.15 mm.	0.30 mm.	0.30 mm.
1.00 mm.	0.15 mm.	0.55 mm.	0.30 mm.
1.25 mm.	0.15 mm.	0.80 mm.	0.30 mm.

S.C.W.	B.L.R.	I.C.R.	P.C.R.
0.50 mm.	0.60 mm.	1.6 mm.	12.50 mm.
0.65 mm.	0.60 mm.	1.4 mm.	12.00 mm.
0.75 mm.	0.60 mm.	1.2 mm.	11.00 mm.
1.00 mm.	0.60 mm.	1.0 mm.	10.50 mm.
1.25 mm.	0.60 mm.	0.8 mm.	10.50 mm.

S.C.W. = Secondary Curve Width
B.L.W. = Blend Width
I.C.W. = Intermediate Curve Width
B.L.R. = Blend Radius. Add this value to the base curve radius and order to the nearest 0.10 mm.
I.C.R. = Intermediate Curve Radius. Add this value to the base curve radius and order to the nearest 0.10 mm.
P.C.R. = Peripheral Curve Radius. Order as shown in table.

DIAGNOSTIC CONTACT LENS SETS

Set No. 1

−3.25 D:C.T. = 0.15 mm.

L.D.	O.Z.D.	S.C.W.
7.5 mm.	6.5 mm.	0.50 mm.
8.0 mm.	7.0 mm.	0.50 mm.
8.5 mm.	7.5 mm.	0.50 mm.
8.5 mm.	7.0 mm.	0.75 mm.
9.0 mm.	7.5 mm.	0.75 mm.
9.5 mm.	7.5 mm.	1.00 mm.

Set No. 2

−3.25 D:C.T. = 0.10 mm.:Minus 6 D carrier lenticular

L.D.	O.Z.D.	S.C.W.
8.0 mm.	6.5 mm.	0.75 mm.
8.5 mm.	7.0 mm.	0.75 mm.
9.0 mm.	7.5 mm.	0.75 mm.

Set No. 3

−1.25 D:C.T. = 0.15 mm.

L.D.	O.Z.D.	S.C.W.
7.5 mm.	6.5 mm.	0.50 mm.
8.0 mm.	7.0 mm.	0.50 mm.
8.5 mm.	7.5 mm.	0.50 mm.

Set No. 4

+2.50 D:C.T. = 0.21 mm.

L.D.	O.Z.D.	S.C.W.
7.5 mm.	6.5 mm.	0.50 mm.
8.0 mm.	7.0 mm.	0.50 mm.
8.5 mm.	7.5 mm.	0.50 mm.

Many laboratories have "loaner" diagnostic sets that the practitioner may borrow. Unless the practitioner does a large amount of contact lens fitting, it is more economical to borrow "loaner" lenses for special design fitting. Many practitioners prefer to purchase contact lenses on a per lens basis. Lenses which prove to be undesirable for a patient can then be made into a supplementary diagnostic lens set.

CARE. For effective use, lenses must be cared for properly. The lenses may be stored in 2 × 2 inch cases having two wells—that is, "Slim Jim" cases—or in a single-well case (Fig. 2–33). Stickers listing the lens specifications are placed on the rear of the case, and the cases are systematically arranged by ascending order of base curve in slide trays (Fig. 2–34).

Diagnostic lenses may be stored dry or wet. Dry storage is preferable because hydration often changes the base curve, and it is troublesome to change fluid every few days. Before diagnostic lenses are used, they are thoroughly wetted to reduce discomfort and to increase cleanliness. After they are used, they are thoroughly cleaned with wetting or cleaning solu-

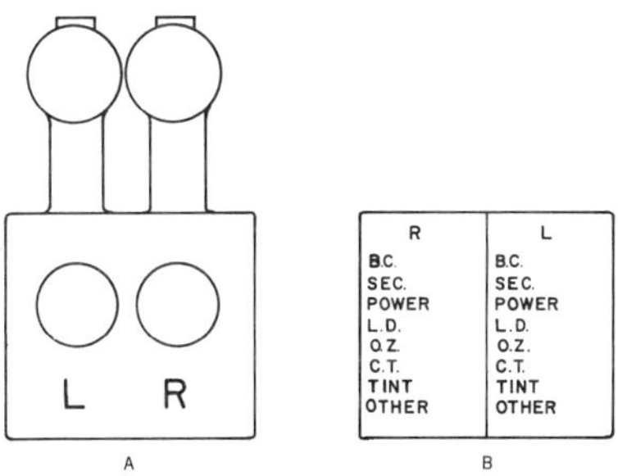

Figure 2–33. A, *Double-well "Slim Jim" case.* B, *Sticker listing lens specifications placed on rear of case.*

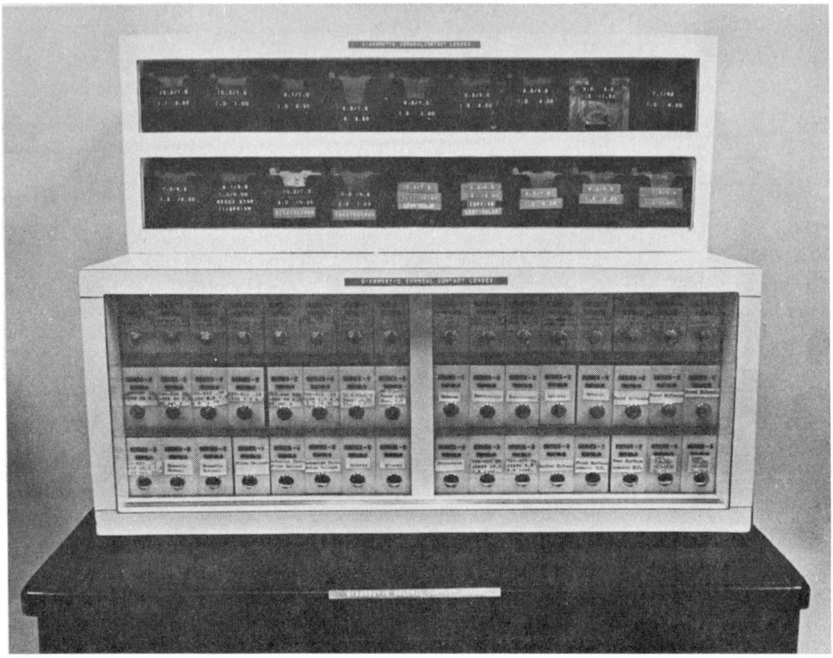

Figure 2–34. Diagnostic contact lenses in slide trays.

tion, which is then rinsed off with water. The lens is air-dried or blotted dry with a facial tissue. Rubbing is avoided because it may scratch the lens surface. Storage without cleaning and drying is not advised because mucoid material and pathogens may be transferred to and irritate a patient subsequently.

Diagnostic lenses are checked periodically to make certain they have not been accidentally switched. If diagnostic lenses are switched, findings based on them are erroneous. They should be checked periodically to make certain that neither the surfaces nor the edges have become marred. If they have become marred, they must be refinished so that no unnecessary discomfort is produced. It is important that the edges of diagnostic lenses be satisfactory, so that no undue discomfort is caused.

Technique. The first placement of lenses on the patient's eyes is an important experience for him. A proper insertion technique is necessary to minimize excessive lacrimation and blepharospasm.[65] Every patient is somewhat apprehensive about having contact lenses placed on his eyes. Because excessive lacrimation and blepharospasm are precipitated or accentuated both by psychic and physical factors, the technique must minimize these factors. Proper technique is begun during the general examination. Discussion is aimed at reducing apprehension and developing rapport with the patient. Slit-lamp biomicroscopy of the anterior segment is done with and without fluorescein (see p. 319), and the use of fluorescein is explained. Placing fluorescein on the patient's eye at this point familiarizes him with the process of something being placed on the eye by the examiner. It also enables the examiner to estimate patient sensitivity and apprehension. Because fluorescein produces little or no discomfort when applied properly, patient anxieties are often reduced.

The patient is seated in the examination chair with his head against the headrest. This position prevents any backing away when the diagnostic lenses are used. The headrest is slightly angled so that the top of the patient's head is tilted slightly back and the chin slightly forward. This arrangement helps relieve lid pressure on the lens. A subject of interest not associated with contact lenses may be discussed with the patient partially to distract his attention.

A diagnostic lens with the appropriate specifications is selected. For practical purposes, the following is a satisfactory guide for the selection of the initial diagnostic lens. If the horizontal iris diameter and the vertical palpebral aperture are average—that is, 11 to 11.5 mm. and 9 to 9.5 mm. respectively—initial diagnostic lenses with relatively average lens diameters and optic-zone diameters are used. If a Nodema contact lens is used, average diagnostic lens diameter is 8.0 mm. and average diagnostic optic-zone diameter is 7.0 mm. If a contour contact lens is used, average diagnostic lens diameter is 9.0 mm., and average diagnostic optic-zone diameter is 7.5 mm. When horizontal iris diameter or vertical palpebral aperature are larger than average, a Nodema contact lens with a 8.5 mm. lens diameter and a 7.5 mm. optic-zone diameter is used, and a contour contact lens with a 9.5 mm. lens diameter and a 7.5 mm. optic-zone diameter is used. When horizontal iris diameter or vertical palpebral aperture are smaller than average, a Nodema contact lens with a 7.5 mm. lens diameter and a 6.5 mm. optic-zone diameter is used, and a contour contact lens with a 8.5 mm. lens diameter and a 7.0 mm. optic-zone diameter is used. The base curve radius of the initial diagnostic lens is 0.10 mm. (0.50 D) steeper than flat "K", or flat "K" plus one-third "K" astigmatism, whichever is steeper.

The patient is told that diagnostic lenses for obtaining information are to be used and that he must follow instructions. The patient makes a fist of his right hand with the thumb extended. The hand is then held up high, but below eye level, and 10 to 12 inches in front of the body. The patient looks at his thumb, and he is told to continue looking at it until he is given further instructions. Discussion of the subject of interest is continued while the practitioner washes his hands thoroughly.

The lens is cleaned with wetting solution and rinsed with warm water, which is used because it reduces any physical discomfort from temperature change when the lens is placed on the cornea. The lens is placed on the end of the index finger of the practitioner's right hand. The practitioner continues to talk to the patient and stands on the patient's right side. The lower lid is grasped firmly but gently above the lash margin with the middle finger of the right hand. The upper lid is grasped below the lash margin with the middle finger of the left hand. The lids are held against the orbital bones. The lens is gently placed directly on the cornea. First the lower and then the upper lid is released; the patient should still be looking down. He is told that normal blinking is permissible.

As the contact lens nears the eye, some patients are unable to maintain fixation inferiorly. Their normal defense mechanism causes them to turn their eyes up. Such patients should be instructed to look up, and the practitioner places the lens on the inferior part of the cornea. After the lens is in place, the patient is instructed to look down, and then the practitioner releases the lids.

A diagnostic lens is placed on the left eye by the same procedure. As the lenses settle, the patient gradually fixates at progressively increasing distances along the floor until he is looking straight ahead. When there is need to remove epiphora, the patient is told to blot and not rub with a facial tissue.

To remove a contact lens, the practitioner stands on the right side of the patient, whose head is held by a headrest. The patient cups a hand near his chin to catch the lens. With the index or middle finger of his right hand, the practitioner pulls the patient's lower lid down and holds it against the infraorbital bones, making certain that the lid margin is tight against the globe. With the index or middle finger of his left hand, the practitioner pulls the patient's upper lid up. The patient looks temporally, and the practitioner pushes his upper lid down and in a temporal direction, making certain that the lid margin is tight against the globe.

Usually, within 15 to 30 minutes after insertion, it is possible to obtain reasonably valid and accurate evaluations. When lacrimation and blepharospasm are excessive, it may be necessary to use a large diameter diagnostic lens, even if this lens design probably will not be fitted. The large diameter adheres better to the cornea, and its edge lies under the upper lid, which often results in better initial comfort. As the eye adapts, other lens designs may be applied.

Diameters and Widths. It must be determined whether the desired position, movement, pupil coverage, and blink action are obtained with the initial diagnostic lenses.

Position. The primary vertical and horizontal positions of a contact lens on the cornea occur with primary fixation during the interphase between blinks. The practitioner should choose a position and fit to it.

Primary vertical position can be designated by dividing the cornea into five positions and labelling each position with a letter (Fig. 2–35). An *SL* (superior limbus) position occurs when the upper edge of the lens is near, on, or above the superior limbus, and the geometric center of the lens is above the geometric center of the cornea. An *S* (superior) position occurs when the upper edge of the lens is at least 1 mm. below the superior limbus, and the geometric center of the lens is above the geometric center of the cornea. A *C* (central) position occurs when the geometric center of the lens is approximately coincident with the geometric center of the cornea. An *I* (inferior) position occurs when the lower edge of the lens is at least 1 mm. above the inferior lid or limbus, whichever is higher, and the geometric center of the lens is below the geometric center of the cornea. An *IL* (inferior lid) position occurs when the lower edge of the lens is on the inferior lid—assuming that the lid is at or higher than the inferior limbus—and the geometric center of the lens is below the geometric center of the cornea.

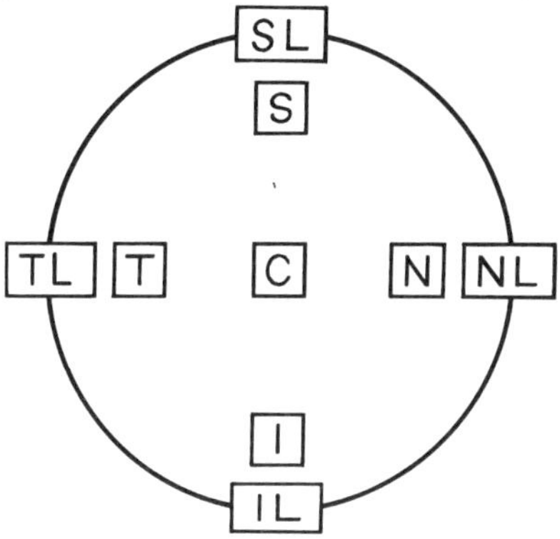

Figure 2–35. Vertical and horizontal positions. Vertical positions: SL (superior limbus), S (superior), C (central), I (inferior), and IL (inferior lid). Horizontal positions: TL (temporal limbus), T (temporal), C (central), N (nasal), NL (nasal limbus).

Primary horizontal position can also be designated by dividing the cornea into five positions and labelling each position with a letter (Fig. 2–35). A *TL* (temporal limbus) position occurs when the edge of the lens is near, on, or beyond the temporal limbus, and the geometric center of the lens is temporalward of the geometric center of the cornea. A *T* (temporal) position occurs when the edge of the lens is at least 1 mm. from the temporal limbus, and the geometric center of the lens is temporalward to the geometric center of the cornea. A *C* (central) position occurs when the geometric center of the lens is approximately coincident with the geometric center of the cornea. An *N* (nasal) position occurs when the edge of the lens is at least 1 mm. from the nasal limbus, and the geometric center of the lens is nasalward to the geometric center of the cornea. An *NL* (nasal limbus) position occurs when the edge of the lens is near, on, or beyond the nasal limbus, and the geometric center of the lens is nasalward to the geometric center of the cornea.

Primary vertical positions *S, C, I,* and *IL*—when the lower lid is at or higher than the inferior limbus—and primary horizontal positions *N, C,* and *T* are usually acceptable. Primary vertical positions *SL* and *IL*—when the lower lid is below the inferior limbus—and primary horizontal positions *TL* and *NL* are usually not acceptable. Lenses in these positions usually bear on the limbus, and may produce problems from tilt, stagnated pools of precorneal fluid, and flare.

Movement. Movement of a contact lens—that is, variance from primary position—is often considered in terms of the lag of the lens relative to the cornea. There are three types of lag.

Dynamic or *blink lag* occurs with primary fixation and normal blinking. *During the interphase between blinks, the lens should be relatively stationary.* When a superior-positioning lens is used, as the upper lid descends in the closure phase of blinking, the lens is moved down slightly. As the upper lid is retracted, the lens is pulled up and released, and quickly assumes its original position. When an aperture-positioning lens is used, as the upper lid descends in the closure phase of blinking, it pushes the lens down and slides over it. As the upper lid is retracted, the lens is pulled up and released, and quickly assumes its original position.

Acceptable vertical movement usually changes position less than a half of one place—that is, a lens pulled up to position *S* would not move as far as position *C*. Movement is, therefore, about 1.0 to 1.5 mm. If there is insufficient movement after the full retraction of the upper lid, the fit is often termed *tight.* If there is excessive movement after the full retraction of the upper lid, the fit is often termed *loose.* Some practitioners term a lens that has apical clearance or a steep relationship *tight* and a lens that has apical touch or a flat relationship *loose.* However, steep is not synonymous with *tight* and flat is not synonymous with *loose.* For example, a lens fitted with apical clearance may be *loose.*

Static or gravity lag is sometimes termed the *sag* of the lens. The upper and lower lids are held away from the lens to eliminate the holding effect of lid to lens. Thus adherence and movement are due only to relationships between lens and cornea. This test is quite significant. Desired movement is about 1.0 to 1.5 mm. Little or no movement indicates a tight fit; excessive movement indicates a loose fit. If there is excessive movement during blink lag but satisfactory movement during static lag, it may be due to excessive lens thickness, improper edge construction, improper lens position, or excessive secondary clearance.

Fixation or *excursion lag* occurs as fixation of the eye is varied; there is a lagging of the lens behind the eye movement. In general, as long as the lag does not cause encroachment of the periphery of the lens over the limbus, stagnated pools of precorneal fluid, or the positioning of too much of the secondary curve over the pupil, the fixation lag is acceptable.

Forces. The major forces that combine to produce lens position and movement are (1) surface tension, (2) friction, (3) gravity, and (4) eyelid adherence.

Surface tension, friction, and gravity combine to produce a certain amount of adherence between the contact lens and the cornea. Another type of adherence is produced between the upper lid and the lens. The balance between these two types of adherence determines lens position and movement.

Surface tension, often called capillary attraction or capillarity, is the force in the precorneal fluid around the edge of the lens. Surface tension is inversely related to the thickness of the precorneal fluid and directly related to the circumference of the lens. If any curve on the posterior surface of the lens is flattened, the thickness of the precorneal fluid layer around the edge of the lens is increased; this effect decreases the surface tension and the adherence of the lens to the cornea. The reverse occurs when any curve on the posterior surface is steepened. If the lens diameter is increased, the circumference of the lens is increased, an effect which increases surface tension and the adherence of the lens to the cornea. The reverse occurs when lens diameter is decreased.

Friction is the force that occurs between the bearing zones of the lens and the precorneal fluid and cornea. Friction is directly related to the viscosity of the precorneal fluid and the area of the bearing zones. Tear fluid from the lacrimal gland is less viscous than precorneal fluid. If the viscosity of the precorneal fluid is decreased by excessive lacrimation, friction and adherence of lens to cornea is decreased. In an apical alignment or very mild apical clearance relationship, the optic zone is the bearing zone. If the optic-zone diameter is increased, the bearing area is increased, increasing friction and adherence of the lens to the cornea. If corneal toricity is increased and spherical lens curves are used, the bearing area is decreased.

Gravity is the force that works on the center of gravity of a contact lens. When the center of gravity of a contact lens moves toward the posterior surface, the adherence of lens to cornea is increased. A decrease of center thickness, an increase in minus power, a steepening of the base curve, or an increase of lens diameter moves the center of gravity toward the posterior surface; and an increase of center thickness, an increase in plus power, a flattening of the base curve, or a decrease of lens diameter moves the center of gravity toward the anterior surface.

Upper eyelid adherence to the lens is directly proportional to upper eyelid tonicity, blink rate and amount, and lens diameter. Upper eyelid adherence is also related to the configuration of the anterior surface toward the edge of the lens. As negative refractive power increases, the anterior surface is flattened, and the edge thickness and base-toward-the-edge prism increase, an effect which increases the adherence of the upper lid to the lens. When edge thickness is more than 0.15 mm., however, it may be difficult for the upper lid to fold over the edge.

A superior-positioning lens tends to move less as the posterior curvatures are steepened, the negative power is increased, the lens or optic-zone diameters are increased, the secondary zone width is decreased, the center thickness is decreased, or the upper lid is tighter—that is, anything that increases the adherence of the lens to the cornea or of the lid to the lens reduces movement. A superior-positioning lens tends to move more as the posterior curvatures are flattened, the negative power is decreased, the lens or optic-zone diameters are decreased, the secondary zone width is increased, the center thickness is increased, or the upper lid is looser—that is, anything that decreases the adherence of lens to cornea or lid to lens increases movement.

Aside from lens diameter and lid tonicity, these factors also apply in the same manner to aperture-positioned lenses. Changes in lens diameter frequently affect aperture lenses in an opposite manner than they do in superior-positioned lenses. As lens diameter is increased for an aperture-positioned lens, the superior edge of the lens is brought closer to the upper lid, and the surface area of the lens is increased. The grasp of the upper lid on the lens is increased, and lens movement is more affected by the blink cycle. As lid tonicity increases, the ability of the lid to grasp and move the lens increases.

Contact lens position can be altered by alteration of the adherence of lens to cornea. Anything that increases the adherence of the lens to the cornea tends to position the lens more nearly central.

Procedure. The practitioner inserts on the patient's eye an appropriate initial diagnostic lens (see p. 71). After lacrimation and blinking become relatively normal, position and movement are evaluated. If position or movement is undesirable, a diagnostic lens with lens or optic-zone diameters or thickness that will theoretically improve position and movement is selected. If the practitioner has the diagnostic unit suggested (see p. 68), lens diameter and optic-zone diameter can be altered in 0.5 mm. increments. The procedure is repeated until satisfactory position and movement are attained. When diameter alteration does not produce desired performance, base curve radius may be altered slightly or minus carrier lenses may be evaluated. It is important to realize that abnormal lacrimation and blinking make it impossible to determine position and movement accurately.

Once a lens is processed, most modifications tend to decrease adherence of lens to cornea and lid to lens. The following modifications can be applied: secondary curves can be flattened, widened, or added, but not steepened; lens diameter can be decreased, not increased; and optic-zone diameter can be decreased, not increased.

Because modification tends to decrease adherence and because initial evaluation is not completely accurate or valid, many practitioners prescribe initial lens characteristics so that they cause a slight excess in adherence. Because the posterior lens curves cannot be altered without altering the relationship to corneal curves, this initial excessive adherence is usually obtained by use of lens and optic-zone diameters 0.2 to 0.3 mm. larger than might otherwise be indicated. Furthermore, when there is uncertainty about which of two secondary radii to use, the steeper one is selected.

CURVATURES. After lens diameter, optic-zone diameter, and secondary widths are determined, relationships between posterior contact lens and the

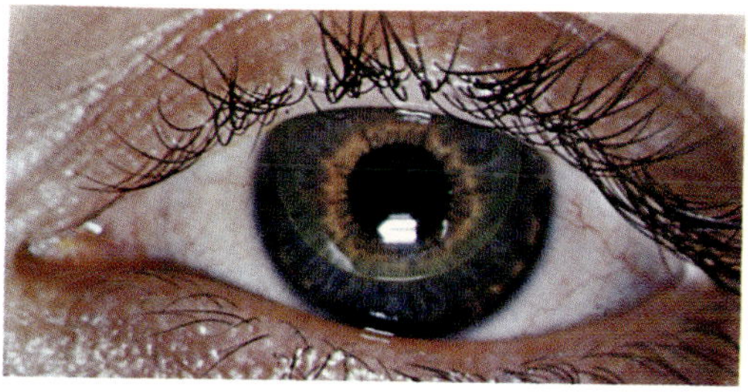

Figure 2–36. Contact lens viewed without the aid of fluorescein and ultraviolet light. (Courtesy of Dr. Donald R. Korb.)

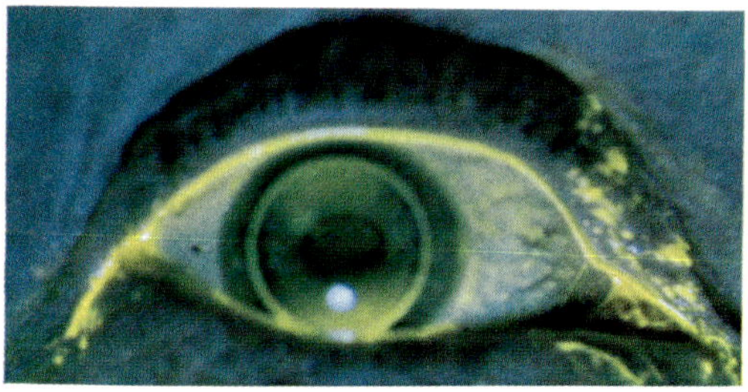

Figure 2–42. The optic pattern on a with-the-rule astigmat when the base curve is selected to produce relative alignment along the horizontal meridians. Note the vertical pooling. (Courtesy of Dr. Charles R. Stewart.)

Figures 2–37, 2–38, and 2–39 illustrate how the optic pattern changes on a nearly spherical cornea when the base curve is changed and the optic-zone diameter is held constant.

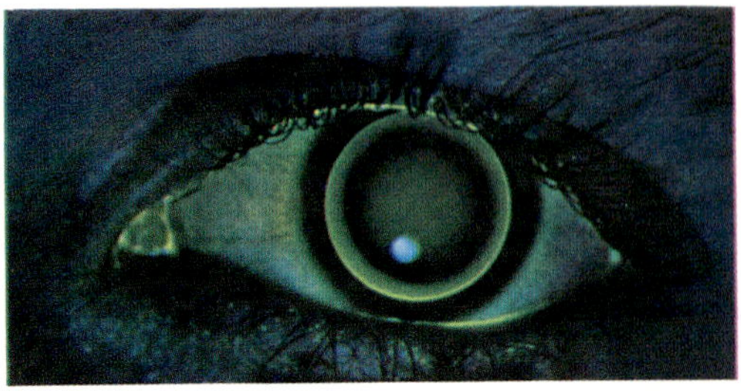

Figure 2–37. Apical clearance or steep relationship. (Courtesy of Dr. Charles R. Stewart.)

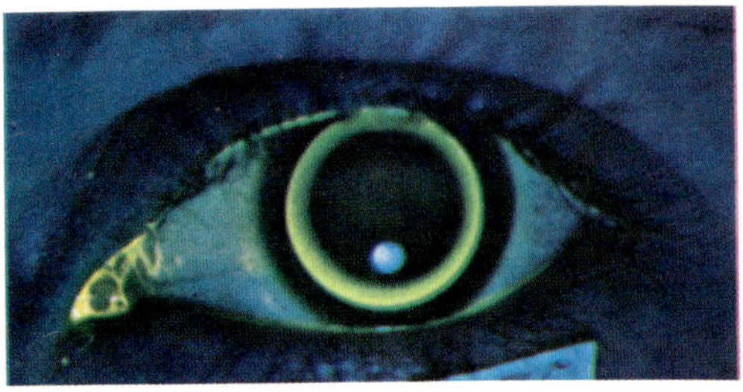

Figure 2–38. Relative apical alignment, parallel, or maximum bearing relationship. (Courtesy of Dr. Charles R. Stewart.)

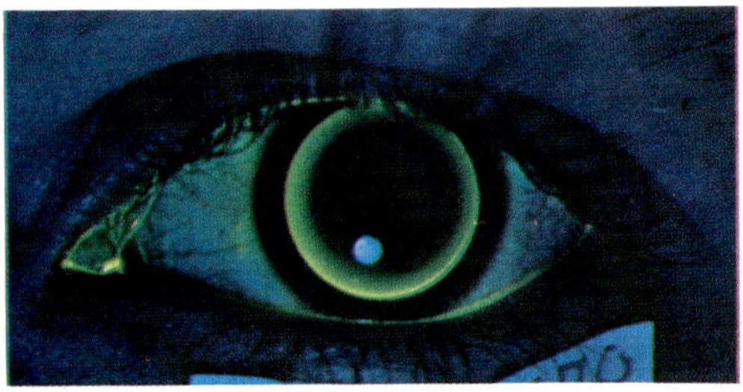

Figure 2–39. Apical touch or flat relationship. (Courtesy of Dr. Charles R. Stewart.)

Figure 2–43. The optic pattern changes on a nearly spherical cornea when the base curve is equal to the ophthalmometric reading and the optic-zone diameter is varied. (Courtesy of Dr. Charles R. Stewart.)

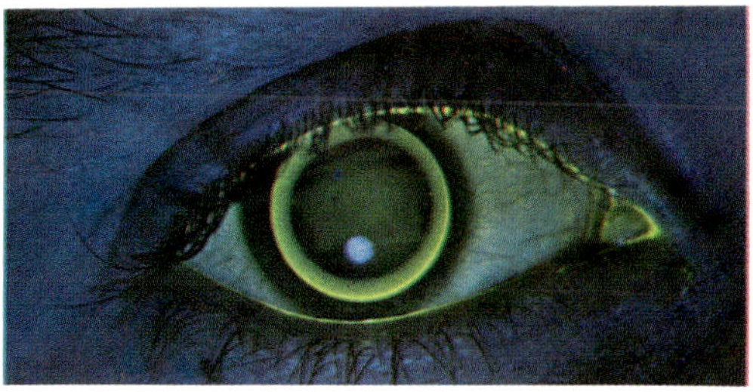

A, *An optic-zone diameter of 7.1 mm. produces a slight to moderate apical clearance.*

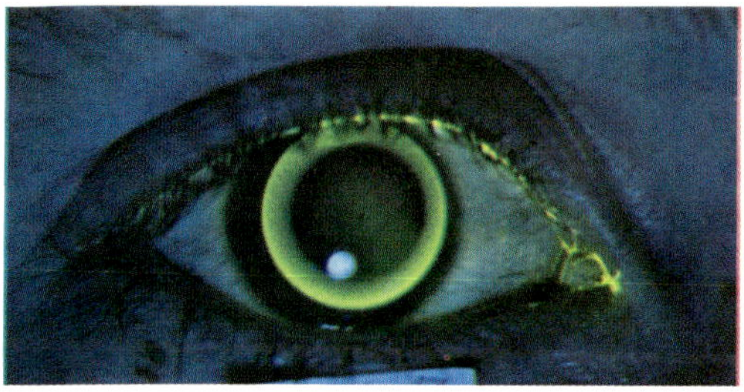

B, *An optic-zone diameter of 6.7 mm. produces very slight apical clearance. A relative apical alignment would be produced with an optic-zone diameter of about 6.5 mm.*

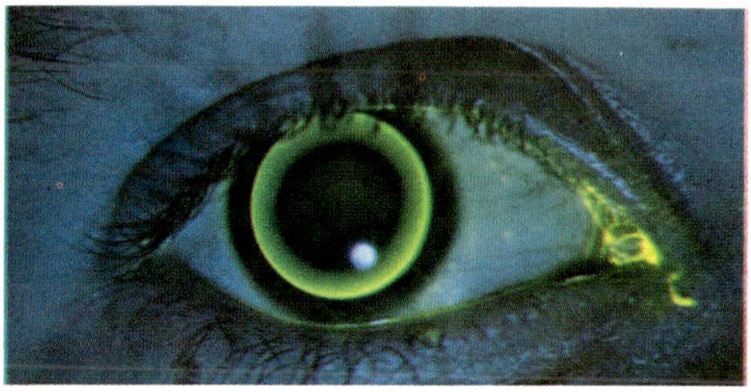

C, *An optic-zone diameter of 6.1 mm. produces apical touch.*

anterior corneal curvatures are determined. As shown in Fig. 2–36, this determination cannot be made unless an additive is mixed with the precorneal fluid. The inert organic fluorescein is the commonly used additive.[66–69]

When fluorescein is mixed with precorneal fluid and activated by ultraviolet light, it glows or fluoresces with a yellow-green color. *Only ultraviolet lights specifically designed for ocular examination should be used.* Because brightness of color depends in part on the depth or thickness of the material, the depth or thickness of the precorneal fluid between a given area of the contact lens and the underlying cornea is estimated from the brightness of the fluorescein.

Assuming that a proper amount of fluorescein is instilled and nothing is impeding the flow of precorneal fluid between the lens and the cornea, a black area indicates that the precorneal fluid is so thin that the brightness is below the level that can be detected. Thus, the curves of the contact lens and the underlying cornea are in close proximity (see the central zone of Fig. 2–39, insert between pp. 76 and 77). A bright yellow-green area indicates that the thickness of precorneal fluid is relatively great, and that the curves of the contact lens and the underlying cornea are separated to a considerable degree (see the secondary zone of Fig. 2–39). A murky or hazy yellow-green area indicates that the thickness of the precorneal fluid is relatively small, and that the curves of the contact lens and the underlying corneal area are separated to a moderate degree (see the central zone of Fig. 2–43A). The brightness of the fluorescein can vary from seeming nonexistence, or black, to a very bright yellow-green. Degrees of brightness between these two extremes help to approximate the amount of separation between the posterior surface of the lens and the anterior corneal curves. This approximation in turn helps in the selection of the radius needed in a given area of a contact lens to achieve the desired degree of brightness and thus the desired amount of clearance. Large bubbles of gas trapped under a lens have no fluid in them and appear black (Fig. 2–45C). Small bubbles may appear yellow.

The yellow-green color is a product of the particular additive and activating light. Other additives may be developed that result in other colors. The basic principle, however, will still be the same.

Terminology. Appearance of the precorneal fluid with the fluorescein between a contact lens and the cornea when activated by ultraviolet illumination is termed the *fluorescein pattern.* In regard to areas of the contact lens, there are two patterns—one between the base curve and the underlying corneal area, termed the *optic pattern,* and the other between the secondary curves and the underlying corneal areas, termed the *secondary pattern.*

In regard to eye movement and blinking, there are two types of patterns. The first occurs when the patient maintains primary fixation and blinking is held in check either by the patient staring or by the practitioner holding the lids; it is termed the *static pattern.* The second occurs when the patient fixates at various distances and angles, and blinking is allowed to function freely; it is termed the *dynamic pattern*.

The fluorescein pattern permits an appreciation of those aspects of bearing and venting due to the relationship of the posterior lens and underlying corneal curvatures. The black areas, which indicate a close apposition of lens and corneal curves, are the bearing areas. Bright yellow-green areas indicate a separation of the lens from the corneal curves. In a secondary clearance lens, the degree of brightness of the secondary pattern indicates the depth of the precorneal fluid reservoir and the interchange potential.

Fluorescein Problems and Insertion. There are several problems involved with the use of fluorescein. Usually, they can be satisfactorily resolved.

1. Fluorescein becomes easily contaminated by the ocular pathogen *Pseudomonas aeruginosa*. This pathogen cannot harm the cornea unless it gains entrance into the corneal tissue through a break in the epithelium. If it does gain entrance, it may cause considerable damage, even leading to rapid blindness. No effective chemical preservative for eliminating *Pseudomonas* contamination has been discovered for liquid fluorescein. Once a container with liquid fluorescein has been opened, it is readily susceptible to *Pseudomonas* contamination, and therefore should be used only once.

Dry fluorescein on strips of filter paper and autoclaved in individual packages remains sterile as long as the package is sealed.[70, 71] To use dry fluorescein strips, a drop of *sterile* solution with a proper pH value, such as an irrigating solution, is placed on the strip. It is important that the mouth of the bottle does not touch or come into very close proximity with the strip. If it does, some fluorescein may be drawn into the bottle, and the irrigating solution may become contaminated with *Pseudomonas*. Subsequent use of the bottle may introduce *Pseudomonas* on the eye. Strips used once with a proper solution are by far the safest means of applying fluorescein. The strips are clinically effective in establishing a good fluorescein pattern and are usually more economical than other methods.

2. Excessive lacrimation, when exhibited the first day by patients, affects the brightness of the fluorescein pattern. The viscosity of lacrimal fluid is less than the viscosity of precorneal fluid. When excessive lacrimal fluid mixes with other components of the precorneal fluid, the combined viscosity is reduced. *The decreased viscosity and increased speed of flow may make it difficult or impossible to interpret the fluorescein pattern accurately.* This condition can be minimized by proper insertion of the lenses and proper patient management.

3. The amount of fluorescein used affects the pattern. Brightness depends partially on the amount or degree of saturation. For a given thickness of precorneal fluid, as the amount of fluorescein is increased the brightness of the pattern increases. Excessive brightness from too much fluorescein can be controlled by employing proper techniques.

4. The type of ultraviolet light used affects the pattern. The degree of

fluorescein activation and brightness depends in part on the wavelength and intensity of the ultraviolet light. The wavelength and intensity of the ultraviolet lights produced by different companies vary somewhat. The practitioner should use an ultraviolet light that adequately activates the fluorescein. Experience then will enable the mental establishment of a standard of brightness variations produced by this light.

5. The type of magnification and accompanying field affects the pattern appearance. Up to a certain point, as magnification increases, the ability to discern between various levels of brightness increases. Magnification enabling proper appreciation of detail within an adequate field should be used. Some ultraviolet lamps are equipped with a plus lens, which produces magnification (Fig. 2–40). Head loupes may be used. The magnification system of the slit lamp may be used, with an ultraviolet filter (p. 307). Use of a slit-lamp biomicroscope is *essential* for proper fluorescein pattern evaluation.

Fluorescein is placed in the precorneal fluid in two ways. The first method involves placing a contact lens on the eye and allowing initial adaptation to take place. The patient then looks down, and the upper lid is grasped firmly by the practitioner below the lash margin and securely held against the superior orbital bone. An area on the superior sclera slightly above the superior limbus about one-eighth to one-quarter inch long is gently "painted" with fluorescein (Fig. 2–41). It is important to standardize the area painted as much as possible to establish a relatively uniform basis of comparison. The patient is requested to blink several times so that the fluorescein is mixed with precorneal fluid and flushed between the lens and the cornea.

The second method involves placing fluorescein on the inner surface of the lens and then placing the lens on the eye. The authors prefer the first method because it is neater, and it provides better control of the amount of fluorescein.

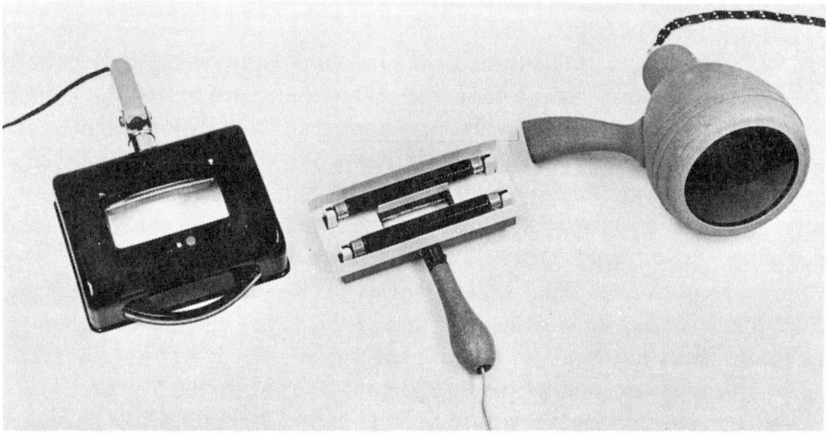

Figure 2–40. Types of handheld ultraviolet lamps.

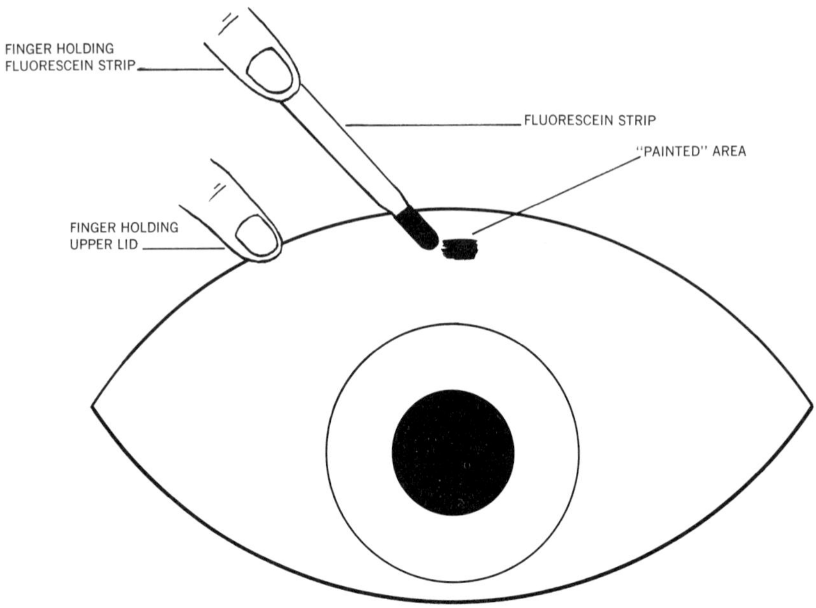

Figure 2–41. Area on superior sclera "painted" with fluorescein.

For simplicity, assume that a rigid contact lens is placed on a rigid, spherical, symmetrical cornea. Under these conditions, there are three possible *static optic fluorescein patterns* and three *basic static secondary fluorescein patterns.* Initially, separate observation of optic and secondary patterns should be considered with the use of a lens that has both optic and secondary zones.

Spherical Static Optic Fluorescein Patterns. In determining the optic fluorescein pattern, it is *imperative* to have clearance between the secondary curves and the underlying corneal area. If there is no clearance, the lens rests on these secondary areas, and the optic area is pushed away from the cornea. This situation gives a false optic fluorescein pattern, for the pattern appears to have either more or less clearance than the relationship of given base to corneal curves should show. It shows more clearance if the lens is pushed away and the fluorescein is able to flow under the lens (Fig. 2–45C, insert between pp. 82 and 83). It shows less clearance if the close apposition of secondary and corneal curves binds the periphery of the lens and impedes the flow of precorneal fluid under the lens. The lack of precorneal fluid under the lens produces a black optic area, which may erroneously be interpreted as close apposition of lens and corneal curves.

Three possible basic optic patterns should be considered.

1. A uniform black pattern through the entire optic-zone area indicates a relative alignment of this base curve to the underlying corneal curves in

this optic-zone diameter. Such a pattern is termed a *relative apical alignment,* or a *parallel* (or *maximum*) *bearing area* fit (Figs. 2–38).

2. A yellow-green pattern in the optic zone and an annular black ring surrounding it between the optic and secondary areas indicate there is clearance of the base curve from the underlying corneal areas in this optic-zone diameter (Figs. 2–37 and 2–43A [insert]). The bearing in this case is on the relatively narrow annular band between the optic zone and the secondary zone. Such a pattern is termed an *apical clearance* or a *steep* fit. As the clearance increases, the brightness increases, if binding has not impeded the flow. If flow is impeded, there is a false relative apical alignment pattern.

In a given case, the practitioner does not know if the relationship is due to a steep base curve, a large optic zone, or a combination of these. Note the similarity between Figs. 2–37 and 2–43A. Clinically, it is usually unnecessary to know the cause. It is necessary to know the remedy.

There are two ways to obtain better contiguity of lens and corneal curves. The first involves maintaining a constant optic-zone diameter and using a lens with a flatter base curve (Figs. 2–37, 2–38, and 2–39). The second involves maintaining a constant base curve and reducing the optic-zone diameter (Figs. 2–43A, 2–43B, and 2–43C).

It is clinically more practical to maintain a constant optic-zone diameter and change the base curve. Diagnostic lens sets are usually constructed on this basis, and it is best to determine the pattern with the approximate optic-zone diameter to be ordered for the patient.

3. There is a black pattern in the central optic-zone area with a murky yellow-green pattern between it and the secondary zone. The size of the black central pattern is *less* than the total optic-zone diameter (Figs. 2–3 and 2–43C). As the base is flattened, this central black area becomes smaller, and the area between it and the secondary curve becomes wider and a brighter yellow-green. Such a pattern is termed an *apical touch* or a *flat fit.* In a given case, the practitioner does not know if the relationship is due to a flat base curve, a small optic zone, or a combination of these. The clinical remedy is to use progressively steeper base curves in the desired optic-zone diameter until an alignment fit is obtained.

Spherical Symmetrical Static Secondary Fluorescein Patterns. In determining the secondary fluorescein pattern, it is imperative to have clearance between the base curve and the underlying corneal area. If there is no clearance, the lens rests on the central area, and the secondary area is pushed away from the cornea, giving a false secondary pattern. Total secondary clearance under such conditions is the sum of the clearance produced by the secondary curves and the base curve pushing the lens away from the cornea. Three basic possible secondary patterns should be considered:

1. A uniform black pattern through the secondary-zone area indicates a relative alignment of the secondary curve to the underlying corneal curves. It is termed *secondary alignment.*

2. A black annular band around the periphery of the lens indicates that the secondary curve is steeper than the underlying corneal curve. It is termed *secondary touch.* Central to this band, there is either a yellow-green pattern, showing the clearance of the lens, or a black pattern, showing that the precorneal fluid has been sealed out.

3. A yellow-green pattern throughout the secondary area indicates that the secondary curves are separated from the corneal curves. It is termed *secondary clearance* (Figs. 2–37, 2–38, 2–39, 2–43A, 2–43B, 2–43C, 2–44A, 2–44B, 2–44C, 2–44D, 2–45A, and 2–45B).

Clinically, the practitioner starts with a base curve that ensures apical clearance in a given optic-zone size. The secondary pattern is observed. When a secondary alignment or touch pattern is present, a lens with a flatter base curve is used. When the secondary clearance pattern is excessive, a lens with a steeper base curve is used.

Simultaneous Interpretation. Optic and secondary fluorescein pattern interpretation have been presented in two steps. The following method is clinically quicker and more efficient. The initial lens is selected with a base curve radius 0.10 mm. (0.50 D) steeper than flat "K", or flat "K" plus one-third "K" astigmatism, whichever is steeper. This usually provides a slight apical clearance. It is easier to evaluate the optic-zone pattern when one is working from apical clearance to apical alignment rather than from apical touch to apical alignment. To a large degree, this is because an apical alignment relationship often looks similar to a very mild apical touch relationship. The basic difference is that the apical alignment relationship extends over the entire optic zone, whereas the very slight apical touch relationship does not. Because there is no marking of the optic-zone periphery, it is difficult or impossible to determine whether the relationship extends over the entire optic zone (Figs. 2–38 and 2–39).

The initial lens is placed on the cornea, and fluorescein is instilled after lacrimation, blinking, and contact lens performance stabilize. The secondary curve is checked for clearance all around, and an approximation is made of any excessive clearance.

When the secondary curve does not show clearance with a given base curve, a lens with a smaller diameter in the same base curve and optic-zone diameter may be used. The narrower secondary curve will then be closer to the center of the cornea and will often clear the underlying corneal areas.

The base curve is determined by the use of diagnostic lenses with base curve radius increments of 0.10 mm. until minimum apical clearance is obtained. Refinement can be made in base curve increments of 0.05 mm., or interpolation to the nearest 0.05 mm. can be made. Because a change of 0.05 mm. in the base curve radius in the case of optic-zone diameters of approximately 7.0 mm. changes sagittal depth only about 0.006 mm., further refinements are seldom clinically significant.

Figure 2–44. Change of lens diameter (L.D.), optic-zone diameter (O.Z.D.), secondary curve width (S.C.W.), secondary curve–corneal curve relationships, and lens positioning. (Courtesy of Dr. Donald R. Korb.)

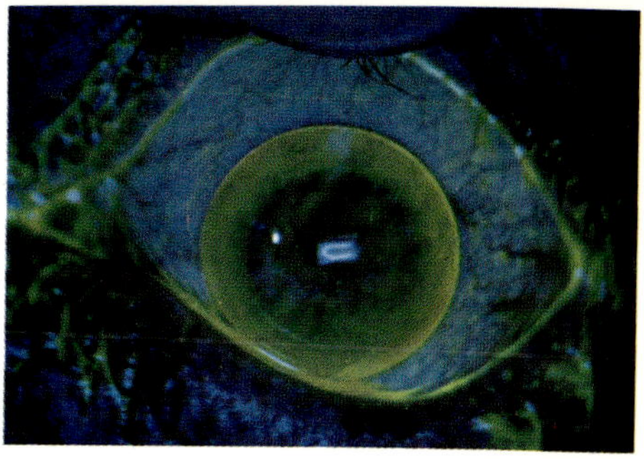

A, *L.D. is 13.8 mm., O.Z.D. is 8.8 mm., and S.C.W. is 1.5 mm. This extremely large lens covers the cornea and extends onto the sclera. Such a lens is usually worn only for 3 to 4 hours during sports activities. Note the centration of the optic zone with the pupil, and also note the secondary clearance.*

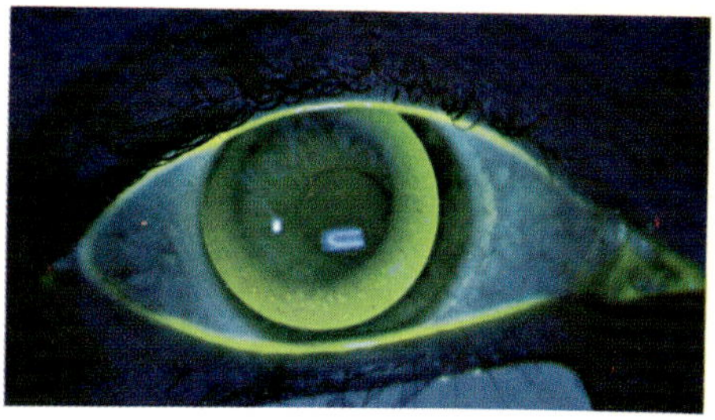

B, *L.D. is 10 mm., O.Z.D. is 6.6 mm., and S.C.W. is 1.7 mm. Because of the large L.D., the small O.Z.D., and the wide and flat S.C.W., the upper lid pulls the lens superiorly and temporally. Note the secondary fluorescein pattern, the bubbles under the secondary curve, the infringement of the secondary curve onto the pupil, and the bearing on the superior temporal limbus.*

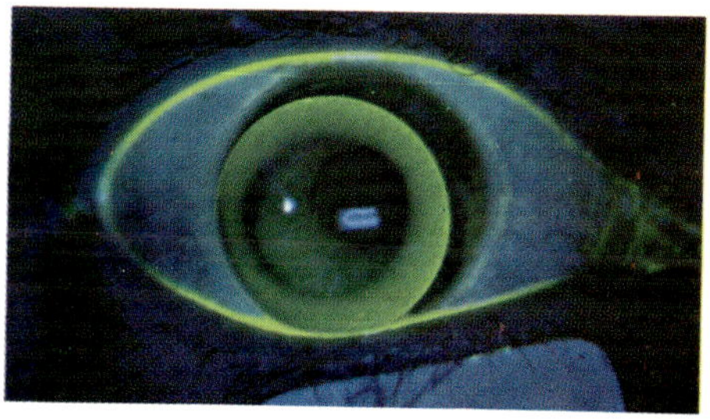

C, *The same lens as in* B. *Because of its small O.Z. and wide, flat secondary curve, the lens has poor adhesion to the eye. As a result, it lags down to the lower lid between blinks. Note the corneal staining above the superior temporal edge of the lens, and the limbal and scleral conjunctival irritation from movement.*

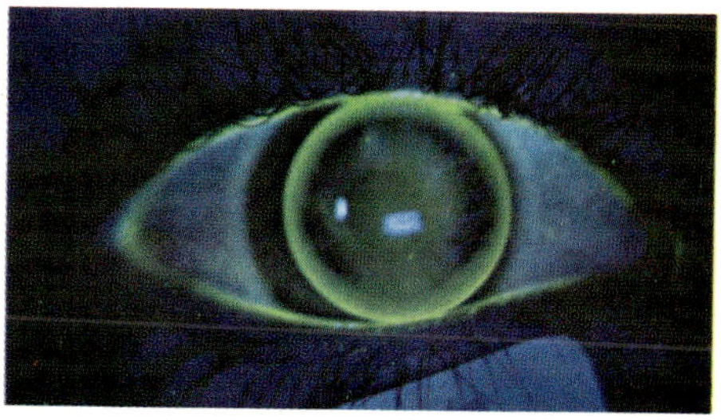

D, *L.D. is 9.0 mm., O.Z.D. is 7.0 mm., and S.C.W. is 1 mm. The lens completely fills the median palpebral aperture. This is a with-the-rule cornea fitted steeper than the flatter ophthalmometric meridian and flatter than the steeper ophthalmometric meridian. Note the wide nasal and temporal optic zone–secondary zone transition bearing areas. The apparent secondary-curve width and clearance are greater vertically than horizontally. Note the vertically oval optic-zone clearance pattern.*

Figure 2–45. Change of lens diameter (L.D.), optic-zone diameter (O.Z.D.), secondary-curve width (S.C.W.), secondary curve–corneal curve relationships, and lens positioning. (Courtesy of Dr. Donald R. Korb.)

A, *L.D. is 8.6 mm., O.Z.D. is 6.8 mm., and S.C.W. is 0.9 mm. Note the 0.2 to 0.3 mm. separation between the upper lid and the top of the lens. The lens has migrated temporally slightly. The secondary pattern is wider and brighter nasally and superiorly than temporally and inferiorly because of corneal asymmetry.*

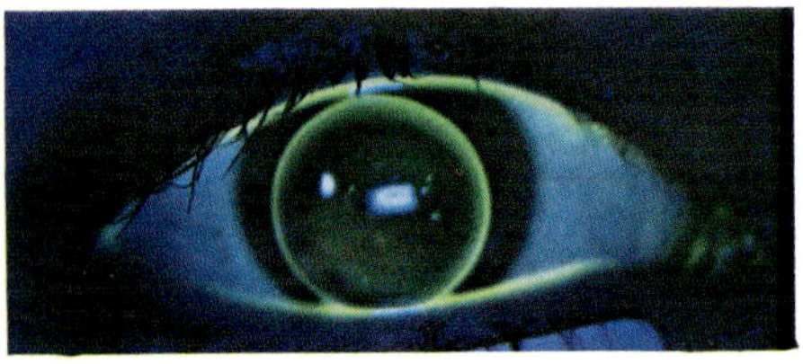

B, *L.D. is 8.0 mm., O.Z.D. is 6.6 mm., and S.C.W. is 0.7 mm. Note the considerable separation between the upper lid and the top of the lens. The secondary pattern shows a narrow peripheral clearance.*

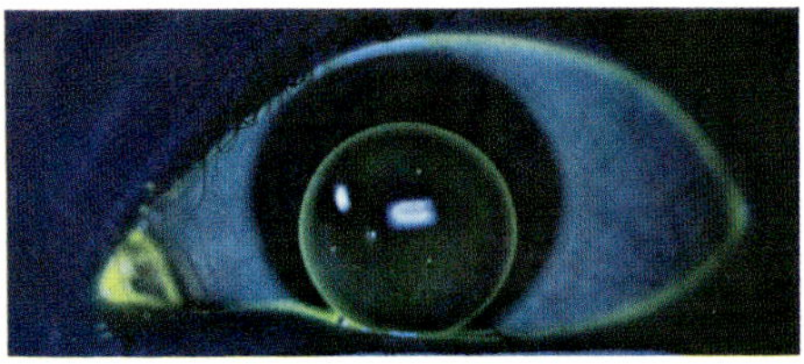

C, *This is the same lens as in* B, *but a steeper secondary curve is used. This pushes the lens away from the cornea and produces central clearance. Note the dark bubble.*

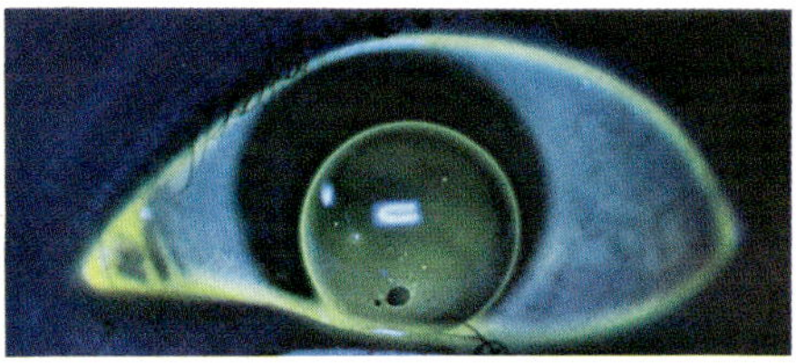

D, *L.D. is 7.6 mm., O.Z.D. is 6.2 mm., and S.C.W. is 0.7 mm. This small lens is fitted steep to bring it from an inferior to a more nearly centered position on the cornea. Note the central, inferior fluorescein pool. The fluorescein at the top of the optic zone is on the anterior surface of lens.*

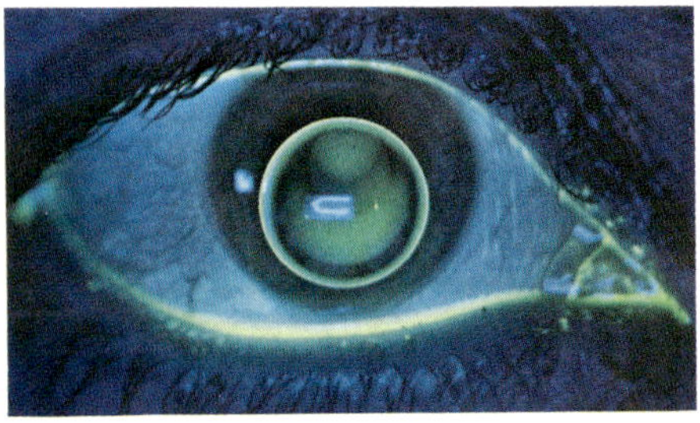

Figure 2–47. The determination of toric base curve radii by diagnostic lens procedure. (Courtesy of Dr. Donald R. Korb.)

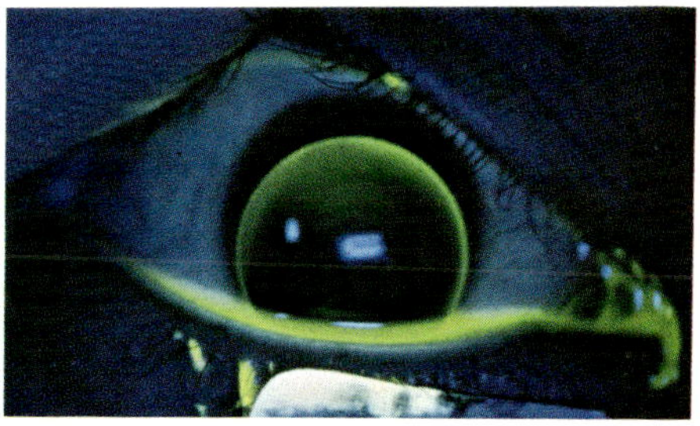

A, *A spherical base diagnostic lens is used to obtain relative apical alignment along the flatter meridian of a with-the-rule astigmat. Note the superior pooling.*

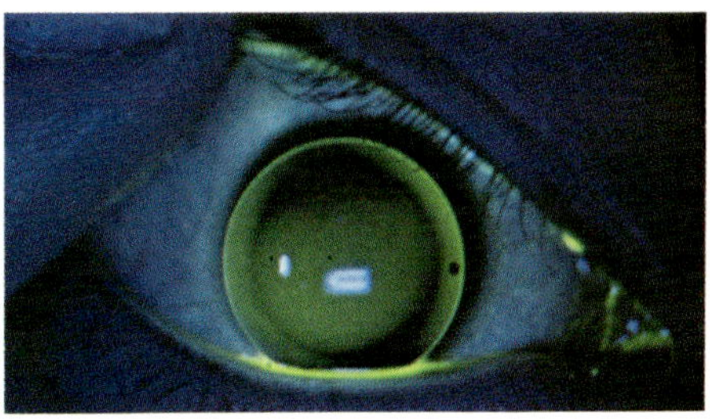

B, *A toric base diagnostic lens. The horizontal radius is the flatter meridian, as found in* A. *The base in the vertical meridian is too steep and bears heavily around the superior and inferior edges of the optic zone. This lifts the optic zone away from the cornea and produces an apparent against-the-rule fluorescein pattern. The black dot toward the nasal edge of the lens marks the axis.*

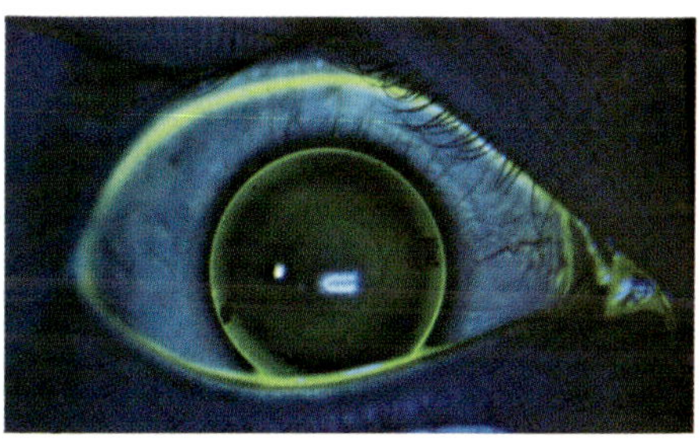

C, *The horizontal radius is kept constant, and the vertical radius is lengthened from that used in* B, *producing a satisfactory optic fluorescein pattern.*

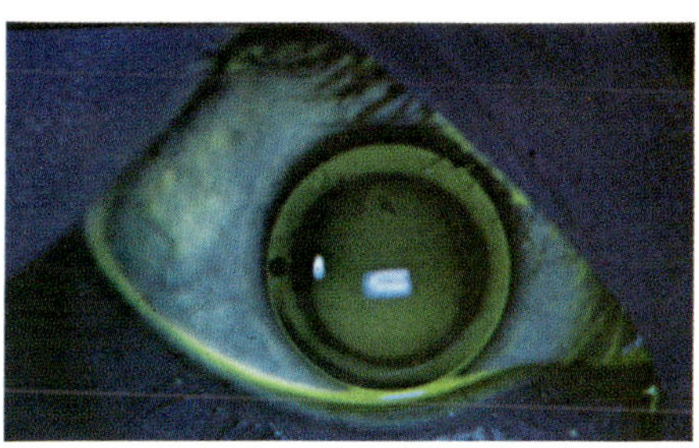

D, *To verify the horizontal radius, the vertical radius is the same and the horizontal radius is shorter than that used in* C. *The base in the horizontal meridian is too steep and bears heavily around the nasal and temporal edges of the optic zone. This lifts the optic zone away from the cornea and produces an apparent with-the-rule fluorescein pattern.*

In each diagnostic set, there is a constant difference between base and secondary curve radii; and secondary curve radii on the diagnostic lenses have been selected so that they usually produce adequate or slightly excessive clearance. Secondary curve radius can be determined by using lenses of various base curve radii in a given diagnostic set. For example, a 7.70 mm. base curve radius the secondary curve radius of which is 1 mm. longer (8.70 mm.) shows excessive secondary clearance. A diagnostic lens from the same set with a 7.50 mm. base curve radius whose secondary curve radius is 1 mm. longer (8.50 mm.) is used and shows satisfactory secondary clearance. This 8.50 mm. secondary curve radius is ordered. To determine secondary curve radius, it is adequate to change base curve radii in 0.2 mm. increments and to interpolate to the nearest 0.1 mm. Although this procedure has theoretic deficiencies because of the geometry of contact lenses (see p. 39), it is clinically adequate as long as the diagnostic lenses have been manufactured with accurate secondary curve radii.

The authors' diagnostic lenses have standard secondary curves (Table on p. 67). Unless fluorescein pattern shows them to be unsatisfactory, these standard curves are ordered. After the patient's lenses are received these standard curves may need to be modified.

Dynamic Fluorescein Pattern. Basic possibilities with a dynamic fluorescein pattern are the same as with a static fluorescein pattern—that is, there may be relative alignment, clearance, or touch between lens and corneal curves. Static and dynamic patterns differ in that the characteristics of the dynamic pattern change with eye movements and blinking. As a result of these factors, the lens moves to various parts of the cornea or assumes different angles of tilt, often changing the appearance of the pattern.

As fixation is varied, the lens moves with the eye to a degree (Figs. 2–44B and 2–44C). The more it moves with the eye, the more consistent are the relationships of lens and eye. Aperture-positioned lenses often follow the eye better than superior-positioned lenses do. Dynamic patterns give a truer overall picture than do static patterns. When lenses are worn, the relationships of lens to corneal curves change with eye movements and blinking. Because of this continuous change, the dynamic pattern is not easy to evaluate. Furthermore, a lens can be designed with only one set of curvatures. It is therefore impossible to design a lens with desired relationships for all fixation positions. The best compromise is to design the lens to have the desired relationship for the most frequently used fixation positions.

Clinically, the static pattern with the lens located where the practitioner feels it will finally position with primary fixation is the basic determination. After the curvatures that provide a desired static pattern are determined, the diagnostic lens most nearly containing these curvatures is placed on the eye. Then the dynamic pattern may be used to modify slightly the static pattern.

Fitting a Lens to the Area over Which It Will Position. The lens curves needed to produce desired relationships depend in part on the lens position and tilt. On a given eye, when the lens positions superiorly, different curves may be needed to produce a desired relationship than when the lens positions inferiorly. In determining curvatures of the posterior surface of the lens, it is important that the practitioner positions the diagnostic lens where he feels that the patient's lenses will finally position. Final positioning is predicted on the basis of experience and diagnostic lens performance.

Toric Fluorescein Patterns. When central corneal toricity is not too great, the proper single spherical base curve often produces a relatively good relationship. When central corneal toricity increases, it becomes more difficult to produce a desirable relationship with a single spherical base curve. The best relationship obtainable between a single spherical base curve and an appreciably toric corneal curve is a decided compromise. This relationship is achieved by using a base curve with a radius equal to flat "K" plus one-third "K" astigmatism.

When a lens with a large diameter and a single spherical base curve with a radius on K is fitted to a cornea having a with-the-rule toricity of 1 to 3 D, the lens usually positions superiorly. The superior part of the lens is tilted back against the cornea, limbus, or sclera. There is a bearing area at the superior edge of the lens and another along the horizontal meridian. Between these two bearing areas is a pool of fluorescein, which is often at least partially sealed off. The inferior part of the lens is tilted away from the cornea, often resulting in excessive inferior secondary clearance, and bubbles are frequently seen in the inferior secondary region because of decreased surface tension. When with-the-rule toricity is greater than this, adherence between lens and cornea and between lid and lens is so poor that the lens frequently positions inferiorly or has excessive movement (Fig. 2–42). When there is considerable against-the-rule toricity, the lens usually positions inferiorly or has excessive movement. When a lens with a small diameter and a single, spherical base curve is fitted to a cornea having considerable toricity, the normal tendency for the lens to position in the palpebral aperture is increased.

When the optimum relationship is achieved with a spherical base curve in a with-the-rule astigmat, the fluorescein pattern resembles an elongated I, or a vertical dumbbell (Fig. 2–27). When the optimum relationship is achieved for an against-the-rule astigmat, the fluorescein pattern resembles an elongated H, or a horizontal dumbbell (Fig. 2–27).

If the toric corneal periphery is symmetrical, a secondary curve aligned along the flatter corneal meridian results in clearance along the steeper meridian. If the secondary curvature is flattened to provide the desired clearance along the flatter meridian, there will be the same amount of change along the steeper meridian.

Because this meridian started with secondary clearance, there will now be excessive clearance. In a with-the-rule astigmat, if the lens remains centered, excessive clearance and standoff of the edge in the vertical meridian will result. This condition may cause lid discomfort and excessive rocking of the lens on the cornea. As secondary curvature width is decreased, there is less clearance difference in the two principal meridians.

Additional Factors. To simplify the discussion of fluorescein patterns, up to this point the cornea has been assumed to be spherical and symmetrical. However, the cornea is generally both aspherical and asymmetrical. In practice then, we try to relate circular (spherical), symmetrical posterior contact lens curvatures to aspherical, asymmetrical anterior corneal curvatures. The best relationships are, therefore, only compromises.

Because of the aspherical anterior corneal curvature, at times a fluorescein pattern of the optic zone may show a small area of central touch, an adjacent annular clearance area, and an annular touch between optic and secondary zones. Because of the asymmetrical anterior corneal curvature, at times a fluorescein pattern of the secondary zone may show alignment in one or more quadrants and clearance in the other quadrants.

Fluorescein patterns can be recorded for diagnostic, research, and legal purposes by drawings with colored pencils or crayons on the patient's record or by photographs.

Pools of fluorescein in the optic zone area are undesirable. The pattern should be evaluated when gaze is depressed for reading to detect potentially stagnated pools. Fluorescence of the crystalline lens must not be misinterpreted. To compensate for flattening from hydration, base curve radius should be ordered steeper by about 0.03 mm. for *all* plus and minus less than 6 D and 0.05 mm. for over −6 D than indicated by fluorescein pattern evaluation.

Center Thickness. This value is computed as in the method of measurements and standards to produce an edge thickness of 0.13 ± 0.02 mm. for a finished but unedged lens (see p. 43).

Refractive Power. After excessive lacrimation subsides and the diagnostic lens position stabilizes, static retinoscopy and subjective lens acceptance tests are performed over the diagnostic lenses. Both a spherocylindrical and a spherical equivalent refraction are used. When the cylindrical component is less than 0.75 D, the spherical equivalent refraction usually produces satisfactory acuity and comfort. When the cylindrical component is greater than this value, a contact lens with an anterior toric surface may be needed (see p. 93).

The spherical refractive power to be prescribed is the algebraic sum of the diagnostic lens power and the phoropter or spectacle trial lens power. When the phoropter power is more than +3 or −3D, vertex distance compensation must be made (see p. 62). When the base curve to be prescribed differs from that of the diagnostic lenses used, compensation must be made (see p. 63).

To obtain reasonably accurate findings, it is often necessary to have the patient blink to flush away excessive lacrimal fluid and provide a better lens position.

Combination

In this method of selection of lens specifications, both the preceding methods are used. The information from the measurements and standards method is used as a basis for selecting the initial diagnostic lens. Then the diagnostic lens procedure is used. The accuracy and validity of each method are evaluated, and the determination of lens specifications is based on the more accurate and valid method for a given case.

The lens specifications to be ordered are based on the seemingly more valid and accurate findings. For some patients, some specifications are based on one method and some on the other. For example, base and secondary radii may be based on fluorescein interpretation, and lens and optic-zone diameters may be based on measurements and standards.

Thickness is a computed value in either method. Refractive power is determined each way, and the two results are compared. Usually the refractive power determinations agree closely if everything has been done properly. This problem is discussed in more detail on page 338.

The authors always use the combination method to select lens specifications because it provides the most information.

SPECIAL DESIGN LENSES: THEORY AND CLINICAL PROCEDURE

Contact Lenses in High Corneal Toricity and Residual Astigmatism

A great deal has been written about the use of contact lenses when high corneal toricity and residual astigmatism are present. Contact lenses with toric surfaces or prism ballast are sometimes used. Much difference of opinion about their clinical effectiveness exists. Some practitioners consider them to be an answer to many contact lens fitting problems; others consider them to be more trouble than they are worth. The truth probably lies somewhere between the extremes.

There are three categories of toric contact lenses. When the anterior surface is toroidal and the posterior is spherical, the lens is termed an *anterior, front,* or *outside surface* toric lens. When the posterior surface is toroidal and the anterior is spherical, the lens is termed a *posterior, back,* or *inside surface* toric lens. Toric posterior curvatures may exist in the optic or secondary zones. When both the central anterior and posterior surfaces are toroidal, the lens is termed a *bitoric* lens. The axes of the central toroidal anterior and posterior surfaces may coincide or be oblique to one another. Usually they coincide.

Posterior Toric Surfaces

Function. When central ophthalmometric astigmatism is considerable, it is often difficult or impossible to produce a desired bearing relationship between posterior spherical lens and toric anterior corneal curvatures. Optic or secondary posterior toric surfaces may be considered to produce primarily better bearing relationships. As a result of the closer coincidence between lens and corneal curves, secondary advantages may be obtained. These are improved centration, decreased lens rocking, decreased lens movement, and decreased edge standoff.[72]

NEED. It is generally accepted that a central ophthalmometric astigmatism of 2 D is the point at which consideration of posterior toric surfaces should start.[73–79] Studies indicate that about 5 per cent of the population has an astigmatism of 2 D or more. Some patients with an ophthalmometric astigmatism of more than 2 D may be satisfactorily fitted with lenses having inside spherical curvatures. Although the percentage of patients best fitted with lenses having posterior toric surfaces is small, it is imperative to understand such fittings to serve these individuals adequately.

CLINICAL POSSIBILITIES. When there is a central ophthalmometric astigmatism of 2 D or more, the practitioner may use a lens with spherical base and secondary curvatures, spherical base and toric secondary curvatures, toric base and spherical secondary curvatures, or toric base and toric secondary curvatures. Clinically, the practitioner evaluates each of the surface types for a given patient and decides which will probably produce the best results.

As a clinical guide, patients having a central ophthalmometric astigmatism of up to 2 D are usually fitted with lenses having spherical base and spherical secondary curves. In a central ophthalmometric astigmatism of 2 to 3 D, lenses having spherical base and spherical secondary curves, spherical base and toric secondary curves, or toric base and spherical or toric secondary curves, are usually used. In a central ophthalmometric astigmatism of more than 3 D, lenses with toric base and spherical or toric secondary curves are usually used. When toric base curves are used, the authors always use toric secondary curves so that a circular optic zone is produced.

ADVANTAGES AND DISADVANTAGES. To understand these guides better, the possible advantages and disadvantages of spherical and toric posterior lenses on toric corneas should be considered.

First, consider the possible disadvantages of spherical posterior curves on corneas that are considerably toric.

The relative contiguity of lens and corneal curves is restricted to a small area. As a result, poor bearing is established, and all pressures are transmitted to this small area. Excessive alteration of corneal topography, mechanical trauma of the corneal tissue, and mechanical stimulation to the nerve endings can result.

Because the area of contiguity between lens and corneal curves is small, the adherence of the lens to the cornea is less. Excessive lens rocking, excessive lens movement, and poor lens position can result. These conditions in turn can produce excessive alteration of corneal topography, mechanical trauma to the corneal tissues, mechanical stimulation to the nerve endings, and insufficient coverage of the pupil by the optic zone.

When clearance along the flatter corneal meridians is satisfactory, clearance along the steeper corneal meridians is excessive. Excessive edge standoff along the steeper meridians can result in marked lid irritation and discomfort. This factor is more significant for a with-the-rule astigmat.

Second, consider the possible advantages of spherical posterior lens curves on corneas that are considerably toric. These advantages are best expressed in terms of the possible disadvantages of toric posterior lens curves.[80, 81] It is difficult to select the radii of the posterior surfaces and the proper optic- and secondary-zone widths to establish a desirable bearing. Further, when close contiguity between lens and corneal curves is present over a considerable area, fluid and gaseous interchange may be impeded. This effect is accentuated by the decreased rotation of a posterior toric contact lens.

When a toric base curve lens is on the eye, an astigmatic refraction occurs at the interface between the base curve and the precorneal fluid (see p. 352). This refraction usually must be corrected by the use of an anterior toric surface, complicating the fitting procedure. This is accentuated by the fact that although lens rotation is decreased, it is often not completely eliminated. As a result, a swinging cylindrical effect is produced.

Fabrication quality is not as good in toric surfaces as in spherical surfaces. Power, axis, and optical quality are often poorer than those desired. Verification and modification are somewhat difficult. Laboratory costs are higher and fitting time is longer than in spherical surface lenses.

In light of these factors, clinical application of the surface types to toric corneas should be considered in greater detail.

Spherical Base and Secondary Curves. When satisfactory bearing, venting, position, movement, comfort, and vision can be obtained with spherical lens curves on toric corneal curves, the spherical curves should be used. This recommendation is based on the belief that the simplest lens construction that fulfills the basic goals is preferable. Complex designs are auxiliary aids to be used only when necessary.

Many practitioners possess spherical posterior surface diagnostic lenses, but relatively few have toric posterior surface diagnostic sets. When central ophthalmometric astigmatism is more than 2 D, the performance of lenses with spherical posterior surfaces should be evaluated first.

In general, the flattest ophthalmometric principal meridian is shortened by about one third of the ophthalmometric toricity to determine base curve radius. The procedure of fitting the base curve steeper than the flatter, but flatter than the steeper ophthalmometric principal meridians is known as *splitting K*. This procedure attempts to neutralize the disadvantages of a spherical base curve on a toric corneal curve. Lens and corneal curve contiguity thus extend over a larger area (see p. 41). This modification improves the bearing relationship. The fluorescein pattern for a with-the-rule astigmat resembles an elongated I, and the fluorescein pattern for an against-the-rule astigmat resembles an elongated H (see p. 42). Adherence is increased, and lens rocking, movement, position, and edge standoff are improved. The appropriate diagnostic lens is placed on the eye and observed. The diagnostic lens procedure is used to obtain the best possible bearing, rocking, movement, position, and edge standoff.

Whenever possible, the authors prefer to use aperture-positioning lenses when spherical posterior lens surfaces are used on corneas that are considerably toric. The reasons for this preference are discussed on page 54. Also, on a with-the-rule astigmat, there is often a superior stagnated pool of precorneal fluid when a superior-positioning lens is used. Often an inferior pool of fluid occurs on a with-the-rule astigmat, wearing aperture-positioning lenses. The optic-zone diameter of an aperture-positioning lens can be decreased slightly without affecting overall performance, this action also decreases the depth of the fluid between the lens and cornea. Finally, aperture lenses often have narrower secondary widths than superior-positioning lenses. A narrower secondary width makes it easier to obtain a satisfactory relationship with the toric and asymmetrical peripheral corneal curves, and it decreases edge standoff.

After the most logical initial design specifications with spherical posterior surfaces are determined, the diagnostic lenses most nearly approximating these values are placed on the patient's eyes. They are worn for an hour or two, and performance is evaluated periodically. Slit-lamp biomicroscopy is especially important.

When performance indicates that the construction used may be successful, lenses are ordered for the patient. Frequent periodic examinations are used to obtain maximum control over the case. As adaptation progresses and lacrimation and blinking become more nearly normal, performance is again evaluated. A determination is made as to whether spherical posterior surfaces will be successful or whether toric posterior surfaces must be used.

It should be remembered that spherical posterior lens surfaces applied to toric corneal surfaces often tend to decrease corneal toricity through a molding process. This phenomenon changes the relationships and may necessitate lens modifications. Often overall performance is enhanced by the decrease in corneal toricity. When adaptation and fit are reasonably stabilized, it is often necessary to provide a new spectacle correction because of the eye's decreased astigmatism.

When it seems that a lens with posterior spherical surfaces will not be successful, the use of posterior toric surfaces should be considered. Much helpful information has been gained for application of posterior toric surfaces by evaluation of posterior spherical surfaces.

Spherical Base and Toric Secondary Curves. It is possible to use a lens with a spherical base and toric secondary curves, especially when central corneal astigmatism is between 2 and 3 D.[82] The base curve is fitted in the manner just discussed, and the secondary curve is fitted with secondary alignment. This procedure places the major bearing on the secondary-zone area and the minor bearing on the optic-zone area.

Because the area of lens and corneal curve contiguity is increased, bearing is improved. Adherence is increased and lens rocking, movement, position, and edge standoff are improved. However, precorneal fluid interchange may be impeded by the secondary alignment and apical clearance. Venting is often further decreased because the lens diameter for a superior-positioning lens is often about 0.6 mm. larger than usual to decrease lens rotation. An aperture-positioning lens with secondary alignment and apical clearance is often preferable. Venting is relatively better as lens diameters and optic-zone diameters are typically small.

It is quite difficult to determine the proper secondary radii. Peripheral measurements of corneal topography are not sufficiently accurate and cannot be converted properly into lens curves. The corneal periphery is often quite asymmetrical, and fabrication of toric secondary curves is not sufficiently accurate in many cases. Diagnostic lenses with toric secondary curves give the best information. Note that a toric secondary curvature on a spherical base lens produces an oval optic zone. The shorter chord width of the optical zone is along the flatter meridian of the secondary curve (Fig. 2–46).

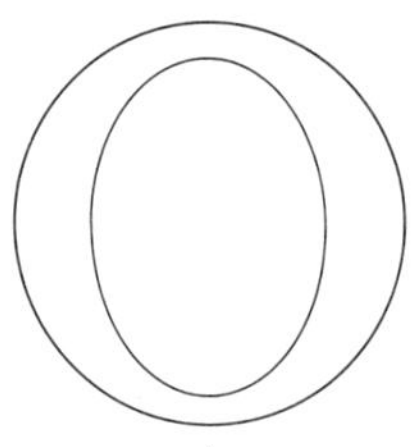

Figure 2–46. An oval optic zone is produced by a toric secondary on a spherical base. The shorter chord of the optic zone is along the flatter meridian of the secondary curve.

The advantage of a toric secondary curve over a toric base curve lens is that no induced residual astigmatism is produced in the optic-zone area. Just the same, a toric base curve lens is often preferable.

Toric Base and Spherical or Toric Secondary Curves. The disadvantages of toric base curves are discussed on page 88. They should be reviewed as a basis for understanding clinical procedure.

Curvatures and Diameters. Posterior lens curves are determined by the method of measurements and standards, by diagnostic lens procedure, or by the combination method. The goal is to achieve a relationship between the posterior surface of the lens and anterior corneal curves that provides satisfactory bearing, adherence, lens rocking, movement, position (both in terms of centration and rotation), and edge standoff. Because perfect bearing and venting are usually mutually exclusive—that is, as one is enhanced, the other is decreased in effectiveness—achievement of these relationships may produce poor venting.

To establish a clinically satisfactory balance, lens and optic-zone diameters are often 0.3 to 0.4 mm. less than would otherwise be used. Base curves are not selected to obtain complete alignment, but rather they are slightly flatter, especially in the vertical meridian in a with-the-rule astigmat. In a 7.0 mm. optic zone, the flatter base curve is about 0.25 D flatter than the flatter ophthalmometric principal meridian. The steeper base curve is flatter than the steepest ophthalmometric meridian by 0.25 D for each diopter of ophthalmometric astigmatism over one diopter. For example, it is 0.25 D flatter when there is 2.00 D of ophthalmometric astigmatism and 0.50 D flatter when there is 3.00 D of ophthalmometric astigmatism.

There are two important considerations. First, fitting with less than full toricity tends to increase lens rotation, and may cause the lens to position at an undesired meridian. Both bearing and visual problems may be produced. Second, the central ophthalmometric astigmatism may not accurately depict the true toricity of the central cornea. Also, true toricity varies in terms of the optic-zone diameter used.

It is preferable to use these guides as starting points; then diagnostic lens procedure can be followed to establish more accurately the desired radii. Because two base curvature radii are involved, the problem is quite complex.

The practitioner should use spherical base diagnostic lenses first to determine the desired curvature of the flatter meridian in a given optic-zone diameter. Toric base diagnostic lenses are then selected with this flatter radius and the approximate amount of toricity indicated by the central ophthalmometric or Keratometric reading. The diagnostic lens procedure is used to determine the radius for the steeper meridian and to verify the radius for the flatter meridian (Fig. 2–47, insert between pp. 82 and 83).

If the practitioner does not have toric diagnostic lenses, he may order appropriate "loaner" lenses from his laboratory. Such lenses should have the base curve for the flatter meridian, as determined by spherical diagnostic lenses. The lens diameter, optic-zone diameter, and secondary radius of these lenses should approximate what the practitioner feels will finally be prescribed. The base curve toricity is the variable. Often, three lenses are sufficient to enable evaluation and interpolation. The first lens should have a toricity 0.10 to 0.15 mm. more than that indicated by the central ophthalmometric reading—that is, it should be 0.10 to 0.15 mm. steeper than the steepest principal meridian. The second lens should have the same amount of toricity as that indicated by the central ophthalmometric reading. The third lens should have a toricity 0.10 to 0.15 mm. less than that indicated by the central ophthalmometric reading.

A lens with a toric base curve and a spherical secondary curve has an oval optic zone. To fabricate an approximately circular optic zone, a secondary curve with about the same toricity as the base curve is used.

Refractive Power and Rotation. When a lens with a spherical base curve is placed on the eye, the anterior precorneal fluid assumes this spherical shape, producing a *stigmatic* refraction of light at this interface. When a lens with a toric base curve is placed on the eye, the precorneal fluid assumes a corresponding toric shape.[83–86] Because the radii of the principal meridians differ, at this interface an astigmatic refraction of light is induced.

The power of this astigmatic refraction on the eye is equal to about 31 per cent of the cylinder of the rear surface of the lens in air. This value can easily be determined from the surface power table, Appendix VI. Either the keratometric or ophthalmometric power of each principal lens meridian may be determined from Column 3 or 4, respectively, or its true radius is located in Column 1 of the surface power table. On the same line for each power or radius at Column 6 or 7, the power of each principal lens meridian is found. The difference between the two powers in Column 6 *or* the two powers in Column 7 is the amount of astigmatic refraction on the eye. This astigmatism is always a minus cylinder with its axis corresponding to the flatter principal lens meridian. For a with-the-rule astigmat, it is generally a minus cylinder axis of about 180°.

When a lens with a toric base and spherical anterior surface is placed on the precorneal fluid, two components cause residual astigmatic refraction—that *induced* at the interface between the toric base and the anterior precorneal fluid, and that contributed by all components and interfaces of the eye *internal* to this. This internal astigmatism is generally a minus cylinder axis of about 180°.

There are two methods of compensating for the astigmatism that is residual—that is, remains—when a lens with a toric base and a single spherical anterior curve is placed on the eye. In both methods, compensation is effected by the placement of an anterior toric surface on the lens. In one method, only the induced astigmatism is compensated for, and the internal astigmatism remains uncorrected.[87] This method may be used when it is felt that the internal astigmatism is not sufficient to cause visual acuity problems or discomfort. In the second method, the sum of the induced and internal astigmatisms is compensated for.

When only the induced astigmatism is compensated for, the axis of the cylinder on the anterior surface is the same as that on the posterior surface. The power is equal in amount but opposite in type. For example, assume the induced cylinder is −1.50 axis 180. On the anterior surface is placed a cylinder +1.50 axis 180. One cylinder neutralizes the other, and the lens has a spherical power *on the eye.* The advantage of this arrangement is that fluctuation of the meridional orientation of the lens does not produce visual problems caused by tilted cylinder. The disadvantage is that when internal astigmatism is considerable, visual acuity problems and discomfort may be produced.

To determine the refractive powers to prescribe, either computation or refraction over diagnostic lenses is done.[88] When computation is used, the needed power for the flatter meridian is found as for a spherical lens not having spherical equivalent power. The power needed for the steeper meridian is equal to the algebraic sum of the power needed in the flatter meridian and the difference in *ophthalmometric* diopters of the principal meridians of the toric base. When diagnostic lenses are used, the needed power for the flatter meridian is found by refraction over diagnostic lenses. The power needed for the steeper meridian is found by the computation just discussed.

When the practitioner corrects for both induced and internal astigmatism, the power on the eye will not be spherical. Part of the cylinder on the anterior surface of the lens will neutralize the induced astigmatism. The rest of the cylinder will neutralize the internal astigmatism.

To determine the refractive power to order, either computation or refraction over diagnostic lenses is used. When the computation method is used, the first five steps, as used for a spherical single-vision lens, are employed (p. 62). The relationship of each principal meridian of the toric base curve to the corresponding central ophthalmometric principal meridian is considered. Allowance (discussed in Step 8 for a spherical single-vision lens, p. 63) is made for each meridian. When diagnostic lenses are used, either toric base-spherical anterior or toric base-toric anterior lenses can be used. The diagnostic lenses should have a dot at the edge of the flatter base principal meridian. The lens most nearly approximating the lens to be ordered is placed on the patient's eye. After the lens is settled, meridional orientation is noted by the placement of a spectacle trial frame containing a low-powered ophthalmic trial cylinder on the patient. A line connecting the axis markings of the ophthalmic trial cylinder is drawn, and is aligned with the axis dots on the diagnostic contact lens. The axis reading is then taken from the trial frame. The trial frame is then removed, and a spherocylindrical refraction with the diagnostic contact lens on the eye is done. This power is combined with the power of the diagnostic lens to determine total power needed. Compensation is made for any variance of ordered base curve radii from those of the diagnostic lens.

Unless the diagnostic lens used is almost identical to the lens to be ordered in all respects but refractive power, meridional orientation often differs. This difference produces an erroneous refractive power. It is often preferable to order a pair of lenses with all desired specifications but with a spherical anterior surface. Refraction is done over these lenses, and the needed power is determined. Either these lenses may be returned to have the appropriate anterior cylindrical surface placed on them, or a new pair may be fabricated.

Anterior Toric Surfaces

Need. Although anterior toric surfaces are used to correct the residual astigmatic error when central posterior toric surfaces are used, an area of greater clinical need is the correction of the residual astigmatic error when central posterior *spherical* surfaces are used.[89–93]

When a spherical base curve is placed on the eye, the precorneal fluid assumes this spherical shape, producing a *stigmatic* refraction of light at this interface. That is, the central ophthalmometric astigmatism (AO) is eliminated. The total astigmatism of the eye (AT) is represented by the spectacle prescription having a full astigmatic correction referred back to the corneal plane. AT is composed of AO and the astigmatism produced by all aspects of the eye internal to the interface between air and the precorneal fluid. This internal astigmatism (AI) is not corrected when a lens with central posterior and anterior spherical curves is used. A clinically practical formula for the prediction of the amount of internal residual astigmatism is $AI = AT - AO$. When internal residual astigmatism is great enough (0.75 D or more), visual acuity or comfort may be affected significantly.

The formula for the prediction of internal residual astigmatism assumes that the ophthalmometric readings are valid and accurate, that the cornea is not tilted relative to the line of sight, that the contact lens will not tilt on the eye enough to induce an astigmatism, and that the contact lens will not become warped.

When the formula for the prediction of internal residual astigmatism is used, AT is in minus cylinder form and AO is considered as a minus cylinder with its axis coinciding with the flatter ophthalmometric principal meridian.

Example:

Spectacle correction: −1.00 −1.00 x 90
Ophthalmometric reading: 43 SPh
AI = AT − AO
AI = (−1.00 a x 90) − (0)
AI = −1.00 a x 90

About 35 to 40 per cent of patients fitted with spherical base contact lenses have an internal residual astigmatism of 0.75 D or more. With very few exceptions, the internal residual astigmatism is against-the-rule, having a plus axis at or near 90°. Residual internal astigmatism is a significant clinical problem.

The optical need for astigmatic correction is neutralized in some cases by three factors:

1. Visual performance with contact lens correction compared to spectacle correction is aided by a slight increase in light transmission (assuming a tinted contact lens has not been used), a slight increase in usable field, and a retinal image of better quality. The quality of the retinal image is improved by the reduction of aberrations and by more consistent fixation through the optical center. With high refractive powers such as are used in aphakia or high myopia, all these benefits are increased. The high myope also receives a considerably larger retinal image. These factors in some cases

tend to outweigh the residual astigmatic error, and the patient's total visual performance is better. As a result, some patients feel that they see better when central acuity with contact lenses is 20/20 to 20/25 than when best-corrected central acuity with spectacle lenses is 20/20.

2. Many patients come for contact lens fitting wearing an old spectacle correction that does not produce best-corrected central acuity. Best-corrected contact lens acuity is often better than the patient's accustomed spectacle acuity.

3. Visual discomfort is often not too great when the residual astigmatic error is not over 0.75 D. This is especially true in younger people, who constitute the great percentage of contact lens wearers. Their accommodation and physiologic reserves are often sufficient to permit function with good acuity and little or no discomfort.

Clinical Possibilities and Guides. Three methods are used in the correction of internal residual astigmatism when corneal contact lenses are used.[94]

1. The first method involves the use of the spherical equivalent principle and a contact lens with *spherical* central posterior and anterior surfaces. The spherical equivalent principle is based on the fact that there is one position between the focal lines of an astigmatic refraction of light that produces the best image—the circle of least confusion. The circle of least confusion can be placed on the retina by taking half the value of the minus cylinder needed and combining it with the needed sphere. This procedure produces an equivalent sphere, to place the circle of least confusion on the retina. Such a spherical equivalent correction is particularly effective when the amount of needed cylinder is relatively small compared to the amount of needed sphere.

2. The second method includes use of a contact lens with a *spherical* base curve and an anterior *toric* surface. Because a contact lens tends to rotate on the eye owing to lid action (see p. 32), the meridional positioning of the toric surface is altered. It is necessary to incorporate something into the lens construction that neutralizes this rotational tendency and produces desired, stable meridional orientation. Currently, the most common means of fulfilling this condition when central ophthalmometric astigmatism is less than 2 D is by placing prism in the lens.[95–99] The heavier prism base is oriented inferiorly on the eye owing to the effect of gravity. This ballast effect is often combined with truncation to further stabilize orientation. Research is being done to find a way to provide ballast by impregnation of metallic strips into a nonprismatic lens. Lenses truncated on two sides and lenses with a scleral flange have occasionally been used clinically[100–103] (Fig. 2–48).

When central ophthalmometric astigmatism is greater than 2 D, a posterior toric surface is usually preferred to stop rotation and to provide better overall performance. An anterior toric surface that corrects the total of induced and internal residual astigmatism is used, producing a bitoric lens.

3. In the third method, a contact lens with central posterior and anterior

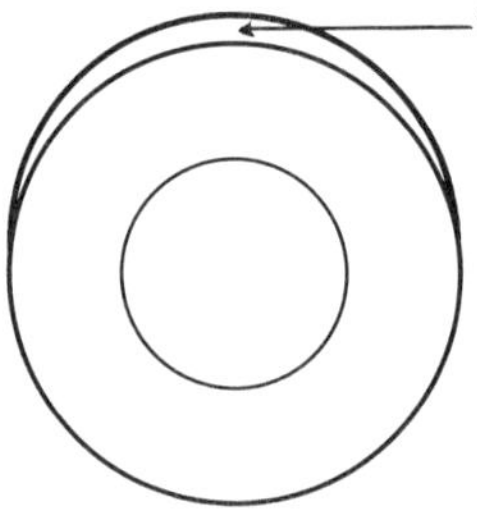

Figure 2–48. A contact lens with a superior scleral flange.

spherical surfaces is used. Spectacles with the needed astigmatic correction are worn with the contact lenses for highly demanding visual tasks. Although the use of auxiliary spectacles is easy for the practitioner and optically sound, it is often not acceptable to the patient, because most patients desire contact lenses to enhance their appearance by eliminating the need for spectacles. Auxiliary spectacles are more readily accepted when the basic patient motivation is to improve vision, such as in aphakia or keratoconus, or to protect the eye, such as when a patient has scarred inner lid surfaces.

The following may be used as a clinical guide. Internal residual astigmatism of less than 0.75 D is usually corrected by a spherical contact lens using the spherical equivalent principle. Internal residual astigmatism from 0.75 to 1.12 D is corrected with a spherical contact lens using the spherical equivalent principle or an anterior toric prism ballast lens. Internal residual astigmatism of 1.25 D or more is usually corrected with an anterior toric prism ballast lens.

Scleral contact lenses have excellent meridional stability. A scleral contact lens with an anterior toric surface may be used to correct internal residual astigmatism. Scleral contact lenses are discussed on page 265.

Advantages and Disadvantages. To better understand these guides for the correction of internal residual astigmatism, let us recapitulate the possible advantages and disadvantages of a spherical nonprismatic lens with the spherical equivalent power and an anterior toric prism ballast lens.

A prism ballast lens is relatively thick and heavy. Excessive movement and eccentric positioning may result, making it more difficult to obtain satisfactory bearing, venting, stability, and visual performance. This problem is accentuated when there is a central ophthalmometric astigmatism of more than 2 D. When the central ophthalmometric astigmatism is more than 2 D, a bitoric nonprismatic lens is preferable.

The optical quality of an anterior toric prism ballast lens is often considerably poorer than that of a spherical nonprismatic lens because of the technical problems in producing a toric surface, and because of the variation in spherical power and aberration due to the increase in lens thickness from apex to base. Furthermore, although meridional orientation is usually stabilized to a large degree by the use of prism as a ballast, often there is still some fluctuation of axis position.

Often the base of the lens is truncated to stabilize further meridional orientation. Additional meridional stability is basically produced by the friction established between the truncated portion of the lens and the lower lid on which the lens rests. As contiguity between the configuration of the truncation and the margin of the lower lid is increased, friction and stable orientation are increased. Truncation makes modification and any subsequent duplication more difficult. Because of thickness variation, it is often more difficult to produce a satisfactory edge finish.

When internal residual astigmatism exists only in one eye and is corrected with a prism ballast lens, an equal amount of prism must be incorporated in the lens used for the other eye. If it is not, a vertical phoria is induced.

The only true theoretical advantage to using an anterior toric prism ballast lens is the satisfactory correction of the internal residual astigmatic error. The practitioner must determine whether this theoretical advantage can be obtained by anterior toric prism ballast lenses. He must further determine whether this advantage outweighs the disadvantages. In general, a spherical nonprismatic contact lens is used whenever satisfactory visual acuity and comfort are produced by it.

The Spherical Lens and Spherical Equivalent. Determination of all lens specifications is done in the usual manner. The refractive power determined either by the method of measurements and standards or by refraction over diagnostic lenses produces the spherical equivalent power.

When spherical refraction over spherical diagnostic lenses produces a central acuity of 20/25 or better, such lenses should be ordered. As adaptation progresses and lacrimation becomes more normal, acuity of 20/20 or better is often obtained with concurrent visual comfort. If satisfactory visual acuity and comfort do not result in about two weeks, an anterior toric prism ballast lens may be considered.

Anterior Toric Prism Ballast Lenses. The specifications are determined by the method of measurements and standards or by the diagnostic lens procedure.

Measurements and Standards Method. The base curve is selected 0.05 mm. longer than indicated in Table 2–7, because a prism ballast lens usually positions inferiorly and tilts with its apex toward and its base away from the cornea. This arrangement often produces an apical touch and inferior pooling (Fig. 2–49). Slight lengthening of the base curve radius tends to decrease the pooling and increase the bearing area. The secondary curve radius is determined by use of Table 2–10.

The weight, center of gravity position, and edge construction of the lens tend to make it position inferiorly on the eye. The lens diameter is selected so that with primary fixation either there is clearance between the apex and the upper lid or the apex is tucked under the upper lid. Thus, the diameter is either less than the vertical palpebral aperture, or it is slightly greater (about 0.5 mm.) than the vertical palpebral aperture size. When the diam-

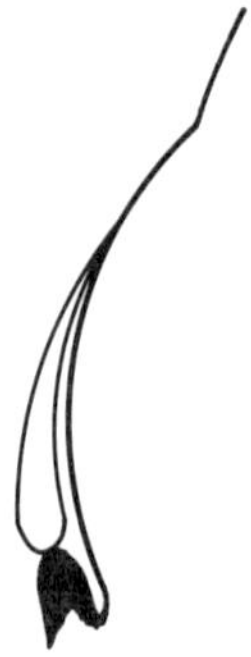

Figure 2–49. A prism ballast lens is tilted by the lower lid to produce apical touch and inferior pooling.

eter is approximately equal to the vertical palpebral aperture size, the upper lid bears heavily on the lens in blinking. Discomfort, lens displacement, and physiologic insult frequently result.

Both smaller and larger diameters have certain advantages. Use of a smaller diameter results in less meridional instability produced by the upper lid. Also, there are a relatively thinner lens for a given amount of prism diopters, less lower lid irritation, and greater corneal exposure.

With a larger diameter, there are better optic-zone centration in front of the pupil and less tendency for lens displacement, and there may be less initial upper lid irritation. The authors prefer to use small diameters which have better clinical performance.

Average lens diameter for a circular aperture-positioning lens is 8.5 mm. and average lens diameter for a circular lens whose apex is tucked under the upper lid is 9.5 mm. When inferior truncation is used, the horizontal lens diameter is usually 0.5 to 0.7 mm. greater than the vertical lens diameter. Average lens diameter for an aperture-positioning truncated prism ballast lens is 8.5 mm. vertically and 9.0 mm. horizontally. The authors order circular lenses and truncate them when indicated by clinical performance.

Superior truncation to reduce rotation may also be used.

The optic-zone diameter is selected as in spherical nonprismatic single-vision lenses. The optic zone is geometrically centered or decentered upward, an arrangement which results in a better coincidence of the optic zone and central cornea, and may produce a better bearing relationship and pupil coverage. The disadvantage of upward decentration is production of an unequal secondary width, resulting in a thinning of the prism base from the wide inferior secondary curve. This thinning results in three possible problems: some of the ballast effect is eliminated, tending to increase lens rotation; the thinner base has a greater tendency to slip below the lower lid, causing discomfort, and vision and bearing problems; and it is more difficult for the practitioner to make modifications of the secondary curves. Generally, the authors prefer to use a centered optic zone with a 7.0 to 7.5 mm. O.Z.D.

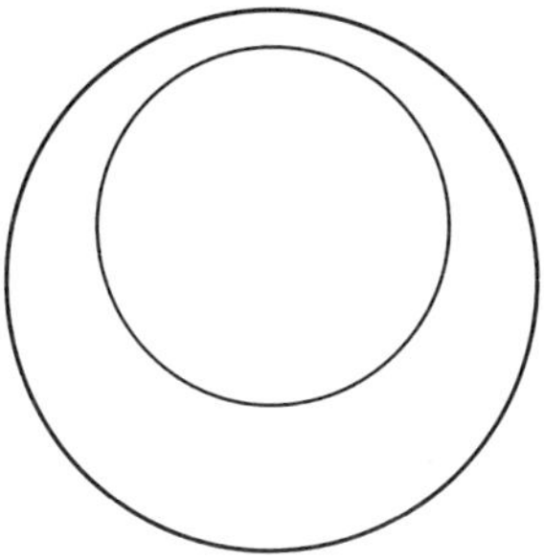

Figure 2–50. Secondary width varies with a decentered optic zone.

The secondary width is half the difference between the circular lens diameter and the centered optic-zone diameter. When a decentered optic zone is used, the secondary width varies from a maximum at the base to a minimum at the apex. This condition makes determination of the secondary radius more difficult (Fig. 2–50).

To keep overall thickness at a minimum and to enhance lid comfort, apex thickness after application of secondary curves should be about 0.10 to 0.12 mm. Other thickness factors are computed to obtain the apex thickness. A thin apex also reduces the ability of the upper lid to rotate the lens. A 0.3 mm. *superior* truncation may also be used to reduce the ability of the upper lid to rotate the lens.

For *refractive power,* the first six steps are the same as those used for a spherical lens (p. 62). Spherical power is determined in Step 5 and cylindrical power in Step 6. Finally, any necessary compensation for the relationship of the base curve to the flatter ophthalmometric meridian is done as discussed previously (p. 63).

Among *auxiliary features,* prism is used as the primary means for stabilizing meridional orientation. Because of possible discomfort, and vision and physiologic problems which may be produced by a prism ballast lens, the desired amount of ballast is the minimum that will produce proper orientation. Although it varies with each patient, 1.25 to 1.5 ΔD often provides sufficient ballast to establish reasonably good meridional stability. The base of the prism may be down, or down and in. The reason for placing the base down and in is that the effect of the upper and lower lids often tends to pull the lens up nasally 10° to 15°. Placing the base down and in by a similar amount tends to reduce this tilting action somewhat. When the practitioner desires to center a prism ballast lens on the eye, the weight of the lens must be decreased by decreasing the amount of prism to about 0.75^{Δ}. Such small amounts of prism, however, may not produce satisfactory meridional orientation.

Inferior truncation as a secondary means of stabilizing meridional orientation is often used in conjunction with prism ballast. To obtain maximum contiguity, the truncation is made to conform to the margin of the lower lid. This construction produces maximum friction to impede rotation and allows the pressure on the lower lid to be spread over a relatively larger area. Corners of the truncation are well rounded to prevent excessive lower lid irritation. The bottom of the truncation is flat to maintain a maximum width for preventing slippage beneath the lower lid, and the sides are rounded, but not thinned, to prevent irritation to the cornea or lid.

When a truncated prism ballast lens is ordered, both the vertical and horizontal lens diameters should also be ordered. It is often helpful to include a sketch of the desired shape of the truncation. When a circular prism ballast lens that is to be truncated by the practitioner is ordered, the lens diameter ordered is the finished horizontal diameter.

Diagnostic Lens Procedure. Either spherical nonprismatic or spherical prismatic diagnostic lenses, which provide more information, are used. The optic zone is centered in nonprismatic diagnostic lenses. The authors prefer centered optic zones in prismatic diagnostic contact lenses.

The appropriate base and secondary curve radii to provide the desired relationships are determined by fluorescein pattern interpretation. When nonprismatic spherical diagnostic lenses are used, the base curve to be ordered is lengthened by 0.05 mm. to compensate for the tilt that usually occurs when prismatic contact lenses are used.

Lens diameter is determined by placing of diagnostic lenses on the eyes of a patient who is fixating at distance. When nonprismatic lenses are used, they are manually placed in the inferior position that a prismatic lens usually assumes. The patient maintains normal aperture size and refrains from blinking, and the lens diameter is determined so that it provides clearance from or tucking under the upper lid. It is important to make certain that the lens is not pushed under the lower lid. The same procedure is used with prismatic lenses, but they usually assume the inferior position without manual positioning.

The optic-zone diameter is usually the same as in nonprismatic lenses, and the secondary curve width is half the difference between the lens diameter and the optic-zone diameter.

Lens thickness should be computed so that a thickness at the apex of 0.10 to 0.12 mm. is produced.

A spherocylindrical refraction is done. The cylinder axis indicated on the phoropter or trial frame may not be completely accurate, because a prismatic contact lens on the eye may tilt in terms of the vertical axis.[104]

Assume, for example, that the lenses have prism base down. When placed on the eye, however, the lens positions so that the base is tilted up 15° nasally rather than directed straight down (Fig. 2–51). Further assume that a minus cylinder axis 90° is read from the phoropter. If the laboratory fabricates a lens minus axis 90° and this lens is placed on the eye, the axis positioning will be in error by 15° because of the tilt. In the case of a 15°

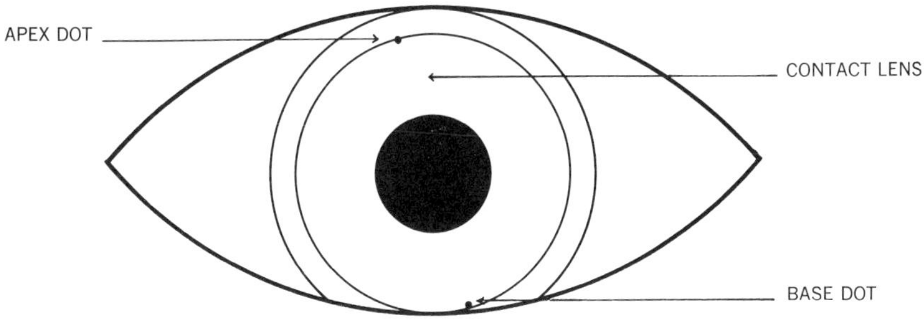

Figure 2–51. A prism ballast lens tilted on the eye. Dots indicate base and apex of lens.

tilt up nasally, the axis will effectively be 105° on the right eye and 75° on the left eye.

Clinically, the following steps may be taken to compensate for tilting. A dot is placed directly at the base and apex of the lens. It is extremely important that this be done accurately or an error will be introduced. An ophthalmic trial lens of ±0.12 D cylinder is used, and a line connecting its axis markings is drawn. The trial lens is placed in a trial frame, and the line on the ophthalmic lens is then aligned with the base apex dots on the contact lens on the patient's eye. The axis reading of the ophthalmic trial lens is then read from the trial frame (Fig. 2–52). Appropriate compensation is made on the final ordering.

The compensation is simple to determine. If we assume that there is a 15° tilt up nasally in each eye, aligning the ophthalmic trial lens with base

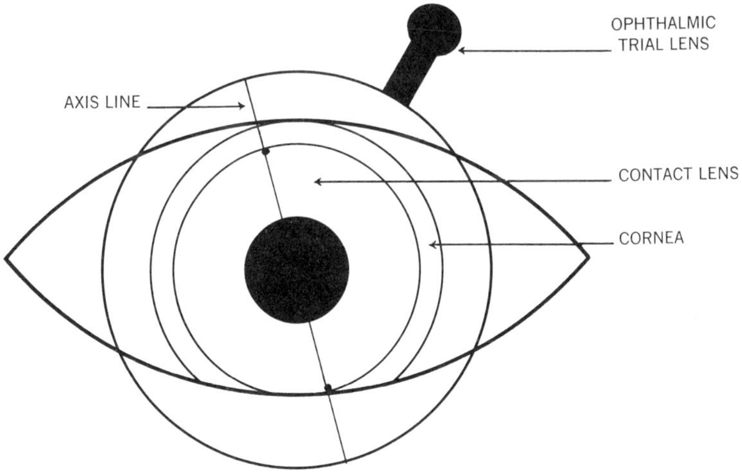

Figure 2–52. An ophthalmic trial lens with a line connecting its axis markings is aligned with dots on contact lens to determine amount of tilt.

apex line of the contact lens will show us a reading of axis 105° on the right eye. Minus axis 90° is needed for proper correction behind the phoropter. To establish this value with the lens on the eye tilting 15° up nasally, minus axis 75° should be ordered ground on the lens. When this lens is placed on the eye, it will tilt 15° up nasally, and the cylinder will position at the needed minus axis 90°. For the left eye the same procedure is followed. This time minus axis 105° should be ordered to produce a minus axis 90° when the lens is on the eye.

The amount of tilt may vary with distance and near fixation. Usually, axis positioning should be for the more critical visual tasks.

Auxiliary Features. The minimum amount of prism that maintains proper lens position is determined. When nonprismatic diagnostic lenses are used, the minimum amount of prism is determined by averages—that is, 1.25 to 1.5 ΔD. When prismatic diagnostic lenses are used, performance is evaluated.

A critical determination of the lens position is necessary to fit properly an anterior toric prism ballast lens. The necessary accuracy can usually be obtained only after adaptation by the patient has become well established; lacrimation and blink action must be stabilized.

Clinically, it is often best initially to fit nonprismatic spherical contact lenses containing the appropriate spherical equivalent power. This method is used even when it is thought that anterior toric prism ballast lenses will be applied finally. The patient usually adapts to nonprismatic lenses more easily and more quickly than he does to prismatic lenses. The patient should be placed on a wearing schedule for one week. At the first weekly progress examination, visual acuity and comfort are evaluated. When necessary, the spherical equivalent power is altered or temporary auxiliary cylindrical spectacle lenses are provided. The patient's wearing time is appropriately increased over the next two weeks, and progress is observed weekly. By the end of the third week, adaptation is usually well established.

A reasonably valid and accurate determination can then be made as to whether spherical nonprismatic lenses with the spherical equivalent power, spherical nonprismatic lenses with auxiliary spectacles for specific tasks, or anterior toric prism ballast lenses are indicated. When anterior toric prism ballast lenses are indicated, much more valid and accurate determination of lens specifications can be made on the well adapted eye. Also, there is better patient acceptance of permanent use of auxiliary spectacles when this procedure is used. Many patients find that they are not as greatly inconvenienced by the intermittent use of auxiliary spectacles as they had assumed they would be.

Spherical Prism Ballast Lenses

Occasionally, a spherical prism ballast lens is used. Generally, this type of lens is used when aperture positioning is highly desired but cannot be accomplished by use of a nonprismatic lens, and as a last resort to lower high-riding superior-positioning lenses. This type of lens is also used occasionally to eliminate the sliding of nonprismatic lenses underneath the lower lid. Such sliding may cause visual or physiologic problems.

Verification of Refractive Power

The contact lens is centered with its posterior surface against the lensometer or vertometer stop, and the contact lens is rotated until the displaced target image is aligned at the proper base-apex meridian. Cylinder axis and power are then determined in the usual manner. Because of technical problems involved with manufacturing the anterior toric surface, aberrations inherent in such lenses, and the 0.25 D. change of spherical power for each 0.10 mm. change of thickness, the image of the lensometer or vertometer target is usually hazy.

Contact Lenses for Subnormal Vision

A visually efficient person is able to perceive the form, position, and color of objects in his environment. Perception of form and position depends to a large degree on the ability to distinguish details satisfactorily—satisfactory visual acuity—over a large field of view. As visual acuity or field of view is reduced, an individual becomes visually less efficient. Ability to function in his environment is impaired.

As a clinical and legal guide, standards of visual acuity and size of field have been established to categorize patients whose performance is subnormal. When visual acuity with the best-correcting lens is less than 20/20 but better than 20/70 in the better eye, the patient may be said to have *mildly subnormal vision.* When visual acuity with the best-correcting lens is better than 20/200 but less than 20/70 in the better eye, the patient may be said to have *moderately subnormal vision.* When visual acuity with the best-correcting lens is less than 20/200, it may be termed *severe subnormal vision* or *legal blindness.* Legal blindness also occurs when the visual field is less than 20° at its greatest diameter, regardless of how good visual acuity is. Thus, a person with 20/20 visual acuity and a visual field of less than 20° is legally blind.

Reduced visual acuity is generally caused by ametropia and the resultant out-of-focus retinal image. The proper refractive power in either a spectacle or a contact lens produces a focused retinal image, and this image allows normal visual acuity and efficiency.

When reduced visual acuity or reduced field of view is caused by an ocular pathologic condition, provision of only a focused retinal image may not restore normal visual acuity and efficiency, because of poor quality or faulty reception, transmission, or interpretation of the focused retinal image. Poor quality may be caused by aniridia, albinism, opacities, or irregular surfaces. Poor reception, transmission, or interpretation may result from retinal, optic-nerve, or cerebral malfunction.

Aid for subnormal vision is based on first producing the best retinal image focus. Then either the quality of the retinal image is improved, or the retinal image is enlarged. Enlargement of the retinal image produces stimulation of more cones, and the neural summation often aids in distinguishing details. As the size of the retinal image is increased, however, the field of view is decreased. There is practically no way to aid subnormal vision by increasing the field of view. However, when an aid is used to enlarge the retinal image, the field of view should not be decreased more than is absolutely necessary. This point is especially important if the aid is to be used while the patient moves about. Sufficient field of vision is more important than acuity for spatial localization and traveling.

A patient with subnormal vision is successfully aided only when his needs are satisfied. Thus, the ability to function in his environment must be improved to a degree *acceptable to him*. Basically, the practitioner must determine whether the amount and type of residual vision can be improved to this degree. This determination depends on three general considerations: subjective considerations, such as the patient's motivations, expectations, intelligence, cooperation, and work demands; the cause of the subnormal vision and the amount and type of residual vision; and the practitioner's knowledge and understanding of these factors and of the advantages and limitations of contemporary aids to subnormal vision. Contact lenses may be used to focus, improve the quality of, and enlarge the retinal image.[105–107] The practitioner must determine which method or combination of methods is to be used and whether the best results can be obtained with contact lenses or other aids. The use of contact lenses as aids for subnormal vision may be considered in three categories: contact lenses may be used to provide an artificial, regular refractive surface at the interface between air and the eye; an artificial aperture for the eye's optical system; and an enlarged retinal image.

Provision of a Regular Surface

When the central anterior corneal surface is irregular, spectacle correction cannot provide a focused, high-quality retinal image. Although there is regular refraction of light between the spectacle lens and air (Fig. 2–53), light is refracted irregularly both at the interface between air and pre-

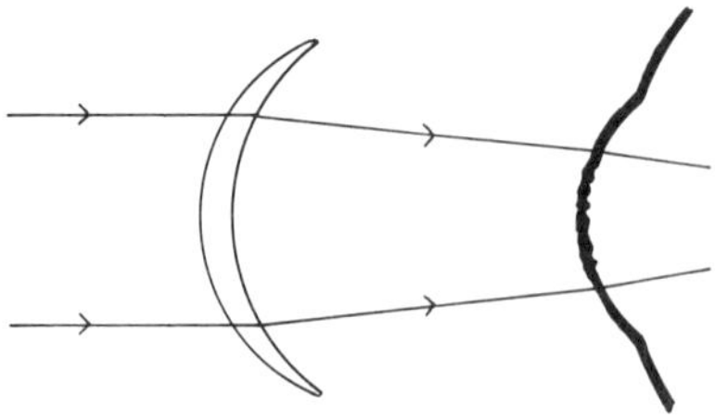

Figure 2–53. Spectacle correction of an irregular cornea. The spectacle surfaces are regular and produce regular refraction. The corneal surfaces are irregular and produce irregular refraction.

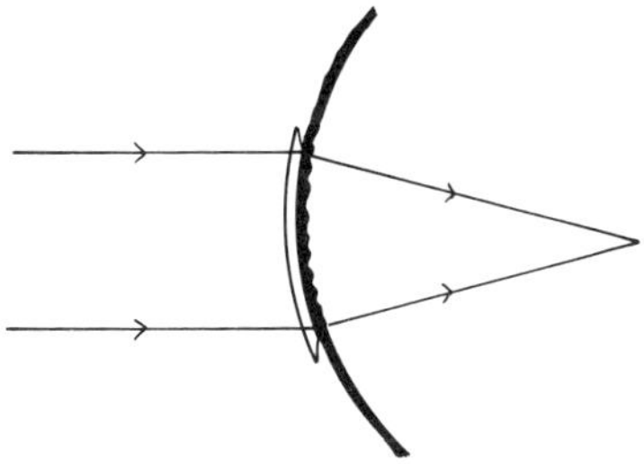

Figure 2–54. When a contact lens is on an irregular cornea, there is only a small residual refractive irregularity.

corneal fluid and the interface between precorneal fluid and anterior cornea.

When a contact lens is placed on the eye, light is refracted regularly at the interface between air and the anterior contact lens surface. Conformation of the precorneal fluid to the contact lens base curve produces a regular surface, and as a result a regular refraction of light, at this interface. The interface between the precorneal fluid and the anterior cornea remains irregular, and irregular refraction of light results. Because the index of refraction of the precorneal fluid is about 1.336 and that of the anterior cornea is about 1.376, there is a small (0.040) indicial difference. This interface, therefore, contributes only a very small percentage of the eye's refractive power (Fig. 2–54). Placing a contact lens on the eye considerably reduces irregular refraction from the irregular anterior corneal surface, thus vastly improving the focus and quality of the retinal image.

An irregular anterior corneal surface may be congenital or caused by certain ocular pathologic conditions. In most cases of corneal irregularity, determination of contact lens specifications is done in the usual way. Because of the irregularity, it is somewhat more difficult to obtain the desired relationships between the posterior surface of the lens and anterior corneal curvatures. Because spectacle refraction is inaccurate in the case of an irregular corneal surface, refractive power must be determined by refraction over diagnostic lenses.

KERATOCONUS. One category of irregular anterior cornea presenting unique contact lens fitting problems is that related to keratoconus.[108–116] In such cases, not only is the cornea irregular, but the apical portion also protrudes in a conelike manner (Fig. 2–55).

Incidence and Etiology. Keratoconus is defined as a degenerative, noninflammatory disease of the cornea marked by conical protrusion. The inci-

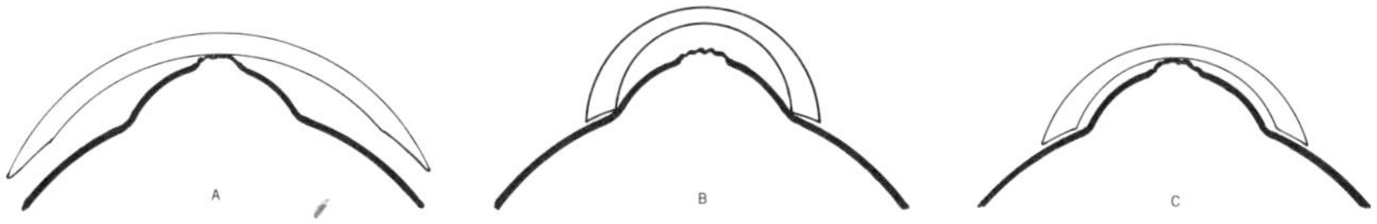

Figure 2–55. Curvature relationships in keratoconus. A, *Distinct apical touch and peripheral clearance.* B, *Apical clearance and secondary alignment.* C, *Slight apical touch and secondary alignment.*

dence of keratoconus in the general population is probably between 0.003 and 0.03 per cent. Incidence in terms of patients coming for professional service is probably about 0.23 per cent.[117] Until fairly recently, it was thought that the incidence is greater in females, but there is now evidence to the contrary.

Etiology is uncertain. The literature mentions endocrine imbalance, hereditary tendency, calcium disturbance, malnutrition, and increased intraocular pressure as possible causative factors. Some consider it to be a dystrophy, and others consider it to be a developmental anomaly. Generally, keratoconus manifests itself during ages ten to 20, a fact which has led some to believe that there is a relationship to puberty. Eye rubbing may contribute.

Progression and Topographic Changes. In some cases, the condition progresses for about six years and then remains relatively stationary. In other cases, it follows this pattern with periodic relapses or it continuously progresses.

As the disease progresses, there is usually a conical protrusion of the apex of the cornea, producing a steep central corneal area, and relatively speaking, an appreciably flatter peripheral corneal area. The protrusion also produces a highly irregular, toric, asymmetrical corneal surface, and the corneal apex often points inferiorly and nasally.

All these problems gradually become worse as the disease progresses. It is therefore mandatory that keratoconus be detected as soon as possible. Early detection permits a better fit of contact lenses to be made, because the corneal topography is more nearly normal. There is difference of opinion on whether contact lenses can retard the progress of the protrusion.

Early Detection. Detection of keratoconus is based on certain symptoms and signs. The patient may present some or all of the following symptoms: monocular diplopia or multiple images of recent onset, especially around lights; poor vision in spite of an acuity value of 20/20 and recent prescription change; increased photophobia; increased corneal sensitivity *at first;* distortion of vision with resultant squinting; progressively decreasing vision at distance and near; frequent prescription changes, especially for one eye; and marked increase of cylindrical power and shifting of cylindrical axis.

The examiner may note some or all of the following signs with slit-lamp biomicroscopic examination: corneal thinning at the apex to about one half to one fifth of normal thickness; the pulse beat from intraocular pressure; vertical stretch lines in deep stromal layers; an endothelial reflex at the apex of the cone; an increased visibility of nerve fibers; Fleischer's ring—a line around the base of the cone; ruptures in Descemet's membrane and superficial linear scarring in advanced disease; and protrusion of the cone itself, often down and nasal; and hydrops, or severe edema.

Using ophthalmometry, the examiner may note a variance in miral image size between the eyes and in various meridians of the same eye; changes in amount or axis of astigmatism; high readings (it is possible, however, to have readings of 48 D or more and not have keratoconus, just as it is possible, especially in the early stages, to have readings of 44 D or less and have keratoconus); and the impossibility of aligning images and principal meridians not 90° apart. This last indication must be differentiated from irregular astigmatism. One basis for differentiation is the relative variability in keratoconus and the relative stability in irregular astigmatism over a period of time.

Other signs include distortion of the images of Placido's disk or of room objects from the cornea; the protrusion of lower lid with depressed gaze—Munson's sign (more apparent in later stages); difficulty in seeing the fundus clearly with an ophthalmoscope; and a scissors motion in skiametry, making it extremely difficult to evaluate reflex motion.

Contact Lens Application. Because of the unique corneal topography in keratoconus, it is difficult to produce contiguity of the posterior surface of the contact lens and the anterior corneal curvatures over a large area. As a result, bearing and adherence are relatively poor. The greatest problem in fitting corneal contact lenses to a keratoconic eye is the provision of a large enough area of contiguity to produce satisfactory bearing and adherence. Toric posterior lens surfaces may be needed.

The value of ophthalmometry for determining corneal topography in keratoconus is markedly limited. At best, ophthalmometry indicates a starting point for diagnostic lens evaluation. Often the reading is steeper than the range of the Ophthalmometer or Keratometer. When this occurs, the range can be extended (p. 331). The diagnostic lens procedure is necessary to determine the appropriate curvature of the posterior surface of the contact lens. Because spectacle refraction is inaccurate for an irreguar cornea, the diagnostic lens procedure is also necessary to determine refractive power.

It is impossible to obtain alignment through the optic zone on a marked keratoconic eye. In the optic zone, therefore, there may be distinct apical touch and peripheral clearance, there may be apical clearance and distinct peripheral touch, or there may be slight apical and relatively heavier peripheral touch (Fig. 2–55). (Good alignment is obtainable in *early* keratoconus.)

The distinct apical touch and peripheral clearance relationship is used in an attempt to halt the progressive cone protrusion, or even to return it to a more normal configuration. Because all pressures are transmitted to this small central area, central abrasions are frequent. This problem is aggravated by the fact that this fitting relationship often produces excessive movement and rocking. It is further complicated because the corneal apex is relatively thin, and often stains before contact lens wear.

The *distinct* apical clearance and peripheral touch relationship is used in an attempt to remove all pressure from the relatively thin corneal apex. This approach often produces a steepening of corneal curvature and physiologic insult. A veiling of vision (Sattler's veil) and decreased visual acuity and wearing time frequently result. *Minimum* apical clearance is often used.

The light apical touch and relatively heavier peripheral touch relationship —an attempt to provide the best balance—is a very widely used contemporary relationship in keratoconus. Slight apical touch produces the best compromise central bearing relationship. *Intermediate curve alignment* provides a secondary bearing on a thicker corneal tissue area for further pressure disbursements. The total optic- and intermediate-zone bearing is often sufficient to reduce considerably excess lens movement and rocking. Venting is still satisfactory, because the area of noncontiguity between the lens and corneal curvatures provides sufficient flow channels. A peripheral curve is used to assist venting.

The base curve radius of the first diagnostic lens should be about 0.15 or 0.20 mm. shorter than the mean of the ophthalmometric principal meridians. This lens usually produces apical clearance. The base curve of subsequent diagnostic lenses is lengthened in 0.10 mm. increments until light apical touch is obtained. This produces the maximum central bearing area, without compression of the central cornea. The authors frequently steepen the base curve by about 0.50 D. to produce mild apical clearance.

Because the intermediate curve radius can be ascertained only when there is apical clearance and because the peripheral cornea is relatively flat, intermediate curve radii on diagnostic lenses with either large or small lens diameters are usually 2.0 mm. longer than the base curve radius. There is also a peripheral curve with a radius about 1.0 mm. longer than the intermediate curve radius and with a width about one third of total secondary width. There is a blend between intermediate and base curves as well as one between intermediate and peripheral curves. The diagnostic lens procedure is used until intermediate curve alignment is obtained. This procedure yields the necessary information for selecting the intermediate curve radius. The peripheral curve radius is arbitrarily 1.0 mm. longer than this value to provide a fluid reservoir without excessive clearance. Blended lenses should be ordered. With large lenses, narrow annular bearing around the optic zone is preferable to intermediate alignment.

The lens diameter for a superior-positioning lens is usually 9.5 to 10.5 mm. A larger lens diameter is used to decrease lens movement and eye rubbing as an aid to bearing.

The optic-zone diameter for a superior-positioning lens is usually smaller than would ordinarily be used, or 6.0 to 7.0 mm. A smaller optic-zone diameter is used to obtain a better relationship with the underlying cornea.

The lens diameters for an aperture-positioning lens are the same as would be used ordinarily. The total secondary width is half the difference between the lens and optic-zone diameters. About two-thirds of this value is intermediate curve width, and one-third is peripheral curve width. Optic zone diameters are often 5.5 to 6.5 mm.

Lenses with a 0.08 mm. center, a 0.10 mm. edge, a plus carrier lenticular, and a bowl 0.3 to 0.5 mm. larger than the optic zone are used to decrease pressure on the cornea, increase adherence, and allow normal blinking. If enough minus is needed, even this construction may have thick areas that cause poor performance. Part of the refractive power can then be placed in the contact lens and the rest in auxiliary spectacles.

The refractive power can be determined only by refraction over diagnostic contact lenses. The best spherical equivalent power is determined. Often visual acuity is slightly subnormal, even with the best contact lens correction, often owing to the residual irregular refraction or to corneal opacities.

Anterior toric prism ballast lenses to correct internal residual astigmatism seldom perform well on an abnormal keratoconic cornea. When it is necessary, auxiliary spectacles with the proper cylindrical correction are used to improve visual acuity and comfort. Bitoric contact lenses may be needed.

As an auxiliary feature, a light tint often aids the patient in handling and locating the lenses.

The advantages of an aperture-positioning lens are that it is smaller and lighter, and relatively free of upper lid pressures. These factors aid bearing. The disadvantages are that there may be more lens movement, upper lid discomfort, and lens displacement. Because of the poor uncorrected vision, handling of small lenses may be somewhat more difficult. Whenever it is possible, the authors strongly prefer to use an ultrathin aperture-positioning lens because of its better bearing. These are more successful with mild or moderate keratoconus. Large corneal lenses or scleral lenses may be needed for marked keratoconus.

The authors initially attempt to fit all keratoconus patients with corneal contact lenses. Because of the atypical corneal topography, the patients' lenses usually have to be modified and custom designed before they can be dispensed. When satisfactory performance cannot be obtained with corneal contact lenses—as may occur with marked keratoconus—molded fluidless scleral lenses are fitted with minimal apical clearance. Scleral lenses move less and bear on the sclera rather than on the thin cornea. The corneal portion of the sclera lenses is kept small—about 8.0 mm.—to reduce the size of the air bubble that develops between the contact lens and the eye below the base of the cone.

Because of poorer tissue strength and reduced corneal sensitivity, the keratoconic patient must be examined quite frequently during the initial fitting period and for the duration of contact lens wear. A normal gradual increase of wearing time may be used to allow lacrimation, blink action, and lens movement to become stable as quickly as possible. During the first few weeks, it is often advisable to see the patient twice a week.

After the initial fitting period, the patient should be seen at least once every three months. The fit may become altered either because the pressure of the lens has flattened the cornea or because the condition has progressed, producing a steeper cornea. In both cases, the patient must be refitted.

When the need for refit is frequent because of progression of the disease, there is often an associated thinning of corneal tissues. If this thinning is allowed to continue, an almost keratoglobic condition may result, and the possibility of perforation is increased. As the disease progresses, making the cone steeper, corneal opacities often develop, decreasing visual acuity. Whenever there is need for frequent refitting because of conical progression or a significant decrease in best-corrected contact lens acuity, the need for keratoplasty must be critically evaluated. If the condition progresses too far, keratoplasty may become greatly complicated.

After keratoplasty, contact lenses often provide considerably better acuity than spectacles because of the residual corneal irregularity. Fitting of the contact lens is not initiated until the tissues have stabilized and there is no staining or dry spots of either the graft or host cornea. Because the margin of the graft is usually raised, the lens should be fitted so that it is relatively clear of the graft margin. Scleral lenses may be considered.

Provision of an Artificial Aperture

A contact lens may be used to provide an artificial aperture and improve the quality of the retinal image[118] when poor retinal image quality is due to opacities, reduced pigmentation, or malformed pupils.

Opacities. When the refracting media of the eye have opacities, there is often a scattering or absorption of light. This scattering produces a dazzling effect or loss of contrast. As a result, perception is impaired. By reduction of the amount of entering light and by limitation of its entrance to relatively nonopacified areas, perception may be improved.

A pinhole contact lens can accomplish both of these objectives. At the same time, the pinhole reduces the retinal image blur-circle diameter caused by ametropia, irregular eye surfaces, or presbyopia.

Effective pinhole size balances reduction of illumination, diffraction and blur-circle decrease. The optimum pinhole size is usually 1.5 to 2.5 mm. The pinhole area is usually clear so that no additional light is lost, and it may have the desired refractive power. It may be placed in any position in a black opaque or artificial iris—for example, a cosmetic lens (Fig. 2–56).

A pinhole contact lens is preferable to a pinhole spectacle lens, because the contact lens follows eye movements allowing fixation through the pinhole, and it provides a larger field of view (Fig. 2–57). A pinhole contact lens may have better cosmetic effect than a pinhole spectacle lens.

A pinhole contact lens, however, has certain disadvantages:

1. It may be difficult to establish adequate, consistent centration of the pinhole in front of the pupil. Centration is often better accomplished with a scleral contact lens.

2. Appearance is poor when a black opaque lens is used. A cosmetic corneal lens improves appearance when it is large enough to cover all or most of the visible iris. Such a lens, however, may cause physiologic problems. A scleral cosmetic lens is often preferable.

3. A pinhole contact lens cannot be put on and taken off as readily as a

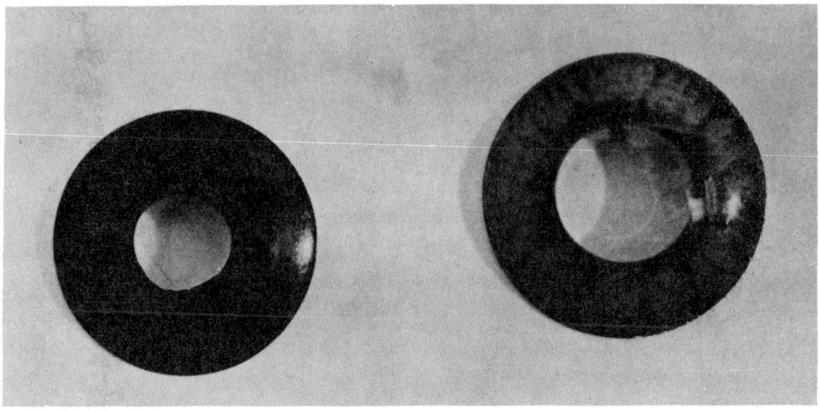

A B

Figure 2–56. Pinhole lenses. A, *Black opaque.* B, *Artificial iris.*

pinhole spectacle lens. This factor may cause problems, especially under conditions of reduced illumination.

Reduced Pigmentation. When there is a reduction of iris pigmentation such as in albinism, the amount of light entering the eye is increased, and there is greater reflection and scattering of light. Some authorities believe this phenomenon is at least partially responsible for reduced visual acuity in albinos. They believe that reducing the amount of entering light by the use of tinted or pinhole lenses improves visual acuity.

Others believe that, because reduced iris pigmentation is usually associated with reduced retinal and choroidal pigmentation, the reduced visual acuity results from hypoplasia of the fovea. They believe that reducing the amount of entering light does not aid visual acuity.

Because the issue has not been finally resolved and because little else can be done for such patients, the authors feel that pinhole spectacle lenses with side shields should be tried. If pinhole spectacle lenses aid acuity, pinhole contact lenses may be considered.

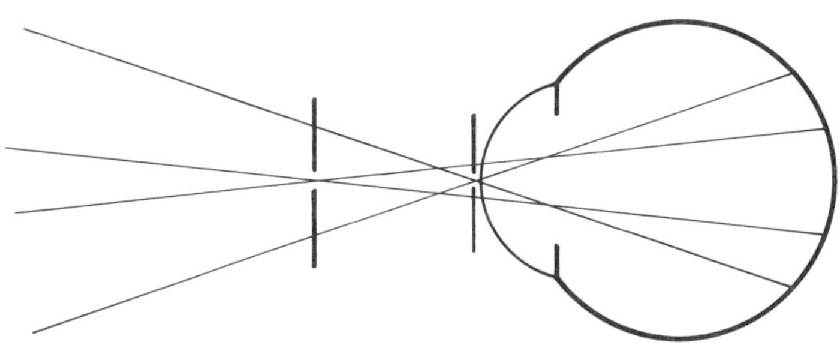

Figure 2–57. As the vertex distance of a pinhole is decreased, the field of view is increased.

Pupil Malformation. Where pupil malformation exists, such as in aniridia, the amount of light entering the eye may be increased. At the same time, aberrations are increased, especially from light entering through the more peripheral corneal areas. Some authorities believe that the increase of light and aberrated retinal image are at least partially responsible for reduced visual acuity. They feel that providing an aperture of 3 to 4 mm. in a cosmetic contact lens to act as a pupil improves visual acuity.

Others believe that reduced visual acuity in aniridia is due to foveal hypoplasia and that a cosmetic contact lens does not improve visual acuity. The authors' clinical approach is the same as that used for albinism.

When there are multiple pupils (polycoria), confused multiple retinal images are formed. A cosmetic contact lens with an optic portion of 2 or 3 mm. may be helpful.

When cataract surgery has produced a malformed pupil, the increase of light and the irregular refraction from the more peripheral corneal areas may reduce visual acuity. A pinhole contact lens may be helpful. At the same time, loss of ability to focus near objects as a result of crystalline lens removal is reduced by the pinhole.

Enlarging the Retinal Image

Methods to Produce an Enlarged Retinal Image. In some patients with subnormal vision due to retinal, optic nerve, or cerebral malfunction, enlargement of the retinal image stimulates more cones and permits a better distinguishing of details.[119–126] Magnification of the retinal image may be produced by a decrease of the object distance or an increase of the object size, or by the use of optical devices.

Decrease of Object Distance. Magnification is expressed by the formula

$$M = \frac{v}{u},$$

where M equals the magnification, v equals the image distance, and u equals the object distance. As long as the image is focused on the retina, image distance is constant. For a focused retinal image, therefore, magnification of a given object is inversely proportional to its distance from the eye. The first and simplest way to obtain magnification is to decrease the object distance while maintaining a focused retinal image. Retinal image focus is produced by correction of the ametropia at distance, and accommodation or the use of auxiliary converging lenses at near.

Increase of Object Size. Magnification is also expressed by the formula:

$$M = \frac{I}{O},$$

where M represents the magnification, I represents the image size, and O represents the object size. As the size of the object is increased, the size of the focused image is increased. Thus, another way to enlarge the retinal image is to increase the object size, such as is done in books with large type.

Use of Optical Devices. When it is impractical to change object distance or size, retinal image size can be increased by the use of optical devices. The optical device used to increase retinal image size of distant objects is the telescope, specifically the Galilean telescope, and the optical device used to increase retinal image size of near objects is the microscope or a telescope with a reading cap.

OPTICS OF A GALILEAN TELESCOPE. The Galilean telescope has a high-power negative ocular and a positive objective. The ocular and the objective are separated by the distance (S) between their first principal focus (F_2) and second principal focus (F_1), respectively:

$$F_1 obj. - F_2 oc. = S$$

Thus, F_1 of the objective and F_2 of the ocular coincide (Fig. 2–58). Parallel entering light is brought to a focus at F_1 of the objective, which is also F_2 of the ocular. Because light from the focal point of a lens is focused at infinity, the emerging light is parallel. Thus, a magnified, erect image is produced (Fig. 2–58).

Magnification is expressed by the formula

$$M = \frac{D_{oc}}{D_{obj.}}$$

$$M = \frac{F_1\, obj.}{F_2\, oc.}.$$

Obviously, the ocular must be stronger than the objective to produce magnification. Figure 2–59 shows how to compute the separation between and

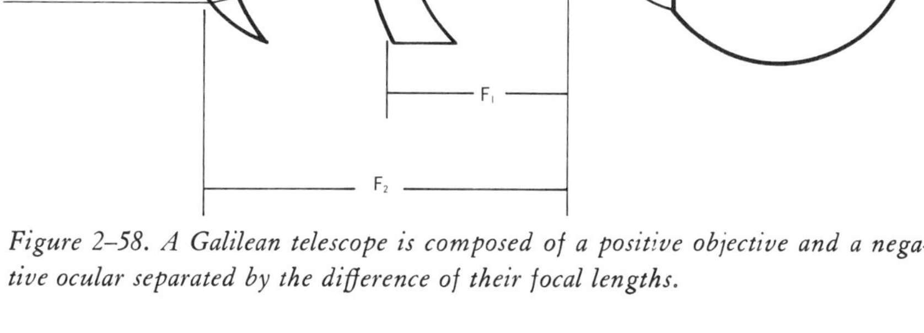

Figure 2–58. A Galilean telescope is composed of a positive objective and a negative ocular separated by the difference of their focal lengths.

(1) F_1 obj. — F_2 oc. = 15

(2) F_1 obj. = F_2 oc. + 15

(3) $M = \frac{F_1 \text{ obj.}}{-F_2 \text{ oc.}} = 1.75$

(4) $1.75 = \frac{F_2 \text{ oc.} + 15}{-F_2 \text{ oc.}}$

(5) −1.75 F_2 oc. = F_2 oc. + 15

(6) −.75 F_2 oc. = 15

(7) F_2 oc. = −20

(8) D oc. = −50

(9) F_1 obj. −(20) = 15

(10) F_1 obj. = 35

(11) D obj. = +28.62

Figure 2–59. Assume that the practitioner wants a 1.75 magnification with a 15 mm. separation between ocular and objective, which is the vertex distance in a contact lens–spectacle lens telescopic system. The effective ocular and objective powers would be found as shown here.

powers of the objective and ocular separated by a given vertex distance for a desired amount of magnification.

A telescopic system is designed for distant fixation—that is, for parallel rays of light. When it is used for near fixation, light is transmitted with a marked divergency. This effect is neutralized by placing over the objective a reading cap the positive refractive power of which is equal to the reciprocal of the near fixation distance. This cap makes the light parallel before it enters the telescopic system—in other words, the light is collimated (Fig. 2–60). If, for example, work is held at 8 inches, a +5 D cap is used—that is,

$$\frac{40 \text{ inches}}{8 \text{ inches}} = 5 \text{ D}.$$

The total magnification is equal to the product of the magnification of the telescopic system and that of the reading cap. The magnification of the reading cap alone is approximately expressed by:

$$\text{Mag} = \frac{\text{D add}}{4}.$$

If a 2.2× telescope is used for an eight-inch working distance and a +5 D

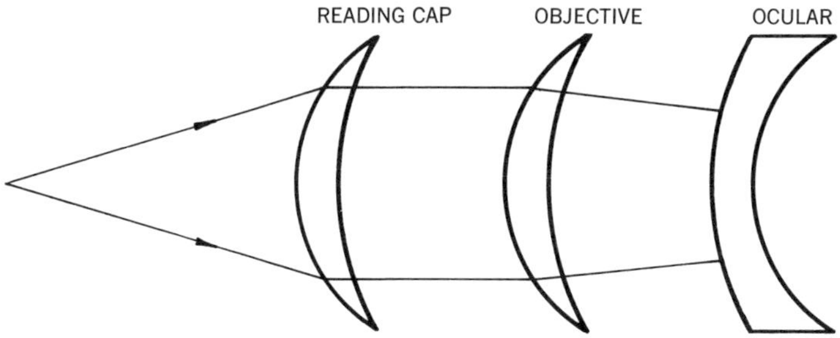

Figure 2–60. When a reading cap with a positive power equal to the reciprocal of the near fixation distance is placed in a telescopic system, parallel light enters the system.

cap is used, approximate total magnification equals $(2.2)\left(\frac{5}{4}\right) = 2.64\times$. Some magnification is also contributed by lens form and thickness.

CONTACT LENSES AND GALILEAN TELESCOPES. A contact lens can be used as the high minus ocular of a Galilean telescope system. The objective is placed in a spectacle frame worn at a vertex distance equal to the difference between the ocular and objective focal lengths.

When a contact lens ocular is used, there must be an appropriate spectacle objective for distance and an appropriate spectacle power for near. If, for example, a −50 D ocular and a 13.3 mm. vertex distance are used, the objective must be +30 D. Near power is the sum of the objective power and the reciprocal of the working distance. If a 13-inch working distance is to be used, the near power must be:

$$+30\text{ D} + \frac{40}{13} = +33\text{ D}.$$

Distance and near spectacle powers are obtained by means of two pairs of glasses, a clip-on over the objective, or a bifocal spectacle.

Because it is impractical to use vertex distances greater than 15 mm., it is difficult to achieve high levels of magnification.

As ocular power increases, optic-zone size must be decreased to permit fabrication. If an optic-zone diameter of 6.6 mm. is desired, the ocular power can be about −40 D. If an optic-zone diameter of 7.0 mm. is desired, the ocular power can be about −30 D. With a maximum practical vertex distance of about 15 mm., an objective of approximately +25 D is used with the −40 D ocular, producing a magnification of 1.6×. With vertex distance of 15 mm., an objective of approximately +20.70 D is used with the −30 D ocular. This arrangement produces a magnification of 1.45×.

There are two ways to establish a Galilean contact lens–spectacle lens system. In the first method, the entire optic zone contains the desired high negative ocular power. There is distant magnification of the entire usable field (Fig. 2–61).

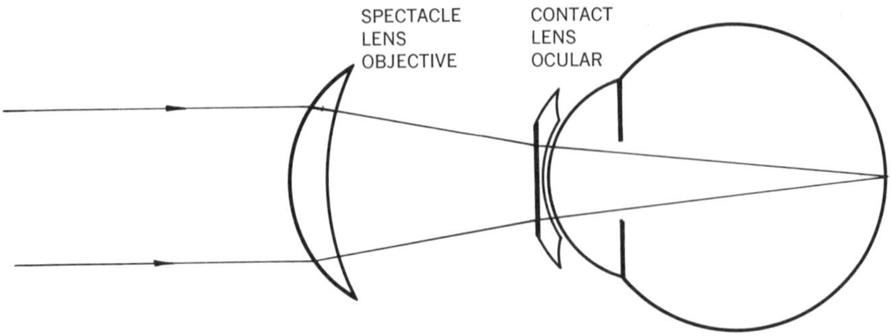

Figure 2–61. A contact lens–spectacle lens telescopic system in which the entire contact lens optic zone acts as a telescopic ocular.

The second method of establishing a Galilean contact lens–spectacle lens system was developed by one of the authors.* It has a small 2.5 to 3.5 mm. optic zone containing the desired high negative ocular power. The anterior curvature may be convex, plano, or concave; around it is an annular optic-zone area containing the power to correct ametropia (Fig. 2–62). Because the ocular zone is always made smaller than daylight pupil size, both the ocular zone and the zone to correct ametropia are simultaneously in front of the pupil. The objective of the system is a spectacle lens having a carrier of plano power ground on a 12.00 D base curve to which is cemented a central segment of 10 mm. diameter with the desired positive objective power. This arrangement produces a magnified central image superimposed on a nonmagnified peripheral image, which aids spatial orientation.

When the anterior ocular curvature is ground plano, the anterior surface of the ocular portion of the telescopic lens system has no power. The ocular power is therefore equal to posterior curvature power. The effective ocular power for a 7.20 D base curve is 68.05 D; for an 8.20 D base curve, it is 59.75 D. This permits higher levels of magnification up to about 2×.

Applicability of Contact Lens Telescopes. Because the basic goal in subnormal vision is to improve the patient's ability to function in his environment to a degree that satisfies his needs, the practitioner must determine whether a contact lens–spectacle telescopic system can fulfill this need for each patient. Consider the disadvantages first.

First, a clinical rule of thumb is that the expected telescopic acuity in subnormal vision is the product of the magnification and the best-corrected spectacle acuity. A contact lens–spectacle lens magnification of approximately 2× is the maximum. This magnification is expected to double best-corrected spectacle acuity. The same effect can be obtained by reduction of the object distance by about one half. Such limited magnification may be insufficient to produce meaningful increased vision for a patient with subnormal vision.

* The Telecon lens system, developed by Dr. Filderman.

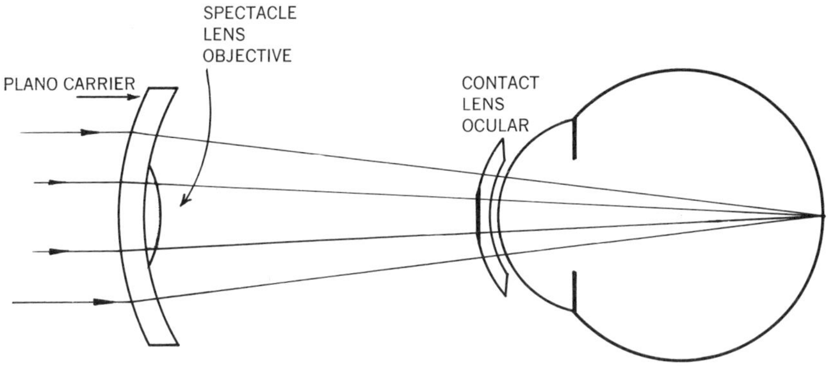

Figure 2–62. A Telecon type of contact lens–spectacle lens telescopic system in which only part of the contact lens optic zone acts as a telescopic ocular.

Second, it is difficult to maintain exact centration of the contact lens ocular in front of the pupil and to maintain an exact vertex distance. When either of these factors is incorrect, blur is produced. Exact ocular centration is often considerably better when a stable aperture positioning lens or a scleral contact lens is used.

Third, magnification is usually most helpful for specific tasks, rather than for general use. A contact lens telescope is a relatively constant aid.

Consider the advantages. First, a contact lens–spectacle telescopic system has a field of view for a given magnification that is about 30 to 50 per cent larger than that of a spectacle telescope. This increase of field is due to the closer proximity of the contact lens to the nodal point. Second, cosmetic appearance is better than with a spectacle telescope.

Clinical Application of Contact Lens–Spectacle Lens Telescopic System. In ametropic correction, before a telescopic system to enlarge the retinal image is considered, the refractive power necessary to produce the best-focused retinal image is determined. It must be remembered that the effective contact lens ocular power is the algebraic difference between its power read in air and the patient's refractive error. If, for example, ocular power in air is -60 D and refractive error as shown by corneal plane refraction is -10 D (i.e., a 10 D myope), effective ocular power is $(-60\text{ D}) - (-10\text{ D}) = -50$ D.

Because of the patient's difficulty in distinguishing details, subjective testing may be difficult. Refractive error is determined by careful static retinoscopy. Astigmatism is often based on the central ophthalmometric findings. Central ophthalmometric astigmatism is eliminated by a spherical base contact lens (p. 350). Internal residual astigmatism of up to 1.50 D usually does not affect subnormal visual acuity to any appreciable degree. Visual acuity with the best ametropic correction is determined.

In telescopic spectacle correction, a telescopic spectacle of approximately

2× is placed in the front cell of the trial frame over the best ametropic correction. This procedure is carried out for each eye separately. Visual acuity is again determined. Because it would then usually be easier for the patient to distinguish details, the ametropic correction may be refined by alteration of the lenses in the rear cell in 1.00 D steps. If refinement does improve acuity, it should be recorded.

About 2× is the practical limit of telescopic contact lens–spectacle lens magnification. If acuity improvement from this level of magnification does not seem adequate to fulfill the patient's needs, the advisability of applying such a system is decreased. Spectacle telescopic lenses of higher magnification may be tried to determine whether application of a telescopic spectacle system is advisable.

If acuity improvement with a 2.0× telescopic lens is satisfactory, a 1.7× or 1.5× telescopic lens is tried. When acuity improvement is still satisfactory, the lower magnifications are preferred. Their use produces a larger field of view and a greater flexibility of lens design.

When it seems that a telescopic contact lens system may fulfill the patient's need, it is often advisable to process the corresponding full diameter telescopic spectacle system with the appropriate reading cap. The patient is asked to use this device and to evaluate whether his acuity needs are adequately fulfilled. If his acuity needs are not fulfilled, the lengthy procedure of fitting a telescopic contact lens system has been avoided. Telescopic spectacles of higher magnification may be indicated in some cases. If the patient's needs are fulfilled by the original telescopic spectacle system, either the case may be concluded at this point or a contact lens–spectacle lens system may be considered. The original spectacle telescopic system is kept by the patient. It may be used when he does not wish to use contact lenses or if his contact lenses are lost.

In nontelescopic contact lens fitting, when a telescopic contact lens–spectacle lens system is ultimately to be fitted, the patient is first fitted with a conventional spherical single-vision contact lens. The patient is allowed to adapt to these lenses, and the basic fit is determined. Fit should be such that there is no appreciable lens movement. When a patient cannot adapt to a contact lens, the case should be discontinued.

After satisfactory adaptation, lens position and movement are relatively stable. The size and position of the ocular can now be determined. Ocular size is based on its power—that is, on the anterior curvature used. As the anterior curvature is flattened to increase minus ocular power, the ocular-zone size is decreased from approximately 8.0 mm. with approximately −10 D to about 2.5 to 3.0 mm. with −60 to −70 D. The ocular zone is geometrically centered in the lens. For a given ocular zone size, the lens diameter for a given lens position must produce proper ocular-zone coverage of the pupil.

In telescopic contact lens fitting, a telescopic contact lens with correct ocular position and with an ocular power to produce the desired magnification with a vertex distance of 15 mm. is ordered. Usually only the better eye is corrected with a telescopic system. Vision in the other eye is usually suppressed.

This lens is placed on the patient's eye. Because it is a slightly heavier lens, positioning may vary somewhat from that of the nontelescopic contact lens. The beginning objective power and resultant magnification for a 15 mm. vertex distance are shown in Table 2–14. This lens is placed in a trial frame

TABLE 2–14

OBJECTIVE POWER FOR 15 MM. VERTEX DISTANCE

Effective Ocular Power	Objective Power	Magnification
−20	+15.37	1.30
−30	+20.62	1.45
−40	+25.00	1.60
−50	+28.62	1.75
−60	+31.62	1.90

set for a vertex distance of 15 mm. Acuity is determined. The objective power then may be refined by trial lens alterations of 1 D.

A bifocal lenticular spectacle lens is used when the entire pupil is covered by the ocular. The distance portion of the lens has the objective power, and the near portion has the sum of this power and the reading addition. The spectacle lens is made up using the segmented construction (p. 116) when the pupil is only partially covered by the ocular. A segment may be cemented inferior to this with the necessary near power or a straight-top bifocal spectacle lens may be used which provides the necessary power.

A frame with rocking pads is used so that vertex distance changes can be made if necessary. Jumbo nose pads are used to disburse the pressure from the heavy spectacle lenses. Cable temples are preferable to maintain a more consistent vertex distance.

All corneal contact lenses move up as gaze is depressed—that is, the lens is translated upward. It is important that the pupil is properly covered by the ocular after translation.

Scleral contact lens fitting is discussed on page 265. Because of a vastly better stability of position, it is often preferable to use a scleral lens as the ocular of a contact lens–spectacle lens telescopic system. Scleral lenses are often easier for a patient with subnormal vision to handle and maintain. When a corneal contact lens is used, a light tint often aids handling and maintenance.

Clinical Application of Near-vision Aids. Most patients with subnormal vision desire aid for near tasks, such as reading. Near aid is provided by moving the working material close to the eye. This enlarges the retinal image because of reduced object distance. To focus the image on the retina, a high plus lens is used. Lens power is the reciprocal of the object distance from the lens surface. The form and thickness of the plus lens also produce angular magnification.

Although not completely accurate, the resultant magnification is expressed by the clinically practical formula $M = \frac{D}{4}$. M represents the magnification, and D represents the power of the lens.

Near tasks, such as reading, are performed only at given periods through the day. Therefore, any optical aid must be easy to remove. In this respect, spectacles are better than contact lenses. Most patients with subnormal vision whose basic need of aid is for near tasks are better aided by spectacles than by contact lenses.

A bifocal contact lens with an appropriately high near add can be used, but it is extremely difficult to fit.

Contact Lenses for the Aphakic

Even when there are no other ocular problems, spectacle correction for an aphakic usually produces a somewhat subnormal visual efficiency. Contact lens correction for an aphakic usually produces almost normal visual efficiency.[127, 128]

Contact Lens Advantages

Magnification. Spectacle correction of aphakia usually produces a 25 to 30 per cent increase in retinal image size. This increase disturbs the spatial orientation of a binocular aphakic, because larger objects appear close. Some binocular aphakics are able satisfactorily to reorient spatially; others are always somewhat troubled.

Contact lens correction of aphakia produces a five to 12 per cent increase of retinal image size, which causes less spatial orientation problems in a binocular aphakic.

A monocular spectacle-corrected aphakic has a 25 to 30 per cent aniseikonia, whereas a monocular contact lens-corrected aphakic has a five to 12 per cent aniseikonia. Because of the amount of aniseikonia, a monocular spectacle-corrected aphakic either has diplopia or suppresses vision in one eye. Many monocular contact lens-corrected aphakics have single binocular vision in spite of a relatively lower but still appreciable aniseikonia.[129–134] A monocular spectacle-corrected aphakic experiences an appreciable vertical prismatic effect when looking away from the optical center. Because a contact lens follows eye movements, there is less vertical prismatic effect.

Aniseikonia in a contact lens-corrected monocular aphakic can be reduced by overplussing of the aphakic contact lens and by compensation for this overplussing with minus in a spectacle lens. Minification formulae can be used. For example, +5.25 D overcorrection in the contact lens and −5.62 D. in the spectacle lens at 12.7 mm. vertex distance decreases magnification by approximately 6.6 per cent. When a contact lens is also worn on the non-aphakic eye, reduction of aniseikonia can be accomplished by overcorrection in minus in the contact lens and compensation for this overcorrection with plus in the spectacle lens.

Visual Field. The size of the visual field for an aphakic is more nearly normal with correction done with contact lenses rather than with spectacle lenses. When spectacle lenses are used, the peripheral visual field is often reduced by about one third because of the prismatic effect produced when the patient looks away from the optical center of a high plus lens (Fig. 2–63).

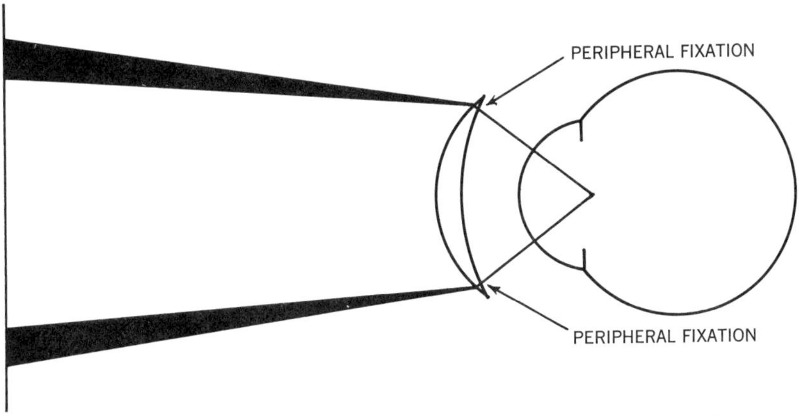

Figure 2–63. The black area illustrates the reduction of usable field of vision caused by the prismatic effect induced by eccentric fixation through a high plus lens.

This reduction of field size is especially troublesome at distances from 20 feet to 15 or 16 inches. In this intermediate distance, objects jump into and out of the peripheral field of vision. This phenomenon is often likened to a jack-in-the-box or a roving ring scotoma.[135]

Spectacle-wearing aphakics usually move their heads rather than their eyes to maintain coincidence of their visual axis with the optical center of the lens. This reduces the problem. Contact lenses follow eye movements to a great degree, resulting in a more normal visual field and neutralizing the jack-in-the-box phenomenon.

Aberrations. In general, the degree of various aberrations inherent in high plus prescriptions is greatly reduced by contact lenses. When there is a reasonable centration of the optic zone to the pupil, peripheral aberrations such as coma, oblique astigmatism, distortion, and curvature of field are relatively slight with contact lenses. Chromatic aberration is about the same with spectacle or contact lens correction, and spherical aberration in air is greater with contact lenses. The eye, however, eliminates much of the spherical aberration, assuming a normal pupil.

Visual Consistency. There is greater consistency of visual performance with contact lenses. A slight adjustment problem with spectacles in terms of vertex distance or tilt is quite common and can be distressing.

Cosmetic Benefits and Comfort. Cosmetic benefits from contact lenses in aphakia are obvious. Spectacle-wearing aphakics are often uncomfortable because of the weight of the frames and lenses. This is especially true in older aphakics whose musculature has lost tone and whose skin is easily irritated by spectacles. Because of reduced corneal sensitivity and relatively flaccid lids, contact lenses are often accepted quite readily by an aphakic.

Need for Special Fitting Procedures

Surgical Considerations. There are three aspects to consider: corneal incision, method of lens removal, and corneal wound healing.[136]

Corneal Incision. Corneal incisions are usually made at or near the limbus, either as a single incision at 12 o'clock, or a double incision at three and nine o'clock. It is important to fit the contact lens so that it does not produce excessive pressure on the scar tissue. Such areas often are less able to withstand pressure.

Method of Lens Removal. The lens is usually removed by intracapsular extraction, extracapsular extraction, or needling (discission).

Intracapsular extraction involves removing the lens within its capsule. Extracapsular extraction involves rupturing the anterior portion of the capsule and expressing the lens cortex and nucleus from the eye. The posterior portion of the capsule is left. Extracapsular extraction is more conservative and easier to perform. A secondary membrane forms, however, in about 30 per cent of the cases. Iridectomy producing a keyhole pupil is thus often necessary in extracapsular extraction. This enlargement of the aperture of the system may produce undesirable visual problems with contact lenses. Whenever possible, a round pupil is preferred.

Corneal Wound Healing. Wounds from the operation usually take about six months to regain normal tensile strength. The rate of wound healing determines when the lens should be fitted. Some authorities believe that lenses should be fitted three to six months after the operation. Others believe that although not normal, the tensile strength of the cornea is adequate so that fitting usually may be started four to 12 weeks after the operation.

One criterion for determining when a contact lens may be fitted is: an uninflamed eye and consistent refractive findings and ophthalmometric readings shown for three consecutive examinations spaced three weeks apart.[137]

Because corneal distortion, corneal astigmatism, and scar tissue are often the sequelae of surgery, it is more difficult to establish desired relationships between the posterior surface of the lens and the anterior corneal curves. Postoperative decrease of corneal sensitivity often occurs. This condition aids

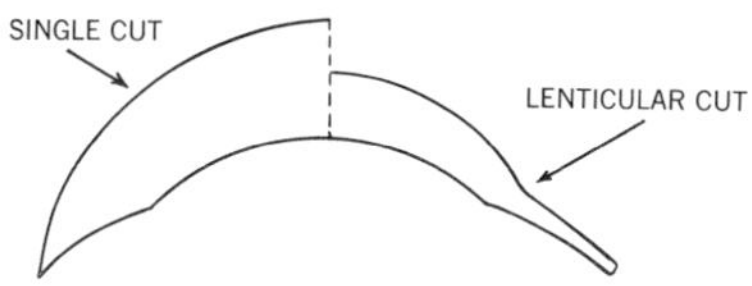

Figure 2–64. Thickness comparison of a lens with a given plus power made in an anterior single cut (left) *and an anterior lenticular cut* (right).

in the physical toleration of a contact lens, but it also reduces the subjective appreciation of any corneal irritation.

Refractive Consideration. The typically high plus refractive power prescription necessitates a thick, heavy lens, producing excessive movement and pressure, and often eccentric lens position. An addition is needed for near visual tasks.

General Consideration. The poor uncorrected visual acuity of a binocular aphakic makes lens handling and maintenance difficult. Most aphakics are relatively elderly, and they may have other systemic or ocular pathologic conditions. Mucus in the precorneal fluid is often a problem.

Clinical Application

Curvatures. *Anterior.* Aphakic contact lenses may have a single or a lenticular anterior curve (Fig. 2–64).[138–142] The lenticular lens has a thinner center thickness than does a lens with single anterior curve for a given lens diameter and refractive power. This thinner center thickness produces a lighter lens and reduces excessive lens movement and pressure. At the same time, a better positioning of the optic zone in front of the pupil is often obtained. Review the discussion of lenticular form on p. 44.

Because there is a considerable difference in the refraction of light through the optic zone and lenticular area, visual problems are produced unless there is proper pupil coverage (Fig. 2–65). It is more difficult to produce proper coverage in a large or keyhole postoperative pupil. In such cases, a single anterior curve may be preferable to a lenticular anterior curve.

Posterior. Base and secondary curvatures are selected in the normal manner, although the base curve radius of an aperture-positioning small lens is often 0.10 mm. shorter than usual. Because of irregular topography, it is more difficult to obtain desirable relationships. Toric bases may be needed.

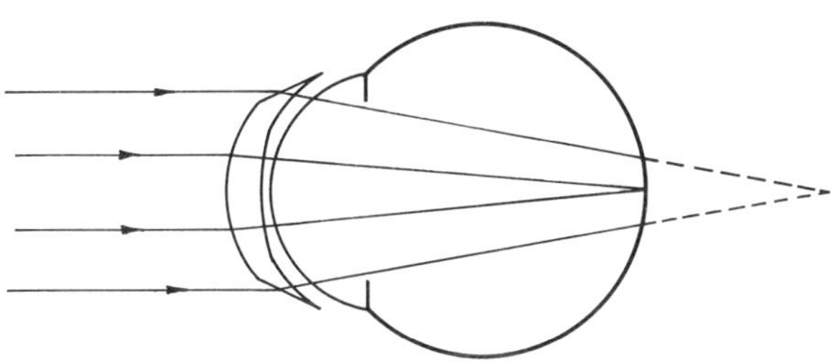

Figure 2–65. A dual retinal image causing visual problems is produced when the pupil is simultaneously covered by optic and lenticular zones.

Diameters and Widths. Lens diameter for a contour-type lens is usually about 0.4 to 0.5 mm. larger than would ordinarily be used in order to increase adherence, reduce lens movement, and provide better optic-zone coverage of the pupil. The posterior optic-zone diameter is usually about 0.3 mm. larger than would ordinarily be used in order to increase adherence, reduce lens movement, and provide better optic-zone coverage of the pupil. When an anterior lenticular construction is used, the anterior optic-zone diameter is usually 0.5 mm. larger than the posterior optic-zone diameter in order to reduce lens weight while making proper retinal image formation possible. The secondary width is half the difference between the lens diameter and the posterior optic-zone diameter. A bicurve construction is used in order to obtain maximum adherence. When it is needed, a peripheral curve can be added. An aperture-positioned lens has normal diameters and widths. Either a single or a lenticular anterior curve is used.

Thickness. Center thickness is best computed by the manufacturer if an anterior lenticular lens is to be used. Because of a smaller lens diameter, an aperture lens with a single anterior curvature is considerably thinner than a superior-positioning lens with a single anterior curvature.

Refractive Power. It is extremely difficult to measure vertex distance accurately to within 1.0 mm. when computation of refractive power is attempted. An error of this amount with the typically high aphakic powers can produce a significantly incorrect refractive power. Refractive power for an aphakic should be determined by refraction over high plus diagnostic contact lenses. The power determined by this method is posterior vertex power.

An aphakic needs a plus add for near. It is best provided in auxiliary spectacles, either single-vision or bifocal. If sufficient residual astigmatism is found, it is best to incorporate the cylindrical element in the spectacles, unless bitoric lenses are used.

Diagnostic lens procedure with high plus lenses is essential to determine the lens parameters that will produce satisfactory position and movement. Excessive secondary clearance must be avoided because it decreases adherence and may produce undesirable position and movement. Centration is essential, especially with a keyhole pupil.

Small, relatively thin single cut lenses are often advisable when the cornea is steep—above 45.50 D or more—and the palpebral aperture is narrow. The authors evaluate diagnostic small single cut and lenticular lenses having −6 D to −10 D carriers to determine the type to prescribe.

Auxiliary Features. Removal of the crystalline lens eliminates some of the eye's light-absorptive ability, especially at wavelengths toward the ultraviolet end of the spectrum. Most tinted contact lenses absorb considerable ultraviolet light (see the transmission graphs on p. 301). Because of the thickness of plus lenses, only the No. 1 shade should be used.

The tint also aids the patient's handling and maintenance of lenses. Because of the decreased corneal sensitivity, the reliability of patient symptoms is decreased and frequent examinations are necessary during the initial fitting period and as long as the lenses are worn.

Contact Lenses for the Presbyope

Structure and Function

Most bifocal contact lenses may be placed in general categories similar to those for bifocal spectacle lenses.[143–145] These include: a two-piece lens with fused plastic of a different index from the carrier for the near portion (Fig. 2–66); a one-piece lens with varying lathed curves giving the desired powers, such as the Ultex (Fig. 2–67); and a two-piece lens using a carrier and an adhered near lens, such as the original cemented bifocal (Fig. 2–68). It is possible to have a central distance portion surrounded by one or more annular near portions (Fig. 2–69).

A successfully fitted bifocal contact lens must permit satisfactory maintenance of tissue integrity, wearing time and comfort, appearance, and satisfactory vision at all distances.

Based on these criteria, there has been a relatively small degree of successful bifocal contact lens fitting. One of the difficult tasks in fitting bifocal contact lenses is satisfactory covering of the pupil by the optic zone for all tasks at all distances.

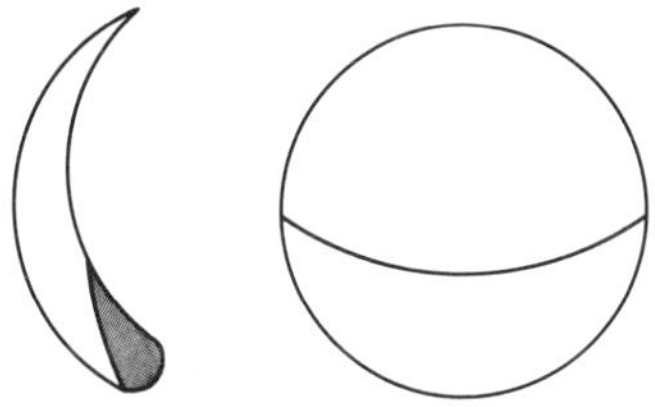

Figure 2–66. Sectional and frontal views of a fused bifocal with prism. (Bi-Site® contact lens—with prism.)

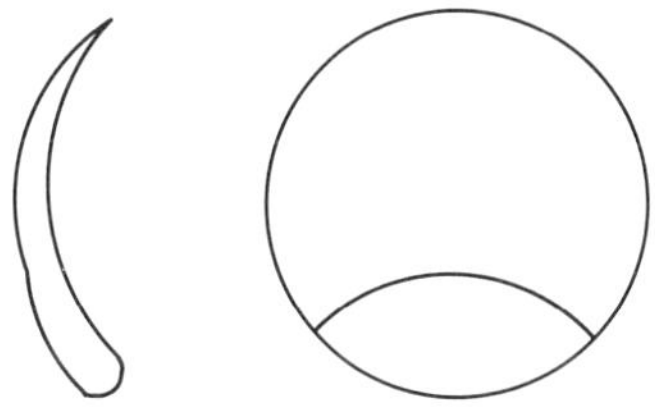

Figure 2–67. Sectional and frontal views of a "one-piece" lathed bifocal with prism.

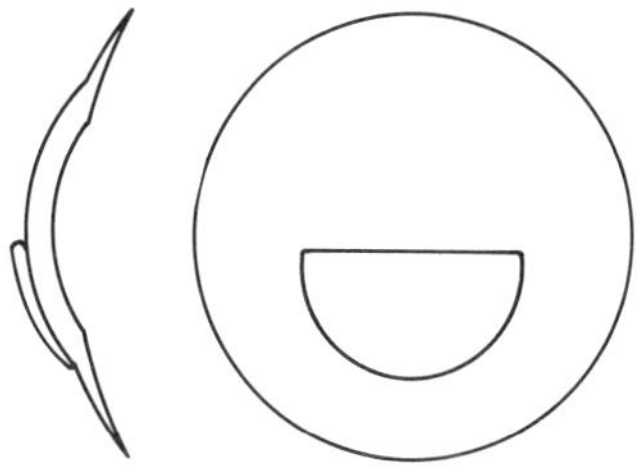

Figure 2–68. Sectional and frontal views of an adhered bifocal.

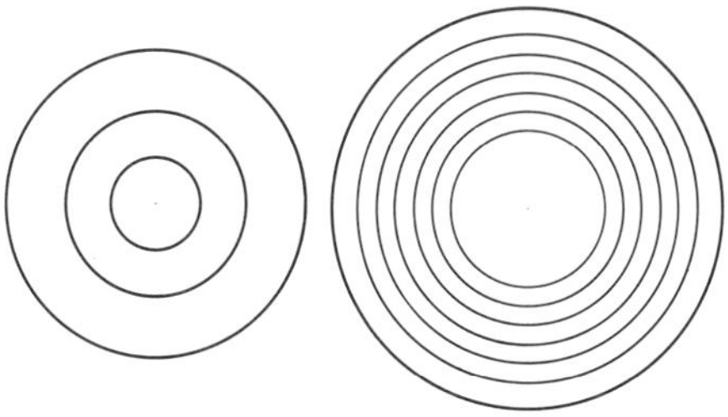

Figure 2–69. Frontal views of uniannular and multiannular bifocals.

Optic-zone Positioning. Bifocal spectacles have large distant and near optic zones. Bifocal contact lenses have small distant and near optic zones, at times smaller than the pupil size. For proper pupil coverage, the optic zones of a bifocal contact lens must be positioned with extreme accuracy. It is difficult to obtain such accurate positioning because of the small optic zones used and because of movement factors.

Because a frame holds spectacles in a relatively constant position, in primary fixation, the distant zone is in front of and completely covers the pupil. Assuming the head is not bent, depressed gaze for near fixation positions the near optic zone in front of and completely covering the pupil. Only the eye and not the lens has moved.

A contact lens is not held in a constant position. Blinking frequently moves the lens up and down. Unless compensation is made, blinking also rotates the lens 360° in about one minute. Rotation is usually counterclockwise on the right eye and clockwise on the left eye. In depressed gaze, two additional movements occur—the lower lid moves down and the lens moves up, or is *translated*.

Rotation and Translation. Bifocal contact lenses are designed to neutralize or to blend in with the rotary effect. The first three categories of bifocal lenses mentioned (p. 127) incorporate a means for neutralizing lens rotation. This neutralization is usually done by prism and truncation in the first two categories, and by the weight of the adhered near lens in the third category. These nonrotating lenses usually have segments for a superior distance optic zone and an inferior near optic zone.

Such *nonrotating segmented* lenses function basically on an *alternating-vision principle,* which theoretically works in the following manner. When fixation is at distance, the distant segment is positioned in front of, and the near segment below, the pupil. When fixation is shifted from distance to near, the lens is translated vertically upward. This translation positions the near segment in front of, and the distant segment above the pupil (Fig. 2–70).

The fourth category of bifocal contact lenses mentioned (p. 125) blends in with the rotary effect. Because the near zone is annular, there is no top or bottom to the lens. Rotation does not, therefore, malposition the near zone. Such *rotating annular* lenses work either on an alternating vision principle or on a *simultaneous-vision,* or *bivision,* principle.

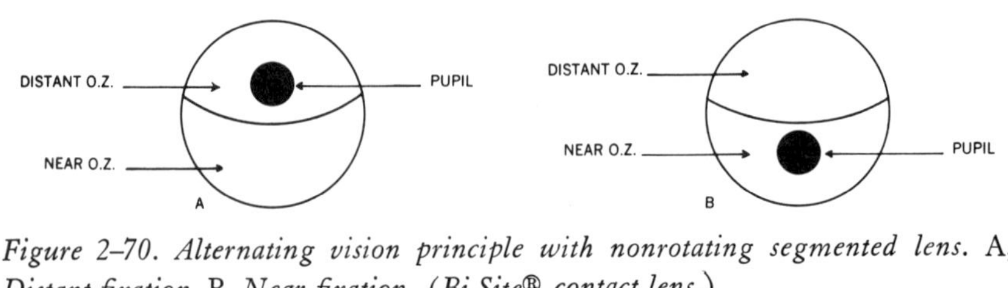

Figure 2–70. Alternating vision principle with nonrotating segmented lens. A, *Distant fixation.* B, *Near fixation.* (*Bi-Site® contact lens.*)

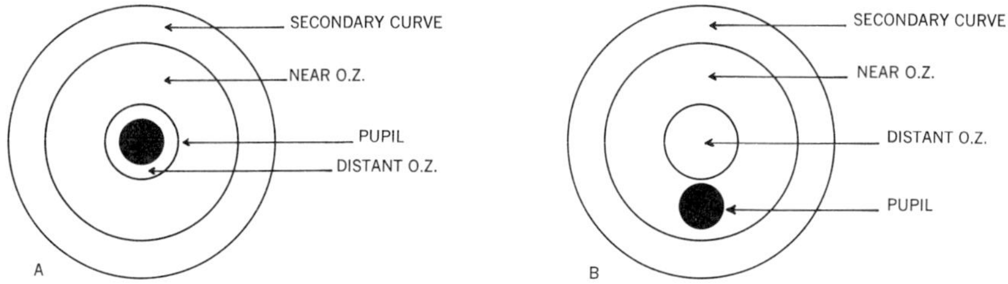

Figure 2–71. Alternating vision principle with rotating annular lens. A, *Distant fixation.* B, *Near fixation.*

When the alternating vision principle is used, distance optic-zone diameter is equal to or larger than pupil size. When fixation is at distance, the pupil is theoretically completely covered by the distance optic zone and surrounded by the annular near optic zone. When fixation is shifted from distance to near, the lens is translated vertically upward. Theoretically, this positions the near zone in front of, and the distance zone above, the pupil (Fig. 2–71).

When the simultaneous vision principle is used, distance optic-zone diameter is smaller than pupil size measured under ordinary room illumination. Distance and near zones are simultaneously positioned in front of the pupil. Rays of light enter through both these zones simultaneously, and produce two superimposed retinal images at the fovea centralis. In distant fixation, the distance image is focused on the retina and is relatively clear, and the near image is focused in front of the retina and is relatively blurred. In near fixation, the near image is focused on the retina and is relatively clear, and the distance image is focused behind the retina and is relatively blurred. The wearer must direct his attention to the clearer image and ignore the hazing effect of the blurred image (Fig. 2–72).

A brief discussion of the more common bifocal contact lenses is presented here, followed by a broader discussion of clinical procedure for the more successful constructions.

Alternating-vision Lenses. *Nonrotating Segmented Lenses.* Fused bifocal contact lenses are made of a basic lens having a refractive index of 1.49. A countersink is cut into the rear surface of the lens for the near optic zone. Plastic with a refractive index of about 1.57 is fused into the countersink. A fluorescing additive may be placed in the fused plastic to aid in segment location. The desired anterior and posterior curvatures are placed throughout the total optic zone. Because of the different indices and the curvature of the countersink, there is more plus power in the near optic zone.

Prism ballast is generally used to control meridional orientation. Inferior truncation may be used as an auxiliary aid in controlling orientation. This construction is discussed in more detail on page 132.

Lathed bifocal contact lenses are made entirely of plastic of one index. The different distant and near powers are obtained by the use of different curva-

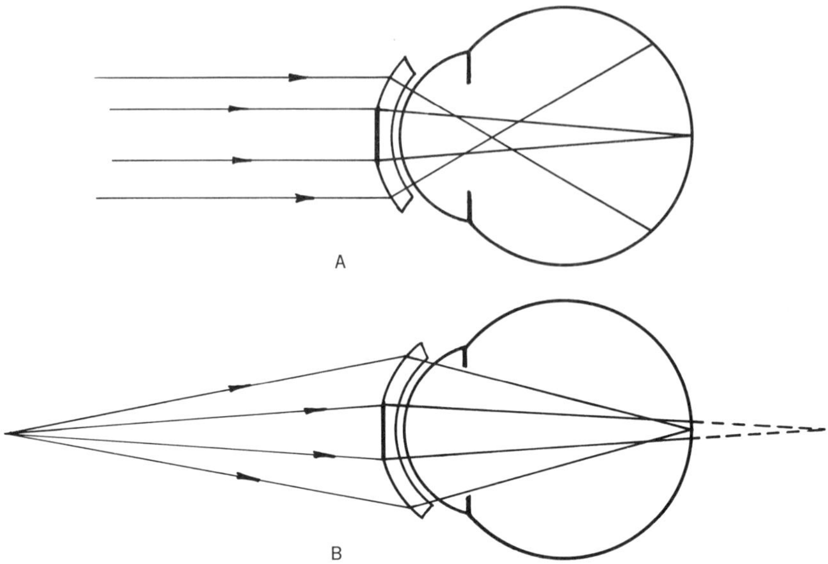

Figure 2–72. Simultaneous vision principle with rotating annular lens. A, *Distant fixation.* B, *Near fixation.*

tures for distant and near zones. These curvatures are placed on the front or rear optic-zone surfaces.[146–149] Usually the distance zone is superior and the near zone is inferior, but there is one construction that reverses this arrangement.[150]

About 1.5 to 2 ΔD is generally used to control meridional orientation. An inferior truncation of 0.5 to 0.7 mm. may be used as an auxiliary orientation aid. Lens diameter ranges from about 9.2 to 10.0 mm. horizontally and 8.7 to 9.5 mm. vertically. Base and peripheral curvature radii are determined as in a spherical single-vision lens.

Total optic-zone diameter is usually quite large—that is, about 8 mm. Distant optic-zone diameter is usually about five eighths to two thirds of total optic-zone diameter. The top of the near segment is placed at, slightly above, or slightly below the inferior pupillary border in distant fixation.

For adhered lenses (piggyback or McKay Taylor) a spherical single-vision contact lens with anterior lenticular construction is used as a carrier. A separate half moon-shaped segment with the required near addition is adhered to the carrier.[151, 152] Adherence is obtained by having the posterior curvature of the segment lens the same as the anterior optic-zone curvature of the carrier lens. The resultant surface tension and the ledge produced by the anterior lenticular construction theoretically hold the segment lens in place. The weight of the segment lens acts as ballast to control meridional orientation and to hold the segment inferiorly.

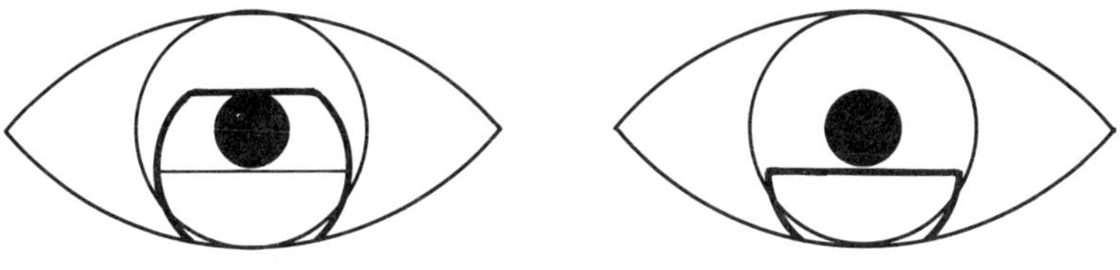

Figure 2–73. Double-truncated bifocals. A, *Distant and near zones.* B, *Near segment only.*

The carrier lens is fitted as a typical single-vision lens. Segment lens positioning is similar to lathed prism ballast, alternating-vision lenses.

Double truncation has been used as the sole means of controlling meridional orientation. There are two types of such lenses.[153–155] The first has both a distance and near optic zone, and has a lens diameter of about 10 mm. horizontally and 7.5 to 8.0 mm. vertically, with the segment line positioned approximately at the inferior pupillary border. The second type, meant for emmetropic presbyopes, is only a near lens, and is fitted with the bottom edge resting on the lower lid and the upper edge infringing slightly onto the lower pupil border in primary fixation. The average lens diameter is about 10.5 mm. horizontally and 4.5 mm. vertically (Fig. 2–73).

Rotating Annular Lenses. Three bifocal contact lens constructions have a central distance optic zone surrounded by a single annular near zone. The first (Bicon) receives its two refractive powers from different *anterior* surface optic-zone curvatures. The distance optic-zone curvature of the Bicon is flatter than the near zone curvature (Fig. 2–74).[156]

The second (DeCarle) and third (Moss-Arner) obtain their two refractive

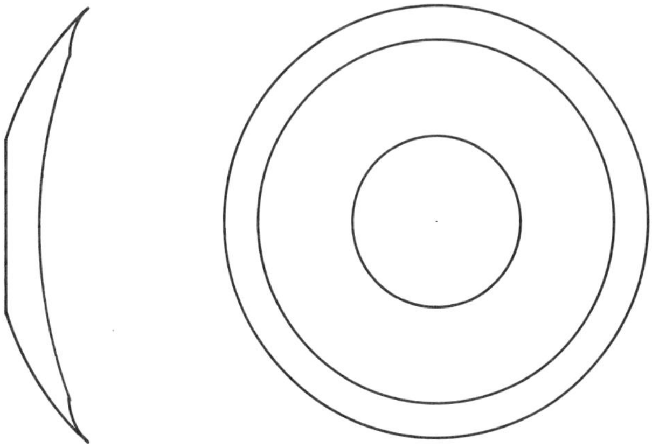

Figure 2–74. Sectional and frontal views of front surface uniannular bifocal. Note the relatively flat anterior central curvature.

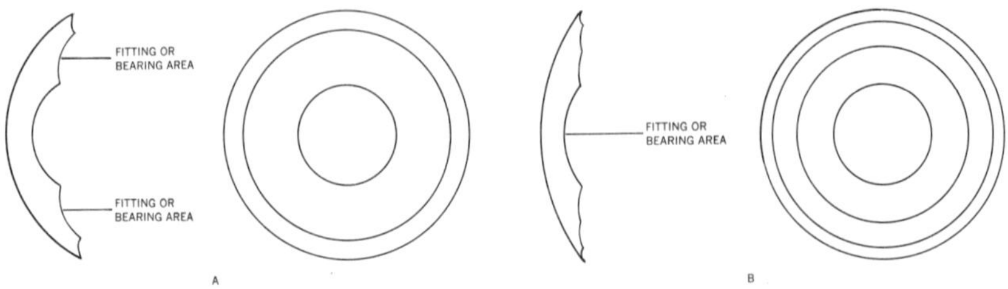

Figure 2–75. Sectional and frontal views of rear surface uniannular bifocals. The junctures are accentuated for diagrammatic purposes. A, *The annular optic-zone curvature is the fitting or bearing area.* B, *The central optic-zone curvature is the fitting or bearing area.*

powers by different *posterior*-surface optic-zone curvatures. The distance-zone curvature is steeper than the near-zone curvature (Fig. 2–75). In the DeCarle, the annular optic-zone curvature is the fitting, or bearing, area, and the central distant optic-zone curvature is made steeper than this to obtain the desired distant power.[157–159] In the Moss-Arner construction, the central distant optic-zone curvature is the fitting, or bearing, area, and the annular curvature is made flatter than this to obtain the desired near power.[160–162]

When rotating annular bifocals are used as alternating-vision lenses, the distant optic-zone size is at least equal to pupil size under ordinary room illumination. These constructions are discussed in more detail on page 134.

There are several bifocal contact lenses (Multifocal Micropupilens) having a central distance optic zone surrounded by a series of annular near zones.[163,164] Anterior optic-zone curvatures are progressively steeper in each annular area, resulting in a progressive increase of plus power. Distance optic-zone size is about equal to pupil size under ordinary room illumination. The lens is fitted in the same way an ordinary single-vision contact lens is, but proper distance optic-zone centration must be obtained (Fig. 2–70) (see also p. 367).

Simultaneous-vision Lenses. *Rotating Annular Type.* The Bicon and the DeCarle bifocals are also used as simultaneous-vision lenses. When they are so used, the distance optic-zone size is made smaller than pupil size under ordinary room illumination. These constructions are discussed in more detail on page 134.

Clinical Procedure

Evaluation. When a presbyope desires contact lenses, the practitioner must make two related evaluations. First, he must decide if the patient's needs can be fulfilled with contemporary contact lenses. Second, if contact lenses are to be fitted, he must decide which clinical course to follow.

For purposes of evaluation, presbyopes may be placed in one of two groups on the basis of their ametropia. The first group is composed of presbyopes who have to wear a constant distance correction. The second group is composed of presbyopes who do not have to wear a constant distance correction. With present knowledge, this second group generally has its needs fulfilled better by spectacles than by contact lenses.

When contact lenses are used, any one of four general clinical courses may be followed:

1. Single-vision contact lenses are fitted. Either one eye is corrected for distance and the other for near, both eyes are somewhat overcorrected in plus at distance, or both eyes are corrected for distance and auxiliary reading glasses are used. Aplanatic lenses may be used (p. 398).
2. Alternating-vision bifocal contact lenses are fitted.
3. Simultaneous-vision bifocal contact lenses are fitted.
4. Pinhole contact lenses are fitted.[165] The pinhole aperture reduces the size of the blur circle of a retinal image that is out of focus. A pinhole contact lens the refractive power of which is the algebraic sum of the distance refractive power and one half the near addition may produce satisfactory distance and near acuity. Optimum pinhole size is 1.5 to 2.5 mm. Such lenses are difficult to fit successfully.

Single-vision Contact Lenses. Whenever it is accepted by the patient, the simplest clinical course is single-vision contact lenses correcting the ametropia and reading glasses compensating for the presbyopia. Frequently, patients who have worn single-vision contact lenses before becoming presbyopic accept this course. It is somewhat less acceptable to patients who have worn spectacles before becoming presbyopic. In many cases, such patients rebel against aging rather than against their cosmetic appearance with spectacles, and they do not want to wear the "tell-tale" bifocals.

When this course is not acceptable, single-vision contact lenses, overcorrecting slightly in plus at distance or correcting one eye for distance and one for near, are considered. Total visual performance is critically evaluated, and such lenses are prescribed when there is satisfactory total performance. Plus overcorrection that reduces distance acuity below 20/25 generally should not be prescribed. It is most helpful, therefore, for low degrees of presbyopia. It should also be remembered that a myope has to accommodate more and a hyperope less with contact lenses than with spectacles (see p. 355).

In the correction of one eye for distance and the other for near, binocularity must be evaluated. Such correction produces images that are dissimilar in size and in clarity at a given fixation distance. Patients have one of four adaptive options: (1) They can fuse these dissimilar images easily and achieve comfortable, efficient, single binocular vision. (2) They can fuse these dissimilar images with difficulty, resulting in uncomfortable, inefficient single binocular vision. (3) They can become diplopic. (4) They can suppress one image and become monocular, usually alternating at distance and near.

Clinically, the authors have seen all these types of adaptation. However, comfortable, efficient, single binocular vision is obtained much more frequently when contact lenses are used in this manner than when spectacles are so used, probably because of the relatively smaller amount of induced refractive aniseikonia with contact lenses. Because contact lenses follow eye movements better than spectacle lenses do, there is also less vertical prism induced at near fixation.

Single-vision contact lenses for a presbyope are fitted as any single-vision lens is. Since precorneal fluid flow may alter with age, this factor should be evaluated when the lens design is determined. The only other difference may be the choice of refractive power.

When a bifocal contact lens is to be used, the practitioner must decide whether alternating- or simultaneous-vision lenses are preferable. Alternating-vision lenses are generally preferable. There is usually a considerable amount of haze produced by the blurred superimposed retinal image in simultaneous-vision lenses. This blur is accentuated outdoors at night when pupil size increases and scotopic vision is used. Pinhole contact lenses decrease illumination and give a vignetted appearance in objects.

ALTERNATING-VISION BIFOCALS. *Fused Lenses.* Evaluation should *always* be done with diagnostic lenses, either fused bifocal or prism ballast single-vision. Because of the prism and weight, fused bifocal lenses typically position inferiorly. The disadvantages of prism should be reviewed (see p. 96 and p. 97). Monocentric bifocals which reduce jump are available.

The vertical lens diameter is equal to the median vertical palpebral aperture size ±0.8 mm. The larger diameter allows tucking under the upper lid and the smaller diameter allows separation from the upper lid. When the upper edge of the lens comes at the margin of the upper lid, there is often considerable discomfort and lens movement. When an inferior truncation is to be used, the horizontal lens diameter in a small lens is usually 0.4 mm. greater than the vertical, and the horizontal lens diameter in a large lens is usually 0.7 mm. greater than the vertical. It may be preferable to order a circular lens in some cases. The authors prefer small lenses.

Diameters of distance and near optic zones should be large enough to provide reasonable pupil coverage, but small enough to provide satisfactory total optic-zone diameter. The near optic zone is placed high enough to provide satisfactory pupil coverage with translation, but low enough to provide relative freedom from near-zone coverage in primary fixation. Table 2–15 is a guide to compromise optic-zone diameters and positioning.

When a circular lens is processed, near segment position is ordered 0.5 mm. higher than indicated by Table 2–15. If subsequent truncation is necessary, this 0.5 mm. allowance compensates for segment lowering due to truncation.

Three conditions reduce the probability of success: (1) When pupil size is larger than 4 mm., pupil coverage is relatively poor, and the total optic-zone diameter is large. (2) When pupil size is less than 2 mm., any infringement of the transition between the two optic zones onto the pupil causes considerable visual problems. (3) A lower lid that is below the inferior

TABLE 2–15

OPTIC-ZONE DIAMETERS AND PLACEMENT
(in mm.)

Pupil Size Under Ordinary Room Illumination	Distance Optic-zone Diameter	Near Optic-zone Diameter	Total Optic-zone Diameter	Top of Near Optic Zone in Relation to Lower Pupillary Margin
5.0	5.0	3.0	8.0	0.5 above margin
4.0	4.5	3.0	7.5	at margin
3.0	4.0	3.0	7.0	at margin
2.0	4.0	3.0	7.0	0.5 below margin

limbus in primary fixation or that moves down considerably in near fixation does not provide a satisfactory supportive barrier. As a result, there is insufficient translation. Such lower lid position and function is quite common when the lid tonus is decreased with age.

Segment position is determined and ordered in terms of the geometric center of the lens. It is desirable that a diagnostic fused bifocal contact lens have the top of the near segment at the geometric center of the lens. This arrangement makes it easier to evaluate segment position and to order it so that the desired positioning is obtained. When prism ballast single-vision lenses are used, a dot is placed at the geometric center of the lens for the same reason (Fig. 2–76).

Because of excessive lacrimation and lens movement, it is difficult to make an accurate determination of segment position the first day. It is often desirable to fit the patient first with single-vision lenses having prism ballast. These lenses should have the characteristics the practitioner feels will be necessary in bifocal contact lenses. Auxiliary reading spectacles are also provided. After the patient has adapted to single-vision lenses for two or three weeks, segment position is determined and bifocal contact lenses are processed.

To produce satisfactory segment position, the optic zone is usually somewhat decentered. Often decentration is upward. Decentration causes unequal secondary widths, and there is more thinning of the edge where the secondary width is greatest.

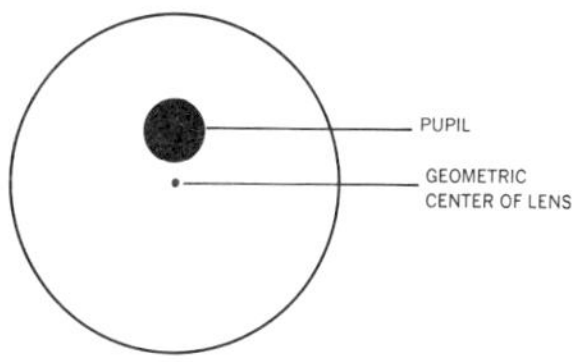

Figure 2–76. A dot at the geometric center (G.C.) *of the lens aids in the determination of the segment position.*

Base and secondary curvatures are determined as in spherical single-vision contact lenses. It is important to compensate the base curve for the relatively large optic zones.

The amount of prism used is the minimum that controls meridional orientation and maintains stable vertical position. Vertical position must be maintained against the upward pull of the upper lid. Also, the base must be thick enough so that it cannot be pushed beneath the lower lid. One and a half prism diopters is an average value. Because the total lens is quite thick, apex thickness is best when it is 0.10 to 0.12 mm.

While bifocal contact lens performance is more readily obtained when the lens orients to the I or IL position, some practitioners seek to center the fused bifocal on the eye. If this is to be attained, it is usually necessary to reduce the amount of prism to about three-quarters of a diopter. Because this may not control meridional orientation, a 0.3 mm. *superior* truncation may be needed to reduce the ability of the upper lid to rotate the lens. In spite of this, meridional orientation may not be satisfactory.

Distance and near powers are determined in the usual manner. When necessary, an anterior toric surface is used to correct residual astigmatism.

Anterior Surface Uniannular Lenses (Bicon). The lens is fitted in the same way a spherical single-vision lens is. Stable lens positioning must be obtained so that the distance and near optic zones are properly positioned. Large lens diameters (10.0 to 10.2 mm.) and a large total optic-zone diameter (8.0 mm.) are often used.

It is often desirable to fit the patient first with a single-vision contact lens having characteristics that probably will be needed for the bifocals. After the patient has adapted, distance optic-zone diameter and position are determined. Distance optic-zone diameter is made equal to pupil size measured under ordinary room illumination. A dot is then placed at the geometric center of the single-vision contact lens. The lens is placed on the eye, and the position of the dot relative to the center of the pupil is measured. Because the distance optic zone must be centered in the bifocal contact lens, lens diameter is ordered to obtain geometric centering (Fig. 2–77).

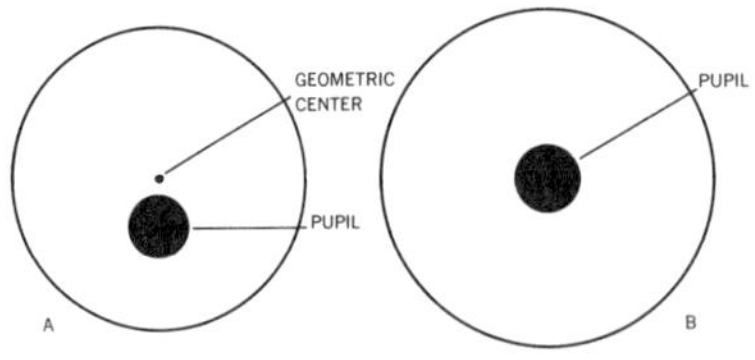

Figure 2–77. A, *The dot at the geometric center* (G.C.) *of a* superior *positioning lens is above pupil.* B, *A larger lens diameter results in centration of the optic zone and pupil.*

Posterior-Surface Uniannular Lenses. The DeCarle is fitted in the same way as the Bicon.

The Moss-Arner bifocal is fitted in the following manner. This lens has three zones from center to periphery—the distance zone, the near zone, and the edge bevel. The central distance zone should be 1.0 mm. to 1.5 mm. larger than the pupil size measured under 15 foot-candles of illumination. When pupil size is greater than 4 mm., satisfactory performance is more difficult to obtain. The average width of the distance zone is approximately 5 mm. The inside curvature of this area is determined by the diagnostic lens procedure to obtain relative alignment. Because the central optic zone is relatively small, the base curve is often steeper than the flatter ophthalmometric principal meridian. An average figure is 0.15 mm. The intermediate curve radius is determined by the needed near addition. The indicial difference between plastic and precorneal fluid adds plus power in this area of relative flattening. A rule of thumb is that a 0.25 D addition is produced by each 0.1 mm. of secondary flattening. The following formula may be used:[166]

$$\frac{100}{r_{sec.}} = \frac{(100 - 0.6494 \cdot \text{Add})}{r_{base}}$$

where

$r_{sec.}$ = Secondary curve radius

r_{base} = Base curve radius

A peripheral curve 0.1 to 0.2 mm. wide with a 10.5 to 11.0 mm. radius is used. The lens diameter is about 9.4 to 9.7 mm. Obviously, if the intermediate curve is used as an optical surface, it must be fabricated to produce regular refraction. This type of surface can be produced by lathe or button cutting and pitch polishing.

Simultaneous-vision Bifocals. The Bicon and DeCarle may be used as simultaneous-vision bifocals. When they are so used, they are fitted as before, with one exception. The distance optic-zone diameter is now made equal to about *two thirds* of pupil size under ordinary room illumination.

3

STAGE THREE

Laboratory Procedures

ORDERING

After the lens specifications have been determined, the lenses must be ordered from the manufacturer. The basic function of a contact lens manufacturer is to fabricate a lens within accepted tolerances. This means that all necessary specifications should be provided by the practitioner on the order form. If the practitioner does not supply all necessary specifications, the laboratory can only use average values for any missing specification. The problems of averages are discussed on page 54. They are compounded here, for the patient is never seen by any of the manufacturer's personnel. The manufacturer is forced by the practitioner's omissions to make decisions determining the fit of the contact lenses.

Lenses may be ordered finished or uncut. A finished contact lens incorporates all necessary specifications. Aside from refinishing of the edge, the lens should need no modification before it is delivered to the patient. An uncut lens has the desired base curvature, refractive power, center thickness, and tint. The lens diameter for an uncut lens is ordered so that it is larger than the desired finished diameter. This excess is needed because material is removed during edging. To finish an uncut lens, the practitioner must place the desired secondary curvatures and edge on it.

Seven specifications must be ordered for each finished lens. These are: base curve(s), secondary curve(s), refractive power(s), lens diameter, optic-zone diameter, center thickness, and tint. In ordering an uncut lens, the width of the secondary curves and the diameter of the optic zone are not needed.

Base Curve(s)

Any curvature of a contact lens should be ordered in terms of radii and not diopters. The radius is a physical constant; the diopter is not. Any given radius may have any number of dioptric powers, depending on the difference in indices of the substance of the lens and that of the surrounding media. If the dioptric power is ordered and converted by an inappropriate table, the radius will not be as desired. This consideration is extremely important.

If a single spherical base is to be used, only the radius need be ordered—such as 7.47 mm. The base may be ordered in 0.01 mm. steps.

If a toric base is to be ordered, both the radii and meridional position of each radius must be designated. For example,

$$\frac{7.50 \text{ ax } 180}{8.00 \text{ ax } 90}.$$

This specification will place the steeper base in the vertical meridian and the flatter base in the horizontal meridian when the lens is on the eye:

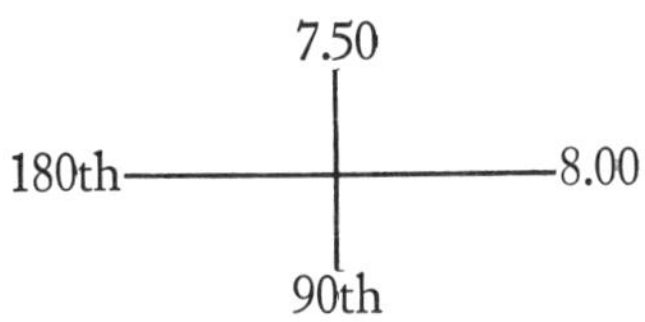

The location of the bases may also be specified by the use of the terms *in* or *at*—for example,

$$\frac{7.50 \text{ in or at } 90}{8.00 \text{ in or at } 180}.$$

Note that there is a 90° difference between *axis* and *in* or *at*.

Secondary Curve(s)

All posterior curvatures, excluding the base curve, are considered secondary curves. The radius and width of each curvature should be specified. Frequently, the width is ordered in terms of its value on each side of the optic zone. When more than one secondary curvature is to be used, they should be listed progressively from steepest to flattest. This is the order in which they are usually fabricated in the laboratory. Some manufacturers are equipped to fabricate secondary curve radii in 0.05 mm. steps. Most are equipped for fabrication in 0.10 mm. steps. All manufacturers are equipped to fabricate secondary curve width to the nearest 0.05 mm. If toric secondary curvatures are to be used, the radii and meridional position of each should be specified.

Refractive Power(s)

The *posterior vertex power* desired is ordered to the nearest 0.12 D. Any compensations for vertex distance should be done by the practitioner. If an anterior toric or bitoric lens is ordered, the posterior vertex spherical and cylindrical powers and the axis of the cylinder must be specified. If a bifocal contact lens is ordered, both the distance refractive power and the near reading add should be specified.

Lens Diameter

The lens diameter is ordered to the nearest 0.1 mm. If the practitioner intends to edge the lens before delivery to the patient, the lens should be ordered large enough to allow for the reduction of diameter due to edging. Usually, 0.1 to 0.2 mm. is allowed for moderate or high minus lenses and 0.2 to 0.3 mm. for plus or low minus lenses. If a truncated lens is desired, both the vertical and horizontal dimensions must be specified.

Optic-zone Diameter

The optic-zone diameter should be ordered to the nearest 0.1 mm. Finished lens diameter minus twice the total secondary curve width on each side equals the optic-zone diameter. If a lens with more than one optic zone, such as a bifocal lens, is ordered, the size and location of each zone must be specified. If a decentered optic zone is desired, the amount and direction of decentration must be specified.

Center Thickness

The center thickness that will produce a desired edge thickness for a finished but unedged lens should be computed. The procedure for doing this is discussed on page 473. Thickness may be ordered in millimeters or inches (0.1 mm. = 0.004 inch). Because all other linear values are ordered in millimeters, it is logical to order thickness in millimeters also.

If a lens with prism in it, or a bitoric nonprismatic lens is ordered, it may be advisable to leave computation of center thickness to the manufacturer. The desired edge thickness at the thinnest point should be specified. This is apex thickness in a prismatic lens, and the thickness at the extremity of the minus axis meridian in a bitoric lens.

Tint

The common tints used in contact lenses are blue, brown, gray, green, and pink. Additional colors such as lavender, yellow, or smoky gray (black) are available. Tints usually come in three shades: No. 1 = lightest; No. 2 = medium; and No. 3 = darkest. It is also possible to obtain a No. 1½ shade in some tints. It should be noted that tints may vary in hue from one manufacturer to another, which may cause a problem when a duplicate lens is ordered as a replacement. See page 298 for further discussion.

Auxiliary Specifications

In addition to these basic specifications, auxiliary specifications are sometimes needed.

Fenestrations or Perforations. Fenestrations in the optic zone may be used to improve the transfer of fluids and gases from between the contact lens and the cornea. Use of fenestrations presents three general problems: they may become clogged with ocular secretions, visual problems may occur from large fenestrations or from the spurting of fluid through small fenestrations that position toward the center of the pupil, and corneal abrasion may occur from improperly fabricated fenestrations or from fenestrations that position on a bearing area.

Optimum fenestration size is 0.10 to 0.20 mm. Positioning is ordered in terms of the geometric center of the lens. Either single or multiple fenestrations are used. Single fenestrations are usually placed at, or 1.0 mm. from, the geometric center. When multiple fenestrations are used, there are usually three, which are staggered 1.0, 2.0, and 3.0 mm. from the geometric center. A diagram to indicate fenestrations is helpful.

Type of Plastic. Contact lenses are typically made of a plastic having an index of refraction of 1.49. Some laboratories also have available plastic of a higher index. If this material is desired, it should be noted. When plastic of a higher index is used, edge thickness must be appropriately computed.

Coating. A coating of titanium dioxide or silicon monoxide may be applied to attempt to improve wetting. If this coating is desired, it should be specified. (See p. 408.)

Truncation. If truncation is desired, the amount must be specified. The shape should also be specified. Because conformation of the truncated area to the margin of the lower lid is often desired, a diagram is helpful. Whether an inferior or superior truncation is desired should be indicated.

Prism Ballast. The amount in prism diopters and the location of the base should be indicated.

Anterior Lenticular. The diameter of the anterior optical zone and any unique characteristics of the front surface of the lenticular should be specified. Figure 3–1 shows two completed order forms with the various lens characteristics discussed.

Identification. It is possible to scribe a small letter on the peripheral part of the anterior surface. Such letters aid in identification of the lenses (Fig. 3–2).

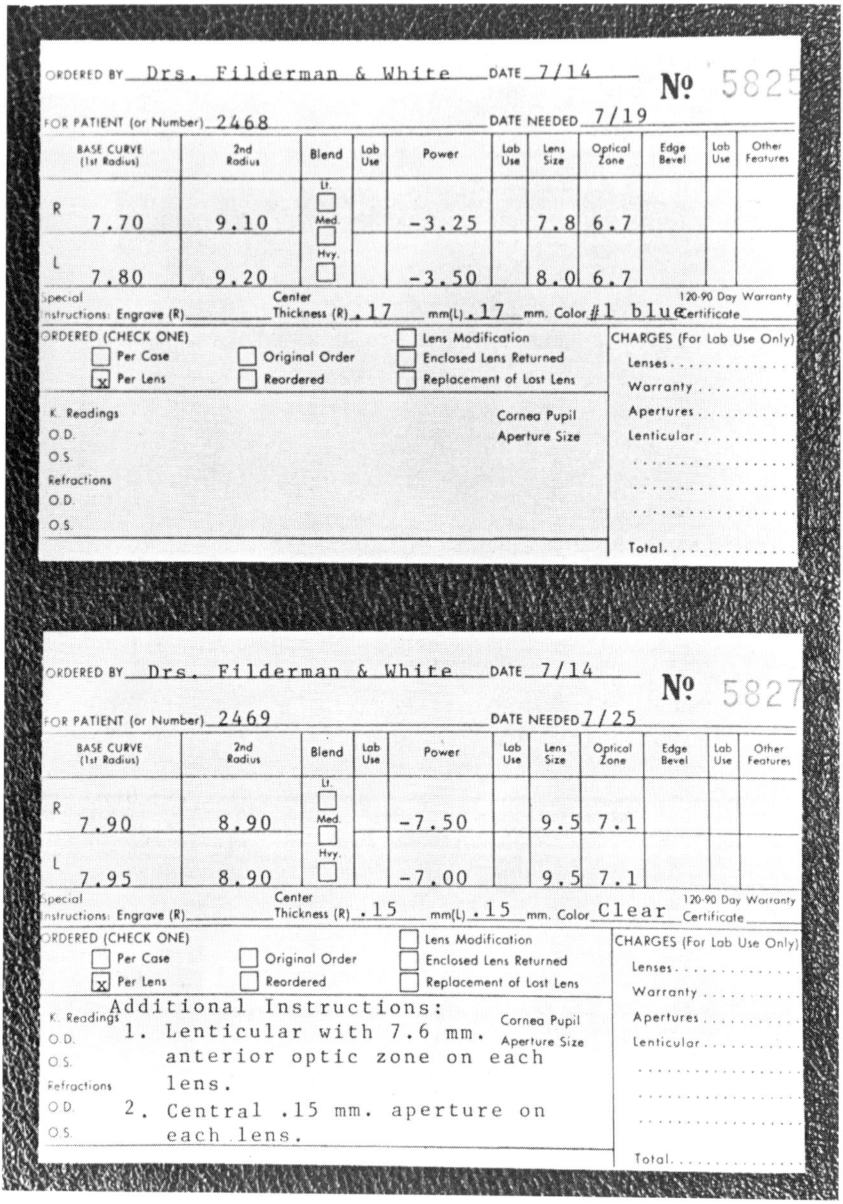

ORDERED BY Drs. Filderman & White DATE 7/14 № 5825

FOR PATIENT (or Number) 2468 DATE NEEDED 7/19

	BASE CURVE (1st Radius)	2nd Radius	Blend	Lab Use	Power	Lab Use	Lens Size	Optical Zone	Edge Bevel	Lab Use	Other Features
R	7.70	9.10	Lt. ☐ Med. ☐		-3.25		7.8	6.7			
L	7.80	9.20	Hvy. ☐		-3.50		8.0	6.7			

Special Instructions: Engrave (R) ____ Center Thickness (R) .17 mm(L) .17 mm. Color #1 blue 120-90 Day Warranty Certificate ____

ORDERED (CHECK ONE)
☐ Per Case ☐ Original Order ☐ Lens Modification
☒ Per Lens ☐ Reordered ☐ Enclosed Lens Returned
☐ Replacement of Lost Lens

K. Readings O.D. O.S.
Refractions O.D. O.S.
Cornea Pupil Aperture Size

CHARGES (For Lab Use Only)
Lenses. . . . . .
Warranty . . . . . .
Apertures . . . . . .
Lenticular . . . . . .
Total. . . . . .

ORDERED BY Drs. Filderman & White DATE 7/14 № 5827

FOR PATIENT (or Number) 2469 DATE NEEDED 7/25

	BASE CURVE (1st Radius)	2nd Radius	Blend	Lab Use	Power	Lab Use	Lens Size	Optical Zone	Edge Bevel	Lab Use	Other Features
R	7.90	8.90	Lt. ☐ Med. ☐		-7.50		9.5	7.1			
L	7.95	8.90	Hvy. ☐		-7.00		9.5	7.1			

Special Instructions: Engrave (R) ____ Center Thickness (R) .15 mm(L) .15 mm. Color Clear 120-90 Day Warranty Certificate ____

ORDERED (CHECK ONE)
☐ Per Case ☐ Original Order ☐ Lens Modification
☒ Per Lens ☐ Reordered ☐ Enclosed Lens Returned
☐ Replacement of Lost Lens

K. Readings O.D. O.S.
Refractions O.D. O.S.
Cornea Pupil Aperture Size

Additional Instructions:
1. Lenticular with 7.6 mm. anterior optic zone on each lens.
2. Central .15 mm. aperture on each lens.

CHARGES (For Lab Use Only)
Lenses. . . . . .
Warranty . . . . . .
Apertures . . . . . .
Lenticular . . . . . .
Total. . . . . .

Figure 3–1. Completed order forms.

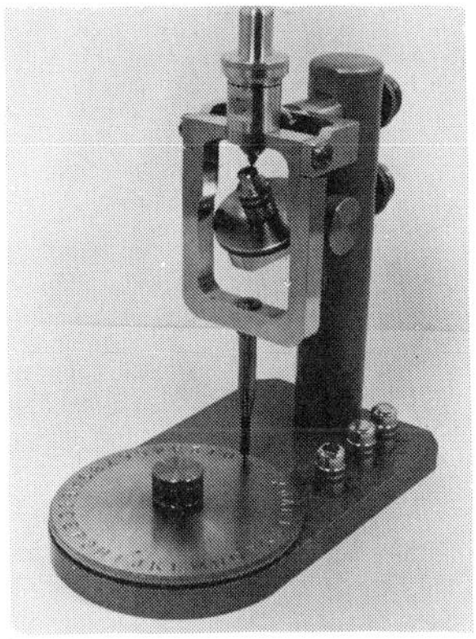

Figure 3–2. Lettering device. (Courtesy of G. Nissel & Co.)

VERIFICATION

By properly inspecting and verifying the contact lens characteristics, each practitioner must assume final responsibility for quality control.[167–170] There are two important reasons. First, because there is no regulatory agency governing contact lens manufacturers, quality level varies. The quality of lenses manufactured by any laboratory depends on individual capabilities and integrity, as well as practitioners' demands. Second, if contact lenses are not inspected and verified, it is impossible to know whether subsequent problems are due to improper fabrication or improper design.

Because manufacturing perfection is impossible, the quality of a product must be judged in terms of acceptable variance from perfection—that is, in terms of tolerance. Tolerance is determined by the degree of manufacturing accuracy that can reasonably be expected and the departure from perfection that can occur before product performance is significantly altered.

To inspect and verify the characteristics of contact lenses, the practitioner must understand the accepted tolerances, the proper equipment, and the proper procedures. All verification instruments should be checked to make sure they are accurate before they are used.

Lens Diameter

Tolerance. A lens diameter can generally be manufactured and verified within ±0.05 mm. of the ordered size. Because a 0.1 mm. variance in lens diameter will usually not alter performance significantly, lenses may occasionally be accepted up to this tolerance. The lens diameter between various meridians should not vary by more than 0.05 mm. for a desired circular lens.

Equipment. The lens diameter may be determined by a V-channel gauge, a measuring magnifier, or a go-or-no-go gauge (Figs. 3–3 and 3–4).

The V-channel gauge has a groove that is graduated in widths of 0.1 mm. The measuring magnifier has a scale (graticule) of 0.1 mm. graduations. The go-or-no-go gauge has openings of 0.2 mm. graduations.

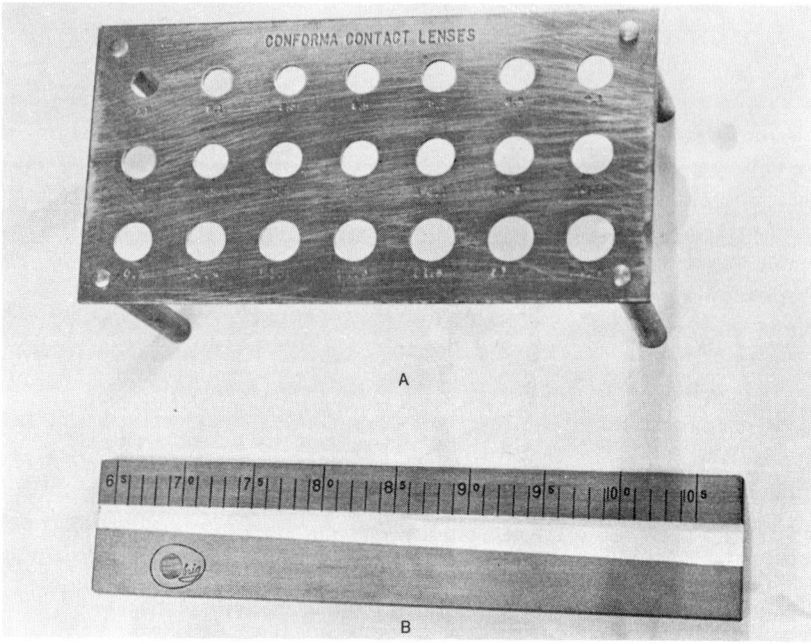

Figure 3–3. A, *Go-or-no-go gauge.* B, *V-Channel diameter gauge.*

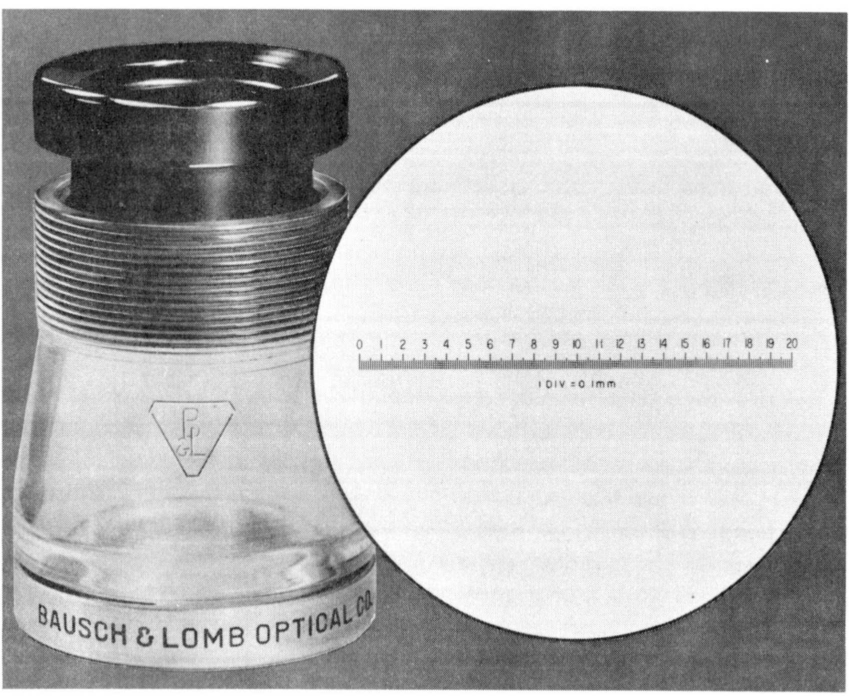

Figure 3–4. Measuring magnifier and its reticle. (Courtesy of Bausch & Lomb.)

PROCEDURES. *V-channel gauge.* The lens is placed concave surface down in the widest end of the gauge. The lens should be dry, and the lens and gauge should be clean to avoid restriction of lens movement, which results in a false reading. The narrow edge of the channel is tilted downward, and the lens slides down because of gravity. When the lens comes to rest, the diameter is read from the scale at the point where two sides of the lens touch the channel edge. Lenses should not be forced along the groove because they may become warped or chipped, or a lowered reading may be established. For removal of the lens, the gauge is tilted with the wide end down. To slide the lens out, the gauge must often be gently tapped with a finger. After rotation of the lens about 90°, the procedure is repeated to make sure the lens is not oval. It is advisable to carry out this procedure over a bench or table; thus if the lens falls, it is easier to locate.

Measuring Magnifier. The magnifier is held close to the eye and a light source is used as a background. The lens is held with its concave surface against the graticule, and it is centered vertically in terms of the scale to provide maximum diameter determination. One edge of the lens is placed at the zero mark. The diameter is read from the zero point to the position where the opposite edge intersects the scale (Fig. 3–5). The lens should then be rotated 90° to determine its roundness. Because it is difficult to center the lens vertically, an erroneous reading may result. An erroneous reading may also be produced because of the meniscus around the edge of a wet lens.

Go-or-no-go Gauge. The lens is placed convex surface down on a hole about 0.2 mm. smaller than the specified diameter. Because the lens should be too large for the hole, it will not go through. It is then placed on progressively larger holes until it does go through. Its diameter is smaller than the first hole it goes through and larger than the preceding hole. Because graduations are in 0.2 mm. steps, the instrument is only accurate to this degree.

OPTIC-ZONE DIAMETER

TOLERANCE. The optic-zone diameter can generally be manufactured and verified within ±0.1 mm. Such a variance from the desired diameter seldom alters performance significantly. If the juncture between the optic zone and the adjacent secondary curvature has been highly blended, verification accuracy is often 0.2 mm. or less. Optic-zone roundness should be accurate to 0.1 mm. for a nonblended or lightly blended lens, and to 0.2 mm. or less for a highly blended lens.

EQUIPMENT. Generally, a measuring magnifier is used (Fig. 3–5). Projection magnifiers may be used, but they are quite expensive.

PROCEDURE. The measuring magnifier is used in a manner similar to that used for checking lens diameter. One edge of the transition between optic and secondary areas is placed on the zero mark at the left side. Optic-zone

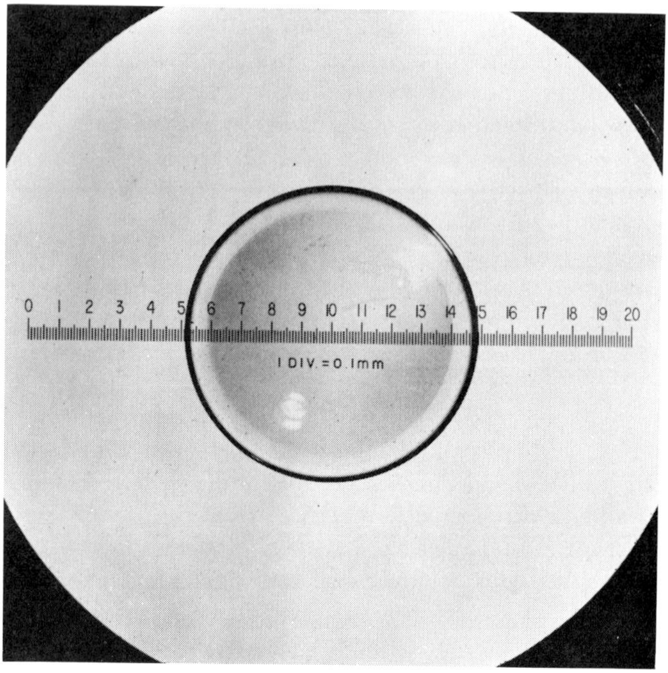

Figure 3–5. Contact lens as seen through a measuring magnifier. (Courtesy of Bausch & Lomb.)

width is read from the zero point to the position where the transition intersects the scale at the opposite (right) end. As in diameter verification, it is important to have the lens vertically centered. After the reading is taken, the lens is rotated 90° to determine its roundness. At times, the zone is most readily determined by moving the head and magnifier from side to side while looking at a bright light source.

Surface Quality

Tolerance. Surfaces should be free of scratches, bubbles, lathe marks, striae, stress marks, and spots of accumulated color. A few very fine scratches on the convex surface may occasionally be accepted.

Equipment. A measuring magnifier, a stereoscopic microscope, or a radiuscope is useful.

Procedure. While the optic-zone diameter is being determined, the lens can be inspected for surface imperfections. Lenses should be cleaned so that dirt or pieces of lint are not misinterpreted as imperfections.

A more detailed inspection may be done with a table stereoscopic microscope or the stereoscopic microscope of a slit lamp (Fig. 3–6). About 20 to 25× magnification is usually adequate. When using the table microscope,

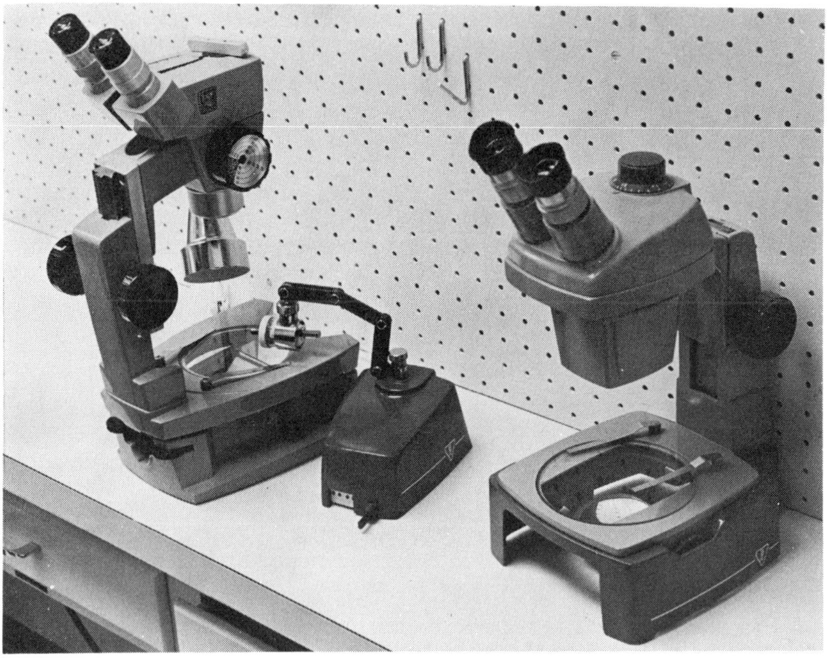

Figure 3–6. Stereoscopic microscopes.

illumination can be provided by a 100 watt bulb in a gooseneck lamp. This illumination may also be used with the slit lamp, or the wide beam illumination of the slit lamp may be used.

The lens must be held steadily in focus. It may either be held between the thumb and index finger or mounted on a holding device such as a suction cup or a stick with double-sided tape. The lens is tilted to reflect the light and rotated so various areas are observed. Surface imperfections reflect the light irregularly. It is often helpful to have a dark background. The practitioner should try not to smudge or dirty the lens because smudges or dirt may be misinterpreted as lens flaws.

The radiuscope sighting tube produces magnification. Surface scratches can be detected while the base curve is being determined.

Secondary Curve Width

Tolerance. The secondary curve width can generally be verified and manufactured to within ± 0.05 mm. on each side of the optic zone. Such a variance usually does not alter performance significantly. If there is little variance between the radii of two adjacent secondary curves or if the juncture between two dissimilar curves is highly blended, it is often difficult or impossible to determine secondary width to an accuracy greater than ± 0.2 mm.

EQUIPMENT. The measuring magnifier is used.

PROCEDURE. The width of a curve on each side is determined by measurement between its two extremities. The secondary curve width on each side of a circular concentric bicurve lens is equal to half the difference between lens diameter and optic-zone diameter. It is often easier to pick up the transition from one secondary curve to another by moving the measuring magnifier back and forth slightly.

REFRACTIVE POWER

TOLERANCE. Lens power can be manufactured and verified within ±0.12 D. *Total meridional refractive error* (the algebraic sum of the refractive power error and the base curve error) should not be greater than 0.25 D.

EQUIPMENT. A Lensometer or Vertometer is generally used.[171,172] It is also possible to determine the central radius of each surface. If the power of each surface and the center thickness are known, the total refractive power can be computed. Because this procedure is time-consuming, it is rarely used clinically.

There are two basic problems with Lensometers and Vertometers in verifying refractive power. The first problem is that the stop of a Lensometer or Vertometer is quite flat, because it is designed to permit conformity with the relatively flat posterior curvatures of a spectacle lens. In the determination of posterior vertex power of a contact lens, the concave or posterior surface is placed against the stop. Because the curves of contact lenses are considerably steeper than those of spectacles, the posterior vertex plane is moved away from the plane of the aperture of the stop. Proper measurement of vertex power demands that the vertex plane be coincident with the stop plane, because the power of a lens, determined by the Lensometer or Vertometer, depends on the distance of its focal point from the stop plane.

When determination of anterior vertex power is desired, the anterior vertex plane should be coincident with the stop plane when the convex surface of the lens is applied to it. The steep curves of a contact lens place the vertex plane in front of the stop plane.

Special inserts have been designed with steep curvatures to allow a relatively better relationship of the posterior vertex plane to the stop plane. If these inserts are used, the anterior surface of the insert against which the posterior surface of the lens is placed must be in the same position as the original Lensometer or Vertometer stop.

The second problem in using a Lensometer or Vertometer is whether posterior or anterior vertex power should be determined. As discussed in detail on page 341 posterior vertex power should be determined, because the lens will be placed on the eye with its posterior surface on the precorneal fluid. Most minus lenses up to 6 D with a center thickness of 0.25 mm. or less have a difference between anterior and posterior vertex power of less than 0.10 D. For such lenses, either posterior or anterior vertex power may be used. From −6 to −10 D, there will be a difference of between 0.10 and 0.15 D. There is always less minus power for anterior than for posterior vertex powers.

There is considerably more difference between the anterior and posterior vertex power of plus lenses because of the greater center thickness. The higher the refractive power and the thicker the lens, the greater the difference is. There is less plus power for anterior vertex than for posterior vertex power. Thus, posterior vertex power should be used.

Before the instrument is used, the eyepiece should be focused by turning it all the way out and then turning it all the way in until the eyepiece reticle is sharply focused. Then the power wheel is turned until the mire target is focused. With no lens in front, the reading should be 0.00 D.

PROCEDURE. A clean lens is gently held in a centered position with its posterior surface against the stop. If the lens is not held gently, it may warp temporarily. If it is not centered, a false prismatic component may be exhibited.

The reading is taken in the normal manner by rotation of the drum. The image of the mires should be clear. Any fuzziness or halo indicates an optical surface of poor quality. The lens should be moved across the aperture, and readings should be taken at various parts of the optic zone. Power and quality should be uniform throughout.

THICKNESS

TOLERANCE. Center thickness of a contact lens can generally be manufactured and verified to an accuracy of ±0.02 mm. Thickness variance of this amount generally does not alter performance significantly.

EQUIPMENT. Thickness gauges are available. A lens clock or Geneva lens measure may be used, but these instruments are more complex to use, often produce less accurate results, and may scratch the lens.

PROCEDURE. Before using a thickness gauge, the practitioner should check to make sure that the hand points to zero (Fig. 3–7). If it does not, it should be properly set. When it is ready to be used, the pin is drawn. The lens is held convex surface downward in the gauge. It is placed so that the pin of the gauge comes to rest in the center of the lens. If placement is improper, a minus lens will measure thicker and a plus lens thinner than its true center thickness. The pin is slowly lowered until it contacts the concave surface. Rapid lowering may scratch or chip the lens. Thickness is read from the scale. To remove the lens, the pin is retracted and the lens lifted out.

Edge thickness may be approximated. The lens is placed convex surface down so that the pin comes in contact with the concave surface as close as possible to the edge. The thickness of various points around the edge may be determined to detect any unequal thickness. A relatively thin pin gives a better approximation of edge thickness.

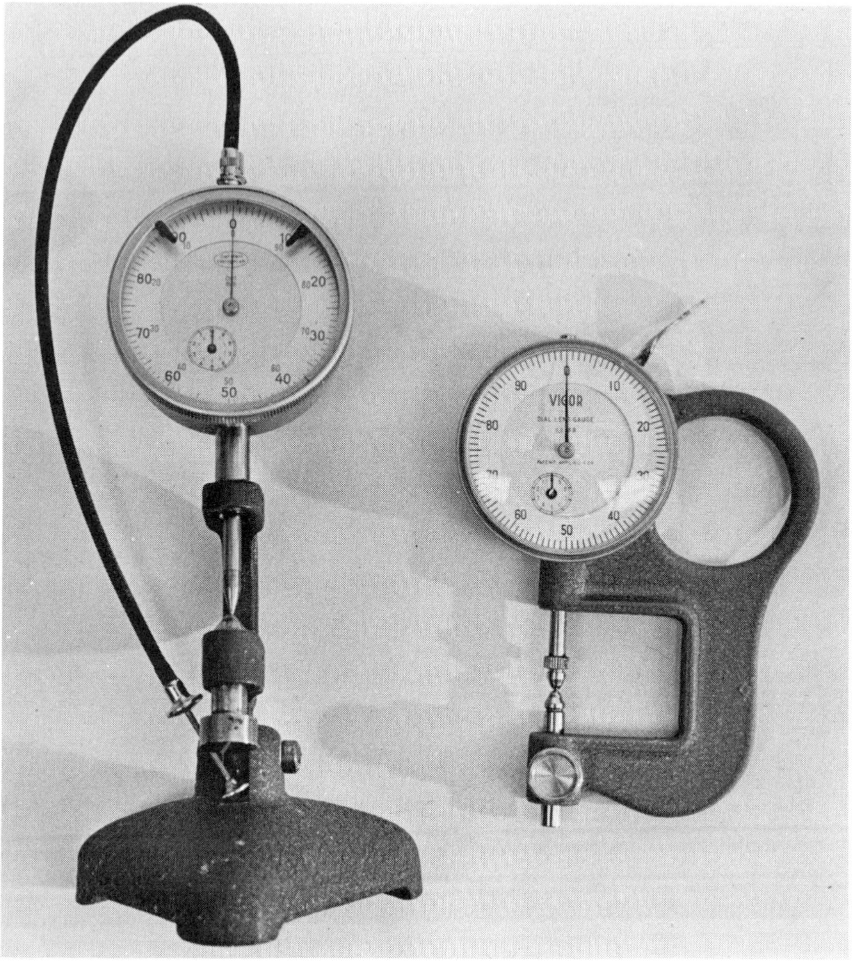

Figure 3–7. Thickness gauges.

Edge Configuration

Tolerance. Proper edge thickness and configuration are two of the more important aspects of contact lens fabrication. They are also two of the most difficult specifications to manufacture and verify.[173]

Before tolerances can be established, the desired edge thickness and shape must be determined. The authors believe about a 0.13 mm. edge thickness is best on a lens finished in all aspects but edge finish. In other words, center thickness should be chosen so that this edge thickness will be produced. Because the tolerance for center thickness is ±0.02 mm., the range of acceptable edge thickness is 0.11 to 0.15 mm.

The edge finishing process alters this thickness somewhat and provides the desired configuration. Configuration should be as ordered (see p. 43).

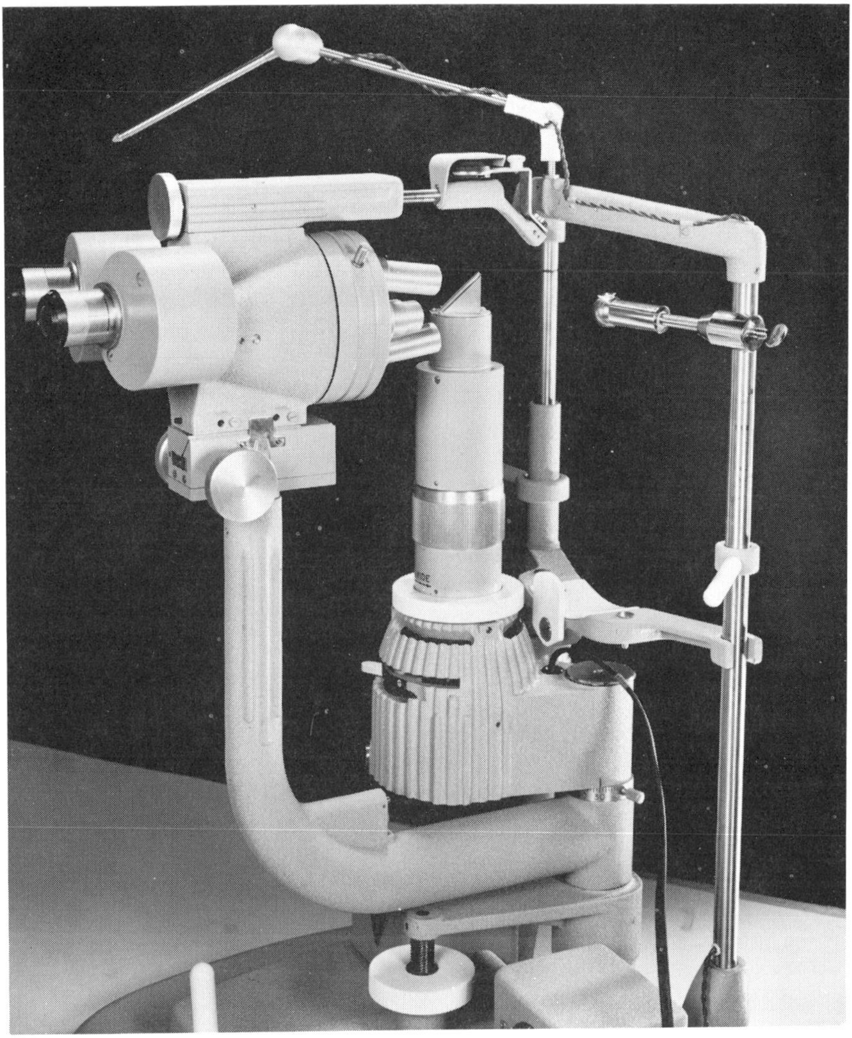

Figure 3–8. Lens mounted for viewing with the stereoscopic microscope of a Thorpe slit lamp. (Courtesy of Lensco Precision Instrument Co.)

EQUIPMENT. A stereoscopic microscope, a projection magnifier, or a molding process may be used to determine edge configuration.

PROCEDURE. All methods for evaluating edge configuration are highly subjective. It takes much training and practice before the observer develops the ability to appreciate desired configuration under the conditions of magnification used.

Stereoscopic Microscope. Either a table stereoscopic microscope or the stereoscopic microscope of the slit lamp may be used (Fig. 3–8). Magnification should be 20× to 25×. With use of a table microscope, illumination may be provided by a 100 watt bulb in a gooseneck lamp above and oblique to the lens. Some practitioners prefer a more focused illumination, which is produced by special commercially available lamps. With use of the microscope of a slit lamp, wide beam illumination may be used. The lens may be held between the fingers or mounted on a special holder.

When the lens is held between the thumb and forefinger of one hand, the apex of the edge is directed toward the practitioner. Before the practitioner looks through the microscope, the lens should be placed so that the beam focuses on it. To overcome the problem of finding the lens, the nail of one of the fingers holding the lens may be brought into focus. Then the lens is found.

The lens is then tilted from front to back for appreciation of contour, polish, and thickness. It may then be rotated by the forefinger of the other hand so that all aspects of the edge are viewed. The surface should be smooth and highly polished.

Projection Magnifier (Shadowgraph). A magnified view of various aspects of the edge is projected on a screen (Fig. 3–9). Because a shadow of the edge rather than the edge itself is seen, edge finish and polish and certain aspects of the posterior edge finish cannot be evaluated properly.

Devices have been made that can be placed on a Lensometer or Vertometer so that a shadow of the edge can be seen through the magnification of the instrument optical system.[174–176] It is also possible to use some slit lamps for this purpose.

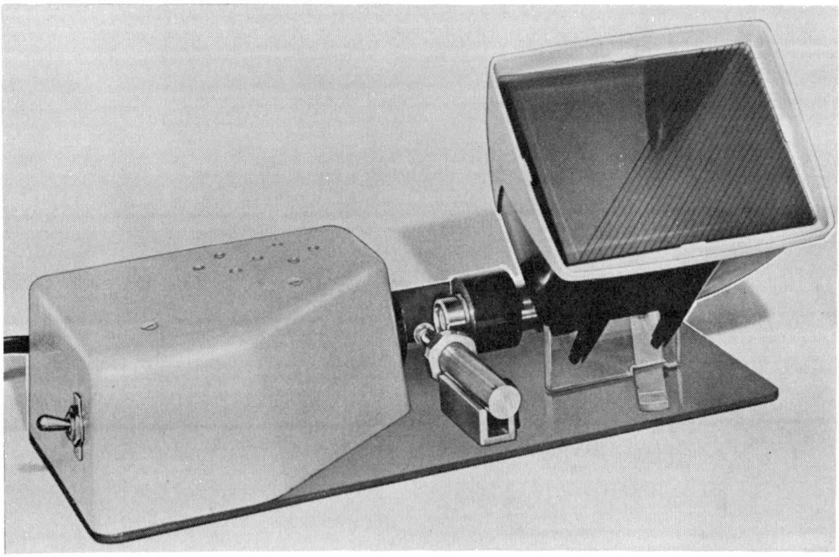

Figure 3–9. Projection magnifier. (Courtesy of Precision-Cosmet Co.)

Molding. Various compounds may be used to make a mold of the edge.[177] After the lens is removed from the mold, a section is cut into it. A profile view of the edge is established and can be viewed with a stereoscopic microscope. This system is advantageous in that a permanent record of the edge is obtained. Disadvantages are that it gives a picture of only one part of the edge, and the procedure must be repeated several times for a composite picture of the entire edge. This method takes considerable time, and even then the polish of the edge cannot be appreciated. Finally, because the mold must be viewed under magnification, it is simpler just to view directly the edge under magnification.

Base Curve(s)

Tolerance. The base curve usually can be fabricated and verified to an accuracy of ±0.02 to ±0.03 mm., or to an ophthalmometric power of about 0.12 D. There should not be more than 0.03 mm. of undesired cylinder. Accurate base curves contribute both to the relationship of lens curves to corneal curves and to the effective refractive power through the optic zone. Variance up to 0.03 mm. usually does not significantly affect performance in either instance. The total meridional power error from a combination of Lensometer reading and base curve reading should not be greater than ±0.25 D.

Equipment. Ophthalmometers, Keratometers, optical spherometers, or an R-C device can be used.[178, 179] If an Ophthalmometer or Keratometer is used, a means for properly holding the lens must be used. Such holders have depressions to which the convex surface of the lens adheres.

There are basically two types of holders.[180, 181] The first is mounted so that its depression is perpendicular to the optic axis of the instrument (Fig. 3–10). When the lens is mounted, the base curve will be relatively perpendicular to the optic axis of the instrument. To prevent slipping due to

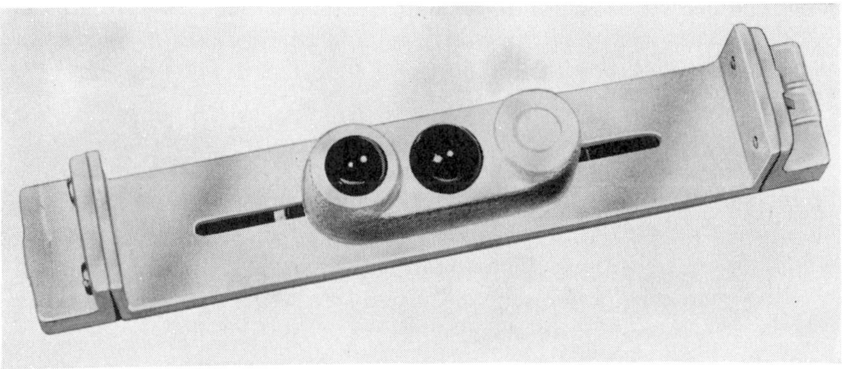

Figure 3–10. Perpendicular contact lens holder. (Courtesy of Plastic Contact Lens Co.)

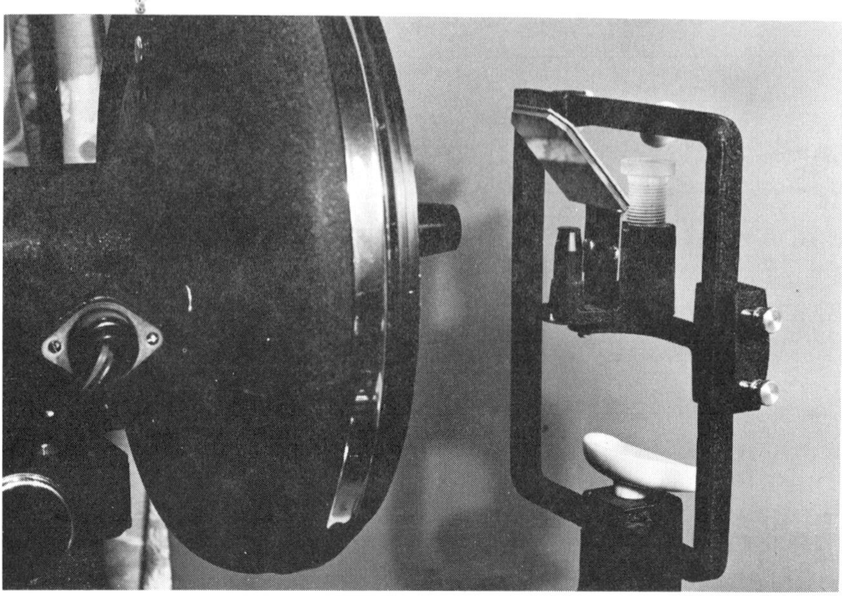

Figure 3–11. A parallel contact lens holder mounting on an Ophthalmometer. (Courtesy of Plastic Contact Lens Co.)

gravitational pull, a somewhat solid adhesive substance, such as double-sided tape, clay, or toothpaste, can be used; or a liquid adhesive, such as glycerine or wetting solution, can be used. The disadvantage of using a somewhat solid adhesive is that the lens may temporarily be warped if the practitioner applies excessive pressure during mounting. A possible disadvantage of using liquid adhesive is that the concave posterior lens surface must be kept dry or the reflection of the mires and the determination of the radius are affected.

The second type of holder is mounted so that its depression is parallel to the optic axis of the instrument. Because of the position of the depression, when it is filled with liquid, none of the liquid will flow out (Fig. 3–11). When the lens is mounted, the base curve is relatively parallel to the optic axis of the instrument. A front surface mirror inclined at 45° to the optic axis of the instrument allows reading of the base curvature. Because the angle of incidence equals the angle of reflection, the incident light from the mires is reflected onto the posterior lens surface. The use of a liquid with an index of refraction similar to that of plastic (1.49) neutralizes the reflecting properties of the anterior surface of the lens. Glycerine (1.47), water (1.33), or wetting solution can be used satisfactorily; the image of the mires, therefore, is produced by the posterior surface only.

PROCEDURE. The instruments should all be checked to ensure that they are working accurately.

Ophthalmometer (Keratometer). The holding device is mounted on the instrument, and the lens is placed as indicated above. Readings should be taken in two meridians of a lens that supposedly has a single spherical posterior curvature. Readings are in terms of diopters. Because the concave surface is being measured, Column 2 of App. VI gives the correct radius value. If a toric central posterior curvature is being measured, the lens must first be aligned for the principal meridians.

Radiuscope. A drop of liquid is placed in the depression of the flat top lens holder to eliminate reflection from the convex anterior surface (Fig. 3–12). A clean dry lens is placed in it with its posterior concave surface up. The holder is placed level on the stage. The target illuminator is turned on. A small beam of green light will appear on the stand or on the lens. Before the observer looks through the monocular microscope, this beam should be reasonably centered on the posterior surface of the lens. This centering helps ensure that the central area of this lens surface is used as the reflector.

The observer looks into the microscope. The adjustment knob is turned until the lowest stellate target is seen. The adjustment knob is turned past the point of best focus. Then it is slowly turned back until the lower target is focused. The dial gauge zeroing knob is turned until zero appears on both the small inner dial and the larger outer dial. The adjustment knob is turned away, and again the lower target is brought into focus. This focus should be at zero. If it is not, the procedure must be repeated. The adjustment knob is turned toward the observer until the aerial image, or the

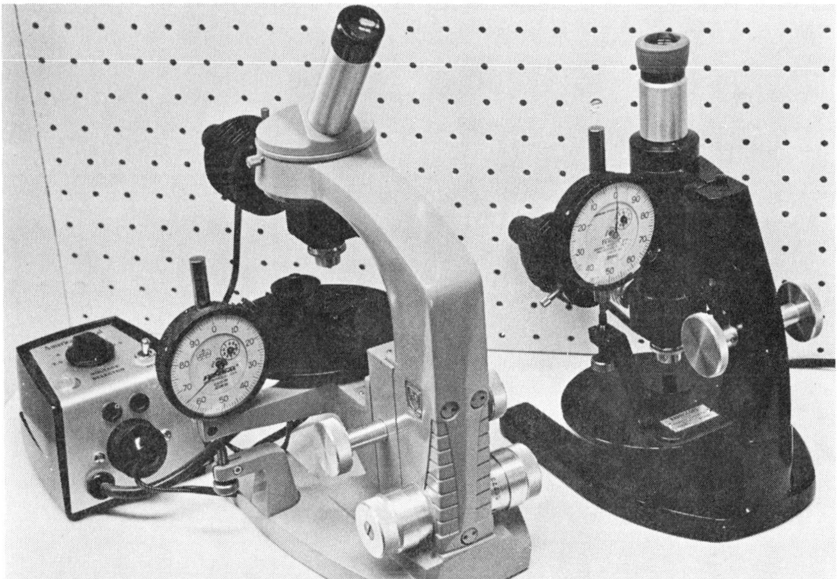

Figure 3–12. Radiuscopes.

higher stellate target, is first brought into sharp focus. The radius is determined first by a reading of the inner dial, which is calibrated in 1.0 mm. increments, and then by addition to this reading of the value from the large outer dial, which is calibrated in 0.01 mm. increments. If the higher or aerial image is not centered, it should be centered by adjustment of the stage. The reading should then be repeated.

If the central posterior surface has a single spherical curve, the eight limbs of the target will come into focus simultaneously. If the central posterior surface of the lens is toric, the limbs of the target will not be simultaneously focused with the higher target reading. For reading a toric surface, the holder should be rotated until one of the limbs representing the principal meridian is continuous. Then the down reading should be zeroed in, and the knob turned until the steeper of the two principal meridians comes into focus. This reading is taken. The knob is turned toward the observer further until the flatter of the two principal meridians comes into focus. This reading is taken.

R–C Device. This device is placed on a Lensometer or Vertometer. The anterior contact lens surface is placed against a liquid (having an index of

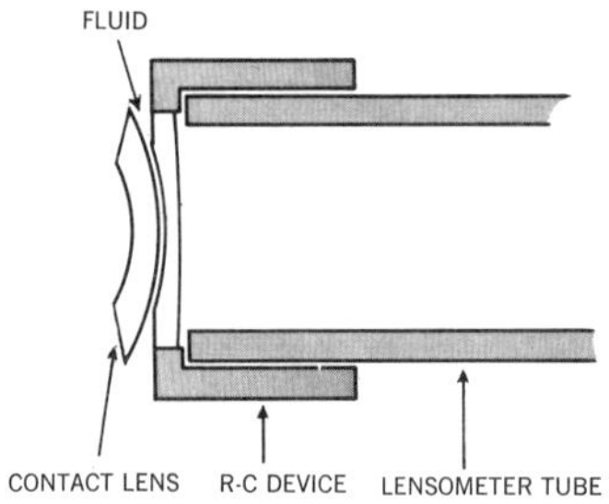

Figure 3–13. Sectional drawing of a contact lens affixed to an R–C device placed on a Lensometer.

refraction of 1.49) that has been placed on the device (Figs. 3–13 and 3–14). The power is read and is converted to base curvature by an appropriate table.

Secondary Radii

With most commonly used instruments, it is difficult or sometimes impossible to verify the radius of a secondary curvature, especially when more than one radius has been used, because the width of a secondary curve is usually quite small, the radius is usually not true throughout, and the optical quality is poor. These factors interfere with the regular reflection of light needed in an instrument such as an Ophthalmometer or Radiuscope. Also, in an Ophthalmometer, the distance between the miral reflection is about 3 mm. This distance is greater than the width of the secondary curve.

Procedures for verifying curvature based on refraction of light may not be applicable because of the narrow width, the poor imagery through the secondary curvature, and the fact that edging affects the anterior curvature.

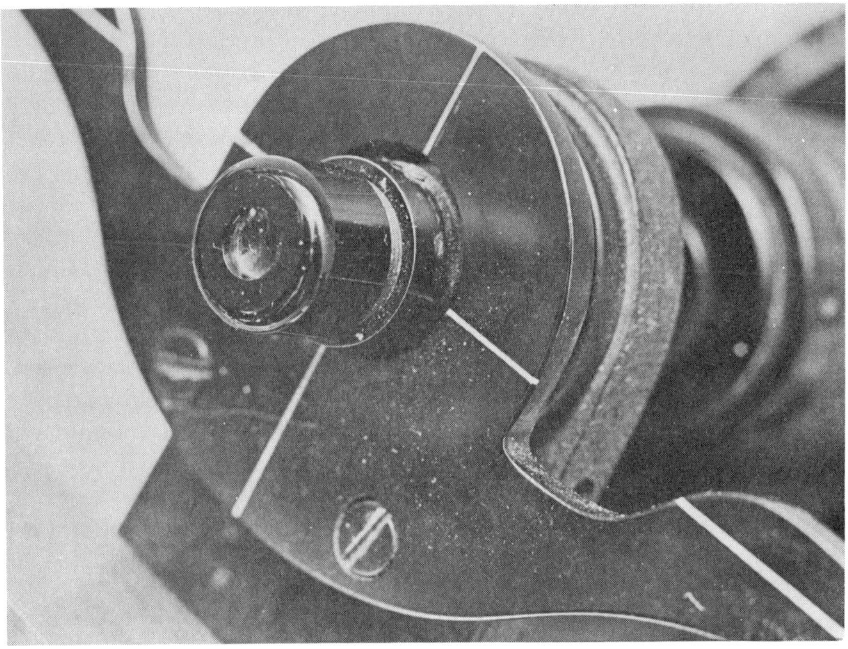

Figure 3–14. R–C device on a Lensometer.

Tolerance. Because it is so difficult to verify accurately secondary radii, it is imperative that they be fabricated properly. The manufacturer's tolerance in his own procedure should be quite strict. Once a secondary curve or series of secondary curves has been applied to a lens, the verification may be limited simply to accepting the fact that they are accurate. Manufacturing procedure should place controlled pressure on the lens, and there should be no undue lens flexing. In the manufacturing process, secondary curvatures may be placed on the thick button before the anterior curvature and final center thickness are fabricated. The thickness of the button provides stability and reduces the possible error from lens flexing. Tools should be checked and care used to ensure that the correct tools are used. They should be labeled in radii so that errors in converting from diopters to radii are not produced. Although this method is not quite so accurate, the secondary curves can be placed on a semifinished (uncut) lens if the pressure is consistent and the lens is mounted so that its anterior surface is securely and uniformly supported. This procedure is discussed more fully on page 170.

If a secondary curvature is about 0.6 mm. or more wide, its radius may be determined. Even then, verification accuracy may be within 0.1 mm. or less for the reasons mentioned above. Because variance of secondary curve radii affects performance, inability to verify these curves accurately is a problem.

The best solution to this problem at present is to employ a laboratory that applies secondary curves on the button or that controls the pressure on the uncut lens. Any diagnostic lenses should be made by the same laboratory using the same procedure, ensuring reasonable consistency in secondary curvatures. When possible, the secondary radius should be verified by one of two methods.

EQUIPMENT. A Radiuscope or a Lensometer may be used.[182,183] It has been suggested that the radius of a single secondary curvature may be determined by placement of the lens on a tool of known radius and evaluation of the fluorescein pattern. It has also been suggested that the secondary area of the lens be coated and then a polishing tool applied to see its grinding action. A third suggestion is that the fluorescein pattern on the eye be evaluated with both a given precision diagnostic lens and a similar lens processed for the patient. In general, none of these suggested procedures is sufficiently accurate.

PROCEDURE. *Radiuscope.* The lens is positioned as it is for reading the base curve. The aperture for the beam of light is reduced to about 3.5 mm. so that a small area can be measured. This may be done by cutting a hole in a piece of tape and placing it on the end of the tube. Reducing the size of the beam of light reduces accuracy somewhat. The lens holder is tilted until the filament doubles. Often the stage must be moved to keep the filament image in the field of view. The adjustment knob is turned until the lower or steeper reading of the two aerial images is brought into focus. This focus is noted. The knob is then turned until the higher or flatter reading of the two aerial images is brought into focus. The difference between the two readings indicates approximately how much flatter the secondary is than the base.

Lensometer or Vertometer. There is more plus power in the secondary curvature than in the optic-zone area. In some cases, the radius of the secondary curvature can be determined on the basis of this fact. Posterior vertex thick lens formulation is used. This procedure is not applicable if the anterior surface of the lens is altered, if the optic zone is larger than 8.0 mm., or if the secondary is not a true curve.

Distance power is read, and the drum is moved in the plus direction until another relatively clear miral image is seen. This is secondary power. It is often necessary to darken the room and to move the lens in front of the aperture of the Lensometer or Vertometer so that more of the secondary curvature is in front of the aperture. The practitioner must make certain not to move the lens too far; otherwise, he might not effectively read the power of some part of the lens. If the lens is moved too far, the reading will be plano, assuming the eyepiece was properly focused initially.

The algebraic difference between the central and the secondary power readings is found. Then the difference between the radius of the secondary area and the base radius is found by the formula:

$$\frac{\text{Lensometer power difference} \times 0.1}{0.75} = R$$

where R is the amount by which the secondary curve is longer than the base curve.

The formula is not completely accurate, because the differences in thickness and the effect of spherical aberration have not been completely considered. The accuracy of the formula is probably no better than ± 0.1 to 0.2 mm.

A verification instrument (Toposcope) based on the principle of moiré fringes has recently been developed. The Toposcope can verify many contact lens characteristics (p. 411).

LENS MODIFICATION

There are two basic categories of lens modification. The first category consists of modifications done before lenses are delivered to the patient, including modifications on uncut lenses to make finished lenses, and modifications done to finished lenses to improve their characteristics. The second category includes modifications done after lenses are delivered to the patient and he starts to wear and adapt to them. Adaptation may indicate that one or more characteristics should be modified to fulfill basic goals better.

Each practitioner should understand modification, even if he does not do the work himself.[184] The practitioner must know what can and cannot be done and what results can be expected. The authors feel that some modification facilities should be available in each office for the following reasons: (1) There is not the delay and resultant inconvenience to the patient that occurs when lenses are returned to the manufacturer for modification. (2) Communication problems between practitioner and manufacturer are eliminated. (3) Results of modification can be quickly evaluated and supplemented if necessary.

Several problems may arise from the practitioner's making his own modifications. Although the work is relatively simple, satisfactory results demand attention to detail, utilization of proper procedure, and sufficient practice. Most fitters have a relatively small volume of contact lens work. They may not develop and maintain the desired level of technical skill. Some modification procedures take considerable time, making it economically unsound for a busy practitioner to do much of his own modification work.

In general, a practitioner or someone in his office should do the work only when the quality will be at least equal to that of the manufacturer's work. Because of the advantages of making modifications in the office, the practitioner or one of his employees should develop the skills needed for making proper modifications.

Equipment

Contact lens modification equipment can be purchased from many manufacturers. All equipment is basically the same, varying only in some details. Initial sets should have the following equipment:

1. There should be a motor-driven spindle mounted in a pan or bucket, which protects the worker from the spray of liquid during operation of the spindle. The motor may have a single speed, usually between 1,000 and 1,500 r.p.m., or it may have varying speeds controlled by a hand or foot rheostat. Because various operations are best done at different speeds, the variable-speed unit is preferable. The spindle may be in the form of a Jacob chuck or a projected spindle (Fig. 3–15).

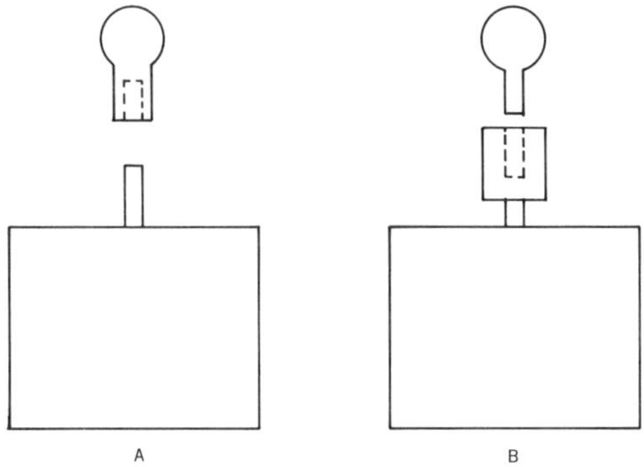

Figure 3–15. A, *Tool being placed on a projected spindle.* B, *Tool being placed in a Jacob chuck.*

2. There should be a series of polishing tools with varying radii for applying secondary curvatures. A beginning set adequate for most needs consists of 23 polishing tools. Radii should range from 7.80 mm. to 9.50 mm. in 0.1 mm. steps and from 10.00 to 12.50 in 0.50 mm. steps (Fig. 3–16). If the practitioner works on uncut lenses, grinding tools from 7.80 to 9.50 mm. in 0.1 mm. steps are advisable.
3. Initial sets of contact lens modification equipment should include implements for holding the lens during various modification procedures. These holders may be chucks, arbors, blocks, spinners, or suction cups (Fig. 3–17).
4. There should be materials to make the lens adhere to the holder and materials to act as polishing surfaces. The adherent material is double-faced tape, wax, or dental impression material; the polishing material is usually single-faced adhesive tape or Mystic tape (used to produce a hard polishing pad) or jewelers' velveteen (used to produce a soft polishing pad).
5. There should be implements for cutting lens diameters and for edging

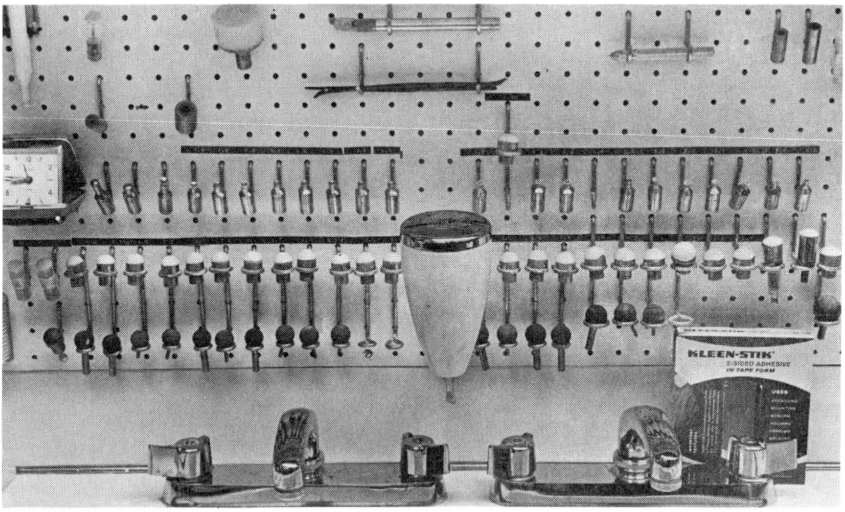

Figure 3–16. Laboratory equipment. Polishing tools are in the next to bottom row, and grinding tools are in the bottom row.

procedures. These may be single-edged razor blades, surgical knives, or files (Fig. 3–23).

6. There should be implements for removing scratches from a lens and for changing power.

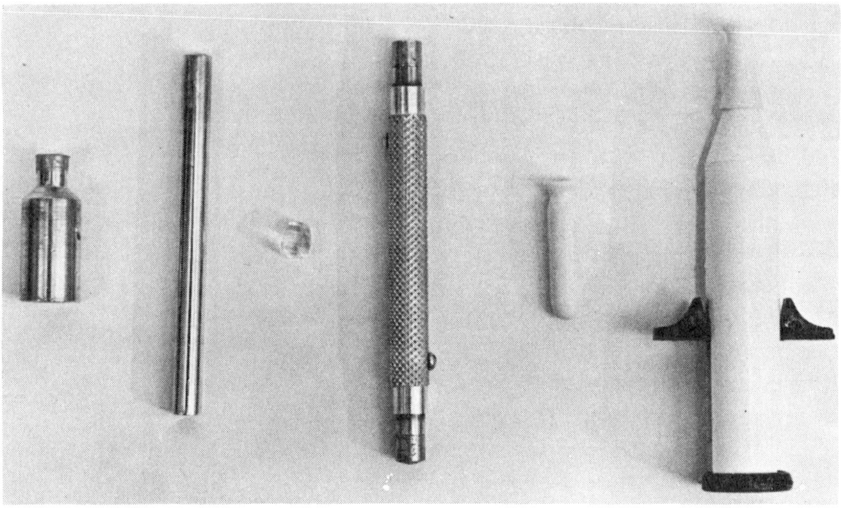

Figure 3–17. Types of holders. From left to right, chuck, arbor, block, spinner, and suction cups.

Mounting and Centering Procedures

For any modification procedure, the lens should be correctly mounted on an appropriate holder. Mounting should result in a lens that is properly centered and securely held throughout the modification procedure. This is extremely important. If the lens is not properly mounted, modification will usually be poor.

In general, the lens may be mounted one of two ways. First, it may be mounted on an appropriate holder placed on the motor-driven spindle. Modification implements are then applied manually. Second, it may be mounted on an appropriate holder that is held manually. Modification implements are then affixed to the motor-driven spindle.

Three materials commonly used to affix the lens to a metallic holder (chuck, arbor, block, or spinner) are double-faced tape, wax, and dental impression material. Chucks, arbors, and blocks may be made of plastic.

Double-faced Tape. This tape usually comes in rolls, although it is possible to purchase circular cutouts of various sizes. In either case, one side has a protective coating. When a roll is used, a rectangular piece of tape slightly larger than the head of the holder is cut off.

Before tape is applied to the holder, the head of the holder should be cleaned (see p. 169). The cleaning fluid is then wiped from the head. The exposed adhesive side is firmly attached to the lens holder, and the protective coating is left on the other side. The protective coating is then peeled off. It is important that the tape completely covers the head of the holder. If it does not, the metallic rim of the holder may mar the surface of the lens when pressure is applied. If a very thin double-faced tape is used, it may be necessary to use two layers. When double-faced tape is used, the lens may be geometrically centered in one of three ways—visually, mechanically, or optically. Mechanical centering is usually best.

Visual Centering. The lens is approximately visually centered and placed gently on a holder covered with double-faced tape. The motor is shut off, and the holder is mounted on the spindle. The edge of the lens is visually aligned with a stationary point such as the edge of the unit. The practitioner holds the head steady, and slowly turns the holder. If the lens is centered, the edge remains aligned with the mark as the holder is turned. If the lens is not centered, the edge does not remain aligned. The lens is gently repositioned until it is aligned. After this is done for 360°, the lens should be centered. Pressure is then applied by the end of a finger so that the lens adheres firmly to the holder (Fig. 3–18).

Mechanical Centering. A centering device is used (Fig. 3–19). The lens is approximately centered visually and lightly affixed to a chuck, having a head about 1 to 2 mm. smaller than the lens diameter. This relatively large head gives more support to the lens and reduces the possibility of the lens flexing. The holder is placed on the spindle, and the centering device is

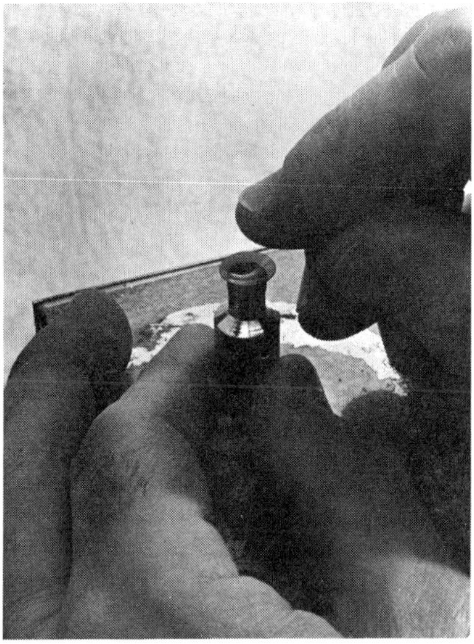

Figure 3–18. Visual centering. Note the alignment of the edge of the lens and the edge of the unit.

gently carried up and tapped down (Fig. 3–20). It should not be released. The holder is rotated about a quarter turn and the procedure repeated. This is done while a turn of approximately 360° is made.

For best results, the diameters of the body of the holder and of the opening in the centering device should be almost identical. There should be only enough difference to permit insertion and removal.

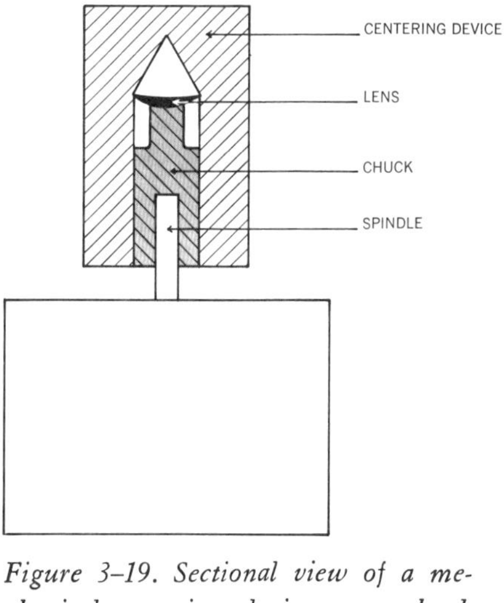

Figure 3–19. Sectional view of a mechanical centering device on a chuck holding a lens.

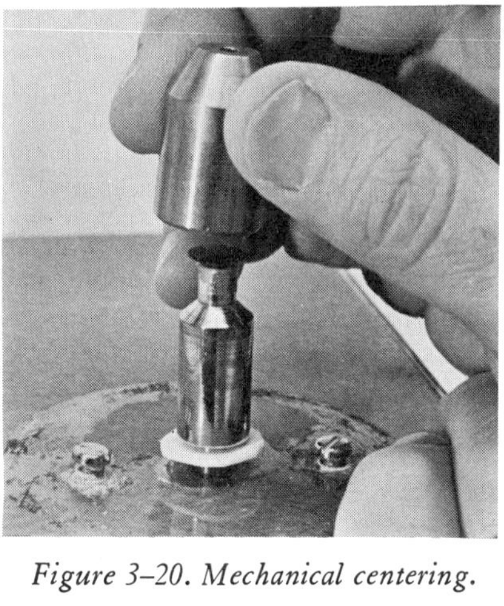

Figure 3–20. Mechanical centering.

Optical Centering. The optical and geometric centers of a nonprismatic lens coincide. If the optical center of the lens is spotted and exactly superimposed on the geometric center of the head of the holder, the lens will be geometrically centered on the holder. The optical center of the lens may be determined by holding the concave surface of the lens against the Lensometer stop. The power drum is set at the appropriate power, and the lens is moved until the target image is centered. The lens is then lightly spotted with the middle dotting pin of the Lensometer.

The geometric center of the head of a holder covered with tape must be determined. This determination may be made by placement of a pointed scribe on the surface of the double-faced tape and adjustment of it toward the center of the holder until there is no wobble. A small indentation is produced in the tape at the geometric center.

It is possible to have the central pin of the Lensometer dotting device removed. An arbor the head of which is covered with tape may be inserted here. The lens is held in front of the aperture stop and moved until the target is centered. The working device is brought into contact with the lens until it is affixed.

To check the centering visually after any of these procedures, the lens holder is mounted on the spindle. A light is placed so that there is a reflection of the bulb from the lens surface. The motor is turned on at a relatively slow speed. If the lens is properly centered, there will be no oscillation of the image of the bulb.

Wax. When wax is used, the holder is placed on a long rod that has a nonconducting material wrapped around one end. The head of the holder is heated by the flame from an alcohol lamp. When the head is hot enough, the wax is held against it. The wax melts and covers the head (Fig. 3–21).

The holder is placed on the spindle, and the lens is approximately centered visually on the holder. The motor is turned on, and a round pencil is gently pressed against the edge of the rotating lens to center it (Fig. 3–22).

Dental Impression Material. A quick-setting, rubber-base dental impression material may be used. As indicated by the manufacturer, the base and the accelerator are spatulated, and the head of the chuck or block is coated. The lens is approximately centered visually, and it is then centered exactly

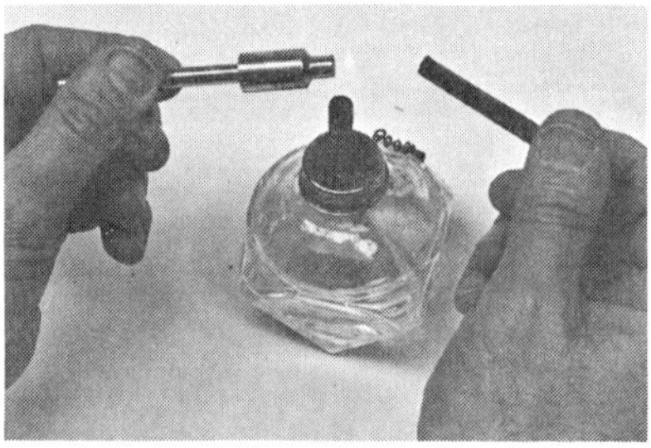

Figure 3–21. Application of wax to a holder.

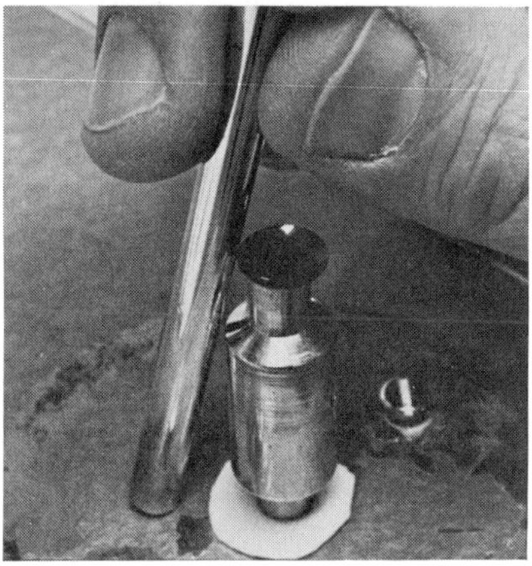

Figure 3–22. Centering a lens on wax.

with a mechanical centering device or with the centering procedure used with wax.

Characteristics That Can Be Modified

Certain aspects of a finished contact lens can be modified; other aspects can be altered only by the processing of a new lens. The following six modifications can be made to a finished lens: (1) lens diameter can be reduced; (2) secondary curves can be flattened, widened, or added; (3) transitional juncture between two adjacent curves can be blended; (4) the edge can be contoured, thinned, or polished; (5) the amount of power can be changed by approximately −0.75 D or +0.37 D; (6) and superficial surface scratches can be polished.

It should be realized that certain procedures modify only one characteristic of the lens, whereas others simultaneously modify more than one characteristic. Those that basically modify only one characteristic are surface polishing, changing the power, and blending between two adjacent secondary curves.

Those that modify more than one characteristic include: (1) Decreasing the lens diameter, which also reduces the width of the secondary area and increases edge thickness. (2) Flattening the secondary curve radius, which may thin the edge of the lens and which produces a more distinct juncture between adjacent posterior lens curves. (3) Widening the secondary curve adjacent to the optic zone, which decreases optic-zone diameter and thins the edge on a bicurve lens. (4) Adding secondary curves with radii longer than the radii of existing curves, which thins the edge and may result in a sharp juncture between two adjacent curves. (5) Blending between the optic zone and secondary curvature, which decreases optic-zone diameter. (6) Finishing the edge, which decreases the lens diameter and may produce an area like a flat peripheral secondary curve.

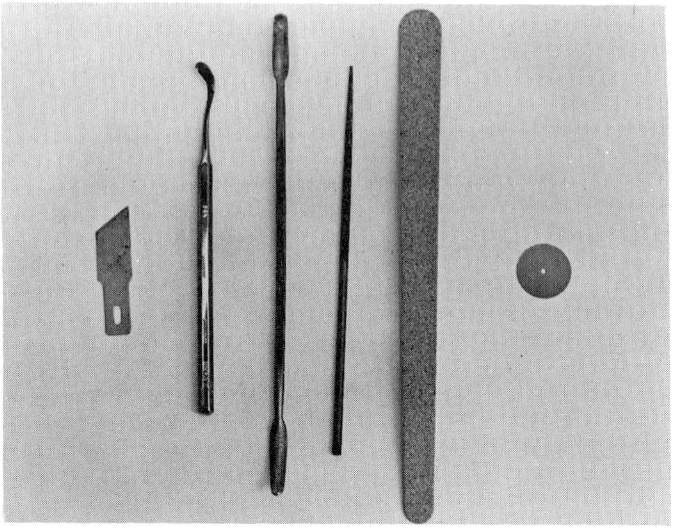

Figure 3–23. Cutting tools. From left to right—single edged razor blade, surgical knife, screw finishing file, rattail file, emery board, and sanding disk.

It is necessary to understand these modifications and their secondary effects. Because modification to change one characteristic often alters another, it is necessary to modify in a certain sequence. If the sequence is not followed, a subsequent modification may alter a previous one. The order is: (1) lens diameter reduction; (2) secondary curvature modification (flattening, widening, addition, or blending); (3) edge finishing, in which the lens diameter is decreased and in which proper allowance must be made; and (4) resurfacing (power change or scratch removal).

Diameter Reduction

Cutting Tool Held Manually. The lens is mounted concave side up on a chuck or arbor. Cutting tools such as single-edged razor blades, surgical knives, files, emery boards, or sanding disks are held manually (Fig. 3–23). The unit is turned on and set to about 1,200 r.p.m.

As the lens rotates, the cutting tool is brought directly to bear on the edge of the lens. Care must be taken not to scratch the anterior or posterior surfaces of the lens. When a file is used, its flat side is placed against the lens. When a razor blade or surgical knife is used, the cutting edge must be slanted in the direction of lens rotation. If it is slanted against the direction of lens rotation, there is a greater possibility of chipping or breaking the lens (Figs. 3–24 and 3–25).

Pressure of the cutting tool against the lens should be light and constant. When the lens is not properly centered, vibration may be felt and a decentered lens will be produced.

In making diameter reductions, it is important to consider edge thickness and amount of reduction desired. The thinner the edge, the quicker it is reduced. When the edge is thin or when small reductions are desired, a fine file or a sanding disk is preferable to a razor or knife. Razors and knives may cut too quickly, and there is danger of too great a reduction. For small reductions and near the completion of large reductions, the cutting procedure should involve an edging motion.

The diameter is repeatedly checked until it is about 0.1 to 0.2 mm. oversize in minus lenses and 0.2 or 0.3 mm. oversize in plus lenses. This excess is needed because of diameter reduction produced as a by-product of edge finishing.

Cutting Tool on Spindle. A *cutdown stone* is an emery tool having a 60 to 90° cone. It is best to use emery having a fine grain. The stone is mounted on the spindle, and the lens is mounted with its convex side secured to a chuck, arbor, spinner, or suction cup.

Before the motor is turned on, the holder is placed in the cone with its axis aligned with the axis of the spindle. This arrangement causes the surface of the lens to be relatively parallel with the floor and not tilted in the cone (Fig. 3–26).

The stone must be kept moist with water throughout the operation to prevent burning and marring of the lens edge. The motor is turned on, and the lens diameter is reduced. It is important to keep the axis of the holder and that of the spindle properly aligned. If this alignment is not maintained, a decentered lens is produced.

Machined Lenses. Some lenses are punched out or cut by a lathe that is set to the appropriate size. The instrumentation for this procedure is somewhat expensive and usually is found only in manufacturing laboratories.

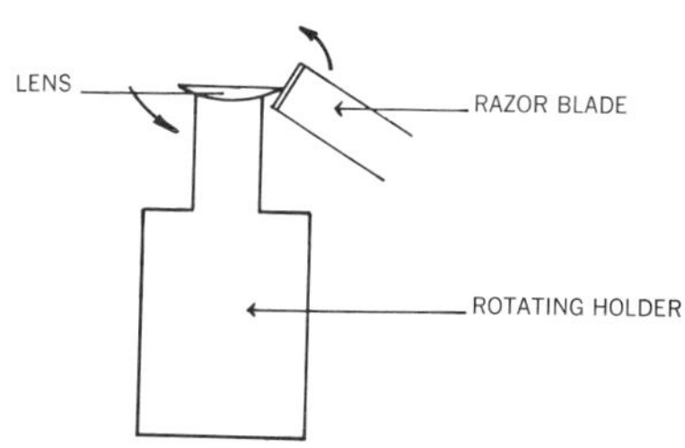

Figure 3–24. When lens diameter is reduced with a razor blade, the cutting edge is slanted with the direction of lens rotation.

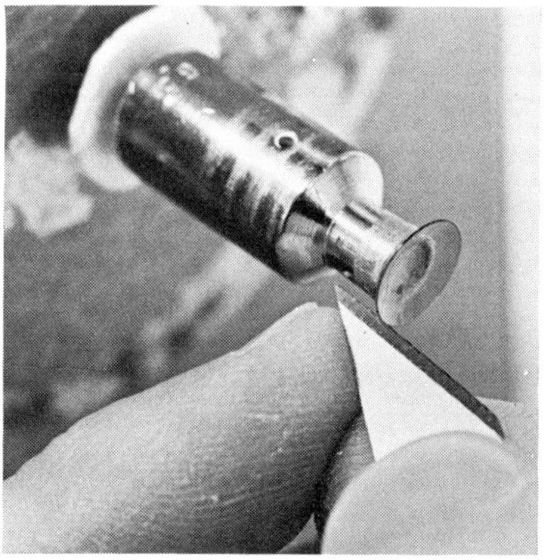

Figure 3–25. Cutting lens diameter with a single-edged razor blade.

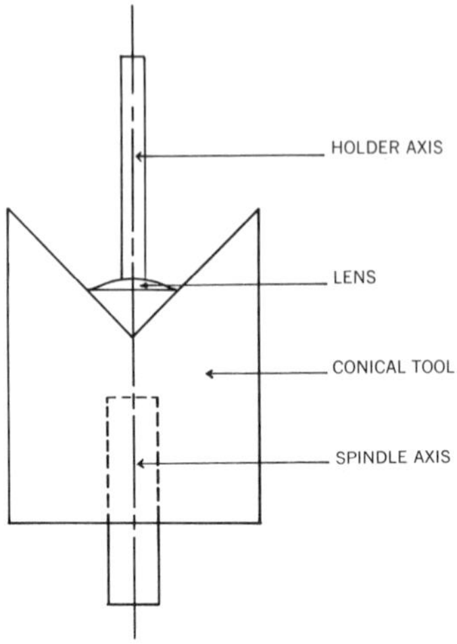

Figure 3–26. Sectional view showing that when lens diameter is cut with a conical tool, the axis of the holder is aligned with the axis of the spindle.

Posterior Curvatures

Because the basic procedures for any application of curves to the secondary area of the posterior surface are similar, they are considered together. These procedures include the placing of one or more secondary curvatures on an uncut lens, and the flattening, widening, adding, or blending of curves on a finished lens.[185]

Tools. Usually, annular spherical curvatures are desired. They are fabricated by spherical tools, or laps, having curvatures of various radii. There are two types of laps. The first has a rough surface and produces lens curvature by grinding, leaving a relatively rough surface. The grinding tool should not have too coarse a grain or the resultant curvature becomes coarse, making it difficult to be properly polished. The second type of lap has a smooth surface and produces curvature by polishing, leaving a relatively smooth surface.

Pads. These are placed on tools for polishing purposes. To produce the proper finish, the surface of the pads should be fine and smooth. To avoid change in the thickness of pads, they should be firm, or noncompressible, and should resist the absorption of water.

Because Mystic tape and nonwaterproof adhesive tape fulfill these criteria, they are the most satisfactory materials for pads. Such tapes also have adhesive backing, which simplifies affixing them to the tools. Pads of this sort are considered hard pads.

The most commonly used material for a soft pad is jewelers' velveteen. Because soft pads are quite compressible and absorb a considerable amount of liquid, they do not generate as true a curve as a hard pad. Thus, they are not recommended for general use. They are recommended for blending, because here the true radius of the curvature is probably less important than the blending action.

When a pad is placed on a tool of a given radius, the radius of the tool is lengthened by an amount equal to the thickness of the pad. Each material used for polishing pads has a specific thickness that can be measured with a thickness gauge. Because the point of the gauge indents the tape, an error is introduced. This error can be eliminated by mounting the tape between two razor blades of measured thickness. Blade thickness subtracted from the thickness of the combination gives the tape thickness. Nonwaterproof adhesive tape has a thickness of about 0.20 mm. Mystic tape has a thickness of about 0.20 mm. Jewelers' velveteen has a thickness of about 0.28 mm. The radius that is engraved on the tools in various modification units may or may not reflect compensated radii. This factor should be determined when the unit is purchased.

When the pad is placed on the tool, it must be uniform. If the pad is stretched more in one area, it is also thinned. Thinning causes the effective radius to vary. The surface of the pad should be smoothed so that there is no bunching.

For a hard pad, the tool is mounted on the spindle. The head of the tool is cleaned (see p. 169), and it is then dried. A rectangular piece of tape somewhat larger than the head of the tool is cut from the roll, placed on the tool, and smoothed down. A single-edge razor blade or an Exacto knife blade is placed at the juncture of the head of the tool and its base (Fig. 3–27).

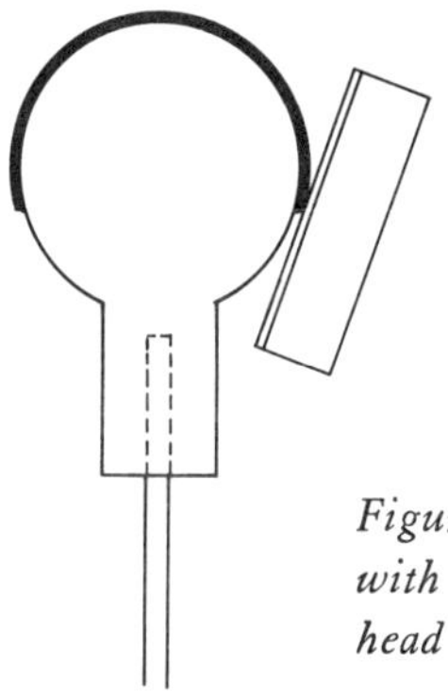

Figure 3–27. Cutting off excess tape with razor blade at juncture of tool head and base.

It is held there firmly, and the motor is turned on at about 2,000 r.p.m. As the tool rotates, the excess tape is cut away. This excess is peeled off. A smooth towel or a contact lens button having a base curve—that is, a semi-finished lens—is then pressed on the tape and rocked back and forth as the tool rotates to smooth the tape out and remove folds and gaps without stretching the tape.

Soft pads may be placed on top of a tool with a hard pad. Velveteen typically does not have an adhesive backing. A piece of velveteen should be cut larger than the head of a tool covered with a hard pad. The velveteen is then stretched over the tool head and is temporarily held with an elastic band wound around the velveteen extending over the base (Fig. 3–28).

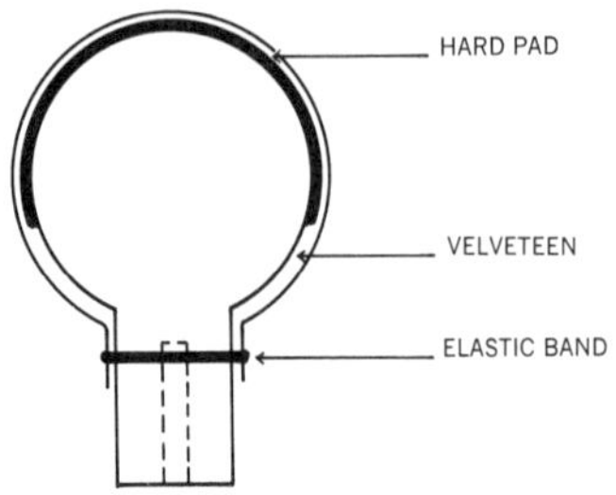

Figure 3–28. Velveteen stretched over hard pad and held by elastic band.

Allowance for both the velveteen and tape thickness must be made. If extreme curvature accuracy and surface quality are desired, a lap having pitch for a polishing surface can be used.

COMPOUNDS. Four types of compounds are used in contact lens work: polishing, grinding, protecting, and cleaning.

Polishing Compounds. Optical grade tin (stannic) oxide or Silvo silver polish is commonly used. To produce a satisfactory polish, the consistency of the compound must be somewhat thick. This thickness helps maintain the compound on the tool head as the tool rotates and helps produce adequate polishing action. Desired consistency is obtained by mixing one to two parts of tin oxide to one part of water. Silvo is used as it comes, or it is thickened slightly by the addition of a little glycerine.

Polishing compounds may be kept in a dish and applied with a fine brush. However, this method may result in several problems. Other compounds may accidentally get into the polish, a hair from the brush may stick to the tool, or lumps of polish may be placed on the tool. It is preferable, therefore, to place the polishing compound in, and apply it from a plastic squeeze bottle. Before the compound is used, it should be mixed to produce a relatively uniform consistency and to eliminate lumps. When it is kept in a bottle, the bottle should be shaken.

Grinding. A tool made of, or impregnated with, an abrasive material can be used. Grinding can also be performed with a tool having a smooth surface by the application of an abrasive material suspended in a liquid medium. It is definitely preferable to use the first procedure.

Rough tools are generally made of Crystolon (silicon carbide) or emery. The Crystolon grade used is no. 70 to no. 400. Lower numbers indicate coarser grades; higher numbers indicate finer grades. The coarser the abrasive, the quicker but rougher the cutting action is. When a coarse abrasive is used, the lens is more difficult to polish. Rough tools impregnated with diamond chips are available. They have a fine, fast-grinding action.

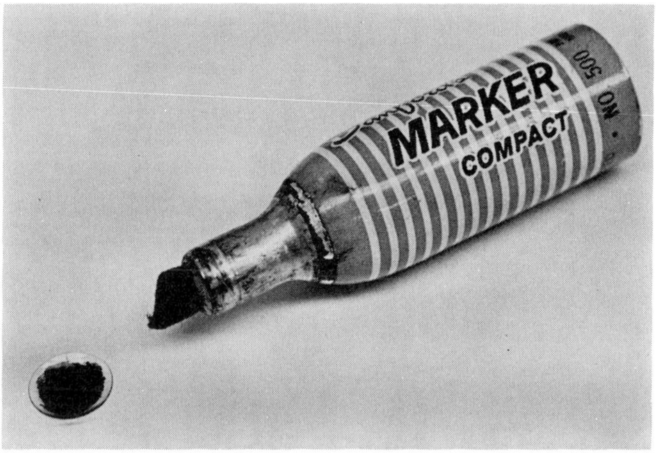

Figure 3–29. The optic zone is coated for protection.

When a rough tool is used, it should be kept constantly wet during operation to prevent burning and marring of the lens surface. Water spread by a brush or ejected from a squeeze bottle is used.

Protection. When secondary posterior curvatures are being fabricated, it is often advisable to protect the posterior optic-zone area. Any commercially available waterproof marking implement with a felt tip (Fig. 3–29) can provide such protection. The optic-zone area is covered with a thin coating, which is allowed to dry for about a minute. To remove the coating, lighter fluid or Tama may be used.

Some practitioners prefer to coat the entire posterior surface of the lens when fabricating secondary curvatures. As the secondary curve is ground into the lens, the coating is ground off. With this method, it is easy to determine the width of the curve. However, such coatings may clog the surfaces of the tools. When clogging occurs, grinding tools should be cleaned with lighter fluid or Tama. Polishing pads should be changed.

Two other protective factors should be considered, although they do not involve protective compounds. If a lens is dropped into the bucket during modification, the weight of the holder may cause the lens to be chipped or scratched. To reduce this possibility, the bucket should be lined with foam rubber. The foam rubber must be placed so that it does not interfere with the movement of the spindle or the modification procedure (Fig. 3–30). Because liquids are used, it is possible for the motor of the unit to become wet. Thus, it is necessary in some units to place a protective cover around the exposed base of the spindle (Fig. 3–31).

Cleaning Compounds. Lighter fluid, Tama, carbon tetrachloride, or benzine can be used to clean the tools and to remove coatings from contact

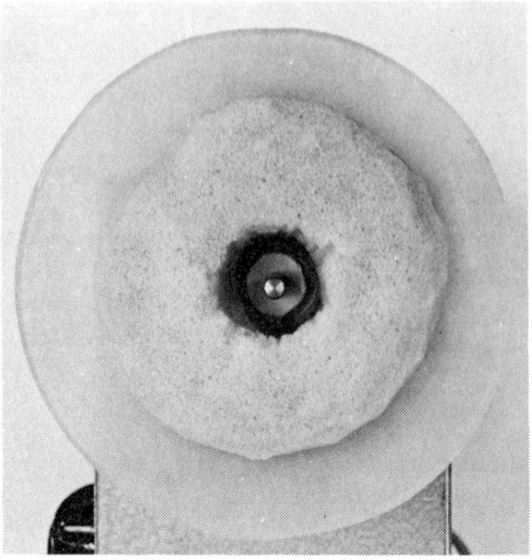

Figure 3–30. Foam protector in a bucket, viewed from above.

lenses. After they are used on a contact lens, the lens must be *thoroughly* cleaned with wetting solution and water before it is placed on the eye.

MOUNTING. Proper mounting and centration have been discussed (p. 160). There is another important related factor. Modification of posterior secondary curvatures is almost always done by the practitioner for relatively thin lenses. Such lenses flex with pressure. When secondary curvatures are added to a lens, pressure is applied to the holder by the practitioner and by the weight of the holder. This pressure may flex the lens and produce secondary curvatures with incorrect radii or even undesired toricity. The problem may be reduced by mounting the lens on an appropriate holder and by controlling pressure. Theoretically, the radius of the concave surface of the holder should equal the radius of the convex surface of the lens, and the diameter of the head of the holder should at least be equal to that of the lens. This

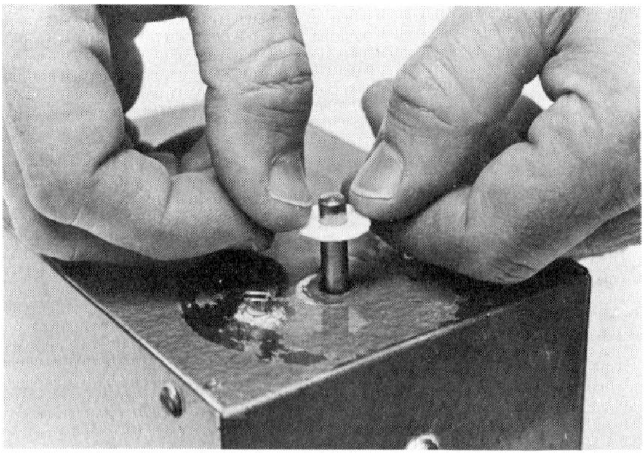

Figure 3–31. Protective cover being pushed down to the base of the spindle.

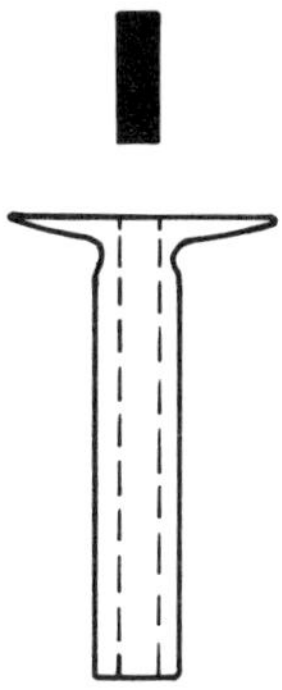

Figure 3–32. Cylindrical plastic tube to be placed in stem of suction cup to reduce flexibility.

procedure would prevent flexing and hold the curves of the lens constant. However, many holders with various heads would be needed.

Satisfactory results can be obtained when a holder with a head about 1 mm. smaller than the lens diameter is used. Flexibility for a given thickness is inversely related to length. Because only a narrow area of the lens is not supported, flexibility is not too great, as long as pressure is not too great. Double-faced tape, wax, or dental impression material is used to affix the lens to the holder. The tape conforms somewhat to the anterior curvature of the lens. Wax and dental impression material conform almost exactly. A series of holders having diameters of 10 mm., 9 mm., 8 mm., and 7 mm. and concave surface radius of 7.00 to 8.00 mm. is usually satisfactory.

It is possible to hold the lens with a suction cup for some operations. Most suction cups are too flexible, both in their barrel and their head, and provide poor support for the lens. Lens flexure can be minimized somewhat by a hollow, cylindrical plastic tube placed in the stem of the suction cup (Fig. 3–32). The tube should be depressed far enough so that it does not touch and mar the surface of the lens. The lens is centered visually. Because of flexure and poor centration, use of a suction cup is recommended only for blending or addition of narrow peripheral curves.

Rotation. As a tool rotates, different areas of the tool move at different velocities. In each revolution, areas closer to the center, or axis, of the tool move a shorter distance than those near the edge of the tool (Fig. 3–33). Thus, the velocity of the peripheral areas must be greater than that of the central areas; the further from the axis of rotation a point is, the greater is its velocity. The greater the velocity is, the greater the grinding action is. For example, in Fig. 3–34, when a nonrotating lens is held against a rotating tool, there is greater grinding action in area *A* than in area *B*. This difference produces an unequal secondary width.

To equalize the grinding action, the lens must also rotate or be rocked back and forth across the tool. The rocking is often done in a figure-eight pattern. When either the lens or the tool rotates, it is a *single-rotation procedure*. When both rotate, it is a *double-rotation procedure*.

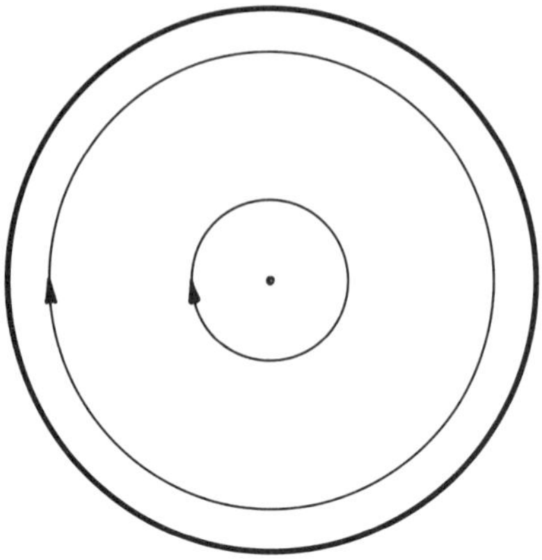

Figure 3–33. For each revolution of a tool, central points travel shorter distances than peripheral points.

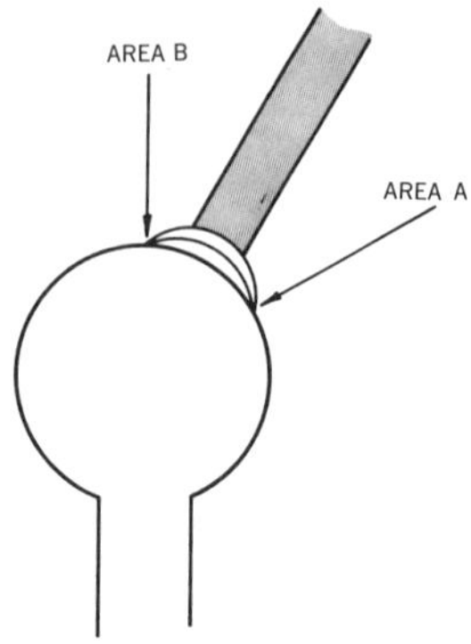

Figure 3–34. When a lens is held without rotation against a tool, there is a greater grinding action in area A *than in area* B.

Procedure. Posterior curvatures may be fabricated in one of two ways. The first involves grinding the desired curve with a rough tool and then polishing it with a smooth tool. The second involves only polishing the curve on with a smooth tool. The authors feel that the first procedure is generally advisable only when the radius of the curvature is at least 0.6 mm. longer than that of the base curve or next steepest curve, and the curvature width is at least 0.6 mm. Following this guideline reduces the possibility of marring the lens, yet permits relatively quick, accurate modification.

Grinding and Polishing. If the unit has a removable bucket, it must be placed on the unit. In some units, the foam pad protector and motor protector are positioned. When a Jacob chuck unit is used, the shaft of the rough tool is placed in the opening. The sides of the chuck are secured against the tool shaft with an Allen wrench or key (Fig. 3–35). When a projecting shaft unit is used, an adapter may have to be placed on the spindle. The tool shaft is then placed in the opening of the adapter (Fig. 3–36).

When a variable speed unit is used, rotation is set between 1,200 and 1,500 r.p.m. The tool is thoroughly wetted with water either brushed on or squeezed from a plastic bottle. The tool must be kept constantly wet to prevent burning and marring of the plastic. The lens is held with its concave surface against the tool. Pressure on the holder should be light enough to prevent lens flexure, but it should be firm enough to prevent lens vibration. The motor is turned on.

As the lens rotates, a figure-eight motion may be used to further equalize grinding action. The lens is periodically checked with a measuring magnifier to determine the width of the ground area. This area will appear hazy or frosted. When a protective coating is applied to the entire posterior surface,

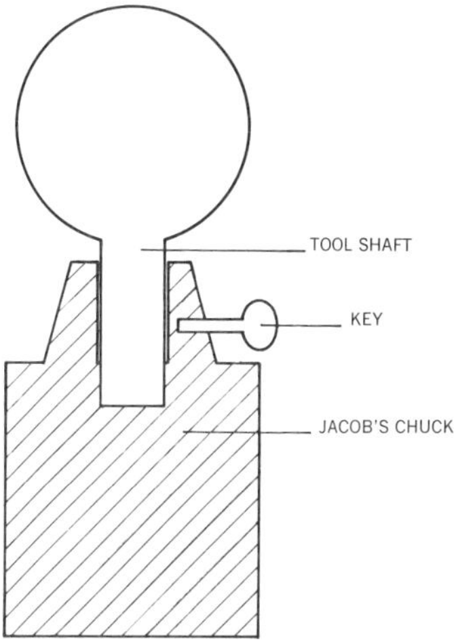

Figure 3–35. A key used to tighten the sides of a Jacob's chuck.

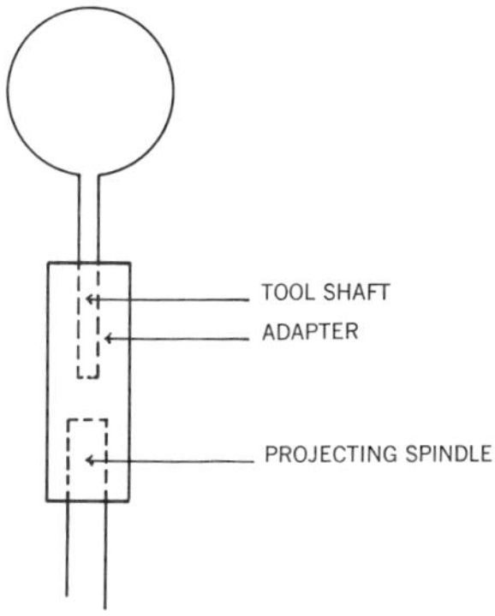

Figure 3–36. An adapter placed on a projection spindle unit to hold the tool shaft.

the area that is ground has had the coating removed during grinding. The procedure is continued until the secondary curve width on each side is 0.15 to 0.20 mm. narrower than that desired. This allowance is for the polishing procedure. When an abrasive compound has been used during a grinding, the lens must be cleaned before polishing.

Polishing. The appropriate tool is chosen (it should be remembered that the radius of the tool has been effectively lengthened an amount equal to the thickness of the pad). When a Jacob chuck unit is used, the shaft of the tool is inserted and secured. When a spindle-type unit is used, the opening in the base of the tool is placed directly on the spindle shaft.

When a hard pad is used, speeds should be relatively slow—1,000 r.p.m. or less—to prevent overheating and warping of the plastic, which may be caused by polishing compound being thrown off and drying of the pad.

Greater speeds, such as 2,000 r.p.m., can be used with a soft pad. A soft pad absorbs more polishing compound and dries less quickly. Even if it dries, there is less tendency for the plastic to burn.

The tool pad is uniformly covered with polishing compound. It must be kept wet by periodic applications of the compound. Generally, the lens is not centered on the tool, but rather it is held at an angle. For blending, however, the lens often is centered (Fig. 3–37). Because blends are narrow and often fabricated quickly, centration assures relatively equal velocity and uniform blending.

The motor is turned on, and the head of the holder is checked to make certain it is rotating.

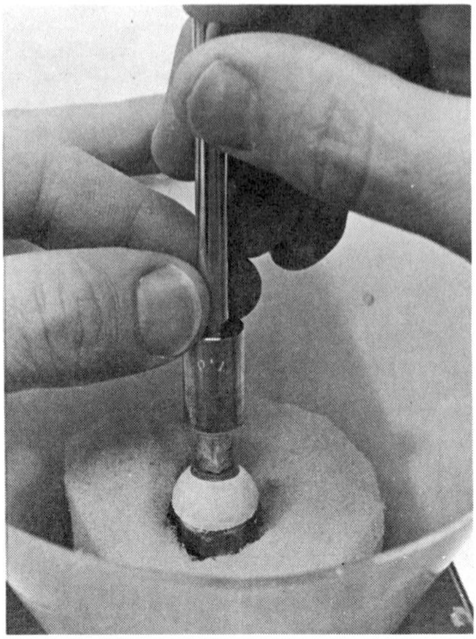

Figure 3–37. Polishing on a secondary curve.

For all procedures but blending, the authors prefer a hard pad for the basic fabrication. A hard pad gives a truer curve than a soft one. Width of the polished area of the curve is checked periodically with a measuring magnifier. The part that has been polished is smooth. Work is continued until the entire area is smooth and the desired width is obtained. When secondary curvature width is about 0.05 mm. less than desired on each side, a soft pad may be used for about 30 to 60 seconds until desired width is achieved. This soft pad produces something of a blending action and improves the luster of the surface polish.

Blending. It is possible to have a sharp transition juncture between two adjacent curvatures. At times, such a juncture may cause problems and must be removed. Removal is accomplished by means of blending. The several types of blends are categorized in terms of the discernibility of the transition between two adjacent curves (see p. 22).

The factors controlling the appearance of the transition are the amount of difference between the two curves, the radius of the blending tool, the type of pad on the blending tool, the speed of the motor, the length of operation time, the polishing compound used, and the pressure applied. Assuming the last two factors are constant, a blend is heavier if the two curves are not greatly dissimilar, if the radius of the blending tool is about half way between the radii of the two curves, if a soft pad is used, if the speed is faster, and if the operation time is longer.

These factors should be controlled to produce the desired blend. They should be recorded for subsequent duplication needs. Usually blends are done best with a soft pad. To avoid marring the base curve, the authors

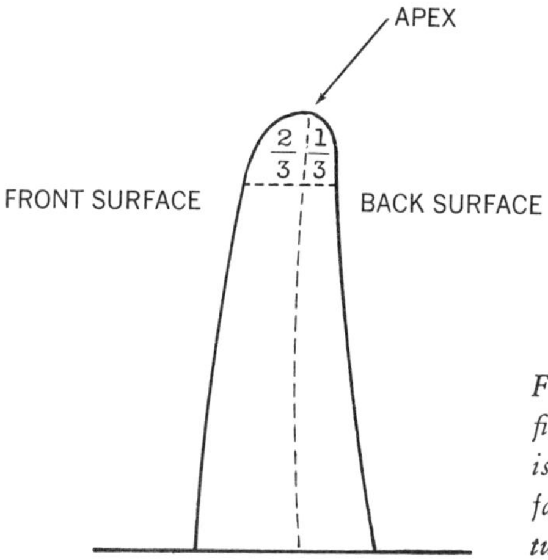

Figure 3–38. A satisfactory edge configuration has a rounded apex, which is one-third nearer to the posterior surface, a taper, and no lips or sharp junctures.

have found that blends between the base curve and a secondary curve must be done carefully.

Edging

A good edge design has proper thickness and configuration. Figure 3–38 shows what the authors feel is a logical and clinically satisfactory edge design. The finished edge thickness at the apex is 0.08 to 0.10 mm., and the edge is tapered. The apex is rounded and it is positioned so that it is about one-third closer to the posterior than to the anterior surface. There are no lips or sharp transition junctures between the edge and the surfaces.

Because verification of edge configuration is highly subjective, it is extremely important that edge fabrication be proper. Proper fabrication involves two basic factors—the theoretic edge design must be proper, and this design must be produced by a relatively accurate and repeatable technique. Edging may be automated or manual.

Automatic edgers are used by some manufacturers and practitioners. Such edgers must be evaluated on the basis of the foregoing factors. The quality of manually produced edges depends not only on the theory behind the technique, but also on the practitioner's technical skill. The skill of the practitioner in turn depends on his knowledge, practice, and attention to detail.

When a minus lens is to be edged manually, the starting lens diameter should be 0.1 to 0.2 mm. larger than the desired diameter. When a plus lens is to be edged manually, the starting lens diameter should be 0.2 to 0.3 mm. larger than the desired diameter. This excess compensates for the reduction in diameter caused by the edging procedure.

Manual edging may be accomplished in one of two ways—the lens may be mounted on the motor unit with the edging implement held manually,

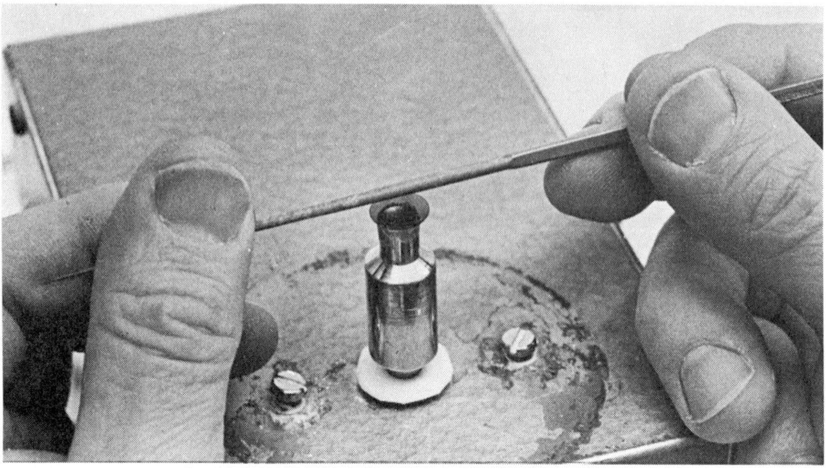

Figure 3–39. File held toward farthest edge of posterior surface of lens. Note position of fingers.

or the edging implement may be mounted on the motor unit with the lens held on a holder manually.

EDGING IMPLEMENT HELD MANUALLY. Two edging implements are used: rattail (needle) file and scalpel.

Rattail (Needle) File. The lens is mounted with its convex surface affixed to a chuck or arbor, which is placed on the motor unit after the splash pan is removed. The motor speed is set between 1,200 and 1,500 r.p.m. A No. 4 file is held with the smooth end between the thumb and the first two fingers of the right hand and the thumb and forefinger of the left hand (or the reverse for a left-handed person). The palms of the hands face each other. To provide stability, the upper arms are braced close to the body and the forearms rest on the counter. The file is held toward the farthest edge of the lens (Fig. 3–39).

The file is kept slowly rotating toward the worker and constantly in contact with a light pressure against the lens; it is brought slowly down and around to about 0.5 mm. onto the anterior surface in an arclike motion. The file is then started and kept rotating away from the worker and constantly in contact with a light pressure against the lens; it is brought slowly up and around to about 0.2 mm. onto the posterior surface in an arclike motion. Rotation of the file is done principally by the right hand, and the arc is controlled principally by the left hand (or the reverse for a left-handed person) (Fig. 3–40).

This procedure is continued until the lens diameter is just slightly greater than the desired finished size. The edge now should have the desired configuration and be ready for polishing.

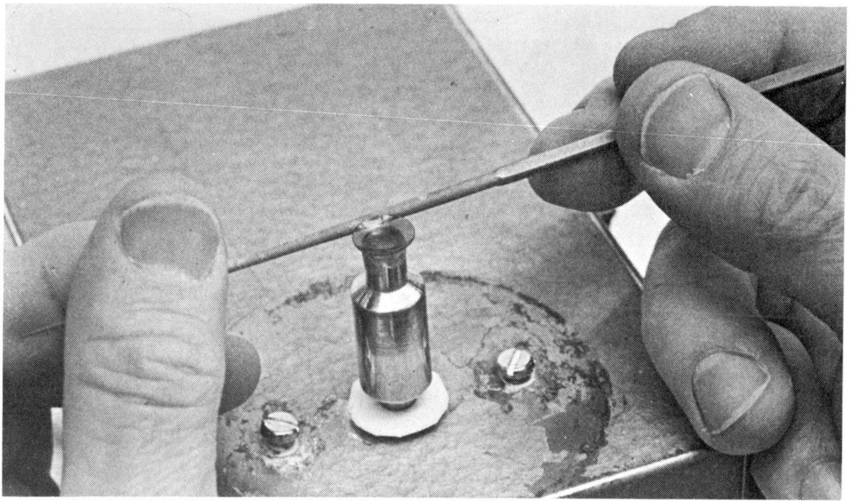

Figure 3–40. File rotated around to anterior surface of edge.

Polishing is accomplished with a hard felt cone which has been soaked in tin oxide or Silvo. The tip of the cone is held against the posterior surface of the lens slightly inside the edge. The rear of the cone is tilted up about 45° and held between the thumb and first two fingers of the right hand (Fig. 3–41). The upper arms are braced against the body and the forearms against the counter top, as before. The middle finger of the left hand is placed on the tip of the cone to guide it.

The cone is rotated slowly away from the worker and gradually brought to the periphery of the posterior surface of the lens. As this is done, the rear of the cone is lowered until it is parallel with the floor. Then the tip of the cone is grasped between the thumb and forefinger of the left hand. The

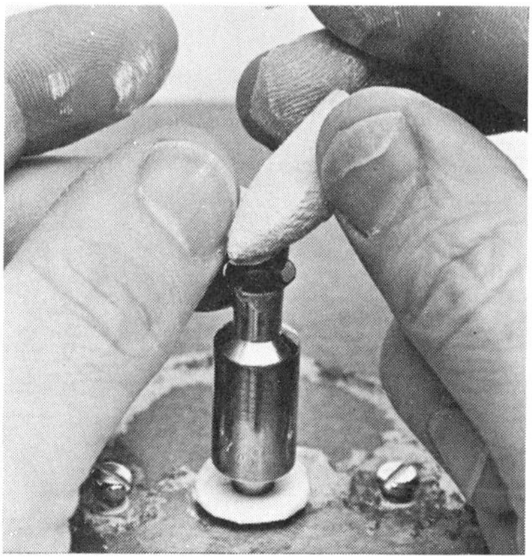

Figure 3–41. Cone held at about a 45° angle with the lens. Note the position of the fingers.

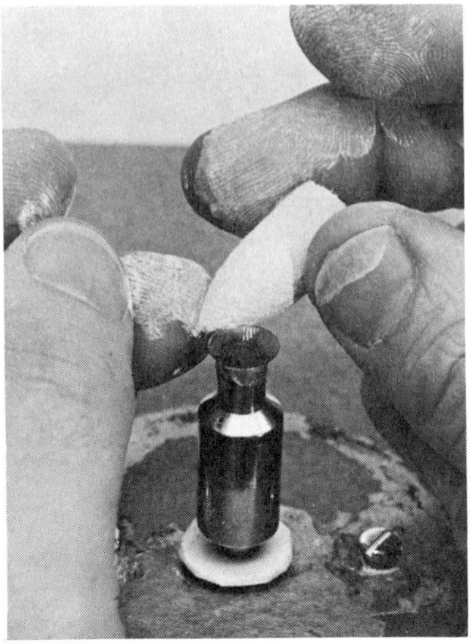

Figure 3–42. Cone being rotated around edge.

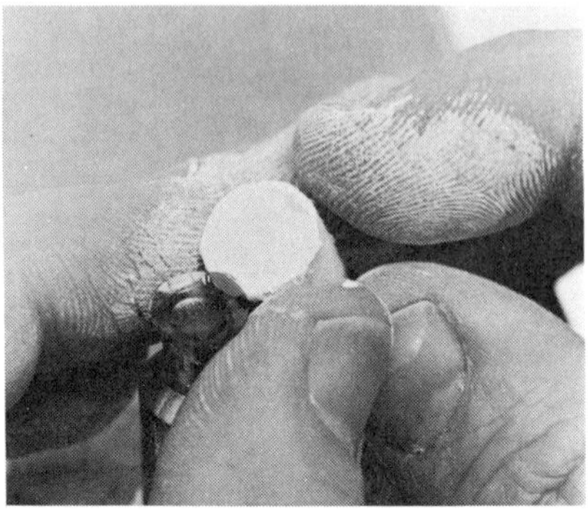

Figure 3–43. Blunt surface of cone held against peripheral part of anterior surface.

broader part of the cone then is in contact with the edge of the lens, and the procedure is the same as that used with the file. The procedure is continued until the edge is completely polished (Fig. 3–42).

The blunt edge of the cone then may be held against the peripheral 0.5 mm. of the anterior surface, and the cone tip is slowly angled up until the cone is almost parallel to the counter top (Fig. 3–43). This step helps polish out any lips on the anterior surface. Then the basic polishing procedure is done several times.

By applying varying amounts of pressure and spending different amounts of time on various areas, the practitioner may obtain many different configurations.

Scalpel. The procedure for a curved, hand-held scalpel is similar to that for a file.[186] Scalpel No. 40–37 with a sharp edge all around the curved cutting part is often used.

The motor is turned on at about 800 to 1,000 r.p.m. The underedge of the blade is placed slightly onto the posterior surface of the lens. The blade is angled so that it faces the same direction as the rotation of the spindle, thus reducing the tendency of the lens edge to chip. The upper arms are braced against the body and the forearms against the table. The scalpel is angled at about 45°. The upper end of the handle is held between the thumb and the forefinger of the right hand and the lower end of the handle is held between the thumb and forefinger of the left hand, the palms facing each other. The scalpel is held firmly against the lens (Fig. 3–44).

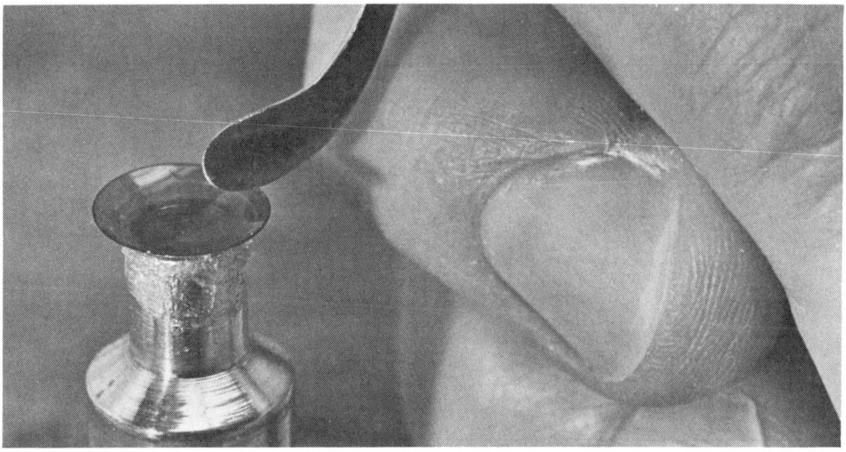

Figure 3–44. Scalpel blade held against posterior surface of edge.

The scalpel blade is brought from the posterior to the anterior surface in an arclike movement (Fig. 3–45). It is important to maintain constant contact between the scalpel and the lens. The scalpel is then brought up from anterior to posterior surface of the lens. This procedure is continued until the lens diameter is slightly less than the desired finished diameter. The edge may be polished with a hard felt cone as before.

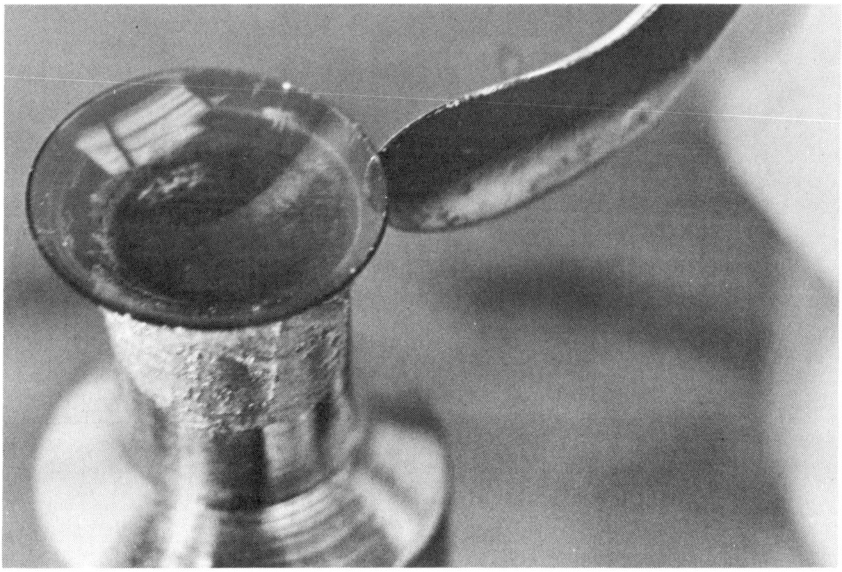

Figure 3–45. Scalpel blade brought around in an arclike movement to the anterior surface of the edge.

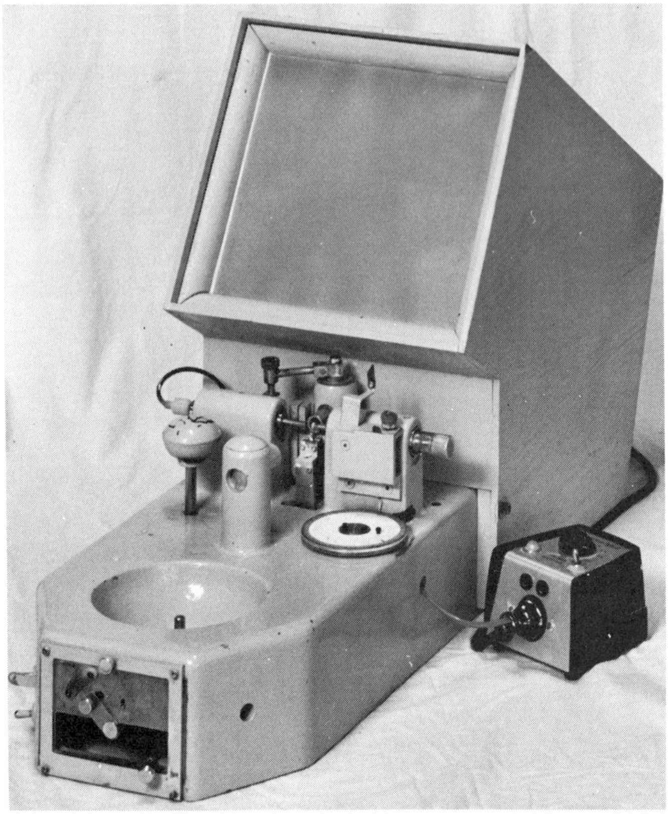

Figure 3–46. Rx-Edger. (Courtesy of Quality Optics, Inc.)

Because a scalpel removes plastic much more quickly than a No. 4 file, the authors prefer to use the file. A file provides better control of the edging procedure and reduces the possibility of error in the fabrication of edge configuration or lens diameter.

Automation. The cutting of the proper configuration on the edge and the polishing procedure can be automated by the use of a template and a cutting tool (Fig. 3–46).

Edging Implement on Motor Unit. Three types of edging implements used in this procedure are the rag or Styrofoam wheel, the polishing pad, and the conical grinding and polishing tools.

Rag or Styrofoam Wheel. A relatively firm, sewn, motor-driven rag wheel is used. The convex surface of the lens is mounted and visually centered on a spinner to produce double rotation. The motor speed is usually between 1,500 and 3,500 r.p.m. The slower speeds are preferable, because there is greater control of cutting, less chance of the lens being thrown off the spinner, and less chance of burning the lens.

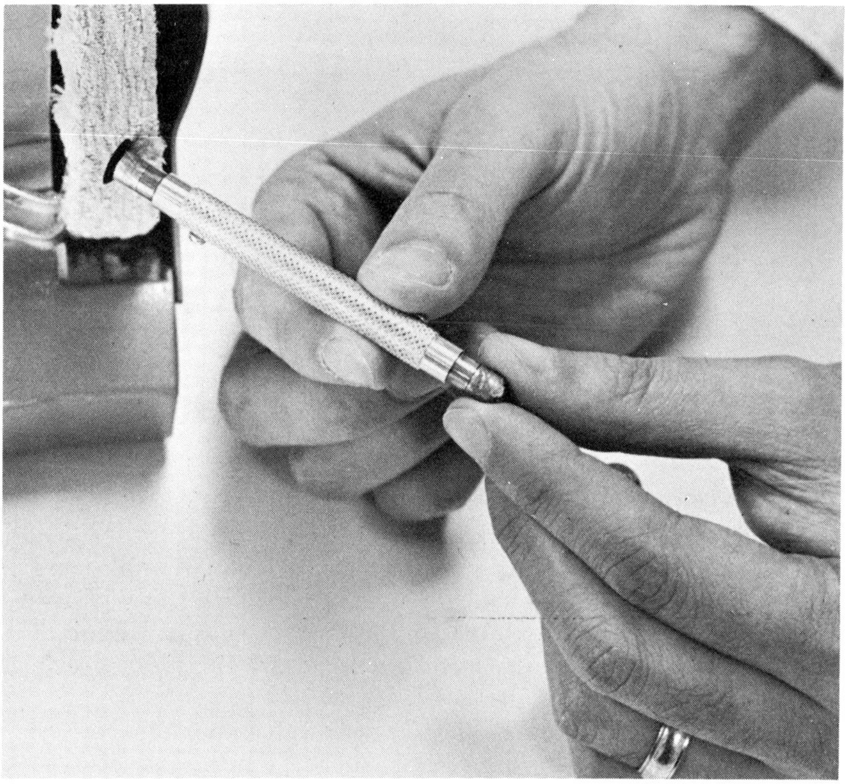

Figure 3–47. Spinner parallel to floor and at a 45 to 60° angle with rag wheel.

Shaping and polishing may be accomplished simultaneously. A polishing compound is placed on the wheel. The polishing compound may be dry, such as Bendeck polish or a fine grade jewelers' rouge, or it may be wet, such as Silvo or tin oxide. A dry compound is advantageous in that it does not splatter and does not clog the head of the spinner and thus retard its rotation. On the other hand, a wet compound reduces the chance of burning and marring of the edge. There are several methods of positioning the lens against the rotating pad. All are meant to produce a rounded edge:

1. The spinner may be held parallel to the floor or counter and at about a 45 to 60° angle to the pad (Fig. 3–47). The motor is turned on, and the spinner is slowly turned until it makes about a 100° angle with the pad. Thus, the edge is rounded from inside to outside (Fig. 3–48).

2. The lens may be held against the rag wheel with a spinner at about a 90° angle with the pad and 45° *above* horizontal. The spinner is maintained at about a 90° angle to the pad and slowly brought down to about 45° below horizontal. This procedure produces a rounding of the edge from outside to inside (Fig. 3–49).

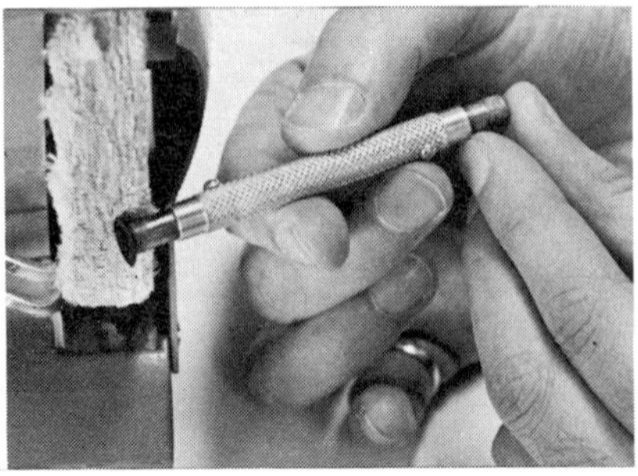

Figure 3–48. Spinner parallel to floor and at about a 100° angle with rag wheel.

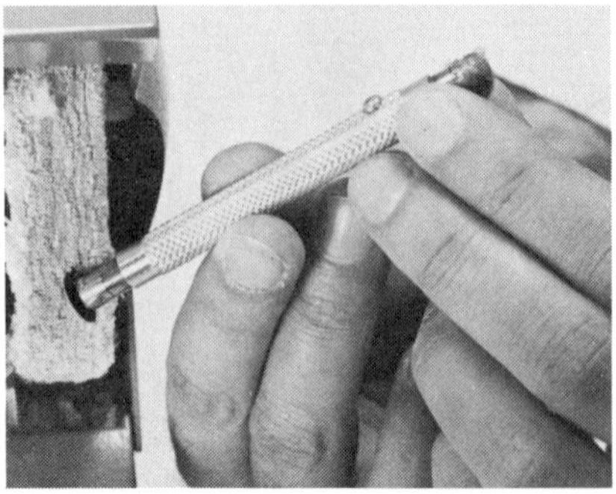

Figure 3–49. Spinner at about 90° angle with rag wheel and about 45° above horizontal.

3. The spinner may be held horizontally at an angle of about 40° to the rag wheel. It is held at this angle and moved back and forth across the rag wheel. The lateral movement provides a grinding action. As the spinner is moved right to left, the posterior edge of the lens is cut and polished; as the spinner is moved left to right, the anterior edge is cut and polished. The back-and-forth motion tends to produce a rounded symmetrical edge. This procedure may be automated (Fig. 3–50).

Automated edge polishing may also be done with a Styrofoam buff wheel (Fig. 3–51). The lens is mounted on a spinning chuck. Final diameter is set on the proper gauge. The wheel turns clockwise for 3½ minutes, and the surface of the anterior edge is polished. The wheel then turns counterclockwise, and the posterior edge surface is polished.

Although some good edges can be produced by a rag wheel—especially an automated one—the desired consistency is not always produced. The spinner may clog and stop rotating, producing an uneven edge. The problems with wet and dry polishing compounds have been discussed (p. 181). Often inside and outside lips are left, and a fine edge polish is not produced.

When the rag wheel becomes frayed, its edging effectiveness is reduced, and the possibility of marring the lens surface is increased. The frayed edges should be worn away by coarse sandpaper held against the rotating wheel.

Polishing Pad. A hard disk covered with moleskin and mounted parallel to the floor may be used.[187] The convex surface of the lens is mounted and visually centered on a spinner. Both the pad and lens rotate, producing double rotation. The spinner is held at an angle of 60° to the pad. The spinner is slowly brought down parallel to the pad, and at the same time it is stroked across the pad toward the center (Fig. 3–52).

At times, it may be indicated to proceed by attaching the concave surface of the lens to the convex head of the spinner and repeating the foregoing procedure. This step removes more plastic from the anterior surface of the

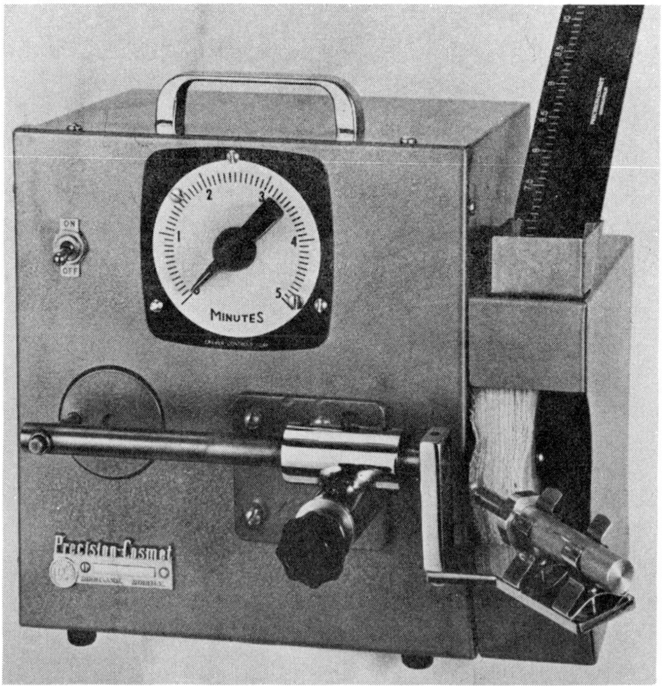

Figure 3–50. Automated rag wheel edger. (Courtesy of Precision-Cosmet Co.)

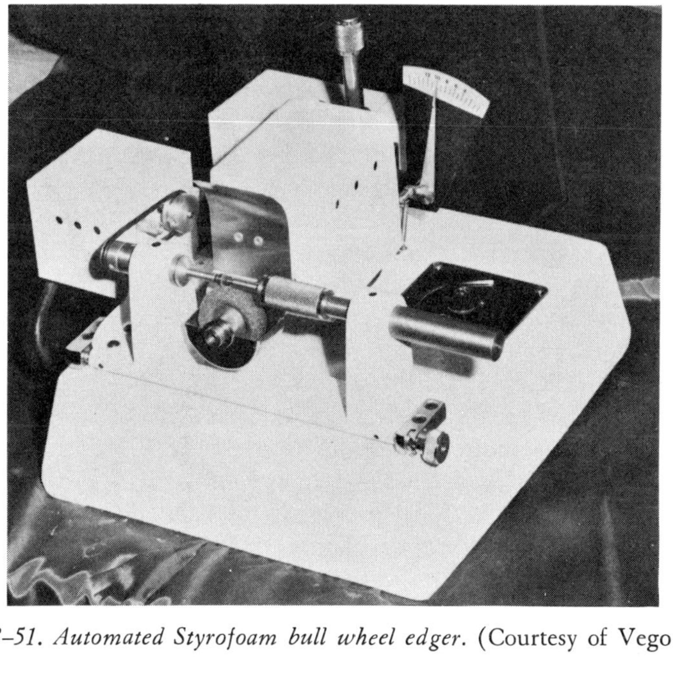

Figure 3–51. Automated Styrofoam bull wheel edger. (Courtesy of Vego Corp.)

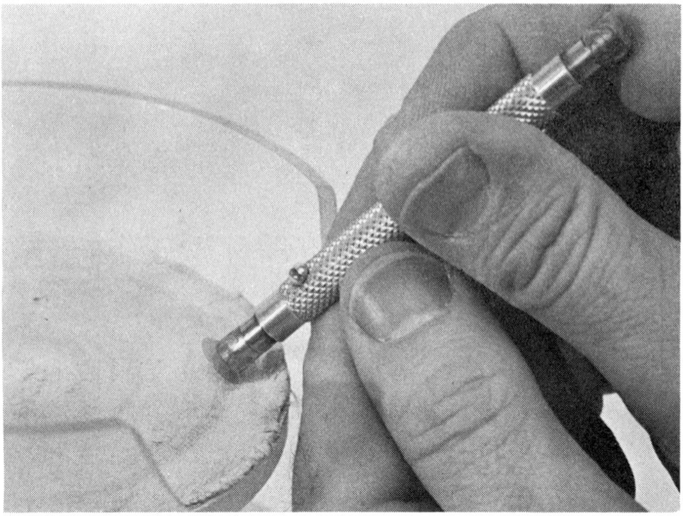

Figure 3–52. Edging with polishing pad. Convex lens surface mounted on spinner.

lens; this effect is useful in high minus prescriptions. The angle of the spinner to the pad on the front surface need be only 40 to 45° at the start (Fig. 3–53). This angle helps keep the anterior curvature in the optic zone from being affected. The anterior surface of the optic zone may be coated with marking compound for further protection.

To help remove inside lips, the spinner may be held perpendicular to the pad at its center when the convex lens surface is affixed to the concave spinner head. The spinner is brought slowly from 90 to 45°.

Concentric Conical Grind and Polish (Con-Lish[188]*).* In this procedure, a

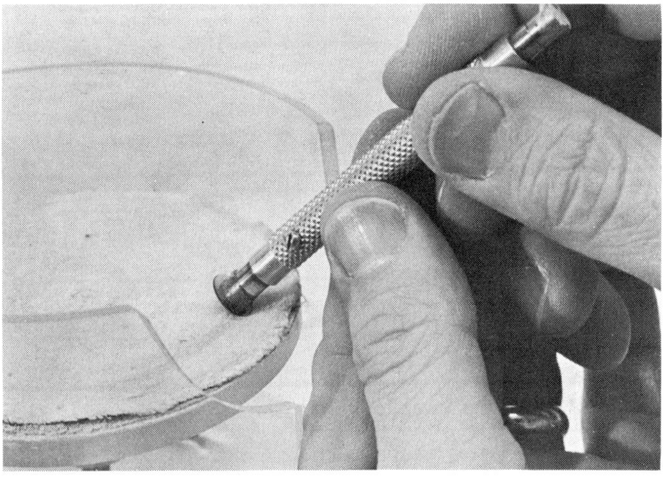

Figure 3–53. Edging with polishing pad. Concave lens surface mounted on spinner.

series of female conical tools of various angles is used to shape and polish the edge. Because the same tools theoretically can be used in the same manner each time, it is claimed that edge duplication is more probable with this technique.

In the original procedure, a 90° conical female grinding tool and 40°, 60°, and 140° female polishing tools were used. A 180° (flat) polishing tool also was used. A more varied selection of tools is applicable with the present method. The 90° conical grinding tool should have a fine abrasive surface so as to avoid deep scratches, which are difficult to polish.

The brass conical polishing tools must have soft pads. Each female conical polishing tool has a corresponding male padding tool. A piece of velveteen large enough to cover the head of the padding tool is cut. The padding tool head is lightly moistened with water, and the velveteen is wrapped around it. Econ-o cloth liquid pad glue is spread evenly and thinly on the inner surface of the female conical tool. When the glue has become slightly tacky, the male padding tool is inserted into the female tool and pressed to secure the velveteen. The two tools should be maintained in this manner for several minutes, after which a twisting motion will remove the padding tool. The glue should then be permitted to set for several more minutes. This procedure is repeated for each polishing tool.

To prepare the flat polishing tool, a velveteen square approximately 2 × 2 inches is cut. The upper, outer sides of the drum are coated with Econ-o cloth glue. The glue is allowed to become slightly tacky, and the velveteen is then stretched over the top and secured to the sides. A rubber band may be wound tightly around the sides of the velveteen, and any excess should be trimmed. The 90° grinding tool is placed on the unit. The motor is set at about 1,200 r.p.m. The stone must be kept wet constantly to prevent burning and marring of the lens.

The lens is mounted and centered with its posterior concave surface against the convex surface of an arbor or chuck. The lens is inserted into the conical tool until all sides touch with the holder exactly aligned with the shaft of the tool (Fig. 3–54). Any tilting about this angle changes the

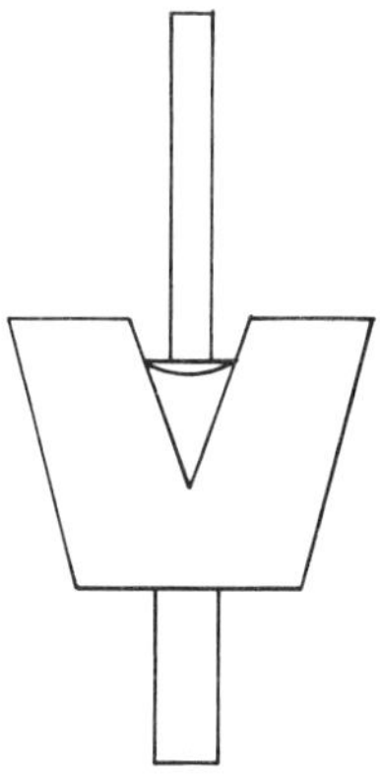

Figure 3–54. Sectional view of edging with a conical tool. All sides of the lens are touching, and the axis of the holder is aligned with the axis of the shaft of the conical tool.

angle of cut and produces an uneven edge. This is true for all subsequent operations. The unit is turned on, and the holder is rotated slowly *against* the direction of rotation of the tool. This procedure is followed for all subsequent operations and is continued until the diameter of the lens is 0.1 mm. larger than the desired finished diameter in plus or low minus lenses, and 0.05 mm. larger in high minus lenses.

The 90° polishing tool is then placed on the unit and used to polish the curvature just ground. The motor is set at 250 to 500 r.p.m. Silvo or tin oxide polishing compound is used on the velveteen pads, which must be kept wet. The lens is inserted properly until polishing is completed. This procedure takes two to four minutes.

Because it is often difficult to polish out all scratches and because it is often difficult to control the alignment of the holder, the technique is often modified to eliminate the use of the 90° conical grinding tool. If this procedure is followed, the lens diameter used at the start should be approximately 0.20 mm. larger for plus, 0.15 mm. larger for low minus, and 0.10 mm. larger for high minus than the diameter finally desired. The 90° conical polishing tool is used until these diameters are reduced 0.05 mm.

No matter which technique is used, touch polishing operations are used to blend sharp junctures and to shape what by then is a knife edge. The 60° conical polishing tool is used for 10 seconds, and the 40° conical polishing tool is used for five seconds.

The lens is then remounted with its convex surface on the concave surface of the holder. This arrangement permits work to be done on the inner concave surface with tools used in the following sequence: 180° tool for 20 seconds, 140° tool for 15 seconds, 90° tool for 10 seconds, 60° tool for five seconds, and 40° tool for two seconds.

This procedure has been modified somewhat and is used by some practitioners in the following manner.[189] In minus and lenticular lenses, the anterior convex edge is ground with a 70° conical tool lined with fine emery at a speed of about 1,500 r.p.m. until a sharp edge is produced. The lenses are then polished with a 70° conical tool with Silvo or tin oxide at a speed of about 500 r.p.m. A blend is produced at the juncture of this curve and the anterior curve with a 90° conical tool lined with plastic tape.

The procedure is started for plus lenses and finished for minus lenses by the following: the lens is mounted with its convex surface on the concave end of the holder, making the inside aspect accessible. The 70° conical tool lined with emery is used to remove the sharp apex. A 60° conical tool, which is lined with mole foam and saturated with water and a polishing compound, is used to polish this area and to blend from anterior to posterior surfaces. Spindle rotation is approximately 1,000 r.p.m. The first movement is a downstroke into the geometric center of the tool, where the lens can be felt to compress the foam rubber. The lens is held in this position for a few seconds and is then brought upward and away from the polishing surface. This motion is repeated several times. The lens is then held in a position near the top of the cone, and the edge is rotated eccentrically a full 360° around the side of the tool. Two or three excursions should be made before the results are examined with a hand magnifier.

The two steps in this procedure are repeated until the desired profile and degree of edge polishing have been obtained.

Resurfacing

It is possible to resurface the anterior curvature of a contact lens to change its refractive power.[190] Anterior and posterior curvatures can be resurfaced to remove scratches. Resurfacing is an extremely delicate procedure and requires considerable practice and skill. A skilled worker can usually alter power up to −0.75 D or +0.37 D and still maintain adequately nonaberrated surfaces. The practitioner is cautioned not to try power alterations until he has developed sufficient skill by practicing with rejected lenses. At first, it is best to establish −0.37 D as the maximum attempted change. Plus changes should not be attempted at the outset. As skill and confidence increase, the maximum changes of −0.75 D and +0.37 D may be attempted.

As background and for purposes of comparison, consider how refractive power is incorporated into the original lens. For the sake of simplicity, neglect center thickness. The radius of the central posterior curvature is established for fitting purposes, and this curvature is cut on a lens with a lathe. The necessary radius of the anterior curvature that will combine with this posterior curvature to produce the desired posterior vertex power is then uniformly cut on the lens with a lathe. As long as the radii of these two curvatures are dissimilar and lie on a common axis, there will be a concurrent uniform change of thickness from the center to the edge of the lens. The anterior curvature for a lens with positive posterior vertex power is steeper than the posterior curvature. The anterior curvature for a lens with negative posterior vertex power is flatter than the posterior curvature. As a result, there is a decrease of thickness from center to edge in plus lenses, and an increase in thickness from center to edge in minus lenses. In this procedure, controlled radii are cut on the lens, and the change of thickness is an inherent byproduct.

When power changes are made in finished contact lenses, an almost reverse procedure is followed. Because the velocity and cutting action increase away from the axis of a rotating tool, the greatest decrease of thickness occurs on the portion of the lens closest to the edge of the tool. Because there is a relatively uniform rate of change of velocity, it is possible to obtain a relatively gradual degree of change in the thickness of the lens. This procedure in effect produces a curvature with a new radius. The control and accuracy of this procedure are considerably poorer than when the radius is cut with a lathe.

Power Changes. Polyester foam tools with concave, convex, or flat shapes are used. When a lens is pressed against the tool, the surface of the flexible polisher conforms to the surface of the lens—that is, it assumes the same radius. Light pressure of the lens into the tool is necessary to ensure that the polisher has conformed to the lens surface. By placement of the lens on the appropriate part of the tool in relation to its center of rotation, a desired change of thickness can be produced that will effectively change the radius.

For adding minus power to the lens, it is necessary to flatten the anterior curvature—that is, decrease thickness in the center more than at the edges. The lens is held so that maximum velocity is applied to the center of the lens with a gradual decrease of velocity toward the edge. If a concave polishing tool is used, this step is best done with approximately one third to slightly less than one half of the lens extending beyond the edge of the tool. The holder should make an angle of about 30 to 40° with the horizontal (Fig. 3–55).

The polishing tool should be kept wet with Silvo or tin oxide. If it is allowed to dry, concentric swirls will be produced by the excess friction and heat. If the tool is too wet, the time needed will be greatly increased, and the stability of the foam toward the edge of the tool will be decreased. The motor is turned on at about 1,000 to 1,200 r.p.m. The upper arms of the operator are braced against the body and the forearms against the table to provide stability. The holder is securely held toward the head with the thumb on one side and the four fingers of the left hand on the other. The base is held between the thumb and fingers of the right hand. The right hand can be used to rotate the holder and lens. This rotation should be against the direction of rotation of the tool. Rotation should be slow and

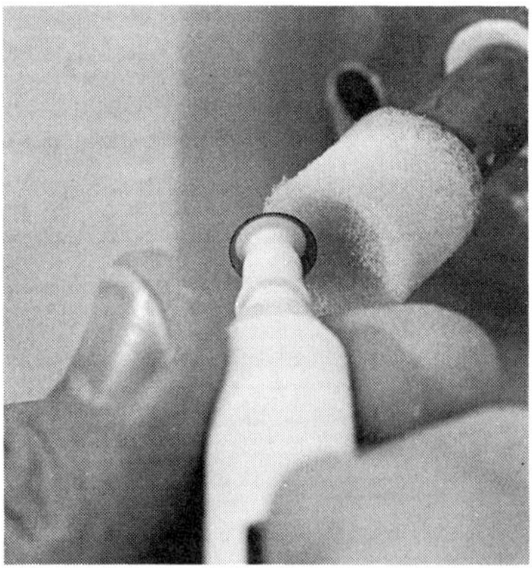

Figure 3–55. Minus power is added by holding the convex surface of a lens with 1/3 to 1/2 of it extending beyond the edge of a concave polyester foam tool.

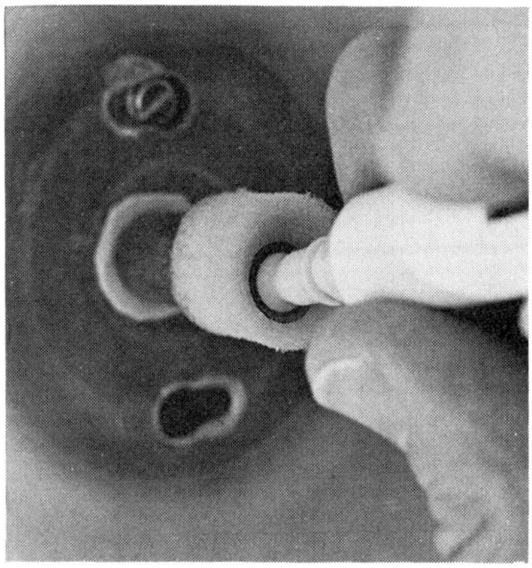

Figure 3–56. Plus power is added by holding the convex surface of the lens approximately coincident with the center of a concave polyester foam tool.

steady, allowing all parts of the lens to be uniformly polished. The lens should be periodically checked for power.

To add plus power to the lens, it is held so that its center coincides with the center of the tool (Fig. 3–56). Slight pressure is applied so that the foam contours the surface completely. The motor is set at about 800 to 1,000 r.p.m. The holder usually need not be rotated. In this case, a small elevation of plastic may form in the center, where there is no cutting action. To avoid this problem, the lens is moved first slightly above center and then slightly below center. Some practitioners prefer a slow, constant rotation of the holder against the direction of rotation of the tool. The authors find that this method increases the tendency for concentric swirls to be produced on the front surface. If hazy optics are produced during the addition of plus power, an extra 0.12 D of plus power may be added. This plus is neutralized by adding 0.12 D of minus power, which may clear up the optics.

If vibrations are felt during the polishing action, results will be poor. Vibration may be due to too high a speed, too much pressure, or too unsteady a polisher. The speed and pressure are easily controlled. The authors have found that the stability of the pad is greatly improved by a ring collar, which is brought up to within about one eighth of an inch of the top of the polishing tool (Fig. 3–57).

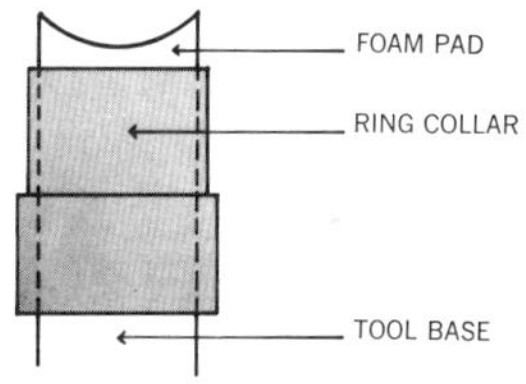

Figure 3–57. A ring collar around a Styrofoam concave polishing tool increases pad stability.

The authors prefer flat pads for power changes. To add minus on a flat polyester foam pad, the concave surface of the lens is attached to a suction cup or other nonrotating holder. The holder is held perpendicular to and slightly inside the edge of the pad. After the motor is turned on at about 800 to 1,000 r.p.m., the lens is slowly revolved around the pad, which is kept moist with polishing compound (Fig. 3–58). To add plus on a flat, slack silk pad, the concave surface of the lens is attached to a suction cup or other nonrotating holder. The holder is held perpendicular to and near the center of the pad. After the motor is turned on at about 600 to 800 r.p.m., the lens is slowly rocked back and forth on the pad, which is kept moist with polishing compound (Fig. 3–59).

Scratch Removal. To remove scratches without changing power, it is necessary to resurface the lens without changing its radius. To do this with a concave pad, the lens must be held midway between the position used in adding plus power and that used in adding minus power. The lens is rotated slowly and steadily against the direction of rotation of the tool. Most

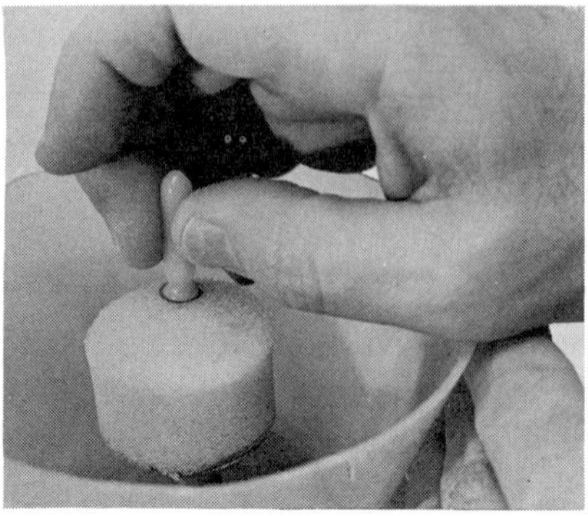

Figure 3–58. Adding minus power on a flat polyester foam pad.

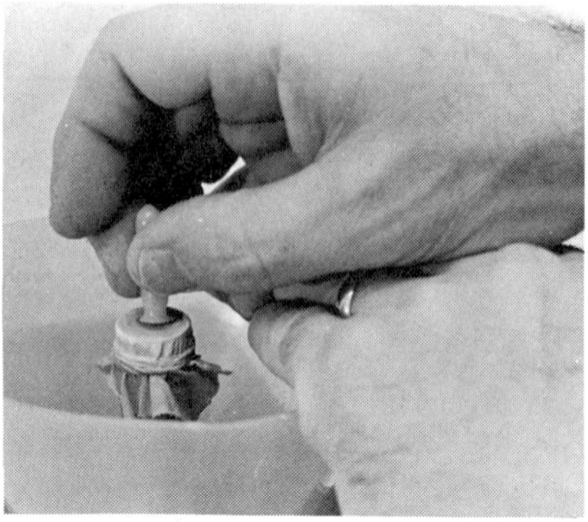

Figure 3–59. Adding plus on a slack tool covered with silk.

scratches are made on the anterior surface as a result of rubbing when the lens is removed from the case, or rubbing along the floor if the lens is dropped. If the lens is dropped concave side down, usually the edges, if anything, are affected.

Scratches may be removed from the posterior surface of a lens by rotating it slowly and steadily about the center of a convex polishing tool.

The best way to prevent scratches is to educate patients so that they handle and maintain lenses properly.

4

STAGE FOUR

Patient Education

For successful contact lens use, the patient must be educated properly. An educated patient has a positive mental set toward contact lenses, and he knows how to handle, care for, and wear them properly.[191–197] Instruction is more effective when the practitioner understands and applies certain principles of educational psychology.

Because the patient may become fatigued or his eyes irritated, short educational sessions are preferable. At least two 30-minute sessions are advisable. The first session is held early in the fitting procedure to help the patient overcome anxieties related to contact lens handling techniques. If diagnostic lenses are available, this session is conducted during the first patient visit. Proficiency in handling techniques is reinforced during the second educational session, which is held when the lenses processed for the patient are ready for dispensing. Contact lens care and guides for wear are taught during the second session. If diagnostic lenses are not available, the first educational session is held when the lenses processed for the patient are ready for dispensing. The second session is held later the same day or on a subsequent day. Because patients are often motivated by the companionship and competition of others, instruction is often more effective if presented simultaneously to several people.

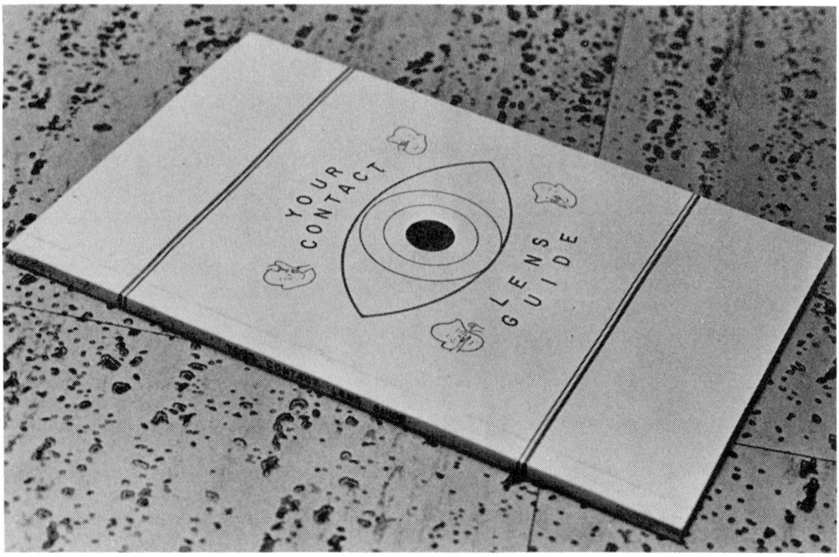

Figure 4–1. Example of instruction booklet for patient.

The practitioner should briefly outline procedures to the patient, and then he should explain each part of the procedure in detail. Because instruction is more effective when information is communicated through more than one sensory mechanism, the practitioner should explain and demonstrate procedures. The patient should then repeat the procedure immediately, and the practitioner should correct any errors immediately. Because instruction should be reviewed, literature should be given to the patient for reference (Figs. 4–1 and 6–1B. See p. 257.)

Psychological factors are extremely important in contact lens care. In four ways, the practitioner can help the patient to establish a positive mental set toward contact lenses. First, he can help to relieve or resolve the patient's anxieties about contact lenses. Second, he can help to maintain patient motivation to use contact lenses at a desirable level. Third, he can help to make the patient aware of the need for responsible contact lens use. Fourth, he can help the patient to fulfill this responsibility by teaching him how to handle, care for, and wear contact lenses.

HANDLING TECHNIQUES

General

The instructor and the patient sit at opposite sides of a small table. A cup of warm water, a contact lens case, a contact lens wetting solution, facial tissues, a mirror, and an appropriate contact lens are on the table. Tinted

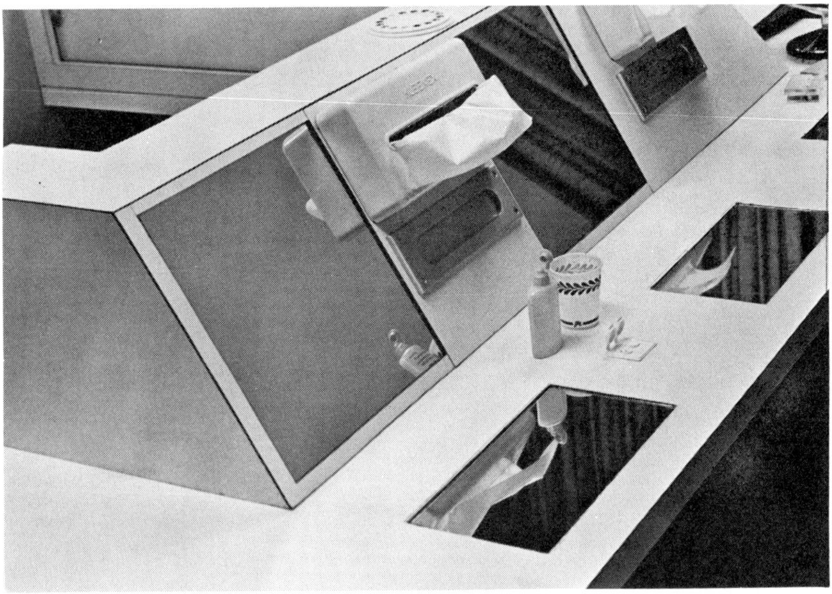

Figure 4–2. Equipment used when teaching handling techniques: cup of warm water, contact lens case, contact lens wetting solution, facial tissues, flat and angled mirrors, and tinted contact lens in case.

contact lenses are helpful in teaching handling techniques. The mirror is placed either flat on the table or at a 45° angle, which permits better observation of the patient (Fig. 4–2).

Although a mirror is an effective initial teaching aid, the patient should learn before dispensing to insert, remove, and when possible, to recenter a contact lens without reliance on a mirror. Most patients must handle contact lenses occasionally when a mirror is unavailable. Inability to do this may cause problems.

Some very young children, very old adults, or people with poor manual dexterity cannot master contact lens handling techniques. When it is necessary to fit contact lenses to such patients, both the patient and a member of his family should be instructed.

Two types of visual aids are used when the patient's uncorrected near visual acuity is extremely poor. First, a flip-up, a semirimless, or a plastic frame with the bottom of the eyewire removed on one side is used. A spectacle lens with a refractive power for about a 20-inch working distance is placed on one side of the flip-up or semirimless frame, or on the side of the spectacle frame with the complete eyewire. The resultant near visual acuity allows the patient to insert a contact lens on the eye not covered by the spectacle lens. Then the frame is removed, and the other contact lens is inserted. Second, a magnifying mirror is used (Fig. 4–3).

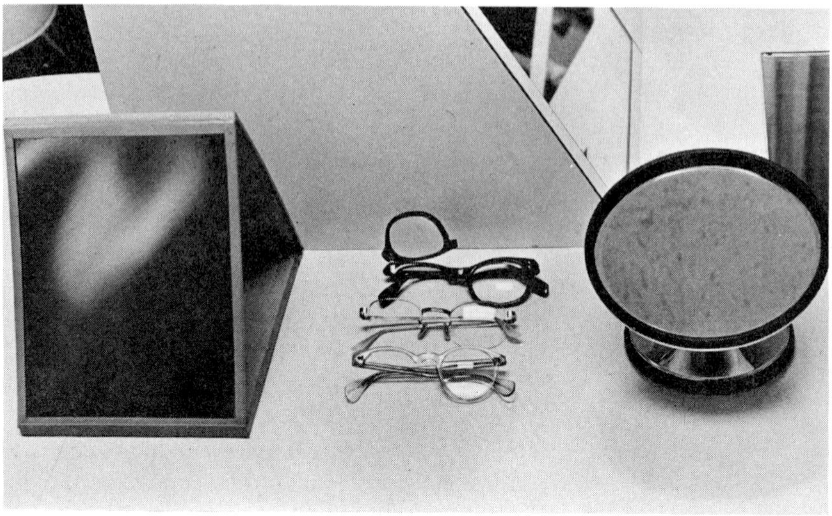

Figure 4–3. Visual aids used when teaching handling techniques to patients with poor uncorrected near visual acuity. (Left) *Angled magnifying mirror.* (Center—from top) *Flip-up, semirimless, and plastic frames with lens on one side.* (Right) *Flat magnifying mirror.*

Devices incorporating suction cups have been suggested as aids for patients who cannot master other techniques of corneal contact lens insertion and removal. Because the patient may place the suction cup on the ocular tissues and thus cause irritation, suction cups should not be used. With proper instruction and sufficient practice, the patient can learn normal techniques.

Insertion

The practitioner's technique for placing contact lenses on the patient's eyes is discussed on page 70. When he is teaching the patient to insert lenses, the practitioner first describes and then demonstrates the insertion technique. The patient imitates each step without a lens, and the practitioner corrects any errors. After these steps are mastered, the patient should insert the lens.

When the patient is extremely apprehensive, he may need to master each step separately. First, the practitioner holds the patient's lids, and the patient maintains fixation and inserts the lens. Second, the patient holds his lids and maintains fixation, and the practitioner inserts the lens. Third, the patient combines the two steps.

The practitioner must teach the patient to take his time, to wash his hands, and to gather all necessary materials before he attempts to insert his lenses. The patient must also work where a dropped lens can easily be found, preferably not over a sink. If the patient does use a sink, the drain should be plugged.

Insertion techniques have common characteristics. First, the patient prepares the lens with wetting solution. Second, he dries his fingers and eyelids because wet lids cannot be held securely. Third, he cups a hand under his eye or places a soft cover on a table top to catch the lens if it drops. Fourth, he fixates a target because looking away causes the lens to be placed off center. Fifth, he grasps his upper lid below the lash margin and presses it firmly against the supraorbital bones because blinking knocks the lens away from the eye. Sixth, he holds his head steady as the lens nears the eye. Seventh, he inserts the lens gently, but nonhesitatingly. Eighth, he releases his lids after the lens has been inserted.

Common Insertion Techniques

The following are the common insertion techniques taught to patients:

Technique 1. Place the wet lens hollow side up on the end of the middle finger of your right hand. Place the forefinger of your right hand just above and toward the middle of the margin of your right lower lid. Pull your lower lid down and hold it firmly against the bone below it. Bring your left hand over your head and place the forefinger or middle finger just below and toward the middle of the margin of your right upper lid. Pull your upper lid up and hold it firmly against the bone above it. Insert the lens. To insert the lens on your left eye, your hands may be used the same way or you may alternate your hands (Fig. 4-4).

Technique 2. This is the same as the first technique, but the lower lid is not held.

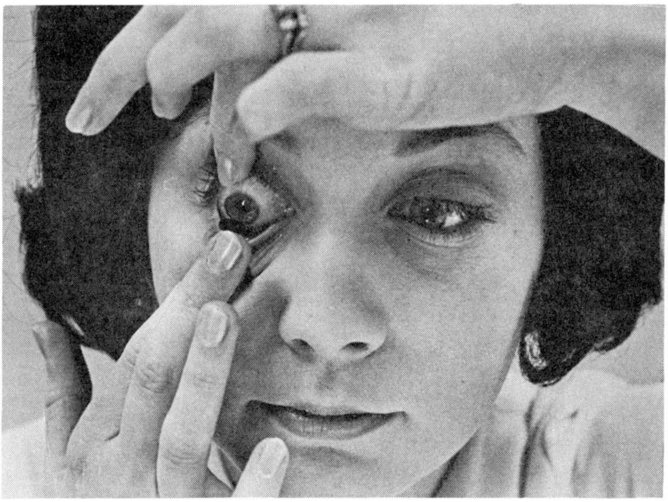

Figure 4-4. Insertion technique number one.

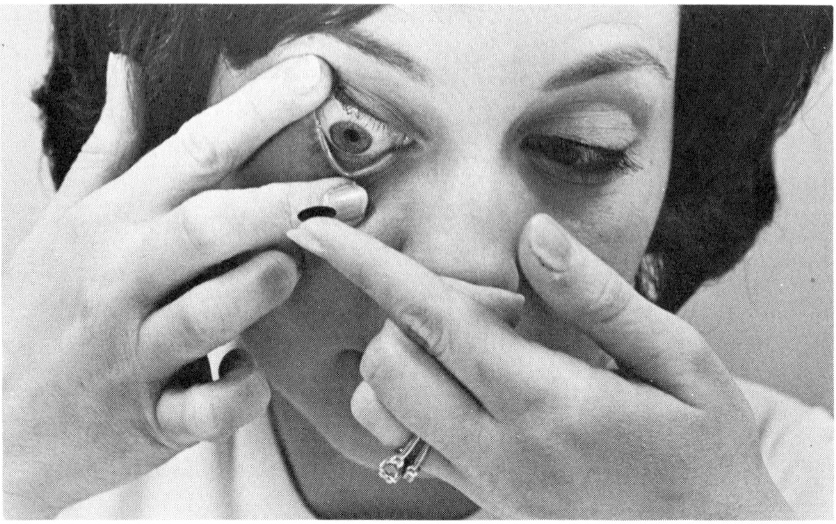

Figure 4–5. Insertion technique number three.

TECHNIQUE 3. Spread the forefinger and middle finger of your right hand in the form of an open pair of scissors. Hold the right lower lid down with the middle finger, and hold the right upper lid up with the forefinger. Place the wet lens with its concave or hollow side up on the forefinger of your left hand. This finger is held relatively parallel to the ground, and the lens is inserted. To insert the lens on your left eye, your hands may be used the same way or you may alternate your hands (Fig. 4–5).

TECHNIQUE 4. Spread the forefinger and ring finger of one hand in the form of an open pair of scissors. Place the wet lens with its hollow side up on the middle finger of the same hand. Hold the lower lid down with the

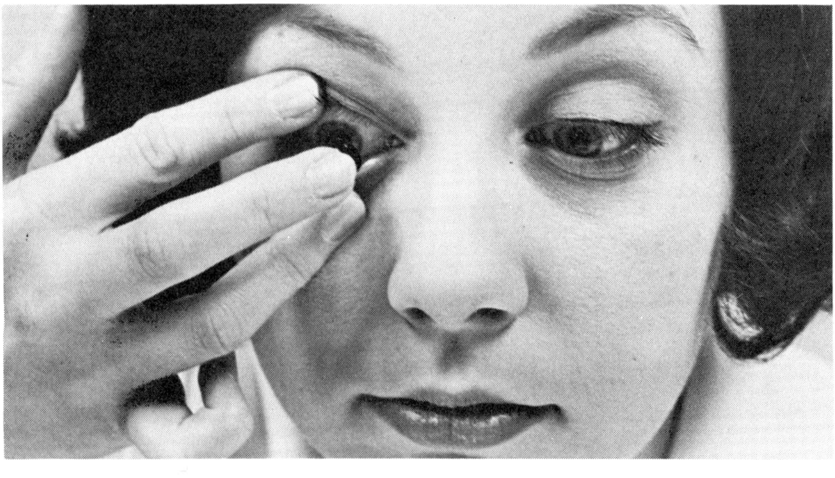

Figure 4–6. Insertion technique number four.

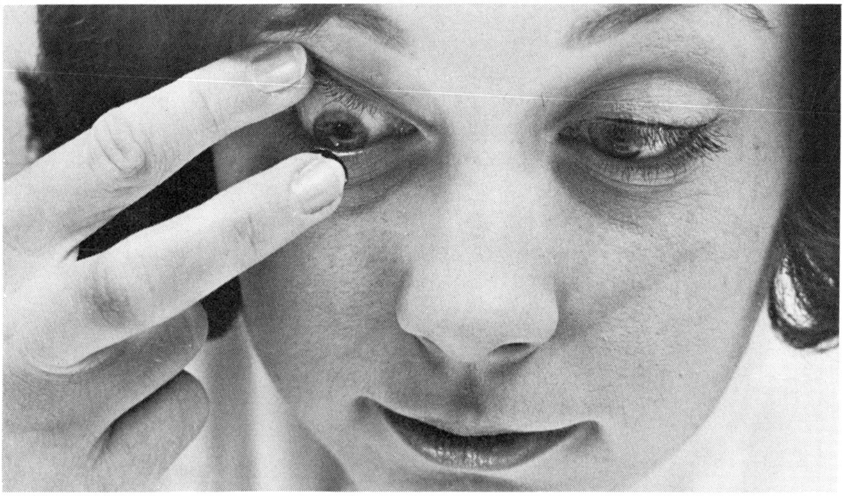

Figure 4–7. Insertion technique number five.

ring finger and the upper lid up with the forefinger. Insert the lens. The same hand may be used for both eyes, or the right hand may be used for right eye and left hand for left eye (Fig. 4–6).

TECHNIQUE 5. Hold the forefinger and the middle finger of one hand relatively parallel to the floor. Hold the upper lid with the forefinger, and place the wet lens hollow side up on the middle finger. Insert the lens. The same hand may be used for both eyes, or the right hand may be used for right eye, and left hand for left eye (Fig. 4–7).

TECHNIQUE 6. The lids are not held. Place the wet lens hollow side up on either the index or middle finger of your dominant hand. Open your eyes wide and insert the lens (Fig. 4–8).

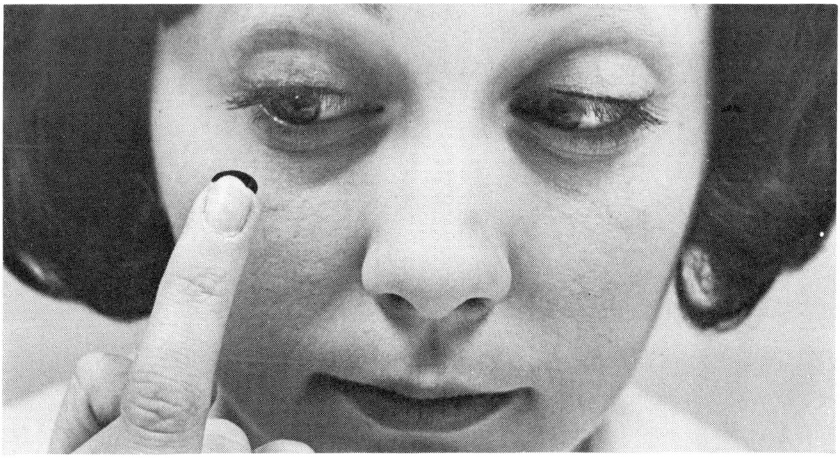

Figure 4–8. Insertion technique number six.

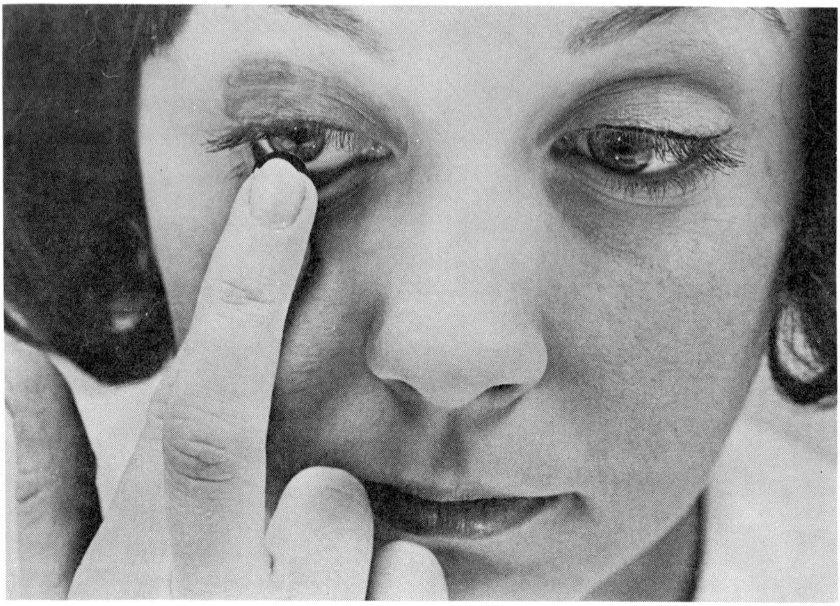

Figure 4–9. Insertion technique number seven.

TECHNIQUE 7. Hold your lower lid just above the lash margin tightly against the bone below it with the forefinger. Place the wet lens hollow side up on the middle finger. Insert the lens. The right hand is used for the right eye and left hand for the left eye (Fig. 4–9).

REMOVAL

The practitioner's technique for removing contact lenses from the patient's eyes is discussed on page 72. Removal techniques used by the patient have common characteristics. First, the patient dries his fingers and eyelids. Second, he prepares to catch the lens when it comes out. Third, he makes certain that the lens is centered before he attempts to remove it. Fourth, he fixates a target. Fifth, he removes his lids from the lens by opening his eyes as if staring or by drawing his lids away from the lens with his fingers. Sixth, he presses his lids tightly against his eyes. Seventh, he draws his lids together.

COMMON REMOVAL TECHNIQUES

The following are common removal techniques taught the patient.

TECHNIQUE 1. Bend over so your head is relatively parallel to the floor. Cup your left hand under your right eye. Place the thumb, index, or forefinger of your right hand at the outer corner of your eyelids. Look straight down and open both eyes wide. Pull the finger in an upward and outward direction. If the lens does not come out, it may be necessary to blink simul-

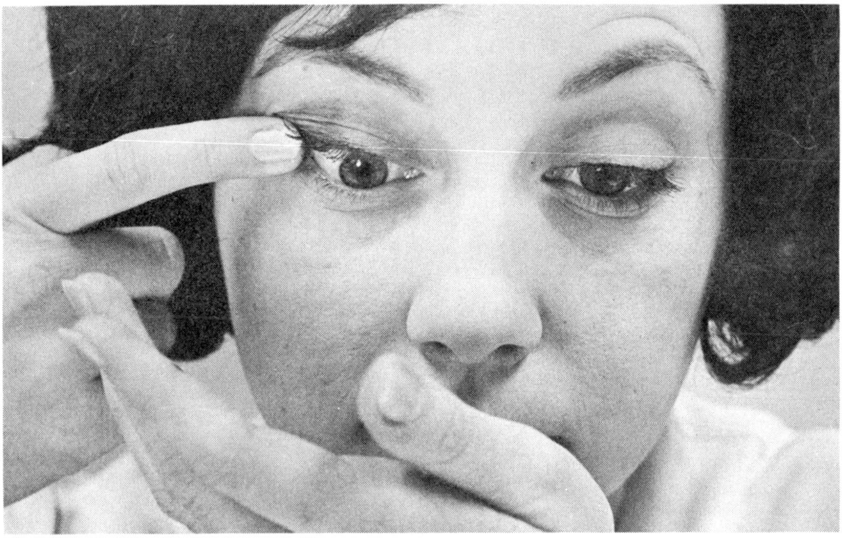

Figure 4–10. Removal technique number one.

taneously while pulling. The opposite hands are used for the left eye (Fig. 4–10).

Technique 2. Bend over so your head is relatively parallel to the floor. Cup your left hand under your right eye, and place the middle finger of your left hand at the outer corner of your right eyelids. Look straight down and open both eyes wide. Pull the middle finger of the left hand in an upward and outward direction. If the lens does not come out, it may be necessary to blink simultaneously while pulling. The opposite hand is used for the left eye (Fig. 4–11).

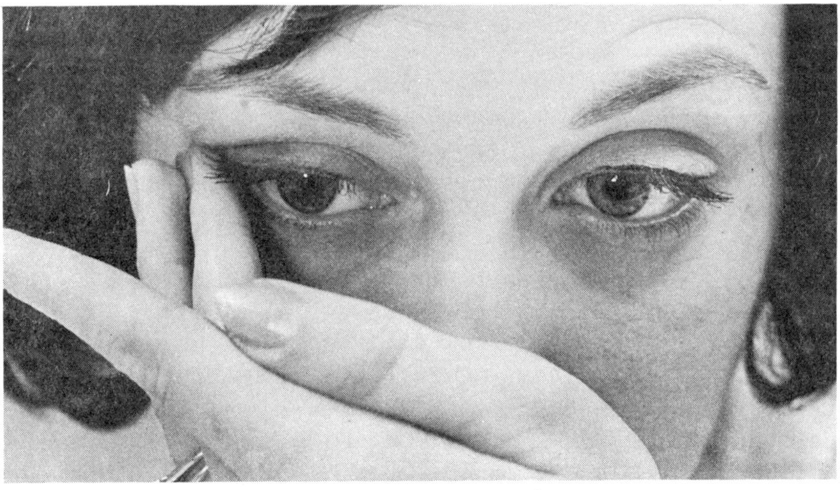

Figure 4–11. Removal technique number two.

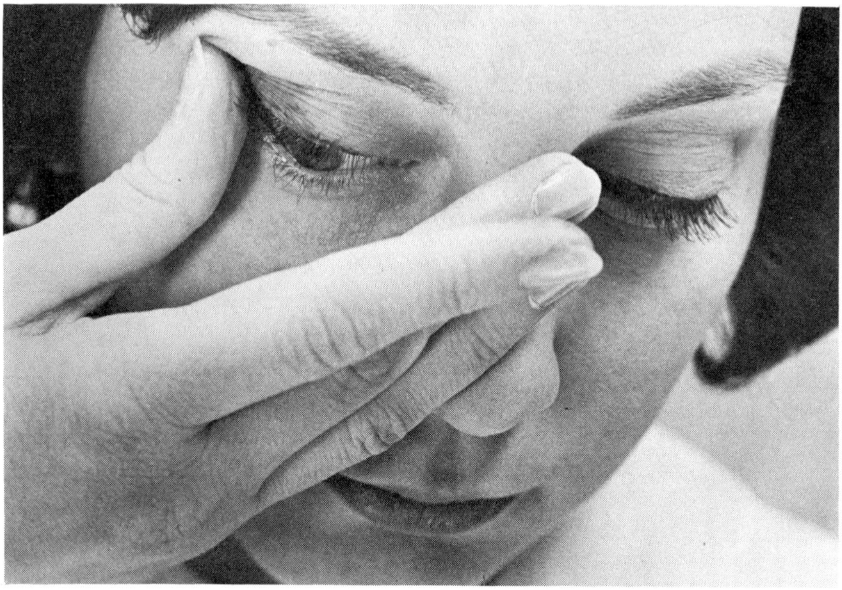

Figure 4–12. Removal technique number three.

TECHNIQUE 3. Bend over so your head is relatively parallel to the floor. Cup your right hand under your right eye and place your right thumb at the outer corner of your right eyelids. Look straight down and open both your eyes wide. Pull the thumb in an upward and outward direction. If the lens does not come out, it may be necessary to blink simultaneously while pulling. The opposite hand is used for the left eye (Fig. 4–12).

TECHNIQUE 4. Bend over so your head is relatively parallel to the floor. Place the middle finger of your right hand along the right lower lid margin and the forefinger of your right hand along the right upper lid margin. Cup your left hand under your right eye to catch the lens. Draw your lids away from the lens, hold them tightly against the eye, and press them tightly together while looking straight ahead. An alternate method is to pull both lids to the side with the forefinger on the lower lid and the middle finger on the upper lid, or with the thumb on the lower lid and the forefinger on the upper lid. The opposite hands are used for the left eye (Fig. 4–13).

TECHNIQUE 5. Bend over so your head is relatively parallel to the floor. Place the forefinger of your right hand on your right lower lid and pull it down while pressing it firmly against the globe. Do not turn the lid margin out. Place the forefinger or middle finger of your left hand against the right upper lid and pull it up while pressing it firmly against the globe. Hold the lower lid in place and push the upper lid down toward the lower lid. Do not release the pressure or let the lid margins turn out. The lens will fall on the table, so it is necessary to have a soft cover on the table. The opposite hands are used for the left eye (Fig. 4–14).

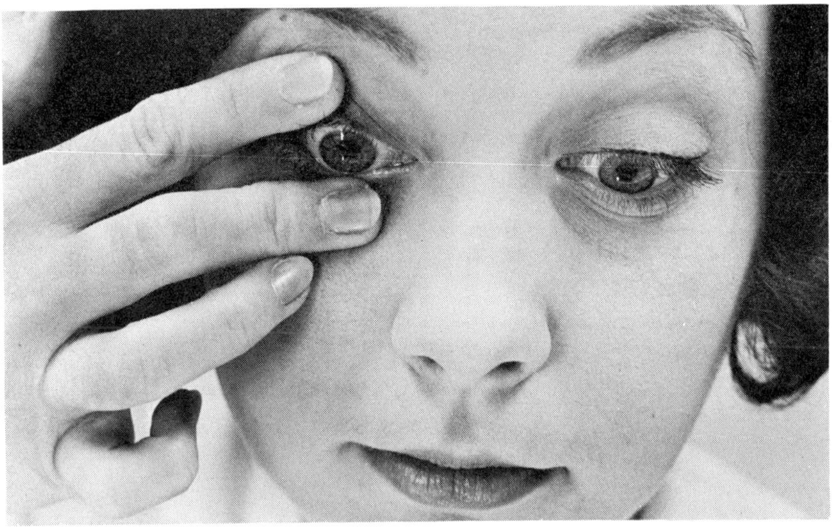

Figure 4–13. Removal technique number four.

Recentration

The practitioner should teach the patient to center a lens from any decentered position. The instructor should place the lens on the superior, inferior, nasal, and temporal sclera, and the patient should center the lens. When it is possible, recentration should be learned without reliance on a mirror.

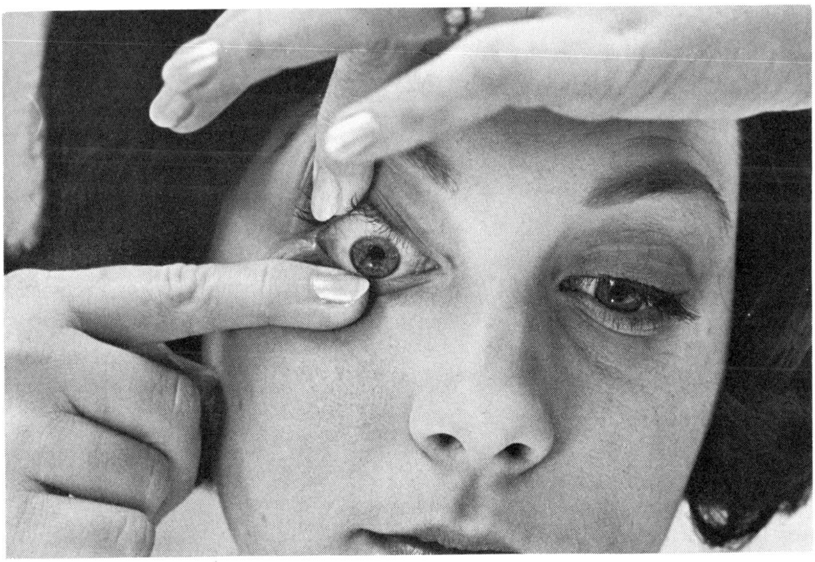

Figure 4–14. Removal technique number five.

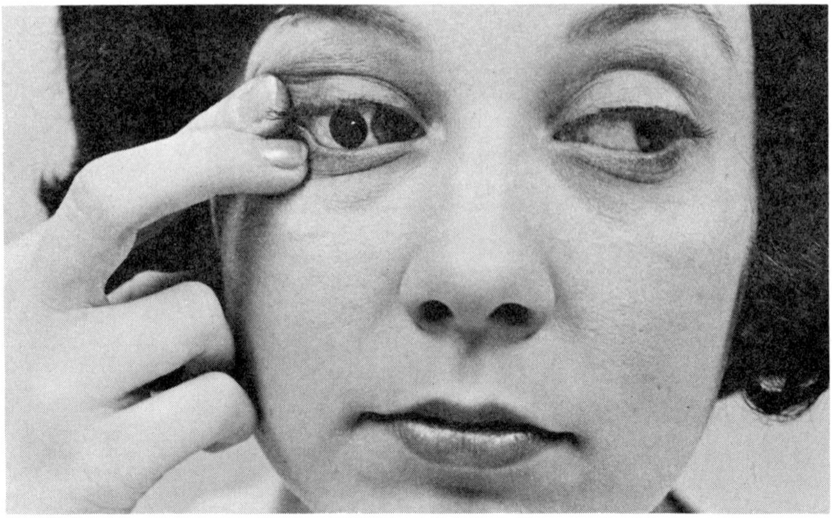

Figure 4–15. Recentration technique number one.

Common Recentration Techniques

The following are common recentering techniques taught the patient.

Technique 1. Locate the lens either by pulling the lids away from the eye and looking into a mirror or by feeling through the closed lids. Once the lens is located, place the forefinger and middle fingers of one hand behind and on either side of the lens (Fig. 4–15). This prevents the lens from slipping to the side. Look directly away from the lens; this frees the lens somewhat. Press your fingers firmly against the eye through the lids. This acts as a barrier to the lens. Then look directly back toward the lens while maintaining pressure on the lens or while sliding the lens toward the cornea. Then shut your other eye. If your vision is good, the lens is centered.

Many patients find it easiest to recenter a lens from the outer corner of the eye. Your forefinger may be used to move a lens from other areas to the outer corner. If the lens is on the upper half of the eye, look down and move the lens with the forefinger through the lid to the outer corner. If the lens is on the lower half of the eye, look up and move the lens to the outer corner. It is advisable to cup the opposite hand under the eye in all centering procedures because sometimes the lens may fall out of the eye.

Technique 2. Close your eyelids. Place the four fingers and thumb of one hand around the eye (Fig. 4–16). Press all the fingers and thumb against the eye and bring them in a clawing action toward the center of the eye.

Technique 3. Hold your lids widely apart and rotate your eyes slowly as far as they will go in all directions. Continue to do this until the lens centers (Fig. 4–17).

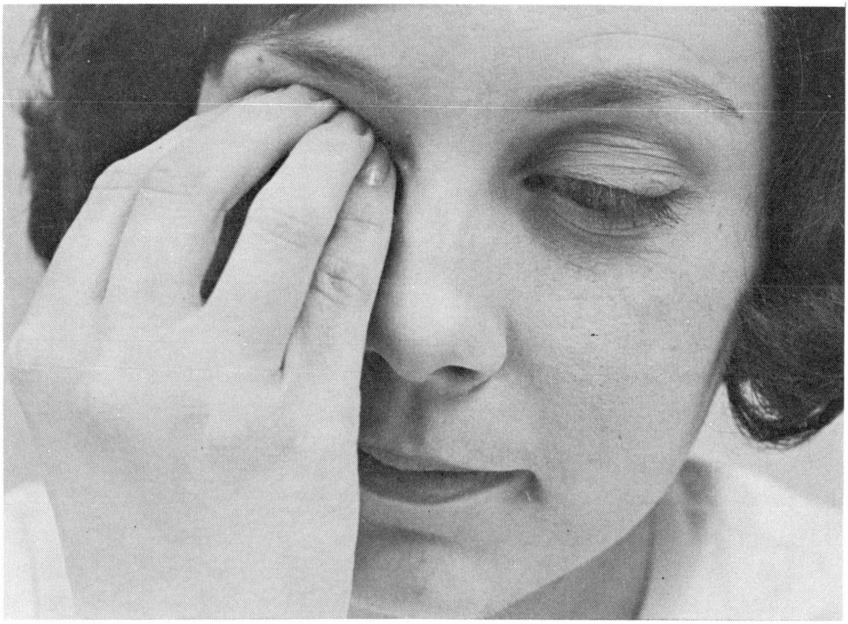

Figure 4–16. Recentration technique number two.

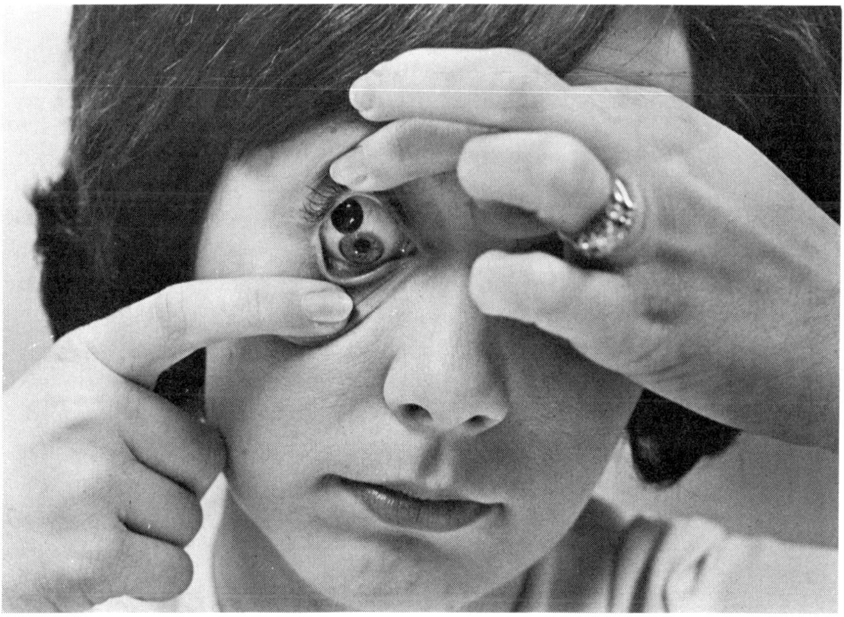

Figure 4–17. Recentration technique number three.

The Dropped Lens

If a lens is dropped, the patient must remain calm and tell everyone in the area to stand still. A contact lens is rarely broken by a fall, but it is invariably broken when someone steps on it. The patient visually scans the adjacent area and examines his clothing, especially cuffs, shoes, and open pockets. If the patient does not find the lens, he moves carefully so that he does not step on the lens. A beam of light is helpful in locating a lens.

After the patient finds the lens, he picks it up without sliding it, so as not to mar the lens. When the lens is concave side up, the patient picks it up by moistening his forefinger and pressing it gently against the lens. When it is concave side down, the same procedure is tried. This method may not work, for a suction may be formed between the lens and the surface on which it has fallen. When this occurs, the patient braces one edge of the lens with the forefinger of one hand and slides a sheet of paper under the opposite edge of the lens. If this method does not work, the patient pours fluid over the lens to loosen it. Fingernails should never be used to pick up a lens, for they may mar or chip it.

If a lens is dropped into a sink, the patient blocks the drain and visually scans the sink. After the patient finds the lens, he picks it up using one of the procedures just discussed. If none of them works, he fills the sink with water and stirs manually to float the lens loose. He then scoops it out with a cupped hand.

The patient must clean and inspect a dropped lens. If it is marred or if it causes discomfort, he should discontinue wear and consult his practitioner.

HYGIENIC CARE

Contact Lens Solutions

Contact lens wear is more successful when the lenses are physically and bacteriologically as clean as possible, when the lenses are wetted properly as the precorneal fluid spreads uniformly over the surfaces, and when the lenses are inserted easily and comfortably.

Proper patient education is of prime importance. Certain bactericidal and wetting actions of the precorneal fluid are also important. The normal physiologic concentration of lyzozyme in precorneal fluid kills some common bacteria, and the protein components of the precorneal fluid are conjugated with highly hydrated polysaccharides, thus providing good wetting of clean plastic contact lenses.[198]

Unless special procedures are used, however, contact lenses become dirty before they are placed on the eye or become dirty when on the eye.[199, 200] Contaminants such as oil, sebum, and bacteria are transferred to the lens by fingers, precorneal fluid, and water.

Dirty lenses do not wet properly and thus disturb vision, tissue integrity, and comfort. Vision is disturbed by the reduction of optical clarity of the lenses. Tissue integrity is disturbed by interference with precorneal fluid interchange beneath the lens and by direct mechanical irritation. Comfort is disturbed by the poor visual performance, tissue irritation, and direct mechanical irritation.

Proper preparation for insertion and proper storage help keep the lenses physically and bacteriologically clean, wet, and easy to handle. The results are better vision, tissue integrity, and comfort. Proper preparation for insertion and proper storage depend in part on the use of certain appropriately formulated solutions.[201–212] The three contact lens solutions commonly used by the patient are wetting solutions, soaking solutions, and cleaning solutions.

A useful and appropriately formulated nonmedicated contact lens solution must have three characteristics. It must meet the requirements of any ophthalmic solution in terms of tonicity, pH, sterility, and preservation. It must be compatible with the ocular tissues, with the other solutions used, and with the contact lens. It must aid in keeping the lenses clean, wet, and easy to insert, while not causing other problems.

WETTING

Because it is important, consider the concept of wetting in more detail.[213–215] Wetting is the spreading of fluid over the surface of a solid. There are three types of wetting processes: adhesion wetting, immersion wetting, and spreading wetting. For simplicity, these are considered together.

Two types of forces of attraction exist between molecules. The force of attraction between molecules of the same substance is termed *cohesion*. The force of attraction between molecules of different substances is termed *adhesion*. When a solid is placed in a liquid, the relationship between cohesion and adhesion determines whether the liquid spreads uniformly over the surfaces of the solid or bunches as drops on these surfaces. When the cohesive force between liquid molecules is greater than the adhesive force between liquid and solid molecules, the liquid forms droplets—that is, it does not wet the solid well. When the cohesive force between the liquid molecules is less than the adhesive force between the liquid and solid molecules, the liquid spreads uniformly. Thus, it wets the solid well.

Each solid has a wetting potential—a given liquid wets certain solids better than it wets other solids. The standard liquid used to determine wetting potential is water, and a solid that does not wet readily with water is termed *hydrophobic* (water-repelling). Polymethyl methacrylate is a relatively hydrophobic solid.

Each liquid has a wetting potential—a given solid is wetted better by certain liquids than by other liquids. Fortunately, precorneal fluid has a good wetting potential for polymethyl methacrylate.

PREPARATION FOR INSERTION

Before it is inserted, a contact lens should be made clean, wettable, and easy to handle. Contact lenses are prepared for insertion with no fluid, with water, with saliva, with synthetic detergents, and with wetting solution.

Alternative Methods

DRY. A dry lens is frequently physically and bacteriologically dirty, and this condition impedes wetting. It may also bear hard, raised particles, which mechanically irritate the ocular tissues. A dry lens is difficult to balance for insertion, and there is no buffer between the lens and the ocular tissues on insertion.

WATER. Water does not clean a lens, and it may even make it dirtier. Tap water is contaminated with bacteria, and its metal ion content favors the deposition of insoluble salts on the lens surfaces. It is difficult to balance the lens for insertion, and there is no buffer between the lens and the ocular tissues on insertion.

SALIVA. Saliva has a good wetting potential for polymethyl methacrylate. It is also viscous enough to allow balance for insertion and to provide a buffer between the lens and the ocular tissues on insertion. Unfortunately, it usually contains much bacteria and is a potential source of ocular infection.

SYNTHETIC DETERGENTS. Synthetic detergents, such as household soaps and cleaning agents, often make polymethyl methacrylate relatively more hydrophobic, and they leave a film on a lens. They also are poorly tolerated by and cause irritation to the ocular tissues.

WETTING SOLUTION. A properly formulated wetting solution prepares a contact lens for insertion by cleaning the lens and making its surfaces temporarily less hydrophobic. As a result of these factors and the temporary viscous coating placed on the lens, it is easy to balance the lens for insertion. The viscous coating also acts as a buffer between the lens and the ocular tissues upon insertion, thus increasing comfort. Because the lens is clean and temporarily less hydrophobic, the wetting ability of the precorneal fluid is enhanced, and it works more efficiently.

Chemistry of Wetting Solution

A wetting solution contains a wetting agent, a preservative, and a substance that increases viscosity. A wetting agent helps make the polymethyl methacrylate temporarily less hydrophobic and helps clean the lens surfaces. One of the wetting agents for contact lenses is a treated, modified polyvinyl alcohol.[216]

Preservatives aid in obtaining and preserving sterility of the solution and in killing bacteria. Commonly used preservatives and their concentrations are benzalkonium chloride (0.004 to 0.02 per cent), thimerosal (0.004 to 0.001 per cent), chlorobutanol (0.3 to 0.5 per cent), disodium ethylene diamine tetraacetate (0.01 per cent), phenylmercuric nitrate, and nitromersol.

Concentration is critical. Too weak a concentration does not provide a sufficient germicidal effect, and too strong a concentration interferes with wetting and may cause ocular tissue irritation.

Substances that increase viscosity also increase contact time and place a temporary mechanical buffer on the lens. Cellulose derivatives, such as methyl cellulose or carboxymethyl cellulose, are used. The viscosity-building substance must be selected carefully because an improper choice may inactivate the preservative.

A wetting solution may be isotonic or slightly hypertonic, which is obtained by the use of sodium chloride or potassium chloride. The pH of the solution should be compatible with that of the precorneal fluid—pH 7.0 to 7.8. Containers should ensure maintenance of solution sterility and should not alter the solution chemically or physically.

STORAGE

Wetting solutions are accepted almost universally as preparations for insertion. There is less acceptance of soaking solutions as storage media. It is generally agreed that storage in a soaking solution helps keep the lenses physically clean, wettable, and comfortable. The controversial point is whether storage in a soaking solution is advisable for bacteriologic cleanliness. Contact lenses may be stored dry, or they may be stored wet in water or soaking solution.

Alternative Methods

Dry. Before a lens is stored dry, it must be cleaned to remove oily and sebaceous materials and bacteria. It is difficult to clean a lens satisfactorily. Water does not eliminate oily and sebaceous materials, and it deposits mineral and bacterial contaminants. Wetting solution eliminates some oily and sebaceous material and some bacteria. Some oily and sebaceous materials remain in the microscopic pores of the lens, however, and the solution is not on the lens long enough to kill all bacteria. A cleaning solution removes oily and sebaceous material reasonably well and may kill some bacteria. Incomplete cleaning allows collection of microscopic and macroscopic material on the lens. Macroscopic material can cause mechanical irritation to the cornea, and microscopic material interferes with lens wetting.

After the lens is cleaned, it must be dried. It is difficult to dry a lens satisfactorily. Drying is usually done with a soft tissue. Frequently, the lens is not fully dried and lint is left on the surface. Even a soft tissue can scratch the lens surfaces. Scratches produce places for matter to collect and interfere with proper wetting.

A contact lens dehydrates in about 12 hours and hydrates in about 48 hours. The normal, or wearing, state for a contact lens is the hydrated state. When a lens dehydrates, debris and sebaceous deposits come out of the microscopic pores and coat the lens; such a coating interferes with wetting.

Hydration usually flattens the base curve of a contact lens; thus, the normal hydrated state should be maintained for best results.

WET. *Water.* Water has bacterial and mineral contaminants, has no preservative, and is a good culture medium for bacteria. Water also does not leach out oily and sebaceous materials from the microscopic pores of a contact lens.

Soaking Solution. A soaking solution maintains lens hydration. It has solubilizers to remove oily and sebaceous material from the microscopic pores, and antimicrobial components to kill bacteria.

Bacteriologic Cleanliness

Advocates of dry storage after cleaning believe that bacterial contamination is greater in wet storage because of the moist, warm, and dark environment.[217–219] Advocates of storage in soaking solution feel that bacterial contamination of lenses, cases, and fornices is less than in dry storage. They contend that bacteria cannot be eliminated by cleaning before storage owing to inadequate contact time. Because lenses are stored for seven or more hours nightly, it is believed that a soaking solution has adequate contact time.[220–226]

Current research indicates that bacterial contamination occurs in either dry or wet storage. It is considerably less, however, in wet storage with a soaking solution. Because of this fact and the general superiority of wet storage, the authors recommend storage in a proper soaking solution. Soaking solution should be changed and the case should be cleaned daily to minimize contamination.

Chemistry of Soaking Solutions

A soaking solution has a solubilizing agent to leach out substances from the microscopic pores of the lens. It also has antimicrobial substances, such as benzalkonium chloride, chlorobutanol, and thimerosal. Some have a chelating agent, such as ethylene diamine tetraacetate (EDTA).

Case

Contact lenses should be stored in a case that has readily identifiable compartments, is easy to clean, permits total immersion of the lenses, is made of lasting materials from which harmful chemicals cannot be leached, and has no sponge material.

Sponge material encourages the growth of bacteria, cannot be cleaned properly, may inactivate the germicidal activity of the soaking solution, and may trap abrasive material that will scratch the lenses.

PREPARATION FOR STORAGE (CLEANING)

Filmy deposits of oily sebum, precorneal fluid proteins, salty perspiration, organic salts, and cosmetic and silicone oils may be adsorbed on the lens surfaces to form a scum. Such a tightly bound accumulation is called *residue.*

Soaking solutions prevent residue from drying on the lenses and leach out some of the residue; wetting solution helps keep the lenses physically clean and wettable. Soaking and wetting solutions, however, do not completely eliminate residue.

Residue is removed by specially formulated contact lens cleaning solutions, by strong solutions, or by repolishing of the lens surfaces. The only safe procedure for the patient is the use of a specially formulated contact lens cleaning solution.

A contact lens cleaning solution usually has a wetting agent to ensure that the solution covers even the dirty surfaces, a chelating agent to tie up and remove insoluble metal ions, and a buffering agent to maintain alkalinity and to dissolve protein-containing deposits. It may also have an antimicrobial agent to kill bacteria.

The cleaning solution is used manually or in conjunction with a hydraulic device that forces jets of cleaner onto the lens. Cleaning solution is also used to clean the case.

Insertion and Storage Procedures

Another important aid to successful contact lens use is organized, unhurried procedures for insertion and storage. These procedures help keep the lenses clean and wettable, and they greatly decrease the possibility of losing, breaking, or switching the lenses.

The following are the insertion and storage procedures taught to the patient and the rationale for them.

Insertion

Step 1. *Thoroughly wash, rinse, and dry your hands, especially the fingertips, with a lint-free towel.* The patient should wash, rinse, and dry his hands to eliminate dirt and contaminants. He should use a nonmedicated soap that has a low oil content, and he should care for his fingertips, for they touch the lenses. Whenever it is possible, the patient should use a lint-free towel to prevent transfer of lint to the lenses.

Step 2. *Work over a safe place and gently remove the right lens in the recommended manner for your case.* The patient should handle his lenses in an area where a dropped lens can be found easily. If the patient must work over a sink, he should plug the drain so that a dropped lens will not fall down it. When the patient is seated at a table, he should move close to the edge of the table to minimize the possibility of a lens falling on the floor. The patient should always handle contact lenses gently, and he should work with one lens at a time to minimize the possibility of switching the lenses. Because a contact lens becomes scratched easily, the patient should never rub a lens along any surface. He should remove the lens from his case so there is minimum sliding of the lens along the case. If a lens does not come out of the case easily, the patient should stop the drain of a sink and flush the lens out with cold running water. He should never pick the lens out of the case with a fingernail or other sharp object.

STEP 3. *Hold the lens by its edges between the thumb and forefinger of one hand, and hold the bottle of wetting solution in the other hand. Apply a drop or two of wetting solution to each surface of the lens. Place the surfaces of the lens between the thumb and forefinger of one hand and gently rub the lens in a circular fashion for 5 to 10 seconds. Hold the lens by its edges, and rinse it with warm water.* The patient should hold the lens by its edges to reduce the transfer of substances from the fingers and to expose the surfaces for solution application. He should cover the surfaces with solution to protect them from the fingertips and to promote cleaning. The patient should rub the lens in a circular manner for about 5 to 10 seconds, or until it appears clean. He should use warm water to rinse loosened substances off the lens. Hot water may mar the lens, and cold water may condense and form a steamy film when the lens is placed on the warmer precorneal fluids.

STEP 4. *Continue to hold the lens by its edges with one hand and cup the other hand under it. View the lens against a light and inspect it for cleanliness. If the lens is not clean, repeat step 3.* Because the lens may fall, the patient should cup his hand under it. If he detects particles on the lens or a poorly wetted surface, he should reclean the lens.

STEP 5. *Insert the clean lens as it is or after applying another drop of wetting solution to it.* The patient should try to insert the lens as it is or after applying additional wetting solution, which may not be rinsed or lightly rinsed with warm water. He should then use the method most effective for him.

STEP 6. *Repeat steps 2 through 5 for the left lens.*

STEP 7. *Wash, rinse, and dry the lens case.* The patient should wash the case daily with nonmedicated soap having a relatively low fat content and no cold-cream base. He may need to use a small tooth brush to clean the case properly. He should thoroughly rinse and dry the case, preferably with a lint-free towel to remove dirt and oils.

STORAGE

STEP 1. *Thoroughly wash, rinse, and dry the hands, especially the fingertips. At the same time, the case may be cleaned and dried again.*

STEP 2. *Working over a safe place, remove your right lens. Hold it by the edges, and place a few drops of wetting or cleaning solution on it. Hold the lens by its surfaces, and rub it gently in a circular fashion between thumb and forefinger for about 5 to 10 seconds. Hold it by its edges and rinse it thoroughly with warm water.* Before storing the lens, the patient should remove elements that have gathered on the lens during the day. He should be cautioned never to place a lens with cleaning solution on his eye; the solution may cause irritation.

STEP 3. *Place the lens in the proper compartment of your case in the recommended manner.*

STEP 4. *Carefully place the cover on the case.*

STEP 5. *Repeat Steps 2 through 4 for the left lens.*

Because rubbing with fingers may scratch a lens, it may be advisable to place the solutions on the lens and to move them over the surfaces with a small cotton swab that has been wetted with water.*

CLEANING AND COSMETICS

CLEANING

Patients should never use anything on their lenses that has not been recommended by the practitioner. Cleaning agents not formulated specifically for contact lenses can harm the patient's lenses and eyes. When the patient uses a soft tissue to dry the lens, he should blot rather than rub it because rubbing may scratch the lens.

When the patient feels that he cannot clean his lenses properly or that his lenses are marred, he should discontinue wearing the lenses and take them to his practitioner. Because some coatings and scratches cannot be removed, the patient should try diligently to prevent their occurrence.

COSMETICS

Women should be careful not to transfer cosmetics to their lenses. Most cosmetics have an oily base that coats the lenses, temporarily irritates the eye, and interferes with vision. Whenever it is possible, the patient should insert contact lenses before most cosmetics are applied. This order reduces transfer of cosmetics to the lenses, and it also reduces marring of the eye makeup. She should apply facial powders with care so that particles do not get on her eyes.

The patient should apply mascara carefully so that it does not flake off into her eyes. Waterproof mascara is preferable, and should be applied before contact lenses are inserted. Some women find it convenient to dye their eyelashes. Liquid eyeshadow should be used. The patient should not permit nail-polish remover, or even its fumes, near her eyes or lenses.

Whenever possible, the patient should apply hair spray before contact lenses are inserted. Some types of hair spray on a lens irritate the eye temporarily and interfere with vision, but they can be removed without permanent damage to the lens. Other hair sprays cause permanent damage. The patient should not apply hair spray with contact lenses on and her eyes closed because the vapor from the spray remains in the air for several min-

* Dr. Harold R. Lutes has contributed much to this area of contact lens practice.

utes and may cause problems after the eyes are opened. If hair spray gets in a patient's eyes, she should wash out her eyes immediately with cold water and continue this washing five to ten minutes. As soon as it is possible, she should consult the practitioner. Plastic shields designed to protect the eyes from hair spray are available in many stores. It is inadvisable to wear contact lenses in a beauty shop.

GUIDES FOR WEAR

Wearing

Initial Adaptation

Because adaptation to contact lenses should be gradual, the practitioner should give the patient a wearing schedule that involves a gradual increase of daily wearing time (see Fig. 4–18 and discussion on p. 225). The patient should never wear the lenses more than the schedule calls for, and the practitioner should discuss the schedule at each progress examination.

WEARING SCHEDULE NEVER EXCEED THIS SCHEDULE		
DAY	SCHEDULE	COMMENTS

WHEN IN DOUBT, TAKE THEM OUT!
Consult with us at:
Office:

Home:

DAY	SCHEDULE	COMMENTS

You must keep your appointments. When this is impossible, consult us for guidance.

APPOINTMENTS			
DAY	DATE	TIME	AMOUNT OF WEAR

CUT OUT CARD

Name: wears contact lenses.
In an emergency, remove these lenses.
If assistance is needed, consult:
Name:
Address:
Office Ph.: Home Ph.:

Figure 4–18. Form related to contact lens wear given to the patient. The practitioner writes the wearing schedule, appointments, and his address and telephone number. The patient writes comments about wear, and he fills in the contact lens identification card.

The practitioner may advise the patient to wear contact lenses at home the first few days. During these initial days of contact lens wear, there is frequently excessive lacrimation. Excessive lacrimation may cause excessive lens movement, hazy vision, and excessive lens decentration and falling out. Wearing lenses at home the first few days makes adaptation easier, interferes least with daily tasks, and makes it easier to center a decentered lens or to find a dropped lens.

For these reasons, the practitioner should advise the patient to avoid tasks at first that involve extreme eye movements or critical vision. Sports, driving, prolonged viewing of television and movies, and prolonged reading are common examples of tasks involving critical vision. Because of associated restricted eye movements, prolonged watching of television or movies and prolonged reading may inhibit precorneal fluid interchange. The practitioner should tell the patient to take frequent breaks when doing such tasks during the initial days of contact lens wear. The patient should also avoid poorly ventilated rooms while adapting to contact lenses.

Amount of Wear

Because patients vary considerably in their ability to adapt to contact lenses, the amount of daily wear should be determined individually. Many people, however, are able to wear lenses 12 to 15 hours a day within two to three weeks. In case of illness or emergency, and as an auxiliary aid, the patient should have a pair of spectacles to wear. He should not be totally dependent on contact lenses.

Maintenance of Wear

After the patient attains a desirable wearing time, he should maintain it consistently. Daily variance should not exceed two to three hours. If the patient does not wear contact lenses for one or more days, he should reinstate his wearing time gradually.

Under such circumstances, the patient should consult the practitioner for a wearing schedule. If he cannot, he should use the following guide. He should subtract three hours for each day lenses are not worn from his average daily wearing time, and he should then add a maximum of 1½ hours a day until he reacquires normal wearing time. For example, assume the patient has not worn lenses for three days and that his average daily wearing time had been 15 hours. He would subtract 9 hours from 15 hours and wear his lenses 6 hours the first day. He would then add a maximum of 1½ hours daily until wearing time is 15 hours. Patients seldom need to start at less than three hours of wear the first day.

Circumstances Causing Problems

Some patients experience discomfort if they insert their lenses immediately on arising owing to the oil, mucus, and edema formation during sleep.

Such patients should wait at least half an hour before they insert their lenses. All patients should wash their faces thoroughly to remove matter from around the eyes.

The patient should not wear contact lenses while he is sleeping because such wear may irritate his eyes. If he accidentally naps with contact lenses on, he should remove, clean, and reinsert his lenses on arising. If unusual discomfort occurs, he should remove the lenses and consult his practitioner.

The practitioner should caution the patient to program his wearing time carefully so that he avoids overwear. During scholastic examination time and during the holiday season, many patients do not sleep sufficiently, and they tend to overwear their contact lenses.

The patient should never rub his eyes while he is wearing contact lenses because rubbing may cause irritation. He should not rest his face against his hand because this may cause a lens to fall out. When he washes and dries his face with his lenses on, he should close his eyes and blot gently. He should place lenses where children cannot reach them, and he should not keep lenses in a very hot place, such as on a radiator.

Occasions Necessitating Removal

Whenever the patient's vision becomes hazy or his comfort decreases, he should remove, clean, and reinsert his lenses. If these steps do not improve his vision and comfort, he should remove his lenses and consult the practitioner.

When a particle gets on the patient's eye while he is wearing contact lenses, he should look down and blink several times to wash the particle away. If discomfort persists, he should remove and clean his lenses. When running water is not available, the patient may use wetting solution alone on his lenses and fingertips. If he is outdoors, he should go into a sheltered area, such as a doorway, before removing his lens so that the lens will not be blown away by wind.

The authors tell their patients to remove, clean, and reinsert their lenses about every five hours.

Identification for Wear

The practitioner should provide the patient with a card indicating that the patient is a contact lens wearer. The patient should carry this card at all times for two reasons. First, in case he becomes unconscious from an accident, someone should remove his lenses. Second, in case his automobile driver's license is restricted by visual correction, he should be able to certify contact lens wear without removing the lenses.

Wear During Sports

As adaptation progresses, the practitioner and patient determine the sports activities in which the patient can participate while wearing his contact lenses. When the patient must engage in a particular sport, the practitioner should try to design lenses that allow such participation (p. 16). If a patient swims while wearing corneal contact lenses, he should narrow his palpebral aperture to reduce the possibility of the lenses falling out.

Wear During Travel

Because water differs in various locales, the patient may find it advisable to use distilled water when traveling. If he doubts the purity of the water, he should not use it. When he is traveling, the patient should not leave his lenses where they may accidentally be thrown away by someone unfamiliar with contact lenses. A patient who travels a great deal should have a spare pair of lenses.

Symptoms

As a patient adapts to contact lenses, he usually experiences certain normal, temporary changes in his appearance, vision, and comfort. If he were not adapting to contact lenses, these same temporary changes would probably cause him to consult his practitioner. The practitioner should guide the patient by explaining in understandable language normal and abnormal contact lens adaptation.

As a general guide, the practitioner should tell the patient that normal symptoms improve as adaptation progresses, and that they are not too severe. Symptoms of abnormalities remain the same or become worse as adaptation progresses, or they are severe. The practitioner should also tell the patient that the number, type, and severity of symptoms vary among individuals and between the two eyes of the same individual. Finally, the practitioner should tell the patient that perseverance is important for contact lens adaptation. However, when the patient experiences abnormal symptoms, he should remove his lenses and consult his practitioner.

Blinking

If contact lens wear is to be successful, the patient must blink fully and with reasonable frequency. A patient with a proper blink must be cautioned not to inhibit his blink, narrow his palpebral aperture, or tilt his head backwards. A patient with an improper blink must be guided to blink properly before contact lenses are dispensed. The patient must be taught to close the eyes gently and fully, to pause briefly before opening, and to blink about 15 times a minute. All patients must maintain clean, scratch-free lenses to allow proper blinking. *Fitting lenses in a manner that allows proper blinking and instructing the patient in proper blinking are two of the more important things a practitioner can do to assure success.*

5

STAGE FIVE

Control and Management of Adaptation

Four general steps have been completed up to this point. In Stage One, the prospective contact lens wearer has been evaluated and judged to be a potentially successful user of contact lenses. In Stage Two, lenses that potentially will attain this basic goal have been custom designed. In Stage Three, these lenses have been prepared for dispensing by proper ordering, verification, and perhaps modification. In Stage Four, the patient has been partially educated. Refinement of patient education before dispensing results in proper use and handling of the lenses.

These four preparatory steps should be completed before the patient is allowed to start wearing and adapting to the lenses. All that can be done is to provide optimum preparation so that adaptation theoretically will occur with maximum ease and a minimum of complications. Controlled, organized management of the patient is then imperative to enable the practitioner to observe and evaluate patient adaptation, and for prompt detection and remediation of undesired reactions. Close management also enables the practitioner to maintain the motivation of the patient at a desired level and to refine patient education. The object of such control and management is to ensure attainment of the basic goals. There are four categories of reasons why lenses cannot be dispensed to a patient without provision for such control and management.

Category one involves preparatory inadequacies. First, contemporary procedures for evaluating and educating the patient, and for designing and verifying the lenses, are not completely accurate. Second, the ability of a given eye to physiologically adapt satisfactorily to any contact lens cannot be completely predetermined. Third, the specific lens design and characteristics that will allow the best adaptation for a given eye cannot be completely predetermined, because each lens design is based on hypotheses of what will be satisfactory for the average patient.

Category two involves changes that occur in contact lens wear. First, temporary corneal topographical changes usually occur with the application of contact lenses. Such changes alter the relationship between the posterior lens surface and anterior corneal surface. Neither the amount and type of these changes nor the ability of the eye to adapt satisfactorily to the range of fitting relationships produced can be predetermined. Second, the base curvature of the contact lenses typically flattens with hydration. Neither the amount of change nor the eye's ability to adapt to it can be completely predetermined. This problem can be eliminated by ordering lenses that are prehydrated to the desired base curve. It is possible that annealing processes which will reduce or eliminate curvature flattening may be developed. Third, the initial environment in which the contact lens functions differs from the final environment. Excessive lacrimation, altered blink action, edema, and hyperemia are often exhibited in the initial environment. As adaptation progresses and these foreign body responses decrease, lens performance stabilizes. Final fitting can be accomplished only when performance is stable.

Category three involves undesired properties of polymethyl methacrylate, from which most contact lenses are made. First, it is a hydrophobic material. Second, it is a hard material. Third, it is impermeable to gases and fluids.

Category four involves signs and symptoms that result as the eye attempts to adapt to the presence of the contact lens. First, normal and abnormal symptoms and signs during the adaptation to contact lenses are often of the same type. They differ mainly in severity and duration. Second, if contact lenses were not being used, these same symptoms and signs would usually indicate to the patient that abnormality exists and professional consultation is needed. Contact lens patients, however, are told to expect these symptoms. Third, undesired reactions can occur without symptoms apparent to the patient.

UNDERSTANDING ADAPTATION

Proper adaptation has two related meanings in contact lens practice. In a physiologic sense, it means the adjustment of the tissues so that they function satisfactorily in the new environment caused by the contact lens. In a mechanistic sense, proper adaptation means the selection and adjustment of the physical characteristics of the lens and the direction of the patient's use of the lens. Proper mechanistic adaptation is meant to provide proper physiologic adaptation, comfort, vision, and appearance. Much of this book is concerned with proper mechanistic adaptation. It is also important to understand what occurs during normal physiologic adaptation and its variations, which form the basis for proper control and management. Only by using such knowledge is it possible to differentiate between normal and abnormal adaptation and then to establish the cause of any abnormality. The cause must be established before the proper mechanistic adaptation of lens characteristics or use can be effected to eliminate the abnormality.

Physiologic Adaptation

The body tends to maintain a balance, or *homeostasis,* between itself and its environment by a process of autoregulation. If an alien element enters the environment, the balance may temporarily be destroyed. Certain responses are made by the body in an attempt to eliminate the presence or neutralize the effect of the alien element and to establish again a balance. The responses may be either positive (stimulatory) or negative (depressive). Positive responses often involve an increase in metabolism, or hyperfunction. Negative responses often involve a decrease in metabolism, or hypofunction.

Most initial responses are simple, immediate, and direct defense mechanisms that act to eliminate the presence of the alien element. If elimination is not achieved, there are secondary responses directed toward adapting to the new environment caused by the presence of the alien element. These secondary responses often are at first relatively simple, immediate, and direct. The prolonged presence of the alien element may produce complex, delayed, and indirect responses.

Anterior Segment Environment

The normal environment of the anterior segment of the cornea has the following basic characteristics:

1. There is a relatively constant exposure to the atmosphere during all hours of wakefulness. This exposure permits atmospheric oxygen to become mixed with the precorneal fluid and produces a satisfactory evaporation rate of this fluid. These factors contribute to a proper metabolic cycle.

2. There is a relatively constant pumping of precorneal fluid across the anterior segment by the action of the upper lid during blinking. This pumping allows the nutrients and oxygen mixed in the precorneal fluid to become available to the cornea for use in its metabolic cycle. It also allows a removal of metabolic waste products.

3. There is external pressure only from the lid against the cornea and limbus during the blink cycle. This condition allows maintenance of the unique anatomic structure of the corneal tissues. It also allows proper blood flow through the limbal vessels, resulting in the availability of nutrients and oxygen, and the removal of waste products of metabolism.

4. There is no excessive mechanical stimulation to the tissues and nerve endings. Thus, a proper metabolic cycle is maintained, and there is no excessive discomfort or secretion.

A contact lens is an external antagonistic force applied in close proximity to some of the tissues of the anterior segment of the eye, thus producing two types of environmental changes. The first type of change is direct chemical interference with the corneal metabolic cycle. This interference is caused by the closure of some of the tissues from the atmosphere and the retardation of precorneal fluid flow. As a result, secondary physical effects such as corneal edema and conjunctival hyperemia may be produced. The second type of change is direct physical interference, caused by excessive pressure on the corneal tissues and limbal vessels from the lens, and excessive mechanical stimulation of the tissues and nerve endings. Secondary chemical effects, such as interference with the metabolic cycle and increased production of the sebaceous glands, may result.

Responses to Contact Lenses

The initial responses to a contact lens on the eye are similar to those produced by any foreign body on the eye. These responses are positive, or stimulatory, and are directed toward eliminating the lens. Hyperfunction of the lacrimal gland produces excessive fluid meant to wash the lens from the eye. Hyperfunction of the lids produces excessive blinking (blepharospasm) in an effort to push the lens from the eye and to flush away excessive lacrimal fluid. That these responses are both physiologic and psychological is demonstrated by the fact that the responses at times occur before the lens is placed on the eye. Adaptation is not complete until lacrimation is normal.

When the lens is not ejected, secondary responses related to the effort to adapt to the new environment are initiated. Active conjunctival hyperemia—an increased flow of blood through dilated vessels toward the affected part—often results. It is probably a result of reflex nervous mechanisms due to direct physical stimulation. Hyperemia may be maintained as a physiologic response due to metabolic hyperfunction or the reduction from other sources of oxygen and nutrient supply, and waste removal. Hyperemia of the lids, especially of the margins, may result from direct stimulation. Pressure of the lens on the limbal capillaries may produce passive hyperemia—that is, decreased flow of blood away from the area—or may prevent blood from flowing to the limbal area.

Corneal metabolism probably changes in this new environment produced by the use of contact lenses, although the exact mechanism is not fully understood. At the same time, the selective permeability of the cells and tissues, especially the epithelium, is probably altered. As a result of these factors and the derangement of the highly organized fibrillar components, the fluid level—degree of turgescence—of the cells and tissues may be changed. The clinical appearance of this condition is called edema.

The corneal tissue in most cases can adapt physiologically so that lenses can be worn for progressively longer periods before corneal or lid edema occurs. In many cases, full-time daily wear (12 to 14 hours) can be achieved without the appearance of edema. The exact mechanism of this physiologic adaptation is not understood. It is known that physiologic adaptation of the tissues is best when mechanistic adaptation of the lens is such that there is relatively little change of environment—that is, when direct chemical and physical interference is within certain limits and the lenses are handled, maintained, and used properly. It is also known that physiologic adaptation is best when duration of wear of the lens is gradually increased and then maintained at a certain level.

Aside from these extrinsic factors, physiologic adaptation probably also depends on intrinsic factors—that is, different corneas probably vary in the way their metabolism and sensitivity adapt to the presence of even a well fitted lens. Research is in progress to find out if this factor can be predetermined (see p. 408).

It is thought that the sensitivity of the cornea and the lid margins, which are richly supplied with free sensory nerve endings, decreases gradually in physiologic adaptation.

Recuperation, Regeneration, and Repair

As a result of the physiologic responses of the cornea, temporary cellular disturbances may occur. These disturbances must be neutralized to establish balance again. This may be done by recuperation, regeneration, or repair.

Recuperation is the recovery to a normal condition of slightly disturbed cells. Regeneration is a replacement of moderately disturbed cells by new cells of similar type and function. Repair is a replacement of markedly disturbed tissue by connective tissue elements—for example, cicatrization leaving a dense scar.

Almost all cellular disturbances from contact lens wear are neutralized by recuperation and regeneration, especially recuperation. It is unusual for permanent scar tissue, or any other permanent injury, to result from contact lens use. Among several reasons for this phenomenon is that, before tissues become markedly disturbed, discomfort becomes so great and vision and appearance become so poor that the lenses are removed. Also, it is unusual that Bowman's membrane, which is incapable of regeneration, is affected.

Edema and hyperemia, manifestations of cellular disturbance, probably are neutralized by recuperation after the lens—that is, the antagonistic force—is removed. Change of the shape or distortion of the elastic corneal tissue by pressure and molding is also probably neutralized primarily by recuperation and secondarily by regeneration. These are the three most common cellular disturbances caused by contact lens wear.

Regeneration of the epithelial tissue is a constant, normal condition to replace cells destroyed by ordinary wear and tear. The life of a corneal epithelial cell is probably less than one week. Regeneration to replace cells destroyed by excessive wear and tear is much quicker. Small or moderate areas (up to 3 mm. in diameter) of epithelial disturbance often are covered with new epithelium within 24 hours. It takes another few days, however, for underlying chemical reactions to stabilize.

Recuperation is usually allowed to occur spontaneously. Regeneration may be allowed to occur spontaneously, or medication or an anesthetic may be used, and the eye may be bandaged. Spontaneous regeneration is usually quicker than regeneration when medication is used, because many medications and anesthetics used on the cornea interfere with regeneration by impeding the migration or the mitotic activity of the cells. However, it may be necessary to use such medication to prevent infection and to relieve discomfort.

Symptoms and Signs Related to Adaptation

As a result of the responses to eliminate the presence or neutralize the effect of the contact lens, certain adaptive signs and symptoms are produced. If their duration is not too long—about three weeks or less—and if their severity is not too great, they are considered to be normal adaptive symptoms and signs. If these same symptoms and signs remain for too long a time or become too severe, they are considered to be abnormal adaptive signs and symptoms—that is, they are partially or completely caused by factors other than adaptation.

In controlling and managing the adaptation of the patient, the practitioner must be able to judge whether adaptive signs and symptoms are normal or abnormal. This judgment is complicated by individual differences, or range, of normal adaptive symptoms. Some patients have relatively many and severe symptoms, whereas other patients have relatively few and mild symptoms. The following is a general guide. Normal adaptive signs and symptoms become progressively better during the first few weeks as wearing time is progressively increased, and they are generally completely gone in two or three weeks. Abnormal adaptive signs and symptoms do not become better or even become progressively worse.

Adaptive symptoms and signs may be placed in three categories: vision, comfort, and appearance.

Vision. Excessive lacrimal fluid may cover and collect on the anterior surface of the lens and cause hazy vision. It may also increase the depth of fluid between the lens and the cornea sufficiently to temporarily alter refractive power. Excessive lens movement may be produced by excessive lacrimation and may cause a fluctuating, or sometimes relatively constant, malpositioning of the lens. As a result, the patient may see reflections, a shadow around objects, and sparklers coming from lights—or objects may have a hazy appearance. Excessive stimulation of the sebaceous glands of the lid and conjunctiva may cause the lens to become coated and the vision to become hazy. A catarrhal exudate may also be formed. As a result of edema, foggy vision or rainbows around lights may be produced. This symptom usually is apparent only when the edema is considerable—greater than in normal adaptation. After removal of the contact lenses, objects may be blurred when spectacles are used—so called spectacle blur—as a result of corneal molding or edema.

COMFORT. Excessive lacrimation and resultant lens movement may cause asthenopia related to poor visual performance. A feeling of nasal congestion may result as the excessive fluid is drained away. The excessive movement may stimulate the sensory nerves of the cornea and lids more, resulting in discomfort and awareness of the lens. Movement, stimulation, or altered metabolic function may produce hyperemia and edema, resulting in sensations of heat, grittiness, itching, and fatigue or vague discomfort. The hyperemia, edema, and nerve stimulation may produce photophobia, or increased light sensitivity. Discomfort may be greater in one eye than in the other. Assuming the fit of the lens in each eye is similar, this unequal discomfort often results because the two halves of the body are usually not neurophysiologically the same. Thus, one eye may physiologically adapt more readily than the other.

APPEARANCE. The patient may be aware of excessive lacrimation and resultant lens movement, and thus he may notice that the lenses position eccentrically or become displaced. He may also notice that he blinks more often in a subconscious attempt to reduce lens movement and flush the fluid away, or that he blinks less often in a subconscious attempt to reduce lens movement or increase his comfort by reducing contact between lens and lid. The patient may notice that he tilts his head back in a subconscious attempt to reduce lens movement and lid contact. He may also notice lid edema, which he reports as swelling of the lids, and conjunctival hyperemia, which he reports as red eyes. At the edge of the lens, bubbles or frothing due to reduced surface tension caused by excessive lacrimation may be noted.

Examination by the practitioner may show excessive lacrimation; increased, decreased, or partial blink action; faulty lens position; excessive lens movement; head tilt; coating of the lens; substandard visual performance; corneal, lid, or conjunctival edema; conjunctival or lid hyperemia; warm lids; altered ophthalmometric readings; and retention of fluorescein by some disrupted cells. These symptoms and signs are considered in greater detail on page 233.

CONTROL AND MANAGEMENT

PREPARATION

Before the patient is allowed to take his lenses home, two points must be verified to confirm that the initial preparation is satisfactory for physiologic adaptation to take place. First, the initial design characteristics must be verified on the patient's eyes. This may be the first time the patient has had a lens with these specific characteristics on his eyes. Often, if diagnostic lenses have not been used, this is the first time the patient has had any lenses on his eyes. In either case, whether predicted results will occur within accepted tolerances must be determined.

Second, the patient must be cooperative and properly informed—a result of proper education. Handling and storage procedures should be repeated until adequate proficiency by the patient is demonstrated. Guides should be reviewed. A wearing schedule that will allow physiologic adaptation to occur with maximum ease and minimum complications must be determined. Finally, an appointment for the next visit must be made.

One week usually is sufficient time to allow between ordering spherical single-vision lenses and the dispensing visit. Lenses of special design may require more time. The practitioner should ask his manufacturer the amount of time to allow.

Verification

At the dispensing visit, the patient's lenses are inserted by the examiner using the method discussed on page 70. After the initial reaction subsides somewhat, the patient sits in the waiting room two to five hours. During this period, the practitioner should make superficial external observations to ascertain that no abnormal discomfort or other reactions are occurring. At the same time, any needed reassurance can be given the patient. The patient may read appropriate material related to contact lenses.

When the lenses have stabilized sufficiently, it is determined whether their performance is adequate. The procedure is substantially the same as that used in progress examinations during the patient's adaptation to and wear of contact lenses. Diagnostic lens procedure is an important part of progress examinations (see p. 72). The seven components to this procedure are patient reports and examiner questioning, general external examination, visual analysis, fluorescein pattern evaluation, tissue integrity evaluation, contact lens physical structure evaluation, and patient responsibility evaluation.

Because of the various factors discussed, findings the first day cannot be expected to fulfill the standards established by the basic goals. Therefore, standards, or tolerances, for first-day findings must be established.

Patient Reports and Examiner Questioning. The patient must be sufficiently comfortable to wear the lenses as directed without the occurrence of tremendous stress. If this is not the case, the patient will become discouraged, and the wearing schedule will not be followed.

General External Examination. Inspection of position and movement of the lenses and the blink action of the patient should be made. Often after the two-to-five-hour waiting period, positioning is reasonably stable. In some cases, lacrimation is still sufficient to produce a considerable lack of stability. Stability of positioning should at least be sufficient so that no frequent displacement of the lens from the cornea occurs, and so that enough of the pupil is covered by the optic zone to permit functional vision.

If the patient has begun to develop backward head tilt or altered blink action in an effort to obtain more comfort, he should be cautioned not to do so. Although better initial comfort may come from these actions, a habit may develop that will retard satisfactory adaptation by the lids to the physical presence of the lens. Development of these habits may also reduce the pumping of the precorneal fluid between the lens and cornea, resulting in metabolic problems. Finally, the precorneal fluid may collect on the anterior and posterior surfaces, hazing vision considerably. If the patient has started to squint in order to hold the lenses more securely, he should be cautioned not to do so.

Visual Analysis. The patient's visual acuity should be satisfactory, so that he can function reasonably well with his lenses. Usually, if the processing has been correct, visual acuity will be 20/25 or better. Often, there is some fluctuation because of excessive lacrimation and lens movement. During the acuity check, the patient should be told to blink fully, or shut and then quickly open his eyes. This procedure usually temporarily flushes away the excess lacrimal fluid and produces satisfactory centration of the optic zone in front of the pupil. Visual acuity should be determined immediately after such a blink.

Fluorescein Pattern Evaluation. Fluorescein is instilled. Excessive lacrimation is usually sufficiently reduced so that a reasonably valid static fluorescein pattern can be obtained. The pattern should be approximately as desired. A central clearance or touch slightly in excess of that desired may be apparent. Assuming the initial design to be accurate, this altered relationship is due to molding or, less frequently, to edema of the cornea, resulting in a change of its shape and therefore in the fitting relationships.

Tissue Integrity Evaluation. At this stage of adaptation, there will seldom be any staining of the corneal tissue. Edema usually is not present or is very mild. Conjunctival hyperemia at the most should be mild. The ophthalmometric readings should have changed by no more than ± 0.50 D, with little or no distortion. The amount of ophthalmometric change may be comparable to the variance of the expected fluorescein pattern.

Contact Lens Physical Structure Evaluation. Evaluation need not be done at this examination unless abnormal reactions have occurred, because the physical structure was verified as part of the preparation for dispensing. If the pertinent factors are within tolerance, it may be assumed that the lenses are satisfactory to dispense for starting adaptation. Otherwise, corrections must be made.

Patient Responsibility Evaluation. Once the physical fit has been verified, further education of the patient is required in the handling, care, and wearing of contact lenses before they are dispensed. The patient is given a wearing schedule and an appointment for the next examination. Many wearing schedules have been suggested. All involve a gradual increase of time during the adaptation period. A frequently used schedule starts with three hours of wear the first day. Wearing time is increased 30 to 45 minutes each subsequent day until the desired total daily wear is attained.

Another common wearing schedule involves two daily wearing sessions that are separated by an interval of nonwear. The first day each wearing session lasts two hours, and the sessions are separated by a two-hour interval. During the first week, each wearing session is increased half an hour daily, and the two-hour interval is kept constant. During the second week, each wearing session is increased to six hours by adding one quarter hour daily, and the interval between the sessions is decreased one quarter hour daily.

These two wearing schedules result in about 12 hours of daily wear in about two weeks. Although these are satisfactory guides, rate of increase and total amount of wearing time must be based on individual patient responses.

Detection, Evaluation, and Remediation

After the patient starts wearing his lenses, the practitioner decides whether the specifications are satisfactory, based on the patient's ability to adapt. Proper adaptation is manifested by fulfillment of the basic goals. When proper adaptation occurs, there is generally no need to modify the lenses, wearing schedule, or patient procedures regardless of other criteria of fit. When proper adaptation does not occur, there is generally a need to modify the lenses, wearing schedule, or patient procedures regardless of other criteria of fit.

During the first two or three weeks of contact lens wear, adaptation is still occurring. The practitioner should not let normal adaptive symptoms and signs force him into making premature modifications. When there is reasonable comfort and tissue integrity the first two or three weeks, modification generally may be delayed. When there are significant abnormal symptoms and signs, however, modifications should not be delayed. Professional judgment is necessary to decide when modifications should be delayed or immediately applied.

Serial examination is necessary to control adaptation. It is used to detect and evaluate signs, to apply proper remediation when necessary, and to follow the progress of the patient. Effective serial examination depends on the practitioner's ability to differentiate between the symptoms and signs of normal and abnormal adaptation. When abnormality exists, the practitioner must differentiate between the possible causes of the abnormality and establish the most logical causes. This process of differentiation, or diagnosis, is an important part of proper management. The following schema shows the general management procedure:

Data gathering + data evaluation → diagnosis → remediation + follow-up

GATHERING DATA

Examination Schedule

Proper serial examination should have adequate frequency, intervals, and duration of coverage.[227] There should be, however, no unnecessary imposition on the patient's or practitioner's time.

The following progress examination schedule is a satisfactory guide: (1) one week after dispensing, (2) two weeks after dispensing, (3) three weeks after dispensing, (4) five weeks after dispensing, (5) eight weeks after dispensing, (6) twelve weeks after dispensing, (7) seventeen weeks after dispensing, and (8) twenty-three weeks after dispensing.

Weekly examinations are indicated during the first three weeks, while adaptation is occurring and wearing time is increasing. When adaptation is satisfactory on the third progress examination, subsequent visits may have the progressively increasing intervals shown. Any significant problems may necessitate deviation from this schedule and more frequent examinations. Traveling problems may necessitate somewhat less frequent examinations.

The basic schedule lasts for six months. In some cases, the last two visits are omitted, providing a three-month coverage. However, the minimum total initial period should be no less than three months. After the initial period, patients should be seen once every six months as long as contact lenses are worn.

Examination Procedure

The examination procedure must be organized and comprehensive so that all necessary data are systematically gathered and recorded (see record form, Appendix X). Symptoms reported by the patient are supplemented by appropriate questioning and testing procedures.

When the practitioner has a thorough knowledge of what is normal and abnormal, patient reports often provide sufficient information to establish several tentative causes of any symptomatic problem. The practitioner then should select tests that aid in determining the causes of the problem. The scope of the testing procedure must be broad enough to determine all possible causes of both symptomatic and asymptomatic problems. It should not be so broad, however, that time is wasted gathering needless data. The components of this procedure are patient reports and examiner questioning, external examination, visual analysis, fluorescein pattern evaluation, tissue integrity evaluation, contact lens physical structure evaluation, and patient responsibility evaluation.

Patient Reports and Examiner Questioning. Patient reports are generally extremely valuable in managing adaptation to and wear of contact lenses. There are several important reasons. First, no tests exist that measure such things as pain or discomfort. Symptoms may or may not be accompanied, therefore, by corroborating objective physical evidence. It is possible for a patient to have a problem that only he can appreciate. Lack of corroborating physical evidence does not automatically indicate that a symptom is of psychological origin, although it is a possibility. Second, the examiner sees the patient for only a short time and in a given environment. Some problems may not be manifest at this time or in this environment. Third, the significance of a symptom to a patient often differs from the significance of the same symptom to an examiner. To a patient, symptoms often are his problem. To an examiner, symptoms are often manifestations of a problem. When a patient relates his symptoms to an examiner, the voicing of these symptoms is often of therapeutic value. Fourth, patient reports in serial examination are a guide to the course of problems and the effectiveness of any therapy.

Meaningful patient reports depend on the rapport between patient and examiner, the examiner's ability to listen, the examiner's knowledge of normal reactions and the etiology and pathogenesis of abnormal reactions, and the examiner's ability to guide the patient by asking pertinent questions in an understandable manner. Patients usually report what they feel is wrong. Practitioners then ask questions about when, where, and how a condition began (onset) and how it acted after it arose (course). It is impossible to establish exact questions to be asked. The patient's initial statement indicates the initial questions to be asked. His answers then indicate appropriate subsequent questions.

The following important questions are often used.

In relation to *onset:*

When: When did you first notice the symptoms?
What time of the day was it?

Where: Which eye or do both eyes bother you?
Were you in any special place when you noticed it?

How: Did it occur suddenly or gradually?
How long had you worn your lenses that day?

In relation to *course:*

Constancy: Is the symptom present all the time or does it come and go?

Duration: If it comes and goes, about how long does it last?

Frequency: If it comes and goes, about how often does it occur?

Severity: How badly does it bother you?

Alteration: Does anything seem to make it better or worse?
Has it become better or worse since you first noticed it?

Associated Problems: Has anything changed about your general health or environment?

Patient reports and examiner questioning usually provide sufficient information to establish several tentative causes of the problem and to select the most logical corroborating tests. The practitioner must evaluate the information in terms of its reliability and corroborating physical evidence. It is important to know the patient's average daily wearing time and the wearing time during the examination day. Patients should generally be seen toward the end of their daily wearing time.

External Examination. While the patient is wearing his contact lenses, an external examination is performed to evaluate appearance, blink action, and contact lens position and movement. External examination of appearance may show excessive lacrimation; narrowing or widening of the palpebral aperture; head tilt; coating of the lenses; lid or conjunctival edema or hyperemia; and catarrhal exudates. External examination of blink action may show an incomplete blink or an excessively fast or slow blink rate. External examination of position and movement may show faulty position, excessive movement (loose), or insufficient movement (tight).

Analysis of Vision. While the patient is wearing his contact lenses, distant and near visual acuity is determined. Spherocylindrical retinoscopic refraction is done over the contact lenses. When the retinoscopic cylinder is less than 0.75 D, spherical subjective refraction is done. When indicated by symptoms, phorometric testing is done.

Refraction involved in the secondary area of the lens must also be considered. There is more plus power, a prism with its base toward the center of the lens, and poorer optical quality in the secondary area than in the optic zone. When enough of the pupil is covered by the secondary zone, two retinal images are produced simultaneously. The clear image is from the optic zone; the blurred, displaced image is from the secondary zone (Fig. 5–1).

When objects appear to have reflections, ghost images, shadows, or fringes around them, *flare* is present. The direction of the flare is opposite to the

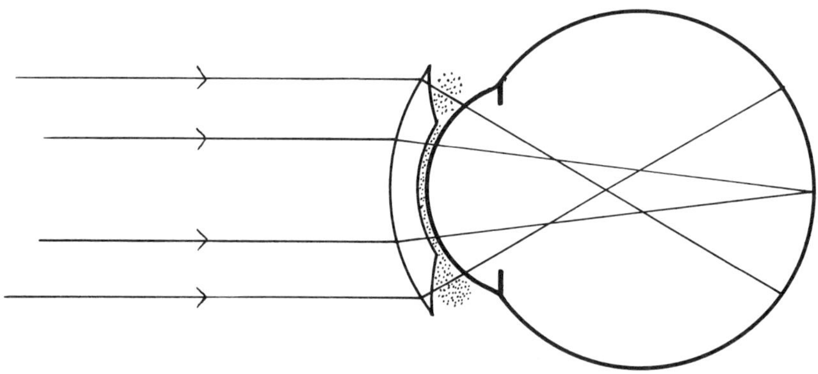

Figure 5–1. Flare (reflections, ghost images, shadows, fringes) is produced when the pupil is simultaneously covered by optic and secondary zones, which produces two retinal images.

decentered position of the lens on the eye.[228,229] For example, a lens positioned superiorly tends to produce flare inferiorly. When indicated by symptoms, flare is checked for at distance by isolation of a letter of best acuity value in a small block of light. The patient is asked what he sees. It may be necessary to ask him if there are shadows or doubling of either the letter or the block of light. When flare is present, its direction should be determined. The test should be done under ordinary room illumination and under dim illumination as pupil size varies. Each eye should be examined separately. The presence of flare may be tested at near in a similar manner by the use of reading material on a near point card.

When indicated by symptoms, hazing of vision is checked for by evaluation of the wetting of the contact lenses, by examination of the corneal tissues for edema, and by examination of the physical structure of the contact lenses.

Fluorescein Pattern Evaluation. While the patient is wearing his contact lenses, fluorescein is instilled, and the fluorescein pattern is studied with a stand or hand-held ultraviolet light and with a slit-lamp biomicroscope. This procedure enables evaluation of those aspects of bearing, venting, and movement due to the relationships of posterior surface of the lens to anterior corneal curves. The procedure is the same as that described on page 80. With the use of a slit-lamp biomicroscope, the interchange of precorneal fluid between the contact lens and the cornea can be evaluated by watching the flow of particles or debris. The flow of precorneal fluid over the front surface of the lens and the wetting of the front surface can also be evaluated by the use of a slit-lamp biomicroscope.

Tissue Integrity Evaluation. The contact lenses are removed, and the tissues of the anterior segment are examined for edema, staining, and injection, which are some of the common objective signs of temporary tissue changes experienced by contact lens wearers.[230–239] The examination is best done by slit-lamp biomicroscopy. The following is a brief discussion of corneal edema, corneal staining, and conjunctival injection.

Edema. This is an increase of the fluid content of a tissue. The water fluid in the body is distributed in three major regions, or compartments. About two thirds of the body fluid is contained within the walls of the individual cells—that is, it is intracellular. The rest is contained extracellularly either in the cellular interstices or in the blood plasma. Because the cornea is avascular, its extracellular fluid is contained in the interstices. On this basis, corneal edema may be considered to be either intracellular or extracellular. The body can accept a reasonable variation of extracellular fluid, but the intracellular fluid level must remain within relatively narrow limits. The cornea is normally in a relatively deturgescent state—that is, it contains less fluid than it is capable of accepting from distilled water or salt solutions. There is no certainty about the mechanism that neutralizes the affinity of the cornea for fluid and that maintains the deturgescent state. It is known that alteration of the physical structure, nerve impulses, nutrition or oxygen supply, waste removal, or evaporation rate may make the tissue edematous. Such changes can be caused by a contact lens.

Corneal edema is best seen with a slit-lamp biomicroscope. There are various appearances of edema with slit-lamp biomicroscopy. One form may be termed *central circular clouding*.[240] It is best seen with sclerotic scatter and the naked eye. It appears as a central, circular, gray area (Fig. 5–2).

Another form of corneal edema may be termed *misting*. It is best seen with retroillumination and the binocular microscope. It gives the tissue a misty appearance similar to frosted glass.

Misting may develop to another form of corneal edema, which may be termed *bedewing*. It is best seen with retroillumination and the binocular microscope. It appears as droplets on the background of the cornea. It resembles small dew drops on the petals of a flower. Some authors use the terms bedewing and edema interchangeably. The droplets may coalesce to vacuoles and then bullae.

Corneal Staining. Cellular permeability and integrity are disturbed by external or internal pressure. External pressure is related to mechanical rubbing (abrasion), and internal pressure is related to increased accumulation of fluid or metabolic waste products. The disturbed areas retain a relatively large amount of fluorescein and become stained. When viewed with ultraviolet light, the disturbed areas are brighter green than the surrounding areas.

Corneal staining may have various appearances, which are often related to the cause. More common types of staining are stippling, foreign body stain, arcuate staining, dimples, and coalesced staining.

Stippling (superficial punctate staining) appears as small, superficial, stained areas spread over various parts of the cornea. It may be caused by poor venting or bearing (Fig. 5–3). When aperture positioning lenses are fitted, a common site of superficial punctate staining is the cornea adjacent to the limbus near three and nine o'clock. This staining is frequently accompanied by a horizontal pattern of bulbar conjunctival injection directed toward the areas of staining. Such staining can be caused by secondary curves that bear on the three and nine o'clock corneal areas. In most cases, however, the lens does not bear on these areas, and staining is due to poor venting and corneal dehydration. It occurs most frequently when there is an inadequate secondary reservoir of precorneal fluid, a large optic zone, insufficient lens movement, inadequate blinking, or lid contact.

Foreign body stain appears as small, superficial, stained areas spread over various parts of the cornea and may be caused by a foreign body moving between the lens and the cornea. The stained areas form a pattern corresponding to the flow path of the foreign body. Usually, a spiral or straight path is formed (Fig. 5–4). When the foreign body lodges between the lens and the cornea, a coalesced stained area is produced (Fig. 5–5).

Arcuate staining appears as an arclike area of small, superficial staining.

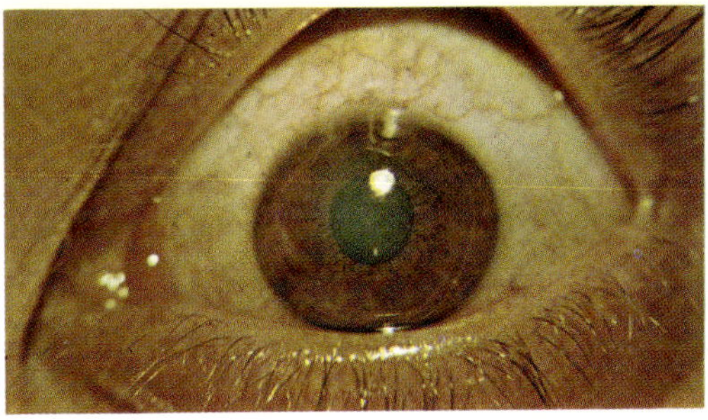

Figure 5–2. Central circular clouding and conjunctival injection. With fluorescein and ultraviolet light, superficial punctate staining is seen. (Courtesy of Dr. Neal J. Bailey.)

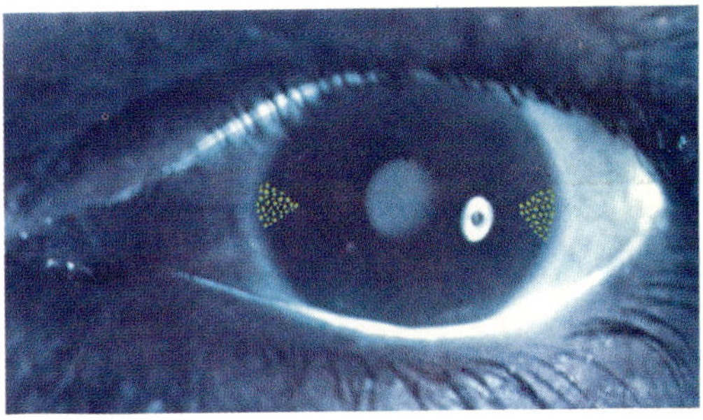

Figure 5–3. Superficial punctate staining.

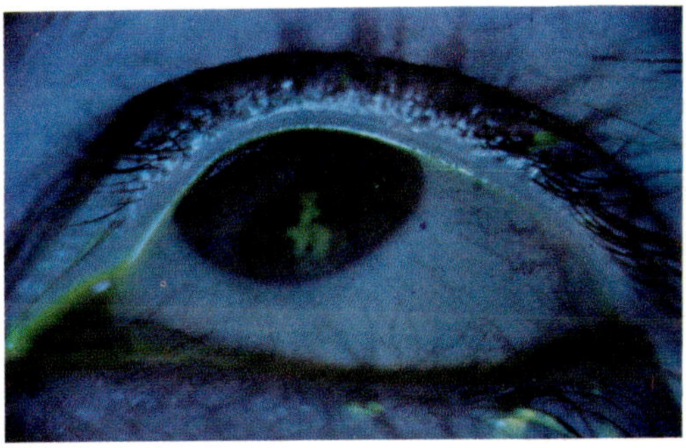

Figure 5–4. Stain pattern caused by a flowing foreign body. (Courtesy of Dr. Neal J. Bailey.)

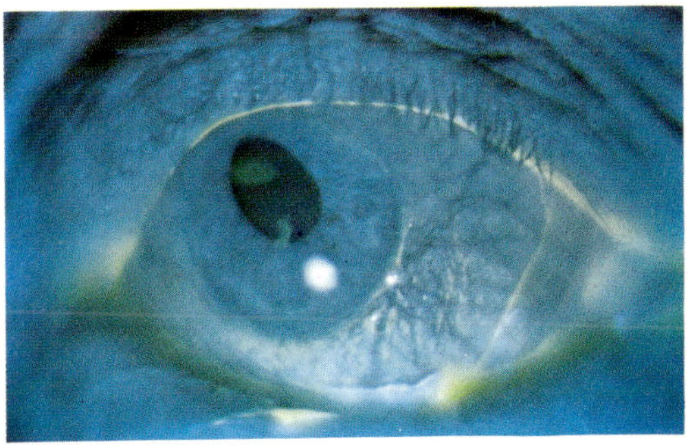

Figure 5–5. Near the bottom of the pupil is a stain pattern caused by a flowing foreign body. Near the top of the pupil is a coalesced stained area caused by a lodged foreign body. (Courtesy of Dr. Neal J. Bailey.)

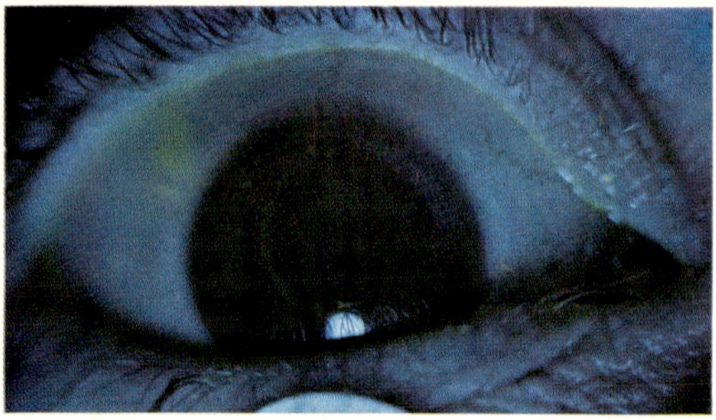

Figure 5–6. An arcuate area of staining caused by excessive pressure from, and poor precorneal fluid interchange under, the secondary zone of a contact lens. (Courtesy of Dr. Neal J. Bailey.)

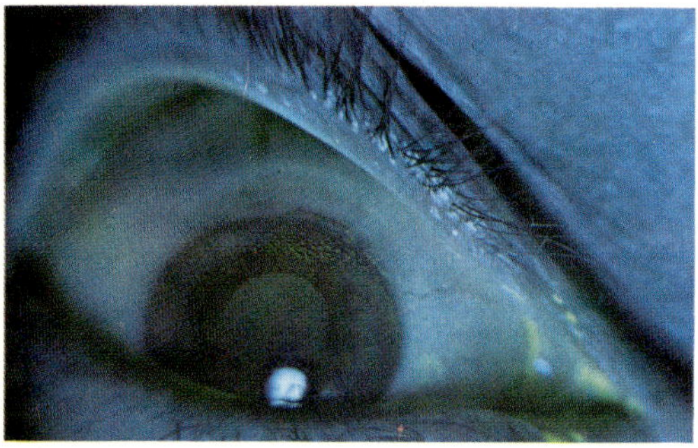

Figure 5–7. Dimple staining of the superior cornea. (Courtesy of Dr. Neal J. Bailey.)

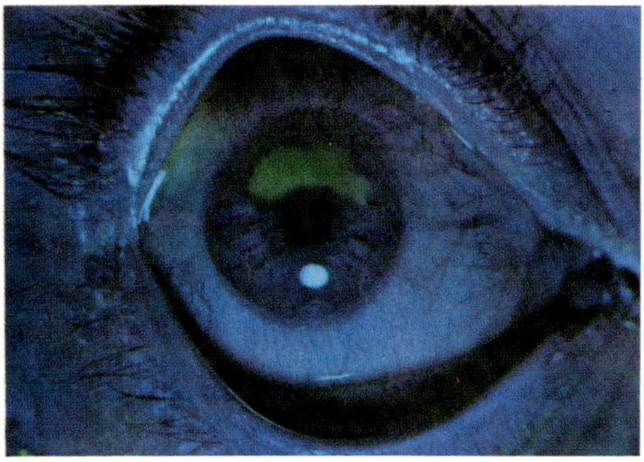

Figure 5–8. Arclike coalesced staining area. (Courtesy of Dr. Neal J. Bailey.)

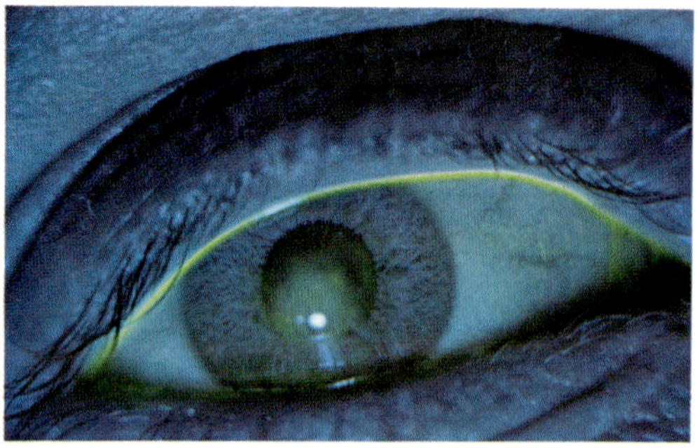

Figure 5–9. Round coalesced staining area. (Courtesy of Dr. Neal J. Bailey.)

It is usually caused by excessive pressure on, or poor precorneal fluid interchange under, a narrow area of a contact lens. Often it occurs in a transition area between two adjacent posterior curvatures (Fig. 5–6).

Dimples—external pressure on an edematous area may cause a pitlike depression. This depression is caused by localized pressure or gaseous bubbles between the lens and the cornea squeezing interstitial fluid into adjacent areas. The pitted area will become stained (Fig. 5–7). Once the pressure is released, the fluid seeps back and the pit disappears. Another type of pitlike depression is Fuchs' dimples or dellen. Dellen occurs at the margin of the cornea at or near the limbus, especially nasally and temporally.

Large, coalesced staining is a large area of relatively deep staining. A large number of cells in this area have been disturbed by external or internal pressure (Figs. 5–8 and 5–9).

Wetting stain—when the corneal tissue is unhealthy, the precorneal fluid may not flow uniformly over it—that is, corneal wetting is poor. The areas that do not wet appear darker than the surrounding areas.

Conjunctival Injection. Because the cornea is avascular, it depends on the conjunctival vessels for part of its nutrient and oxygen supply and waste product removal. When there is sufficient alteration of the corneal environment, the conjunctival vessels may become engorged, a phenomenon which may aid in the supply of nutrients and oxygen to and the removal of waste products from the cornea. Engorgement of the vessels may also be caused by direct irritation or trauma of the conjunctival tissues. Injection associated with contact lens wear is often greatest near 3 and 9 o'clock on the cornea. Such injection may be associated with dellen.

Corneal Curvature Change. Another relatively common sign of temporary tissue change experienced by contact lens wearers is corneal curvature change. This change is best detected by ophthalmometry. The amount of spherical or toric change is determined by comparison of present readings to those taken before the patient was fitted with contact lenses. Distortion of the corneal tissues is detected by study of the regularity of the miral images. Corneal curvature change may be due to molding of the elastic corneal tissues or to edema.

Evaluation of the Physical Structure of Contact Lenses. When indicated by symptoms or signs, it may be necessary to inspect and verify the physical structure of the contact lenses.

Patient Responsibility. When indicated by symptoms or signs, it may be necessary to review the patient's handling, care, and use of his lenses.

EVALUATING DATA AND REMEDIATION

General Causes

There are three general causes of symptoms and signs related to contact lens wear: normal adaptation, patient-related factors, and lens-related factors.[241–243]

NORMAL ADAPTATION. Certain normal symptoms and signs are often found in the patient as his eyes adapt to contact lenses (see p. 221). Abnormal reactions are usually due to patient- or lens-related factors.

PATIENT-RELATED FACTORS. Patient-related factors include environment; handling, care, and use; and psychological reaction.

Environment. An undesirable external environment may result from an atmosphere antagonistic to contact lens wear. An undesirable internal environment results when the atmosphere provided by the patient's body is antagonistic to contact lens wear. Examples of undesirable external environment are windy, dusty, or smoky locations. Examples of undesirable internal environment are colds or allergies. Patient reports and examiner questioning usually provide the necessary diagnostic information for remediation.

Handling, Care, and Use. The patient may be handling, caring for, or using his lenses improperly. Patient reports and examiner questioning usually provide the necessary diagnostic information for remediation.

Psychological Reaction. The patient may have developed anxieties related to contact lens wear. Patient reports and examiner questioning, patient attitudes, and lack of physical evidence corroborating the patient's complaints usually provide the necessary diagnostic information for remediation.

LENS-RELATED FACTORS. Lens-related factors include inadequate initial design selection, refractive power, and physical structure.

Design Selection. Initial lens characteristics may be inadequate for the patient, producing improper bearing, venting, position, and movement. Patient reports and examiner questioning, external examination, analysis of the patient's vision, fluorescein pattern evaluation, and tissue integrity evaluation provide the necessary diagnostic information for remediation.

Refractive Power. Poor visual acuity and comfort may be due to an inadequate refractive power. Patient reports, examiner questioning, and analysis of the patient's vision provide the necessary diagnostic information for remediation.

Physical Structure. The physical structure of the contact lens may be poor, owing to improper initial verification and inspection, to improper patient care and handling, or to some problems inherent in the use of polymethyl methacrylate. Included in the latter category may be spherical or toric curvature changes due to hydration and pressure. Patient reports, examiner questioning, and physical structure evaluation provide the necessary diagnostic information for remediation.

Only problems due to lens-related factors necessitate altering the lens structure. Alteration may be either by the modification of the present lenses or by the processing of new lenses.

SPECIFIC EVALUATION

A patient reports problems in his own words. For example, he does not say that the refractive power is incorrect, but rather that his vision is blurred. A patient reports the effect of a problem; the examiner must establish the cause and remedy, and follow up the case.

Considered here are the most common patient reports of problems in three categories: vision, appearance, and comfort. Then the more common causes, the related onset and course, the appropriate corroborating tests, and the appropriate remediation are discussed.

VISION. The specific evaluation of vision by the practitioner may depend on the patient's complaints of blurred vision with contact lenses; reflections, ghost images, shadows, and fringes around objects; blurred vision with spectacles; rainbows; and discomfort in reading.

Blurred Vision with Contact Lenses at Distance or Near. Causes for blurred vision during contact lens wearing include improper refractive power, coated lenses, switched lenses, excessive lacrimation, and central corneal edema.

Improper spherical or cylindrical power may produce blurred vision. Plus overcorrection produces blurred distance vision. Unless it is great, minus overcorrection usually does not produce blurred vision for a young person with ample accommodation. It usually produces blurred distance and near vision for older people with poor accommodation. Asthenopia may also be produced. High degrees of uncorrected astigmatic error produce blurred distance or near vision. Low degrees of uncorrected astigmatic error frequently produce only asthenopia.

Blur from improper refractive power is constant, starts as soon as the lenses are inserted, and is not helped by removal and cleaning of the lenses. Improper refractive power may be due to improper initial prescription, a change in the patient's ametropia, or a spherical or cylindrical change of the base curve. When the base curve is changed, there is also some change of the bearing, venting, position, and movement of the lens.

Corroborating tests that should be done include visual acuity, retinoscopic, and subjective refractive tests. Also, the base curve should be read to determine any change.

In remediation, spherical power of the original lenses may be safely changed up to a maximum of about $-.50$ D to $-.75$ D, or $+.37$ D. When greater amounts of spherical power change are needed, it is often necessary to make a new lens. When an astigmatic correction is needed, new lenses must be ordered. A base curve change sufficient to produce bearing, venting, position, or movement, as well as visual, problems, necessitates a new lens. Generally, the base curve does not change this much.

Polymethyl methacrylate becomes coated easily and blurred vision results. Oily and sebaceous material can be transferred to the lenses from the fingers or precorneal fluid. Scratches on the lens, infrequent or incomplete blinking, exudates from conjunctivitis, stimulation of the lid glands by a poor lens edge, mucus from a cold or allergy, and improper handling or care also contribute to the coating of a lens.[244, 245]

Blurred vision from coating may be constant or intermittent. Usually, visual acuity is not reduced much, but things look hazy to the patient. Removing and cleaning the lenses often gives temporary relief.

Corroborating tests include external examination with a slit lamp and white light to show coated surfaces. Coating may remain on the lenses after they are removed from the patient. The coating can then be seen with a reticule or stereoscopic microscope. Refraction is usually negative, and there is no corneal edema.

Remediation, as the need indicates, should include cleaning of lenses, removal of scratches, and refinishing of edges. Patient handling, care, and use are reviewed.

Central corneal edema—light is properly refracted through the cornea only when it is of normal transparency and regularity. When the corneal tissue becomes edematous, it does not possess normal transparency and regularity. If central edema is great enough, vision is blurred.

The patient usually reports foggy or hazy vision. It may be accompanied by increased photophobia, the appearance of rainbows around lights, conjunctival injection, hotness, stinging, and itching. Frequently, hazy vision and other symptoms are not noticed until the lenses are worn several hours. Removing lenses to clean them gives little or no relief. If the lenses are removed for several hours and then inserted again, vision and comfort are usually satisfactory for several hours. Then the symptoms recur. Vision may be blurred considerably when the contact lenses are taken off and spectacles are put on (spectacle blur). There may also be pain when the lenses are removed.

Corroborating tests should include slit-lamp biomicroscopy after removal of the lenses to show corneal edema or staining.

Remediation depends on the cause of the edema or staining. There are two general causes of corneal edema or staining due to the relationship of the lens to the cornea. The first includes factors that tend to produce excessive external pressure on a relatively small corneal area. The second includes factors that tend to produce excessive internal pressure on the corneal tissues. Internal pressure often results from retardation of the precorneal fluid flow between the lens and cornea or from too large an exclusion of the cornea from its normal environment.

Many symptoms of excessive external pressure arise almost as soon as the lenses are inserted, and many symptoms of excessive internal pressure arise several hours after the lenses are inserted. Assuming a normal fit and sound physical structure of the lens, improper venting causes most edema and staining.

External examination and fluorescein pattern evaluation are used to evaluate the bearing, venting, position and movement of the lenses and to determine the cause of the edema or staining. External examination permits an evaluation of lens movement. A loose fit tends to produce excessive external pressure on the cornea, but there is usually an adequate flow of precorneal fluid between the lenses and cornea. A tight fit tends to produce excessive internal pressure by inhibiting precorneal fluid flow between the lens and cornea.

The degree of movement is the important factor. To eliminate an undesired type of movement, the possible causes of the excess or insufficiency should be analyzed (see p. 74). Blink action should be evaluated.

Fluorescein pattern evaluation allows for determination of the relationships between the posterior surface of the lens and anterior corneal curvatures. If the fluorescein pattern indicates poor bearing or venting and if there are signs of edema or staining, appropriate lens modification is made. This modification may be done by alteration of the original lenses or by the ordering of new lenses. Alteration of the original lenses may be made when the needed curvature change is a flattening, widening, or addition of secondary curvatures. Any other posterior curvature change can be obtained only by the processing of a new lens.

If considerable edema exists, lens movement and the fluorescein pattern may be misleading. Considerable edema is often accompanied by a steepening of corneal curvature, making the apparent relationship between the posterior surface of the lens and anterior corneal curvatures flatter than it normally would be. Before the fit can be evaluated, lens wear must be discontinued until there is no edema.

It is possible for edema or staining to occur without a blurring of vision when contact lenses are worn. This phenomenon occurs when the edema or staining is toward the periphery of the cornea or when the degree is small. Edema or staining can also be caused by improper wear.

Switched lenses—when the base curve and refractive power of the lenses are the same, visual acuity is not affected by switched lenses. When the base curve or refractive power of the two lenses is different, visual acuity may be affected by switched lenses. Visual acuity is affected when the *total effective refractive power* differs between the two lenses.

Total effective refractive power is based on the refractive power read on the Lensometer plus the base curve relationship to the flattest central corneal meridian. For example, if a right lens has a 7.50 mm. base curve and a −4.00 D refractive power, and a left lens has a 7.40 mm. base curve and a −4.50 D power, the total effective refractive power when the lenses are on the eye is the same. If the lenses are switched, there is no reduction of acuity. Bearing, venting, or movement problems may occur because of incorrect base curve relationships. Total effective refractive power difference causes blurred vision in the same manner as that discussed under improper refractive power (p. 233).

Corroborating tests should include visual acuity, retinoscopic, and subjective refractive tests. The refractive error in each eye would correspond to the difference in total effective refractive power between the lenses. Additional plus would be needed for one eye and an equal amount of additional minus for the other eye. Base curves and/or Lensometer refractive power should be determined.

Remediation is simple. The lenses are switched and worn on the appropriate eyes, and the patient is again instructed in the prevention of lens switching.

Excessive lacrimation—when there is an excess of lacrimal fluid on the eye, vision may intermittently be clear and blurred. The reasons are: (1) excess fluid causes an irregular refraction of light; (2) it increases the thickness of the precorneal fluid layer between the contact lens and the cornea, thus altering the refractive power somewhat; and (3) because of the excess fluid, there may be too much lens movement, causing intermittent malpositioning of the lenses, and a simultaneous pupil coverage by optic and secondary zones. Blinking flushes away excess fluid and temporarily clears vision.

Corroborating tests include an external examination to show excessive lacrimation and lens movement. Visual acuity would fluctuate. Physical structure evaluation of the lenses may show a poor edge, scratches, or foreign substance.

Remediation requires determination of the cause of the excessive lacrimation. Excessive lacrimation may be due to a poor edge, a scratched lens, foreign substances on the lens, or a loose lens. As the need indicates, the edges are refinished, the scratches are removed, the foreign substances are removed, or the design characteristics of the lens are altered. When scratches or foreign substances cause the problem, proper care and handling must be reviewed.

Reflections, Ghost Images, Shadows, or Fringes around Objects. These problems, generally grouped under the term *flare,* are also discussed on page 228. Two causes discussed here are excessive lens movement and too small an optic zone for the lens position.

When flare is due to excessive lens movement, the problem is usually an intermittent one because the amount of pupil coverage by the secondary zone varies.

Corroborating tests include external examination to show excessive lens movement. The flare check test should be used (p. 229). Fluorescein pattern evaluation may show the causes of the excessive movement as well as the pupil coverage by the secondary zone. Physical structure evaluation may show causes for the production of excessive lacrimation, which in turn produces excessive movement. Such causes are poor edge configuration, excessive edge thickness, scratched lens surfaces, or foreign elements on the lens surfaces.

Remediation includes alteration of the lens design to reduce movement, refinishing of the edges, removal of scratches, or removal of foreign substances. When scratches or foreign substances are the cause of the problem, proper care and handling must be reviewed.

When flare is relatively constant, it usually results from too small an optic zone for a given lens position. There is no excessive lens movement, but the pupil is constantly covered simultaneously by optic and secondary zones.

Corroborating tests include external examination to show satisfactory movement. The flare check test would be positive. Fluorescein pattern evaluation would show a simultaneous optic- and secondary-zone coverage of the pupil.

For remediation, the optic zone must be positioned over a larger amount of the pupil. This can be done in one of two ways. First, a lens design similar to that used but with a larger optic-zone or lens diameter is used. Second, a lens design in which the lens will position more nearly centrally is used (see p. 76).

Blurred Vision When Contact Lenses Are Removed and Spectacles Are Worn. When the refractive power of the patient's spectacles does not properly compensate for his ametropia, vision is blurred. Improper compensation may be due to temporary alteration of the corneal curvature or transparency or to an ametropic alteration. When contact lenses are removed and spectacles are worn, vision is blurred. This is termed ***spectacle blur.***

Temporary corneal curvature or transparency change—contact lens wear may temporarily alter corneal curvature, and thus alter the eye's refractive power. Spectacles prescribed for the ametropia before this alteration may no longer provide good visual acuity. Because the cornea is elastic, it may be molded by the pressures from, and curvatures of contact lenses. (There may also be distortion.) The toricity of a toric cornea fitted with a spherical base lens tends to be decreased. A temporary change in corneal curvature and transparency may also be due to edema. After contact lenses are left off for a while, the corneal curvature and transparency return to normal, and vision improves.

In the corroborating tests, ophthalmometric readings would vary from those found before contact lenses were fitted. There may be distortion of the miral images. Spectacle refractive power would vary from that needed before contact lenses were fitted. Needed contact lens refractive power would not be altered. Owing to corneal curvature change, fluorescein pattern evaluation would show a different relationship between the posterior surface of the lens and the anterior corneal curvature. Edema may be detected with slit-lamp biomicroscopy.

In remediation, it is often impossible to eliminate completely spectacle blur due to corneal curvature change. Spectacle blur should be minimized so that the patient does not become entirely dependent on contact lenses. The authors use two criteria concerning spectacle blur during adaptation: spectacle blur associated with significant corneal edema or staining must be eliminated, and spectacle blur not associated with significant edema or staining must be eliminated when the patient becomes overly dependent on contact lenses. The factors of amount of blur and time enter into the discarding of spectacles. Either the amount of blur is so great for any given time that spectacles are not used, or the amount is not great but it takes so long for vision to clear that spectacles are not used.

Corneal curvature change during adaptation of one diopter or more frequently causes prolonged spectacle blur. The physical fit of the lens must be altered to provide better bearing, venting, or movement.

See page 251 for a discussion of long-term spectacle blur.

Ametropic alteration—the basic ametropia in a contact lens patient may change. Spectacles frequently are not changed when contact lenses are prescribed. Often the patient compares visual acuity in an old spectacle with visual acuity in a current contact lens.

In corroborating tests, spectacle and contact lens refraction would have changed from those needed initially, or an old spectacle refractive power may be in use.

For remediation, proper refractive power should be prescribed.

Rainbows Around Lights. When corneal edema is sufficiently severe, the patient may see colored rings around lights. Photophobia, smoky vision, and pain may accompany this phenomenon.

Corneal edema—dispersion and scattering of light through an edematous cornea may cause rainbows.

In corroborating tests, external examination may show conjunctival injection. Visual analysis may show decreased acuity or hazy vision. Fluorescein pattern evaluation may show poor bearing or venting. Tissue integrity evaluation will show edema or staining.

In remediation, the cause of the edema or staining must be determined and eliminated. Because edema often changes corneal curvature, relationships between the posterior surface of the lens and anterior corneal curvatures are altered. Lens wear is discontinued until the edema is relieved. The fit is then evaluated, and the proper modifications are made. Note that the report of rainbows may indicate flare and not edema.

Eye Discomfort in Reading. Residual refractive error—residual astigmatism or hyperopia may cause discomfort during near-visual tasks, even when distant visual acuity and comfort are satisfactory.

Corroborating tests include retinoscopic and subjective refraction tests to show residual astigmatism or hyperopia.

For remediation, the residual astigmatism or hyperopia should be compensated for.

Insufficient accommodative ability—a myopic incipient presbyope uses more accommodative effort with contact lens than with spectacle lens wear (see also p. 355).

Corroborating tests include accommodative tests to show a need for additional plus at near.

For remediation, the patient should be treated as a presbyope.

Poor fluid interchange—when a person reads, only small eye movements are made. Depressed gaze removes some of the pressure from the upper lid on the lens. Because of these factors, there is less lens movement and pumping action. This condition reduces precorneal fluid interchange. Depressed gaze also causes the lens to be translated upward, a condition which may produce stagnated pools of precorneal fluid beneath the top of the optic zone.

Corroborating tests include external examination to show little lens movement in depressed gaze. Fluorescein pattern evaluation would show stagnated pools.

For remediation, the patient may be instructed to move his eyes more, to look away from his close work periodically, and to blink more; or the lens design may be altered. When the basic fit is satisfactory, the former procedure should be tried initially. When the basic fit is not satisfactory, the lens design should be altered.

Flare—when gaze is depressed for near, the contact lens is translated upward. This may produce a simultaneous covering of the pupil by optic and secondary zones, which may result in flare.

That a haze or ghost image is imparted to the letters on a near point card is corroboration of flare.

For remediation, the optic-zone or the lens diameter is altered to provide for proper optic-zone coverage of the pupil in depressed gaze.

Poor binocular coordination—poor binocular coordination may produce discomfort during close work.[246]

Corroborating tests include binocular near point testing procedures to indicate a deficiency in binocular coordination.

For remediation, the refractive power of the contact lens should be altered, visual training should be employed, or auxiliary spectacles should be used.

Comfort. The specific evaluation of comfort by the practitioner depends on the patient's complaints of feeling lens movement; soreness of lids; discomfort in eye movements; sensations of burning, heat, itching, scratchiness, grittiness, dryness, or light sensitivity; pain in eyes; tiredness or headaches; and discomfort in the morning.

Feeling of Lens Movement. Lens movement is probably felt more in the lids and conjunctiva than in the cornea.

Awareness by the patient of lens movement is often due to a loose lens, to a poor edge, to an incorrect secondary curve, to a foreign element on the lens, or to the anxiety of the patient.

Corroborating tests include external examination to show excessive movement. Fluorescein pattern evaluation may show excessive movement, a poor bearing relationship, or touch of some of the secondary curves with the conjunctiva. Physical structure evaluation may show an edge with poor configuration or thickness, or a foreign element on the lens surface. Tissue integrity evaluation may show central edema or staining when the lens is loose, peripheral corneal staining and bulbar conjunctival hyperemia when the secondary curve is too steep, and lid or palpebral conjunctival hyperemia when the edge is inadequate or the secondary curve is too flat.

For remediation, as the need indicates, the lens is altered to decrease movement, to provide a satisfactory secondary curvature, or to provide a satisfactory edge configuration and thickness. Foreign substances should be removed from the lens when present.

Soreness of Lids or the Feeling That They Touch the Lens. Usually, these patient complaints are caused by an improper edge configuration or thickness, or a lid that touches the lens at an undesired position.[247] Undesired contact position may be caused by a secondary curve with excessive clearance. It also may be caused by too close an approximation of the top of an aperture lens to the upper lid. When this occurs, the upper lid hits the upper edge of the lens with considerable force and drives the lower edge of the lens into the lower lid. This type of patient report may also be due to a lens with excessive movement that bangs against the lids.

Corroborating tests include external examination to show excessive movement and banging of the lens into and by the lids or improper lens position. Fluorescein pattern evaluation may show excessive apical touch or excessive secondary clearance. Physical structure evaluation may show improper edge configuration or thickness.

For remediation, as the need indicates, the lens is altered to decrease movement, to produce a desirable edge configuration or thickness, to provide a desirable secondary clearance, or to reduce lid banging.

Discomfort in Eye Movement. This complaint often results from the same factors that cause the patient to feel the lenses move and cause lid discomfort. Corroborating tests and remediation are the same as those in lens movement.

Sensations of Burning, Heat, Itching, Scratchiness, Grittiness, Dryness, or Light Sensitivity. These many symptoms usually are due to disturbance of tissue integrity. Corneal edema or conjunctival hyperemia are the typical associated temporary tissue changes.

Poor bearing or venting may disturb the corneal and conjunctival tissues. Some of these symptoms are more common when there is poor venting or a tight lens. Others are more common when there is poor bearing or a loose lens. Feelings of burning, heat, dryness, and stinging are more common in poor venting or a tight lens. Feelings of scratchiness, grittiness, itchiness, and light sensitivity are more common in poor bearing or a loose lens. There may be additional symptoms with a loose lens, such as an excessive awareness of movement, sore lids, and discomfort with eye movement. There is a tendency for symptoms from poor venting or a tight lens to become evident after the lens is worn several hours. Symptoms from poor bearing become evident sooner than this, especially when there is considerable lens movement. Corroborating tests, not description of symptoms, determine whether the cause is poor venting or a tight lens, or poor bearing or a loose lens.

Corroborating tests include external examination to evaluate lens movement, and fluorescein pattern evaluation to evaluate bearing and venting due to relationships of the posterior surface of the lens and anterior corneal curvatures. Tissue integrity evaluation would be used to evaluate corneal edema and conjunctival hyperemia.

For remediation, the lens design is altered to produce better bearing, venting, and movement. Blink action may have to be altered.

Any foreign substance on the lens can irritate the tissues. Coatings on the lenses from improper cleaning of ocular secretions, soap, or nicotine cause irritation. This irritation may be relieved after the lenses are worn for a while, because some of the coatings are neutralized by the precorneal fluids. Solid and raised foreign substances on the lens usually cause pain, as well as other symptoms.

Corroborating tests include patient reports and examiner questioning to indicate the possibility of improper care and handling of the lenses, and physical structure evaluation may show coated lenses.

For remediation, the lenses should be cleaned, and proper care and handling should be reviewed.

Poor environment—insufficient oxygen, a smoky environment, or fumes in the environment may cause tissue irritation and symptoms.[248]

As corroboration, patient reports and examiner questioning would indicate that such symptoms are evident only when the patient is in a specific environment.

For remediation, when there are no other problems, the patient should avoid such environments or should not wear contact lenses when in such environments. When work demands frequently place a patient in such unfavorable environments, contact lens wear may be contraindicated.

Symptoms of asthenopia are common in residual astigmatism, residual hyperopia, residual presbyopia, or problems of binocular coordination. When caused by these factors, the symptoms are often worse or occur only during protracted close work. Discomfort during reading is discussed on page 238.

Conjunctivitis may cause burning, itching, and stinging. If external examination shows conjunctivitis, it should be treated.

Pain in Eyes. When bearing or venting is sufficiently poor, considerable corneal edema or staining may occur, often accompanied by photophobia, excessive lacrimation, and rainbows around lights. Symptoms may not occur until several hours after contact lenses are removed.

A corroborating test is the tissue integrity evaluation with slit-lamp biomicroscopy, which would show considerable corneal edema or staining.

Remediation consists of waiting until the tissues become normal, after which the fit should be reevaluated and the appropriate alterations made. Medication may be necessary to relieve discomfort and prevent infection while the tissues are healing.

A solid foreign body can cause corneal abrasions and pain. Pain is immediate and accompanied by photophobia and excessive lacrimation. Foreign bodies usually consist of dust particles from the atmosphere or dried secretions on the lens.

Corroborating tests include patient reports and examiner questioning. Tissue integrity evaluation may show corneal abrasion, and physical structure evaluation may show a foreign body on the lens.

For remediation, plano sunglasses may be worn outdoors as a protective shield. Proper care and maintenance must be reviewed.

Overwearing contact lenses or varying wearing time greatly may cause considerable corneal edema or staining (see also p. 251).

Corroborating tests include patient reports and examiner questioning to indicate improper wear. Tissue integrity evaluation would show considerable corneal edema or staining.

Remediation would consist of emphasizing the importance of proper wear to the patient.

A rough or chipped edge can irritate the lids and cornea.

Corroborating tests include a physical structure evaluation to show a rough or chipped edge. Tissue evaluation would show irritated lids or cornea.

Remediation consists of refinishing the lens edge. If the lens diameter is decreased too greatly, a new lens should be processed.

Poor insertion can irritate the cornea. If patient reports and examiner questioning indicate poor insertion, the patient should be reeducated as to proper insertion techniques.

Tiredness or Headaches. When related to contact lens wear, tiredness and headaches are frequently due to the same causes that result in discomfort in reading.

Discomfort from Lenses in the Morning. When the patient awakes, mucus may have collected in the eyes, and the cornea may be slightly edematous. As a result, some people experience discomfort when they insert their lenses immediately upon arising.

If patient reports and examiner questioning indicate no other problems, the patient should be advised to rinse his eyes well with cold water upon arising, and then to wait about half an hour before inserting his lenses.

APPEARANCE. The specific evaluation of appearance by the practitioner depends partly on the patient's complaints of excessive blinking, insufficient blinking, squinting, head tilt back, bubbles around edge of lens, milky fluid on lens, excessive tearing, redness of eyes, swollen lids, improper positioning of lenses, displacement of lenses, and difficulty in lens removal.

Excessive Blinking. Blinking excessively is usually caused by loose lenses. It is an attempt to maintain a stable lens position. A poor edge or a foreign substance on the lens may irritate the lids or cornea and initiate excessive blinking. Occasionally, a patient blinks excessively to try to promote better precorneal fluid interchange.

Corroborating tests include external examination to show excessive lens movement. Fluorescein pattern evaluation may show poor bearing. Tissue integrity evaluation may show corneal edema, lid edema, or conjunctival hyperemia. Physical structure evaluation may show a poor edge or foreign substance on the lens.

For remediation, the lens is altered to decrease movement or to promote better precorneal fluid interchange, the edge is refinished, or the foreign substance is removed from the lens.

Insufficient Blinking. Blink rate or amount may be decreased to reduce contact between the lid and lens. This decrease frequently occurs when there is a poor edge configuration or thickness, when the secondary curve is excessively flat, when the upper edge of an aperture lens positions just at the upper lid margin, or when blinking causes excessive lens movement. Reduced blinking may also result from psychological causes.

Corroborating tests include external examination to show infrequent or incomplete blinking and possibly faulty lens position or movement. Fluorescein pattern evaluation may show excessive secondary clearance. Physical structure evaluation may show poor edge configuration or thickness.

For remediation, edge configuration or thickness is modified, a new lens with a steeper secondary curve is processed, or lens position and movement are altered. When insufficient blinking seems to be psychological in origin, the patient's anxieties should be relieved.

Squinting. Excessive lens movement—the patient may find that excessive lens movement can be reduced by narrowing of the palpebral aperture. Thus, the lids cover a greater part of the lens, pressing it closer to the cornea.

Corroborating tests include external examination to show squinting. When the patient is instructed to widen the palpebral aperture, excessive lens movement may result. Fluorescein pattern evaluation may show poor bearing.

Remediation consists of fabricating a new lens that moves less.

Poor vision—an undercorrected refractive error or improper pupil coverage by the optic zone may cause squinting. In the former instance, the retinal blur circle is reduced; in the latter instance, better pupil coverage is obtained.

Corroborating tests include visual analysis to show an uncorrected refractive error. The flare test and fluorescein pattern evaluation may show insufficient pupil coverage by the optic zone.

Remediation consists of placing the proper refractive power in the present lenses, or processing new lenses that provide needed refractive power or pupil coverage.

Head Tilted Back. Excessive lens movement may cause the patient to tilt the head back. When the head is tilted back, more of the lid covers the lens and presses it closer to the eye.

When the patient holds his head normally, external examination may show excessive lens movement. Fluorescein pattern evaluation may show poor bearing.

Remediation consists of using a lens design that results in less movement.

A poor edge or a flat secondary curve can cause lid irritation, which is relieved by tilting the head back.

Corroborating tests include fluorescein pattern evaluation to show excessive secondary clearance. Physical structure evaluation may show poor edge configuration or thickness.

Remediation consists of refinishing the edges or using a lens with a steeper secondary curve.

Bubbles or Frothing Around the Edge of the Lens. When the secondary curve is too flat, surface tension is decreased, and bubbles may form around the edges of the lens.

Fluorescein pattern evaluation would show excessive secondary clearance.

Unless there are other associated problems, the presence of bubbles may be acceptable. When there are other associated problems, a lens with a steeper secondary curve should be processed.

Milky Fluid on Lenses. If the patient finds a milky fluid on his lenses when he takes them off, the mucus and sebum from the precorneal fluid and normally desquamated corneal epithelial cells may be collecting on the lenses. Any catarrhal exudate adds to the problem.

Unless there are associated problems, remediation is not necessary. When there are associated problems, such as corneal or conjunctival tissue disturbances, the cause of the disturbance must be found and eliminated.

Excessive Tearing. Excessive lacrimation is produced to wash away or neutralize foreign objects on the eye. Proper precorneal fluid disbursement over the eye helps maintain undisturbed corneal and conjunctival tissues. Disturbance of these tissues may initiate excessive lacrimation, which is also elicited by irritation of the ophthalmic division of the fifth nerve and by certain emotions.

Mechanical irritation—a lens with excessive movement, a poor edge, or foreign elements may irritate the anterior segment tissues or nerves of the cornea.

Corroborating tests include external examination, which may show excessive lens movement. Fluorescein pattern evaluation may show poor bearing. Tissue integrity evaluation may show corneal edema or staining, or conjunctival or lid hyperemia. Physical structure evaluation may show a poor lens edge or foreign substances on the lens, and patient responsibility evaluation may indicate improper handling and care.

In remediation, the lens is altered to reduce movement and provide better bearing, the edge is refinished, the lenses are cleaned, and the patient is instructed in lens care and handling.

Poor precorneal fluid interchange can disturb corneal tissue integrity, resulting in excessive production of lacrimal fluid to establish proper function and integrity.

Corroborating tests include external examination, which may show insufficient lens movement or infrequent or incomplete blinking. Fluorescein pattern evaluation may show poor venting. Tissue integrity evaluation may show corneal edema or staining, and conjunctival hyperemia.

In remediation, the lens design is altered to obtain better venting, or the patient is instructed in proper blinking.

Residual refractive error—uncorrected astigmatism, hyperopia, or presbyopia may cause excessive lacrimation due to eyestrain.

Corroborating tests include analysis of vision, which would show residual astigmatism, hyperopia, or presbyopia.

In remediation, the hyperopia is corrected by alteration of the power of the original lenses or by the ordering of new lenses. The astigmatism or presbyopia is corrected as discussed on page 93 and page 125.

Colds, allergies, or sinusitis—these conditions may be accompanied by excessive fluid on the eye.

Corroborating tests include patient reports and examiner questioning, which would indicate whether one of these conditions were present when there is an excess of fluid on the eyes.

For remediation, the basic condition should be treated. Contact lens wear may have to be discontinued until the colds, allergies, or sinusitis improves.

Emotional factors may caúse excessive lacrimation—for example, fear of contact lenses.

If patient reports and examiner questioning indicate fear of contact lenses, the practitioner should discuss the cause of the patient's anxiety in an effort to dispel it.

Redness of Eyes. Irritation to the corneal or conjunctival tissue may cause conjunctival injection.

Poor bearing or venting may irritate the corneal or conjunctival tissues.

Corroborating tests include external examination, which may show conjunctival injection and excessive or insufficient lens movement. Fluorescein pattern evaluation may show poor bearing or venting. Tissue integrity evaluation may show corneal edema or staining and conjunctival hyperemia.

For remediation, the lens design is altered to produce better bearing or venting.

Conjunctivitis is the most common ocular pathologic condition, and it can develop in a contact lens patient.

If external examination shows conjunctivitis, it must be cured.

Poor hygiene or poor wearing habits may cause conjunctival injection.

If patient reports and examiner questioning indicate poor hygiene or wearing habits, patient indoctrination should be reviewed.

A poor edge, a foreign element on the lenses, or an improper secondary curve may irritate the conjunctiva.

Corroborating tests include fluorescein pattern evaluation, which may show a poor secondary curve relationship to the underlying conjunctiva. Tissue integrity evaluation may show corneal edema or staining, or conjunctival hyperemia, and physical structure evaluation may show a poor lens edge or foreign substances on the lens.

For remediation, the secondary curve is altered, the edge is refinished, or the foreign substance is removed.

Insufficient sleep may cause conjunctival injection.

If patient reports and examiner questioning indicate insufficient sleep, the patient should be advised to get sufficient sleep.

Residual refractive error may cause conjunctival injection (see p. 245).

Swollen Lids. Any irritation of the lids may cause edema.

Mechanical irritation from a poor lens edge, excessive lens movement, or too flat a secondary curve may cause lid edema.

Corroborating tests include external examination, which may show excessive lens movement. Fluorescein pattern evaluation may show poor bearing or too flat a secondary curve. Tissue integrity evaluation may show lid and corneal edema, and conjunctival hyperemia. Physical structure evaluation may show a poor edge.

For remediation, the lens design is altered to reduce movement or to produce a steeper secondary curve, or the lens edge is refinished.

Allergies may cause lid edema. Women may be allergic to their cosmetics.

If patient reports and examiner questioning indicate allergies or use of a new brand of cosmetics, the basic cause should be eliminated.

Improper Positioning of Lenses. Many patients believe that contact lenses should be centered on the eye. Many contact lenses do not maintain such a position, and this fact should be explained. Lens design need not be altered unless eccentric positioning produces visual, comfort, or tissue problems (see p. 73).

Improper relationships between the posterior surface of the lens and the anterior cornea—improper base and secondary curve radii, a cornea with considerable toricity and asymmetry, and a decentered corneal cap are all conducive to eccentric contact lens positioning.

Excessively long base or secondary radii decrease adherence between the contact lens and the cornea. If upper lid pull is sufficient, the lens will position superiorly. Its upper edge is tilted back until it bears on the superior cornea, limbus, or sclera. A flaccid upper lid or an insufficient blink action tends to allow the lens either to sag down or to have considerable movement, especially if the lens is small or thick.

When the cornea is considerably toric, adherence between a spherical base curve and the toric corneal curves is decreased. If upper lid pull is sufficient and there is with-the-rule astigmatism of 3 D or less, the lens is often positioned superiorly in the manner just discussed. If there is insufficient upper lid pull, with-the-rule astigmatism of more than 3 D, or against-the-rule astigmatism of more than 1 D, then the lens usually sags down or has considerable movement.

When the cornea is asymmetrical, the lens tends to migrate to the steepest quadrant until it reaches a bearing area. When the corneal cap is not centered geometrically in the cornea, the lens may tend to position near the eccentric corneal cap.

Improper relationships between the posterior surface of the lens and the anterior corneal surface may be due to change of corneal topography caused by contact lens wear. Lens positioning in such cases may change from day to day or in the course of a single day.

Corroborating tests include external examination, which shows eccentric positioning. Fluorescein pattern evaluation shows improper relationships between the posterior lens surface and anterior corneal surface. Tissue integrity evaluation may show edema, staining, and corneal curvature change.

Remediation should consist of the selection of proper base and secondary radii. When the cornea has considerable toricity, a compromise spherical or a toric base curve is often needed.

Improper diameters—lens positioning related to lens diameter is discussed on page 45. An aperture-positioning lens with too large a lens diameter may be pushed by the upper lid into or below the lower lid. This movement causes discomfort, tissue irritation, and flare. A superior-positioning lens with too large a lens diameter may be pushed by the lower lid into or above the superior limbus. This movement is aggravated by a high lower lid or during depressed gaze.

Small optic-zone diameters decrease adherence of lens to cornea. A small optic-zone diameter combined with a large lens diameter produces a wide secondary zone. This combination reduces adherence to the cornea and produces a large surface area to be grasped by the upper lid. Such lenses tend to be pulled up, especially if there is with-the-rule corneal astigmatism and minus refractive power. If there is against-the-rule astigmatism, a flaccid upper lid, insufficient blink action, or plus refractive power, the lens frequently has considerable movement. A small optic-zone diameter combined with a small lens diameter reduces adherence to the cornea and produces a small surface area to be grasped by the upper lid. Such lenses tend to position in the palpebral aperture.

Corroborating tests include external examination, which shows improper lens positioning in primary and in depressed fixation. Fluorescein pattern evaluation may show a small optic zone and a wide secondary zone.

For remediation, the lens diameter or optic-zone diameter is altered. Prism ballast may be used to prevent an aperture lens from being pushed beneath the lower lid.

Improper thickness—the base-away-from-center prismatic configuration of a minus lens makes it easier for the upper lid to pull it superiorly. The base-toward-center prismatic configuration of a plus lens makes it more difficult for the upper lid to pull it superiorly.

As center thickness increases, adherence between lens and cornea decreases.

Thick lenses tend to position inferiorly or to have excessive movement. As center thickness decreases, adherence between lens and cornea increases.

Corroborating tests include external examination, which shows improper lens positioning. Physical structure evaluation shows improper center or edge thickness.

For remediation, if center thickness is improper, a lens with proper center thickness is ordered. If center thickness is proper but edge thickness is not, an anterior lenticular construction is used. A minus lenticular construction may be used to move a plus lens up, and a plus lenticular construction may be used to move a minus lens down. Base-down prism may also be used to pull a minus lens down.

Generally, centration is aided by increasing optic-zone diameter, decreasing center thickness, or shortening the base curve radius (see p. 76).

Lenses Fall Out or Get Onto White Part of Eyes. A loose lens may have a tendency to fall out. If external examination shows excessive movement and fluorescein pattern evaluation shows poor bearing, the lens design should be altered to decrease movement.

A poor edge, especially a thick one, may allow the lid to push the lens onto the sclera or out of the eye. If physical structure evaluation shows a poor edge, it should be refinished.

Improper patient procedure—people often rest their faces against their hand or brush something away from around their eyes. Either of these actions may cause a lens to be pushed onto the sclera or out of the eye. If patient reports and examiner questioning indicate the foregoing to be the cause, the patient must be advised to guard against these actions.

Difficult Lens Removal. The patient may be using an improper procedure, or the lens may fit too tightly.

Corroborating tests include external examination or fluorescein pattern evaluation, which may show insufficient lens movement. Patient responsibility evaluation may indicate a faulty removal technique.

For remediation, the lens should be altered to loosen it, or the removal technique should be reviewed with the patient.

Checklist of Symptoms

The most common patient reports of problems, and the most common causes of these problems are listed in Table 5-1. This table is only a guide, and it must be integrated with the overall procedure for best results.

TABLE 5–1

SYMPTOMS OF CONTACT LENS PROBLEMS

Patient Report	Common Causes
VISION	
Blurry vision at distance or near	Improper refractive power Coated lenses Corneal edema Switched lenses Excessive lacrimation
Reflection, ghost images, shadows, or fringes around objects	Excessive lens movement Too small an optic zone for a given lens position
Blurred vision when contact lenses are removed and spectacles worn	Temporary corneal curvature or transparency change Ametropic alteration
Rainbows around lights	Corneal edema Confusion with flare
Eyes are uncomfortable when reading	Residual refractive error Insufficient accommodative ability Poor fluid interchange Flare Poor binocular coordination
COMFORT	
Feel the lenses move	Loose lens Poor edge Foreign substance on lens Improper secondary curvature Psychological
Lids are sore or patient feels the lids touch the lens	Improper edge Excessive secondary clearance Excessive lens movement Poor lens position
Discomfort when eyes move	Improper edge Excessive secondary clearance Excessive lens movement Poor lens position
Eyes burn, feel hot, itch, sting, feel scratchy, feel gritty, feel dry, or photophobia	Poor bearing or venting Foreign substance on lens Poor environment Asthenopia Conjunctivitis

Pain in eyes	Poor bearing or venting Foreign body Improper wear Poor edge Poor insertion
Tiredness or headaches	Same as discomfort while reading
Lenses are uncomfortable in the morning	Normal secretion and edema collection Abnormal secretion and edema collection Improper handling and care

APPEARANCE

Excessive blinking	Excessive lens movement Poor edge Foreign substance on lens Poor fluid interchange Psychological
Insufficient blinking	Poor edge Poor lens position Excessive secondary clearance Excessive movement Psychological
Squinting	Excessive lens movement Poor lens position Improper refractive power
Head tilted back	Excessive lens movement Poor vision Poor edge or flat secondary Poor pupil coverage by optic zone
Bubbles or frothing around edge of lens	Flat secondary
Milky fluid on lenses when taken off	Normal collection of secretions Exudates from ocular irritation—colds, allergies, sinusitis
Too much tearing	Mechanical irritation (poor edge, etc.) Poor fluid interchange Residual refractive error Colds, allergies, sinusitis Psychological
Redness of eyes	Poor bearing or venting Conjunctivitis Improper care, handling, or wear Mechanical irritation (poor edge, etc.) Insufficient sleep Residual refractive error

Swollen lids	Mechanical irritation (poor edge, etc.) Allergies
Improper positioning of lenses	Improper posterior lens–anterior cornea relationships Improper diameters Improper thickness
Lenses fall out or get onto white part of eyes	Loose lens Poor edge Improper patient procedure
Difficult lens removal	Tight lens Improper patient procedure

AFTER-CARE

After the initial fitting period, a contact lens patient should be examined at least twice a year to prevent, control, or remediate possible long-term problems. The procedure is substantially the same as that used in progress examinations.

Overwear of contact lenses can occur both during and after the three- to six-month initial fitting period. It may take the form of excessive or variable wear. Perhaps because of temporary corneal anesthesia, there is frequently little or no discomfort while the lenses are worn or for several hours after removal. Then the typical symptoms of corneal edema and abrasion appear—blepharospasm, foreign body sensation, pain, photophobia, and tearing. After treatment and return of the tissues to normal, wearing time must be rebuilt as in a new patient. The patient should be seen weekly for about three weeks to control readaptation.

Corneal curvature, regularity, transparency, and organization can be altered by contact lens wear. The degree of change tends to be directly related to both daily and total wearing time. Corneal curvature change can alter bearing, venting, movement, and positioning of contact lenses. All these corneal changes can produce spectacle blur.

If not only the corneal radius but also its regularity and transparency are altered, no spectacle refractive power produces normal visual acuity. Generally, the cornea returns to normal after contact lenses are left off. This process may take a few minutes to a few weeks or longer. Unless spectacle-corrected acuity becomes satisfactory shortly after removal of contact lenses, the patient becomes almost totally dependent on contact lenses. The resultant prolonged wear further increases the corneal changes and may produce edema and abrasion from overwear. Contact lens practitioners should strive to control the degree of corneal changes so that spectacles can be interchanged with contact lenses. Curvature change of 0.50 D. or less is desirable.

The desired spectacle refractive power is one that allows such interchange. It is frequently necessary to prescribe a refractive power that is a compromise between that needed about 30 minutes after removal of contact lenses and that needed if the cornea were to return to normal. Prescribing refractive power only for the normal cornea frequently will not permit interchange.

Although mild degrees of edema or injection are common during the first two to three weeks of contact lens wear, subsequent recurrence of edema or injection must be considered to be abnormal.

6

STAGE SIX

Practice Management

Because practice management is an integral part of contact lens care, various aspects have been discussed. The first five stages are a method for the management and care of contact lens patients. A supplementary discussion of practice management is presented in this stage.

Practice management starts before a prospective patient enters the office, and it continues as long as he remains a patient. Its goals are providing satisfactory service to the patient and satisfactory economic return to the practitioner.[249–255]

It is more difficult to attain these goals with contact lenses than with spectacle lenses. Contact lens application is considerably more complex than spectacle application; thus, there is reduced probability of success with contact lenses. In addition, because of the greater complexity, the fee for contact lens application is generally considerably greater than that for spectacle application. These first two factors simultaneously increase the patient's economic involvement. Finally, because of the complexity of the work, the time and materials consumed, and the acquisition of special equipment, the practitioner's economic involvement is increased.

RAPPORT

It is extremely important for the practitioner to establish a satisfactory rapport with the patient. Poor practice management may cause resentment in one or both parties, which adversely affects rapport. Such a disruption of confidence may be the basis for many problems.

Economics

Economic misunderstandings are the basis for much resentment and loss of confidence by the patient or practitioner. Much disruption of rapport is avoided when financial aspects are clearly established initially. During the first interview, the amount and payment plan of the initial fee, the services covered by the initial fee, and the protection plans covering loss of contact lenses should be discussed.

Amount and Payment Plan of Initial Fee

As a result of the initial clinical evaluation, there are two basic economic possibilities. The first is for patients who are judged to be unsatisfactory contact lens candidates. A fee may be charged for any services rendered.

The second is for patients who are judged to be satisfactory contact lens candidates. Economic arrangements for such patients are handled through one of two approaches, but the total fee for patients carried to completion is usually the same in either approach.

The first approach involves accepting the patient as a contact lens wearer and quoting the total fee indicated. The patient is told the fee, and then arrangements for payment are made. When the case is more complex and special design lenses or more time is required, the fee is increased. All financial arrangements should be discussed and recorded.

The second approach is a *step procedure*. Step One is the initial evaluation. Step Two involves processing lenses and building wearing time for three to four weeks. During this period, a determination is made as to whether a satisfactory fit can be obtained. If it is judged that a satisfactory fit cannot be obtained, the case is discontinued. Either separate fees are charged for each of the first two steps, or a combined fee is charged for the first two steps. If it is judged that a satisfactory fit can be obtained, an additional fee is charged for the duration of the initial three to six months. When a step procedure is used, all elements should be clearly presented in the initial discussion with the patient.

There is a general belief that advance payment of all or a substantial part of the fee strengthens the patient's motivation. In any financial arrangement, it is usually better to receive payment promptly. This arrangement is not always possible, however, and cooperating with the patient establishes better rapport in such cases. Pressure to get maximum payment in these cases results in tension, embarrassment, and discord.

There are three general methods of payment. The first is full advance payment the day of evaluation or the day of dispensing. The second is partial advance payment with the balance carried on the practitioner's books for several months. The third is budgeting payment through a third party, such as a bank.

Services Covered by the Initial Fee

The patient should be told what he is provided in return for this fee. The total period covered, the approximate number of visits, and the included supplies are established.

Contact Lens Loss Protection Plan

Some type of coverage for lens loss should be obtained before the patient takes lenses from the office.[256–258] Many patients are afraid they will lose lenses. Tension resulting from this factor can affect the ultimate outcome of the case. There are several types of loss coverage plans available. It is very important to use a plan that is continuous and will not be canceled at the first loss. To reduce problems due to delay, a close relationship with a laboratory should be established so that lost lenses are replaced quickly.

Subsequent Services

Other economic factors that are discussed either initially or subsequently are probability and cost of refitting, cost of after-care examinations, and arrangements with an unsuccessful patient.

Refitting. Probability of refitting depends on the change of the patient's refractive status, disruption of normal corneal integrity, and change of the physical structure of the lens itself.

Refractive Status. With consideration of the type and amount of ametropia and the patient's age, the probability of ametropic change necessitating a refit can be estimated.

Myopia usually stabilizes in the late teens or early twenties.[259] Ametropic change for such patients generally is not greater than the amount of power change that can be incorporated in their initial contact lenses. Many myopic patients are at least in middle adolescence when they are fitted with contact lenses. Often ametropia is not sufficiently severe until this age to make the patient accept the need for constant correction, nor are social needs sufficient to make the patient dislike spectacles. Also, parents often do not feel children are old enough to be fitted with contact lenses until they are at least in middle adolescence.

Despite the lack of controlled group studies, the progression of myopia seems to be retarded in some patients by contact lens wear. Parents are conditioned to purchasing new spectacles every year or so for their early teen-age children. They are concerned that yearly purchase of new contact lenses will become necessary; this often is not necessary.

Many low and medium hyperopic adolescents function satisfactorily without spectacles for most of their tasks. Acuity is maintained by accommodation. During adolescence, hyperopia often tends to decrease somewhat. Because of these factors and the relatively small percentage of medium and high hyperopes, fewer young hyperopes than young myopes are fitted with contact lenses.

From the early or middle twenties to the late thirties or early forties, ametropia is generally relatively stable. After this age, physiologic changes usually slightly decrease myopia or increase hyperopia. Presbyopia emerges, and the progressive increase of near addition must be considered.

Disruption of Normal Corneal Integrity. When lenses are fitted and used properly, a refit is not necessary frequently on this basis. Lens modifications, however, may be necessary.

Physical Structure of the Contact Lens. When a patient handles, maintains, and cares for his lenses properly and is faithful in keeping his periodic examination appointments, contact lenses usually last many years.

The cost of refitting depends on the amount of the practitioner's service and time involved, and the time lapse since the original fitting. The fee increases as these factors increase. For example, a refit to replace physically unacceptable lenses involves relatively little of the practitioner's service and time.

After-care Examinations. The patient is told the average fee and what is done.

Unsuccessful Cases. There are two philosophies about fees in unsuccessful cases. The first proposes that nothing in life is guaranteed and that the practitioner often spends more time and money on an unsuccessful case. The patient, therefore, is obligated to pay the full fee. The second proposes that it is currently impossible to predetermine with sufficient accuracy which patients will be successful. The patient, therefore, is not obligated to pay the full fee.

The practitioner should decide which philosophy he feels is best and apply it consistently. If one philosophy is used on one patient and the other on a second patient, much ill will may result. When the second philosophy is followed, either a fixed percentage is used for all cases, or the obligation is related to the amount of time and money invested.

PATIENT CONTROL

Patient Selection

Stage One is devoted to patient selection. Proper patient selection is an important control in a successful contact lens practice.

As indicated in Stage Five, there is no guarantee that successful results will be produced, even for a good candidate. The practitioner should indicate this fact to the patient.

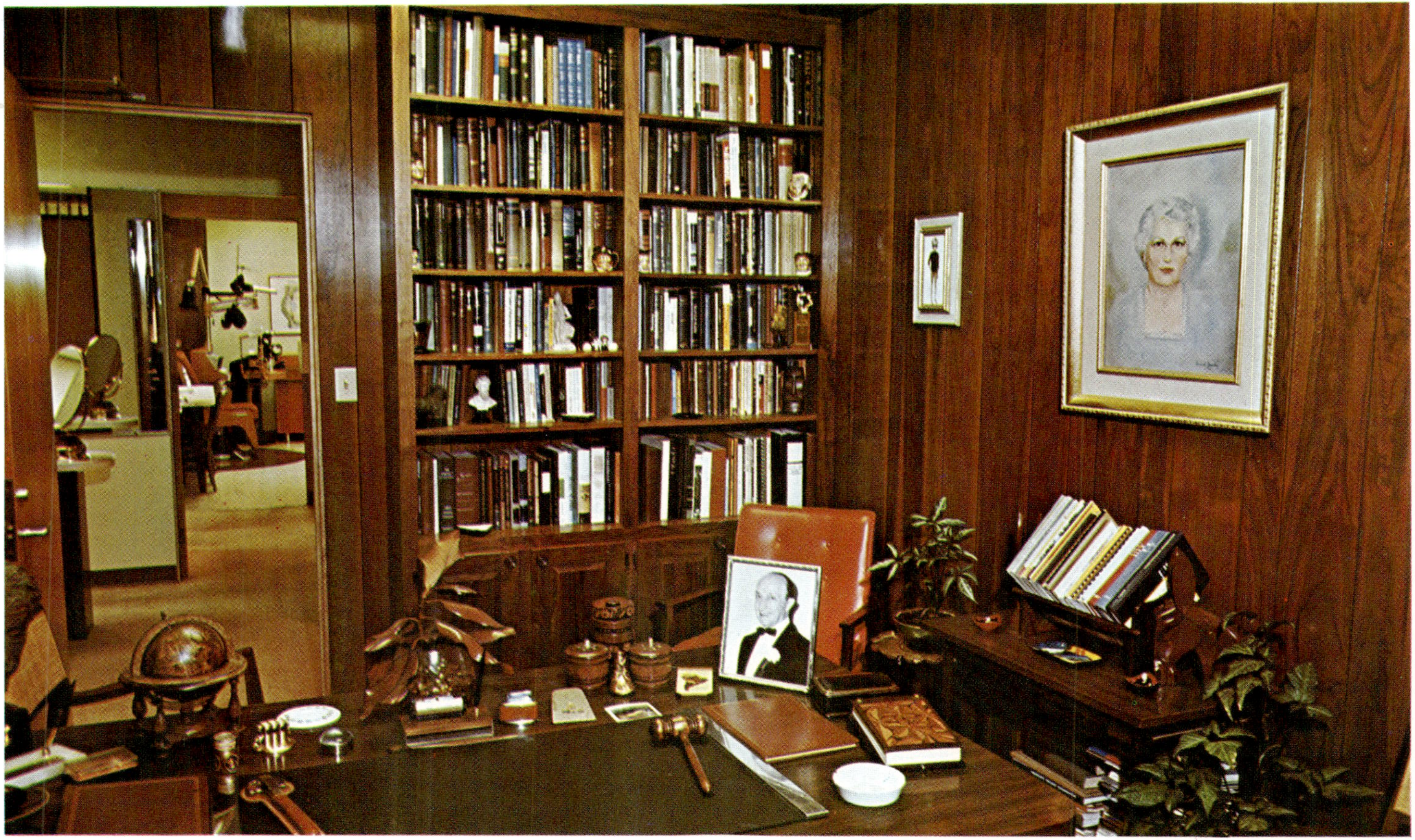

Figure 6–1A. Consultation room.

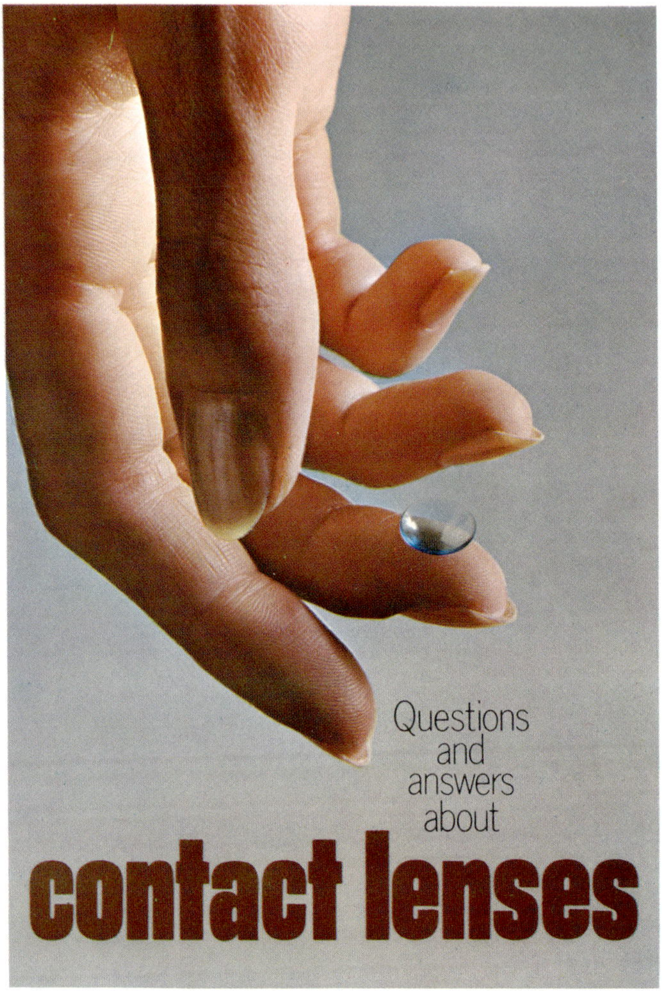

Figure 6–1B. Example of patient education booklet. (Courtesy of Barnes-Hind Pharmaceuticals, Inc., and Dell Publishing Co., Inc.)

Education of the Patient

Stage Four is devoted to patient education. The patient should be taught to handle, care for, and use his lenses properly.

Frequency of Observation

This aspect is discussed in Stage Five (p. 226). Anyone who has not faithfully kept his appointments should be contacted.

Recall

Contact lens patients should be seen at least once every six months after the initial fitting period. Recall cards should be sent out before each six-month periodic examination. If one appointment is not honored, the next card should note this fact. Supplementary telephone call–recalls regarding a specific appointment are part of a sound, continuous, contact lens service.

Getting patients to honor these semiannual checkups may be difficult. A satisfied patient may believe that he does not need to be seen. Patients who have been properly informed during the initial four to six months respond better to recall cards. It is the practitioner's responsibility to educate the patient, thus providing the desired control over the case both from the standpoint of the patient's well-being and from the practitioner's economic standpoint.

Referral

It is important to have a proper referral system in the event that problems needing related aid occur. In our mobile society, people change locality frequently. The patient who permanently or temporarily moves should be given the name and address of a competent practitioner in his new locality.

The practitioner's office and home phone numbers should be given to each patient. Provisions should be made for times when the practitioner is out of town. A list of local practitioners used for referral should be made available to the patient.

Telephone

It is sometimes necessary to communicate with the patient by telephone. The date of such communication, the nature of the discussion, and any advice given should be placed on the patient's record.

RECORDS

Complete records must be kept enabling the practitioner to follow the patient's progress, for legal protection, and as a basis for further research and study. Each entry should include the date, the findings, the course of action, and the instructions. Records should never be destroyed, even after a practitioner has died. His estate may be liable for suits.

FACILITIES

The physical facilities and organization of the practitioner should be such that adequate service is provided with maximum efficiency. When there is sufficient space, separate rooms for training and observing the patient are desirable. Equipment is in this room and the examination room (Figs. 6–1 to 6–7). Equipment the authors consider necessary is discussed in the first five stages.

LEGAL ASPECTS

Malpractice is more accurately termed negligent practice. It is defined as practice in which the degree of learning, skill, care, or judgment is below the average for the locality.

Most malpractice suits are not instituted because of negligent practice, but rather come about through a breakdown of rapport between practitioner and patient. When there is improper patient control and record keeping, or inadequate facilities, the practitioner is more vulnerable to a malpractice suit.[260–262]

The best defenses against a malpractice suit are maintenance of rapport, maintenance of technical knowledge and facilities, proper patient control, and proper record keeping. Because a person assumes a certain risk when he willingly participates in anything, when he does not participate as instructed, he is a contributory party to negligence.

When a malpractice suit is instituted the practitioner should say nothing until he has consulted his personal lawyer and his insurance company. It is important to have sufficient malpractice insurance with a responsible company.

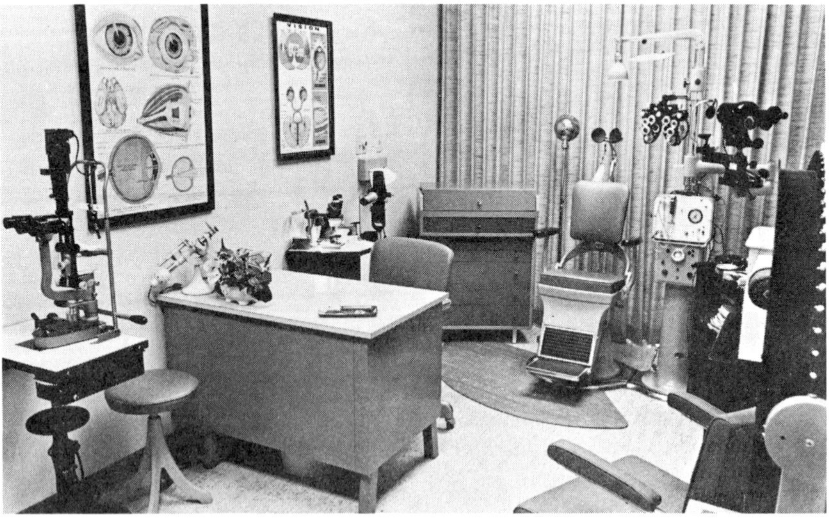

Figure 6–2. Examination room.

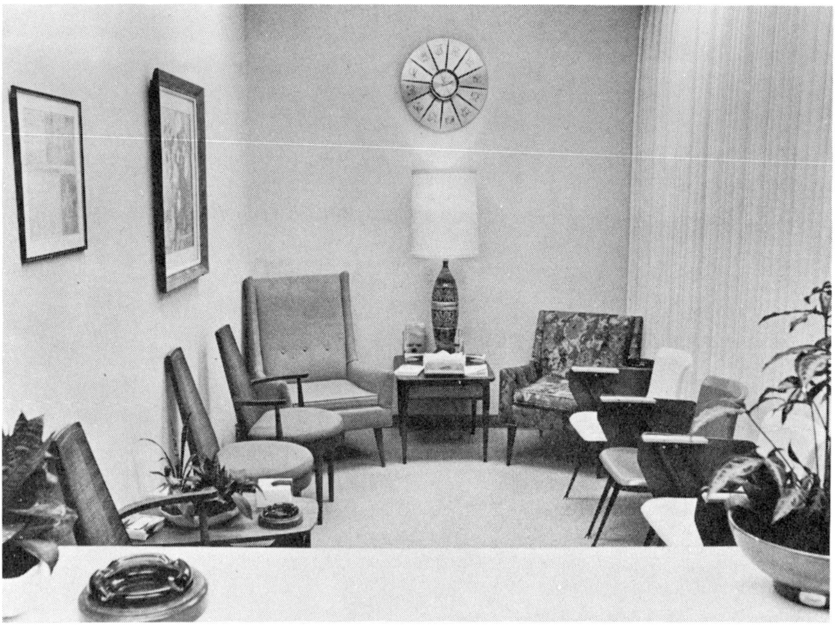

Figure 6–3. Lounge for contact lens patients.

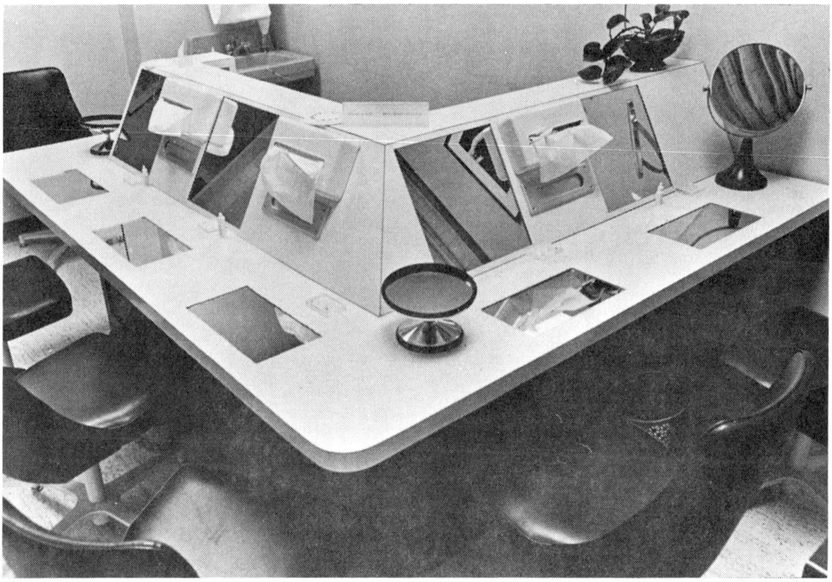

Figure 6–4. Training room for contact lens patients.

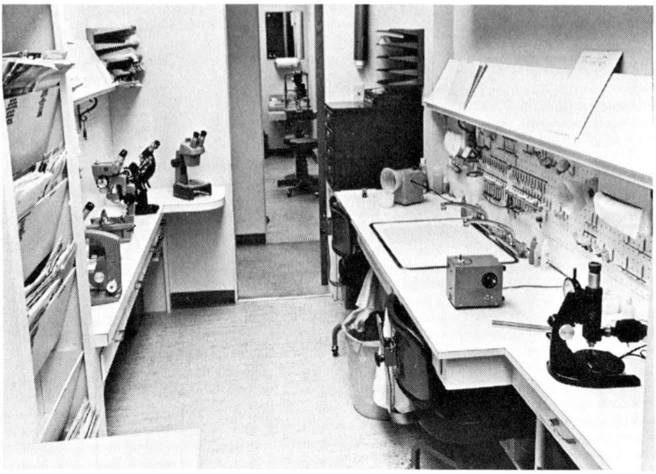

Figure 6–5. Contact lens laboratory.

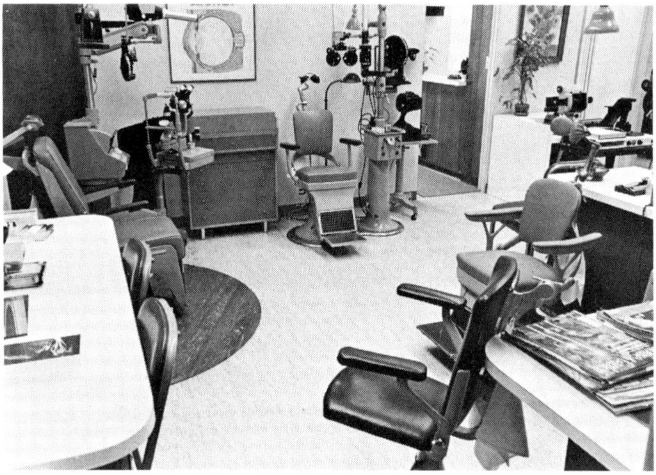

Figure 6–6. Observation room for contact lens patients.

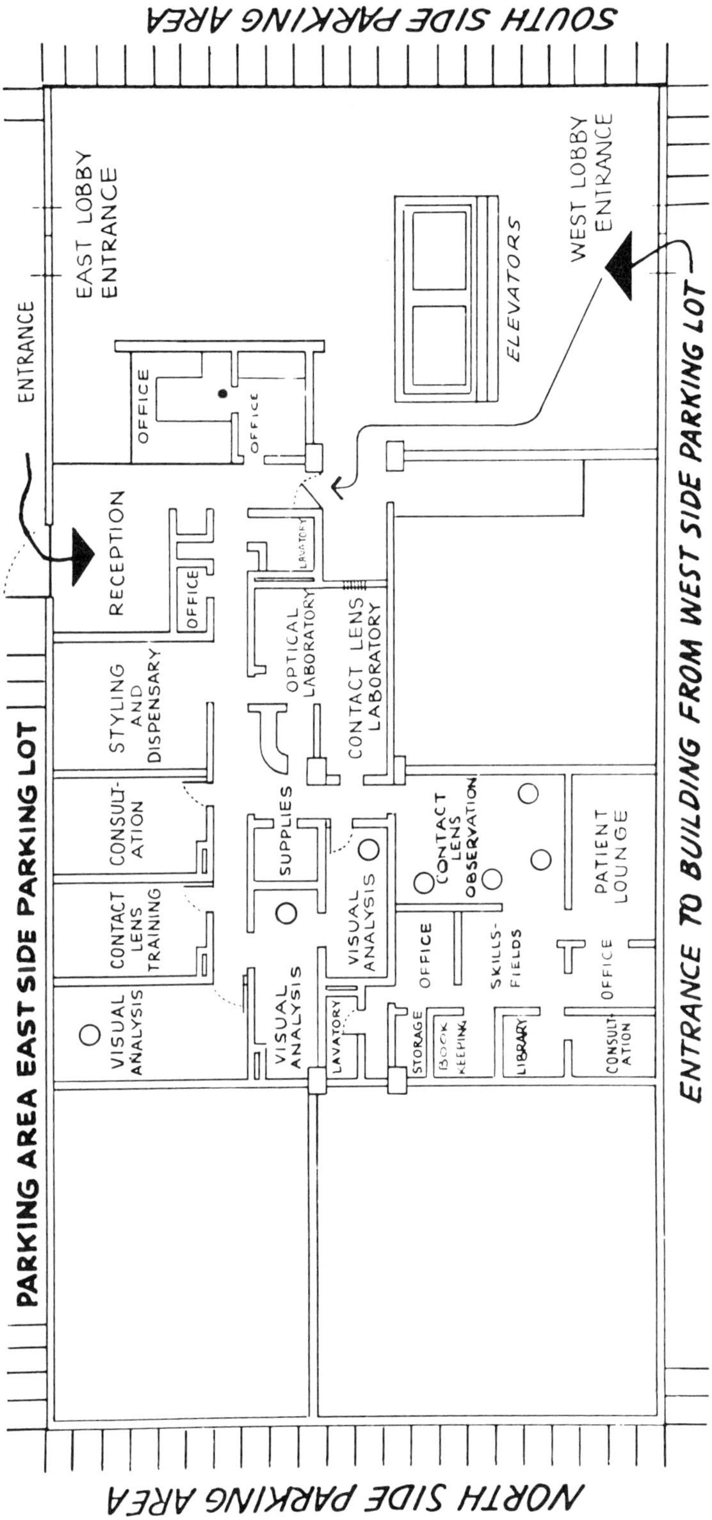

Figure 6–7. Office plan.

PART TWO

Clinical Reference

7

Special Lenses

SCLERAL LENSES

Patient Evaluation

Corneal contact lenses are used more frequently than scleral contact lenses for many reasons. (1) It is generally easier to fit corneal contact lenses. (2) It is generally easier to obtain satisfactory cosmetic appearance with corneal contact lenses. Scleral contact lenses frequently give the eyes an exophthalmic appearance. Many scleral contact lenses have a relatively large fenestration, which produces a large air bubble between the lens and the cornea. This bubble is cosmetically undesirable and causes visual problems when it covers the pupil. The edges of a scleral contact lens may be apparent during extreme rotations. (3) Promotion has led the public to believe that small lenses are preferable to large lenses. (4) The development of corneal contact lenses has practically stopped the research and development of scleral contact lenses in the United States. Because of these and other factors, scleral contact lenses are used to supplement corneal contact lenses. (Fig. 7–1).

Advantages of Scleral Lenses[263–264]

A scleral contact lens exhibits more stable positioning than does a corneal contact lens. This is advantageous to people participating in certain sports.

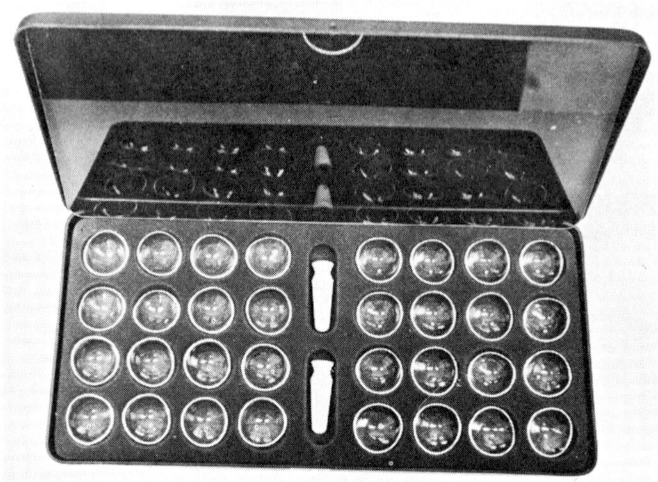

Figure 7–1. Scleral lenses and suction cup in a case.

It also provides more stable positioning of an anterior surface cylinder, prism, the ocular of a telescopic spectacle and contact lens system, an aphakic lens, a keratoconic lens, or a cosmetic lens.

A scleral contact lens covers almost all the eye's anterior segment, making it difficult for particles to enter between the lens and the eye. This is advantageous to people participating in certain sports or having certain occupations, and it also provides better corneal protection from a scarred lid.

A person with considerably reduced uncorrected vision can see and handle the large scleral lens relatively well. This may be advantageous in keratoconus and aphakia, or in a patient with subnormal vision.

Scleral contact lenses may be used to hold medication against the anterior ocular tissues.

Initial Design Selection

General Structure and Terminology

Preformed or Molded Lenses. Scleral contact lenses are fitted by use of preformed diagnostic lenses or by a molding procedure based on an impression of the eye.[265]

Fluid or Fluidless Lenses. The first scleral lenses were fitted with considerable central clearance. An artificial buffered saline solution was placed in the deep central area of the lens. Such lenses usually produce corneal edema, rainbows around lights, and foggy vision (Sattler's veil) after several hours of wear. Fluidless scleral contact lenses are used almost exclusively today, making use of only the normal precorneal fluid.

Fenestrated (Open) or Nonfenestrated (Closed) Lenses. A fluidless scleral contact lens may have a fenestration, which aids in fluid and gas interchange.

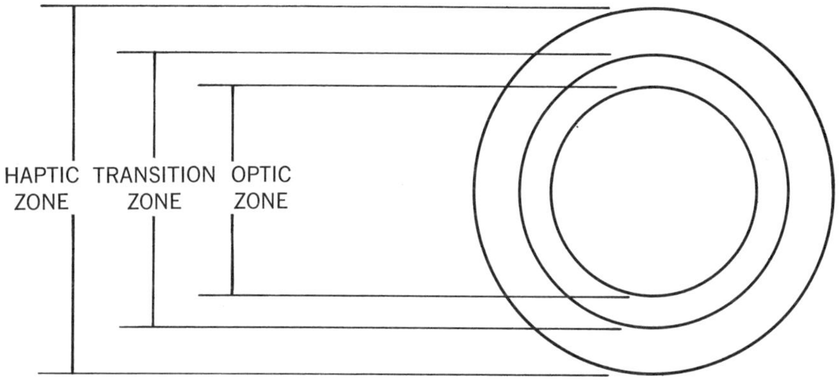

Figure 7–2. Central optic, intermediate transition, and peripheral haptic zones of a preformed scleral lens.

Preformed Lenses

Specific Structure and Terminology. The three basic areas of the rear surface of a preformed scleral contact lens are the *central optic* (corneal) *zone;* the *peripheral haptic* (scleral) *zone;* and the *transition* (limbal) *zone,* between the optic and haptic zones (Fig. 7–2).

Chord value from edge to edge of an optic-zone meridian is termed *optic* (corneal) *zone diameter* or width. Chord value in a given meridian from one outside lens edge to the other is termed *lens diameter,* total lens diameter, or overall size. Chord value in a given meridian from one inside lens edge to the other is termed *back haptic size.* Back haptic size equals the lens diameter minus twice the edge thickness (Fig. 7–3).

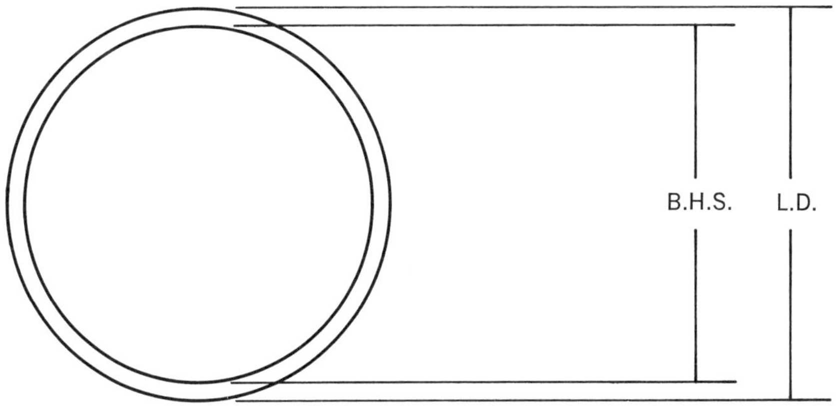

Figure 7–3. The scleral lens diameter (L.D.) (total lens diameter, overall size) is the chord width between anterior surfaces of the edges. The back haptic size (B.H.S.) is the chord width between posterior surfaces of the edges.

The curvature in the optic zone is called the *base* or *back optic curve.* The curvature in the haptic zone is called the *haptic curve.* The curvature in the transition zone is called the *transition curve.*

Posterior curvature in the optic or haptic zones is spherical or toric, and in the transition zone it is spherical or conical. The radius of the transition curvature is between the optic and haptic radii.

When there is considerable scleral toricity, toric haptic curvature and a round lens shape may be used to produce a satisfactory relationship with the underlying sclera. Spherical haptic curvature and an oval lens shape also may be used to produce a satisfactory relationship with the underlying sclera. A vertically oval lens would be used for with-the-rule scleral toricity, and a horizontally oval lens would be used for against-the-rule scleral toricity. Vertically oval lenses are cosmetically poor and are seldom used. Oval lenses are discussed in more detail on page 270.

The distance from the temporal limbus to the outer canthus is almost always longer than the distance from the nasal limbus to the caruncle and plica semilunaris. The caruncle and plica semilunaris should be free of the lens, even during convergence. If the optic zone of a scleral lens is to be centered over the cornea, it usually must be decentered nasally. The amount of decentration is half the difference between nasal and temporal haptic widths, often 1 to 2 mm.

When a fenestration is used, it is usually 0.5 to 0.8 mm. in diameter. To function properly, it must be positioned so that it is not covered by the lids. At the same time, however, it must be close enough to the upper lid so that it is somewhat camouflaged by the eyelashes. Usually, it is placed in the superior temporal transition between the optic and haptic zones of the lens. In this position, the fenestration is free of the lid and somewhat camouflaged by the eyelashes. It is also in an area clear of the underlying tissues, which reduces the possibility of tissue irritation.

The *center thickness* of a lens is the separation between anterior and posterior curvature at the geometric center of the optic zone. The *edge thickness* of a lens is the separation between anterior and posterior surfaces at the edge of the lens.

DESIRED RELATIONSHIPS BETWEEN POSTERIOR LENS AND ANTERIOR EYE CURVATURES. Clinical experience indicates that certain relationships between posterior lens and anterior eye curvatures produce the best results with any fluidless scleral lens.

Optic (Corneal) Zone. Minimum apical clearance is the best relationship between the base curve and the underlying cornea. Apical touch usually produces pain, lacrimation, photophobia, corneal edema, conjunctival injection, and corneal distortion. Excessive apical clearance usually produces poor precorneal fluid interchange, resulting in edema or staining, foggy vision, and discomfort. Bubbles are frequently trapped in the retrolens space, disturbing vision, appearance, and comfort.

The final apical corneal clearance should be about 0.08 mm. Because scleral contact lenses tend to settle toward the cornea during the first month or so of wear, an initial apical clearance of about 0.12 mm. often produces a final apical clearance of about 0.08 mm.

Haptic (Scleral) Zone. Alignment is the best relationship between the haptic curve and the underlying sclera. This relationship distributes pressure relatively uniformly, which reduces force per unit area. Haptic bearing should start about 2 mm. beyond the limbus.

A steeper haptic relationship impedes precorneal fluid interchange, lifts the optic portion away from the cornea, and impedes circulation through the conjunctival vessels. This results in problems in tissue, vision, comfort, and appearance. A flatter haptic relationship produces poor bearing, permits the entrance of many bubbles and causes lens lag and lid discomfort.

When no fenestration is used, the haptic curve is fitted slightly flatter than alignment. This is necessary to produce satisfactory venting.

Transition (Limbal) Zone. Moderate clearance is the best relationship between the transition curve and the underlying limbus. Alignment impedes precorneal fluid interchange through the optic-zone area and circulation through the limbal vessels. Such interference with corneal physiology produces corneal edema or staining, hazy vision, and discomfort. Excessive clearance permits the entrance of many bubbles into the optic zone area, causing visual and physiologic problems.

Diameters. The lens diameter usually ranges from 21 to 25 mm., and it should be as large as possible to reduce edge visibility. The lens diameter should be small enough, however, to prevent edge pressure against the caruncle or plica nasally or the semilunar membrane and fornices superiorly and inferiorly. This relationship must be maintained for all directions of gaze. The longest chord value of an oval lens is often about 1.5 to 3 mm. greater than the shortest chord value.

Optic-zone diameters usually range from 8.0 to 14.5 mm., and they are usually standardized for each lens design.

Bubbles. It is important to have a bubble under the corneal portion to aid venting. Optimal bubble location in primary fixation is temporal, inferior, and slightly inside the limbus. Optimal final bubble size in primary fixation is about ¼ inch by ⅛ inch. Because bubble size decreases with settling, the initial bubble size should be slightly larger than this.

Bubble size and position change with eye movements and lens lag. Bubble movement is opposite to fixation. When a nonfenestrated lens is used, it is often desirable to have several bubbles under the haptic portion to aid venting.

Basic Fitting Procedure. *Diameters and Shapes.* The practitioner must first decide which lens and optic-zone diameters to use. This then enables him to select the needed radii to establish desired posterior lens and anterior eye relationships throughout these diameters.

A 23 mm. round lens is average in size. The patient's eyes are inspected. When they are of average size, a 23 mm. initial diagnostic lens is used; when smaller than average, a 22 mm. lens is used; and when larger than average, a 24 mm. lens is used.

After the initial diagnostic lens is inserted, two important criteria concerning the horizontal meridian are used to determine lens size. The temporal edge should be relatively difficult to see in primary fixation, and the nasal edge should not extend to the caruncle or plica. Therefore, the largest lens diameter that does not extend onto the caruncle, plica, or fornices, even on eye excursions, is used. Various diagnostic lenses are used until the desired diameter is obtained.

The optic-zone diameter is standardized for the various types of diagnostic scleral lenses.

When the sclera is considerably toric, an oval lens with a spherical haptic curvature may be used. A round lens is typically used until scleral toricity is greater than 0.50 mm. Because each 0.5 mm. of oval diameter is used for about each 0.20 mm. of scleral toricity, the minimal diameter difference for an oval lens is usually 1.5 mm. Often considerable corneal toricity is associated with considerable scleral toricity. Although there are frequent exceptions, a cornea with considerable toricity alerts the practitioner to suspect a considerable toricity in the sclera. An oval lens is used with its narrowest lens diameter along the flatter scleral meridians. This allows the lens to settle in closer to the eye, and it also allows the use of a somewhat shorter haptic radius. As a result, undesired excessive clearance along the steeper scleral meridians is reduced, while a satisfactory relationship along the flatter scleral meridians is maintained.

Posterior Radii. After lens and optic diameters are determined, haptic and optic radii are determined to provide the desired relationships throughout these diameters. Radii are determined by fluorescein pattern evaluation, by the blanching of conjunctival vessels caused by haptic pressure, and by the bubble appearance.

Liquid fluorescein is placed on the base curve before the lens is inserted, or in the fornix or through the fenestration after the lens is inserted. The fluorescein pattern is evaluated to determine the relationships between the posterior surface of the lens and anterior eye curves. The diagnostic procedure is the same as that used with corneal contact lenses.

The desired central fluorescein pattern of 8 to 9 mm. in diameter is light green and about 0.12 mm. in depth, which indicates minimum corneal clearance. The remainder of the optic and transition zones is a brighter green, which indicates increased clearance. Clearance diminishes until there is alignment and a white pattern starting about 2 mm. beyond the limbus and extending to the edge of the lens (Fig. 7–4).

A steep base curve causes excessive corneal clearance and often annular touch around the central 8 to 9 mm. zone (Fig. 7–5). A flat base curve

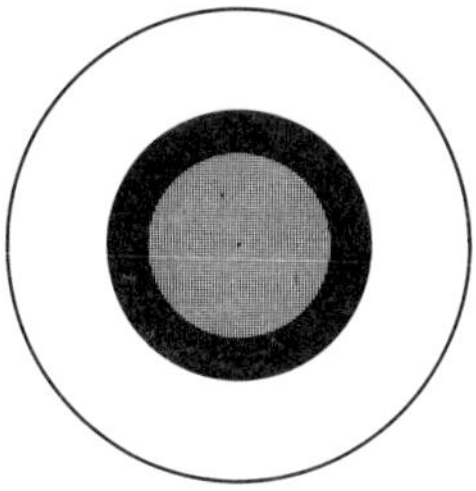

Figure 7–4. The desired fluorescein pattern has a wide central minimum clearance of 8 to 9 mm., an increased intermediate clearance, and an alignment starting about 2 mm. beyond the limbus and extending to the edge.

Figure 7–5. Steep base curve producing central corneal clearance.

Figure 7–6. Flat base curve producing central corneal touch.

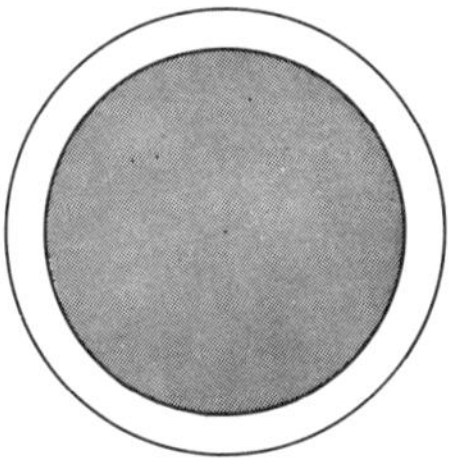

Figure 7–7. Steep haptic producing peripheral touch and a wide area of central corneal clearance.

results in central corneal touch (Fig. 7–6). A steep haptic causes excessive central clearance over too wide an area (Fig. 7–7). A flat haptic curve results in an annular area of touch around the limbus, and there is often clearance of the haptic curve from this point to the edge of the lens (Fig. 7–8).

When there is considerable scleral toricity, two other basic patterns are possible. A vertically oval pattern extending considerably beyond the limbus and toward the edge in the vertical meridian indicates with-the-rule scleral toricity. There usually is tightness along the horizontal meridian (Fig. 7–9). A lens with a toric haptic curvature should be used to obtain the ideal fluorescein pattern. A horizontally oval pattern extending considerably beyond the limbus and toward the edge in the horizontal meridian indicates against-the-rule scleral toricity. There usually is edge tightness along the vertical meridian (Fig. 7–10). A horizontally oval lens or a lens with a toric haptic curvature should be used to obtain the ideal fluorescein pattern.

It is best to have two sets of diagnostic lenses when the fluorescein pattern is to be evaluated. The first set is used to determine the necessary haptic curvature. The optic and transition radii of this set are such that corneal

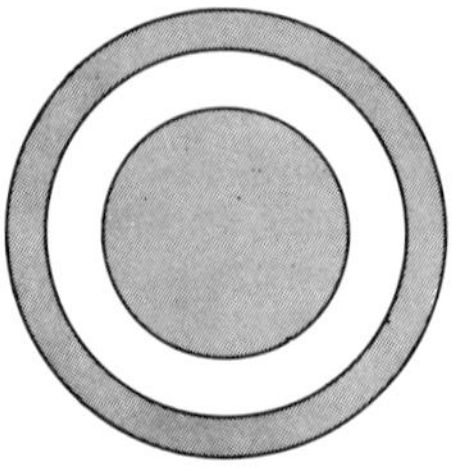

Figure 7–8. A flat haptic produces annular touch around the limbus and excessive peripheral clearance.

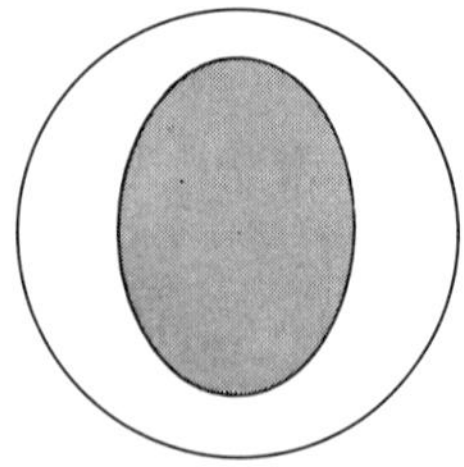

Figure 7–9. A vertically oval pattern is produced when a circular lens with spherical curves is placed on an eye that has considerable with-the-rule scleral toricity.

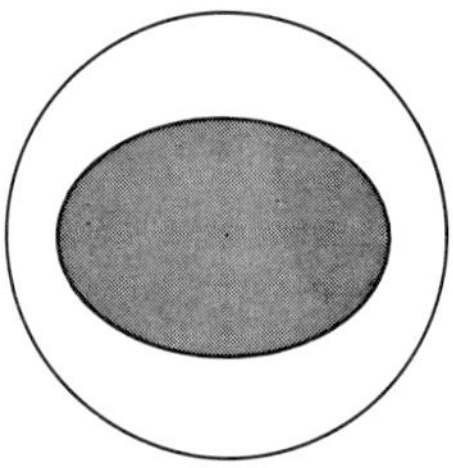

Figure 7–10. A horizontally oval clearance pattern is produced when a circular lens with spherical curves is placed on an eye with considerable against-the-rule scleral toricity.

and limbal clearance is assured. The haptic radius is determined without introduction of an artifact by corneal touch lifting the lens away. The second set is a unit of corneal lenses and it is used to determine the necessary optic radius. Lens diameter is 2.0 mm. larger than optic-zone diameter, and the secondary curves are flat enough to assure clearance. The optic radius is determined without introduction of an artifact by scleral touch lifting the lens away. *When only one set of diagnostic lenses is used, it is important to make sure that no artifact is introduced.* This procedure is similar to that of fitting of corneal lenses.

External examination with the white light and magnification system of a slit-lamp biomicroscope or with a pen light is an aid in evaluating haptic fit. A steep haptic curvature causes pressure on the underlying conjunctival blood vessels, often toward the lens edge. This impedes blood flow and causes a white or blanched area. In this circumstance, the practitioner would see the redness along the course of a blood vessel suddenly disappear under the tight area (Fig. 7–11). A flat haptic zone allows excessive bubbles to collect between it and the underlying cornea. It may also press on the blood vessels underlying the haptic-transition juncture, which causes a blanching (Fig. 7–12).

The size and position of the corneal bubble are studied in primary fixation. Abnormal bubble size or position may indicate an improper base curve. A centrally located bubble is often related to a steep base curve. A large

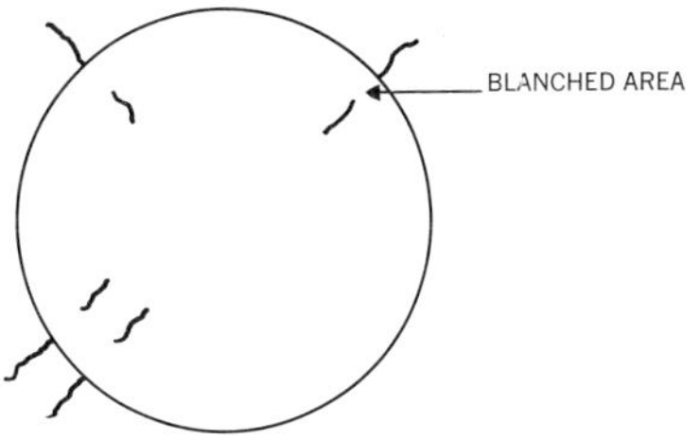

Figure 7–11. Steep haptic zone producing blanching of the conjunctival vessels underlying the edge of the lens.

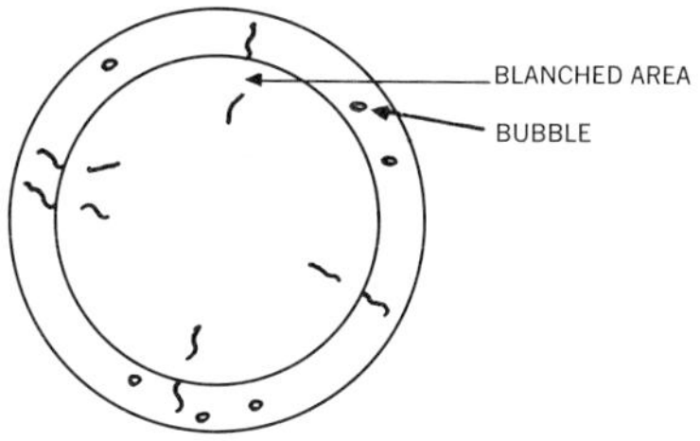

Figure 7–12. A flat haptic zone produces blanching of the conjunctival vessels underlying haptic-transition juncture and allows a collection of bubbles beneath the haptic zone.

bubble, peripherally circulating around and even beyond the limbus, is often related to a flat base curve. Bubble size and position should also be studied as the eye makes moderate rotations. When the base curve is steep, there is relatively little change in the position or size of the bubble with rotations. When the base curve is flat, there is relatively great change of bubble position or size with rotations. Note that too steep a haptic curve or too large a lens diameter simulates a steep base curve.

The base curve of the initial diagnostic lens depends on the central ophthalmometric reading and diagnostic lens optic-zone diameter (Table 7–1).

TABLE 7–1

INITIAL DIAGNOSTIC BASE CURVE

Optic-zone Diameter (in mm.)	Add to Flatter Ophthalmometric Principal Meridian (in mm.)
8.0	0.00
8.5	0.08
9.0	0.16
9.5	0.24
10.0	0.32
10.5	0.40
11.0	0.48
11.5	0.56
12.0	0.64
12.5	0.72
13.0	0.80
13.5	0.88
14.0	0.96
14.5	1.04

About 0.06 mm. is subtracted from the value found in Table 7–1 for every diopter of central ophthalmometric astigmatism after the first one. The haptic curve of the initial diagnostic lens depends on the base curve (Table 7–2).

TABLE 7–2

INITIAL DIAGNOSTIC HAPTIC CURVE

Base Curve (in mm.)	Initial Diagnostic Haptic Curve (in mm.)
8.00 or less	12.75 or steepest available
8.00 to 8.25	13.00
8.25 to 8.50	13.25
8.50 to 8.75	13.50
8.75 to 9.00	13.75
9.00 to 9.25	14.00

In Table 7–2, a lens diameter of about 23 mm. is assumed. Because the sclera seems to flatten from limbus to fornix, a flatter haptic radius is needed when lens diameter and scleral coverage are increased. When lens diameter and scleral coverage are decreased, a steeper haptic radius is needed. The initial diagnostic haptic radius is lengthened about 0.12 mm. for every 0.75 mm. of increase in lens diameter above 23 mm., and it is shortened about 0.12 mm. for every 0.75 mm. decrease of lens diameter.

Refractive Power. This value is determined by refraction over a diagnostic scleral contact lens. It is best to use the diagnostic lens with a base curve closest to what will be ordered, in order to reduce errors from precorneal fluid thickness. Appropriate compensations should be made for the difference between the base curve of the diagnostic lens and that of the ordered lens.

Fenestration. Fenestration location is frequently not determined until after lenses are processed for the patient. These lenses are inserted, marked, and fenestrated by the practitioner.

Overall Procedure. The radius of the haptic curve is determined first. The patient's eye size is approximated, and the initial diagnostic lens size is determined. Central ophthalmometric values are studied, and the initial diagnostic haptic curve is selected from Table 7–2. A lens is selected with the desired diameter and a base curve steep enough to assure central clearance. A base curve 0.25 mm. shorter than that found from Table 7–1 usually assures such clearance.

The lens is inserted and allowed to settle. White light is used to detect an excess of bubbles or transition blanching under the haptic curve, indicating too flat a haptic curve, or edge blanching, indicating too steep a haptic curve. Fluorescein is then instilled. When the haptic pattern shows the lens to be too flat, a diagnostic lens with the next steeper haptic curve in the same lens diameter and having apical clearance is used. The procedure is reversed when the haptic pattern is too steep. Various diagnostic lenses are used until the desired pattern is obtained.

When a sclera with considerable toricity is encountered, diagnostic lenses with oval shapes or toric haptics are used.

To determine the radius of the base curve, when using scleral diagnostic lenses, a lens with the desired diameter, haptic curvature, and base curve, found from Table 7–1, is inserted. When the fluorescein pattern shows the lens to be flat, a diagnostic lens with the next steeper base is used. When the fluorescein pattern shows the lens to be too steep, a diagnostic lens with the next flatter base is used. Various lenses are used until the desired pattern is obtained. Because many diagnostic sets have bases in 0.25 mm. steps, it is often necessary to interpolate to determine the base curve. It is preferable to determine base curve radius by a special diagnostic set (see p. 271).

When the optic-zone diameter of the ordered lens is different from that of the diagnostic lens, appropriate compensation must be made. A rule of thumb is that an 0.08 mm. change in radius must be made for every 0.5 mm. change in optic-zone diameter. This is added to the base curve if a larger optic zone is ordered and subtracted if a smaller optic zone is ordered.

It is preferable to have an initial central clearance of approximately 0.12 mm. because, after the lens settles, clearance is often reduced to about 0.08 mm. It is often preferable to order an optic diameter about 0.50 mm. larger than that of the diagnostic lens. This also helps compensate for settling, and if excessive clearance remains after settling, the optic-zone size can be reduced through modification.

Occasionally, the best fluorescein pattern shows simultaneous central and perizonal touch, possibly because of considerable peripheral corneal flattening. In such cases, a secondary curve should be used in the optic zone. The central optic-zone diameter should be about 8.0 mm., and its base curve should be about equal to the radius of the flatter ophthalmometric principal meridian reading. The secondary curve should have a radius about 0.7 mm. flatter than that of the base curve.

When the size of the ordered lens differs from that of the diagnostic lens, appropriate compensation should be made to maintain the same relationship between the haptic curve and the underlying sclera. A rule of thumb is that the haptic radius is lengthened 0.12 mm. for every 0.75 mm. of increase in lens diameter. The haptic radius is shortened 0.12 mm. for every 0.75 mm. of decrease in lens diameter.

Transition curve radii are usually standardized about halfway between base and haptic radii.

Commonly Used Preformed Scleral Lenses. Various preformed scleral lenses are known by specific names. They are all fitted in basically the same way.

Transcurve Lens.[266] The average lens diameter is 23 mm., and the range of lens diameters is 21 to 25 mm. The average optic-zone diameter is 13 mm., and the range of optic-zone diameters is 12 to 15 mm. The transition width is about 1.5 to 2.5 mm. Transition curvature is spherical, and its radius is often the mean of base and haptic radii. These lenses may be round or oval, and they may have toric haptic curves. A fenestration may be used. Double-curve optic zones may be used. In such cases, the central optic-zone diameter is often equal to about three-fourths of the corneal diameter, and the annular secondary optic-zone diameter is about 2 to 2.5 mm. wide on each side. The secondary optic-zone curvature is 0.5 mm. longer for a steep cornea and 1.0 mm. longer for a flat cornea than the base curvature.

Wide-Angle Lens.[267] The average lens diameter is 23 mm., and range of lens diameters is about 21 to 25 mm. The optic-zone diameter is 11.5 mm. Oval lenses with about a 2 to 3 mm. difference between vertical and horizontal diameters are used. The optic zone is decentered about 1 mm. nasally. Fenestration may be used. A distinguishing characteristic of this lens is that the 2.25 mm. wide transition curvature is formed by a conical rather than a spherical tool. The cone angle used is determined by the base curve (Table 7–3).

TABLE 7–3

TRANSITION CURVES OF WIDE-ANGLE LENSES

Base Curve (in mm.)	Cone Angle (in mm.)
7.50	90°
7.75	93°
8.00	96°
8.25	99°
8.50	102°
8.75	105°
9.00	108°

Offset Lens.[268–269] The average optic-zone diameter is 13.5 mm., and the range of optic-zone diameters is 12.5 to 14.5 mm. The average lens diameter is about 22.5 × 23.5 mm. The optic zone is decentered nasally about 2 mm. The transition curve may be like that of the transcurve or that of the wide-angle lenses. The transition width ranges from 1.5 to 3.5 mm. A distinguishing characteristic of this lens is the aspheric haptic curvature. The haptic curvature radius varies about 0.25 mm. for each 0.75 mm. variance of haptic width (that is, a 1.5 mm. change in lens diameter). This aspheric curvature is obtained by using a tool whose center of curvature is offset to the opposite side of the anteroposterior axis.

Preformed Lacrilens. The average lens diameter is 23.5 mm. A distinguishing characteristic of this lens is the corneal section, which has four

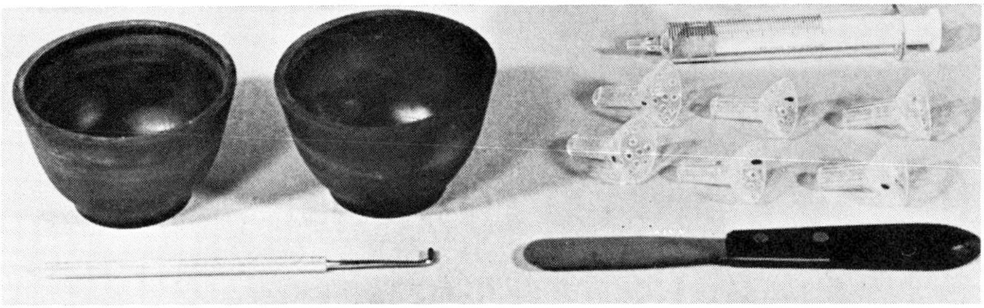

Figure 7–13. Molding equipment. Rubber bowls, syringe, and molding shells (top). *Muscle hook and stainless steel spatula* (bottom). (Figs. 7–13 to 7–25 courtesy of Obrig Laboratories, Inc.)

zones. There is an 8.0 mm. central optic zone surrounded by three annular, concentric secondary zones of 1.0, 1.0, and 1.25 mm. widths, respectively. The corneal section is, therefore, 14.5 mm. wide. The radius of each secondary zone is flatter than the radius of the adjacent, inner zone. The corneal section is decentered nasally. A 1.0 mm. fenestration is placed in the temporal side of the first secondary zone. The suggested fitting set of 16 lenses has base curve radii of 7.50, 7.70, 7.90, and 8.10 mm. each combined with four haptic radii in 0.25 mm. increments.

Molded Lenses

Scleral contact lenses are often fitted by using a molding procedure.[270–272] This is especially necessary in lenses for highly irregular eyes. Figure 7–13 shows molding equipment.

When a molding procedure is used, the impression material is placed in an appropriate shell. This is inserted on the eye, and an impression is obtained. After the shell with the impression material is removed from the eye, a creamy mixture of dental stone powder and water is poured into the negative impression, producing a solid positive cast of the front of the eye. The cast is appropriately marked and sent to the laboratory. It is used as a mold to make the contact lens. A molded lens may have posterior lens–anterior eye relationships similar to those of preformed lenses. A molded lens also may be fitted in an attempt to have it conform exactly to the contour of the eye. These *flush fitting* lenses are usually used on diseased eyes.

Preparation. Moldite, Cosmet, Tissuetex, Zelex, and Zylex are the trade names of the most commonly used eye impression materials. Such materials produce an impression whose consistency is like that of the white of a hard-boiled egg. Directions for use are provided on the containers.

Because the impression material is relatively soft, it must be placed in a molding shell. These shells are shaped like scleral contact lenses. They are perforated, thus permitting the escape of excess material during impression taking and the adherence of the impression to the holder.

Some shells may have handles, which may be hollow. A shell without a handle and containing the impression material is inserted and removed just as a scleral contact lens is. A suction cup may be used to aid removal. When a shell without a handle is used, the procedure is termed *concentric molding*. A shell with a solid handle is used in a similar manner. A twisting action of the handle aids insertion and removal. This type is termed *insertion molding*. A shell with a hollow handle is inserted without impression material. A hypodermic syringe with impression material is placed in the hollow handle, and the impression material is injected. This type is termed *injection molding*.

All equipment necessary for preparing the impression material, taking the impression, and making the cast should be set up in advance. The proper amount of impression powder and distilled water is emptied into a rubber bowl or mortar. The mixture is spatulated according to the manufacturer's instructions, to produce a creamy mixture without particles. The mixture is then poured into the appropriate shell or syringe (Fig. 7–14).

Making the Impression (Negative). The patient is seated with his head tilted slightly back against a headrest. A covering towel is placed under his chin as a bib, and the shell is inserted. When an injection procedure is used, the syringe is cleared of air (Fig. 7–15). The shell is lifted away from the eye, and the impression material is injected (Fig. 7–16).

In all molding procedures, the patient is instructed to maintain fixation at a proper target. If this is not done, a poor impression is produced. Excess

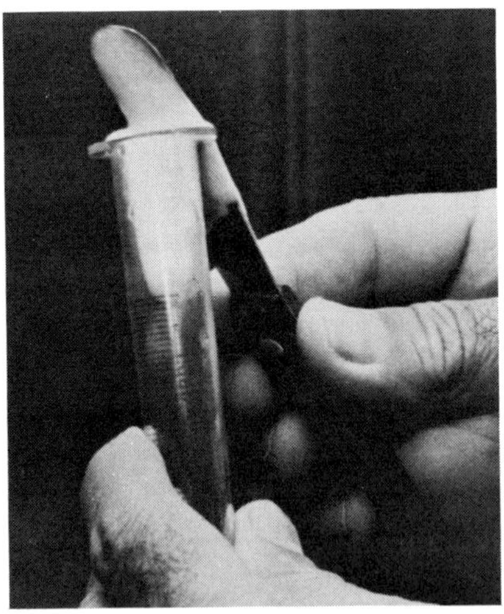

Figure 7–14. Impression material being placed in syringe.

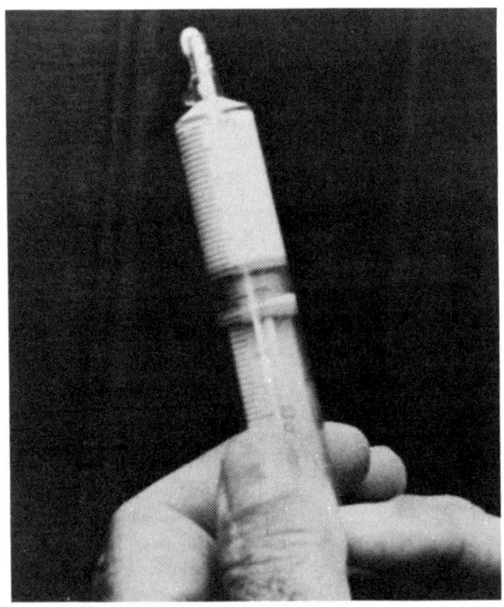

Figure 7–15. Clearing syringe of air.

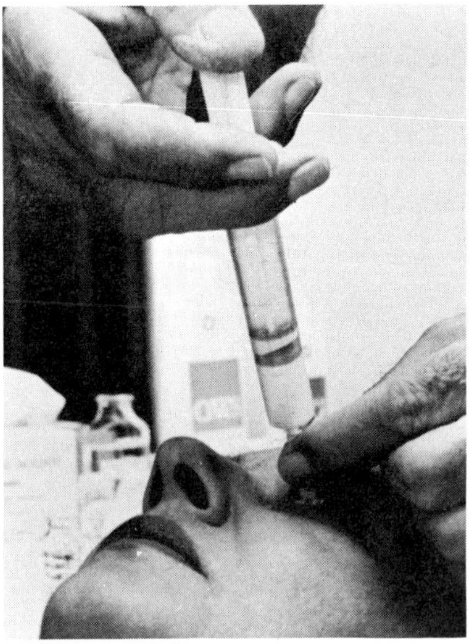

Figure 7–16. Injecting impression material into shell.

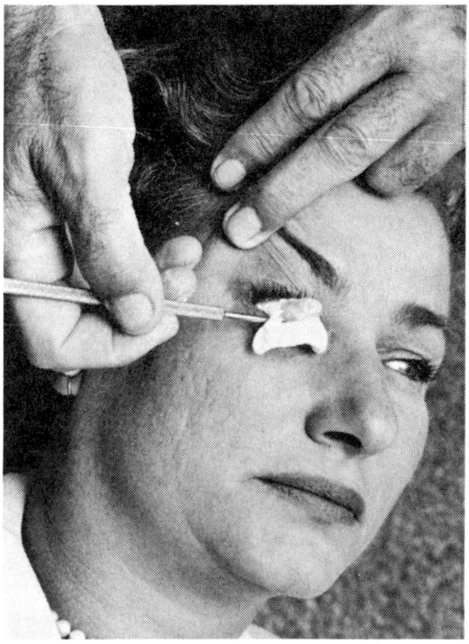

Figure 7–17. Removing excess material.

material is removed from around the lids while the impression is setting, according to the manufacturer's instructions (Fig. 7–17). After the material has set, an *x* is placed temporally and a dot nasally along the 180° line of the shell with an indelible pencil. The adherence of the impression to the eye due to suction is broken when the patient looks temporally and the practitioner pushes nasally against the inner canthus. More precorneal fluid enters behind the lens, and the shell and impression are removed. This is also done by drawing the shell handle toward the eyebrow and pulling the lower lid down with a muscle hook (Fig. 7–18). The shell is separated from the lower lid. Then the patient looks down and the shell is carefully pulled out (Figs. 7–19 and 7–20).

Excessive impression material is removed from around the lids, and the lids are everted to facilitate removal of material trapped under them. The eye is irrigated (Fig. 7–21); it is then examined with a slit-lamp biomicroscope. Finally, the impression is evaluated.

Making the Positive Cast. About three tablespoonfuls of dental stone powder are placed in a rubber bowl. Water is added, and the mixture is spatulated until it becomes creamy. The impression shell is positioned in a holder so that it remains upright at all times. The creamy mixture is poured into the negative impression, making sure that the impression is completely filled and that there are no air bubbles (Fig. 7–22). The mixture is allowed to set as indicated by the manufacturer.

After the mixture has set, the rear of the cast is marked nasally (N) and

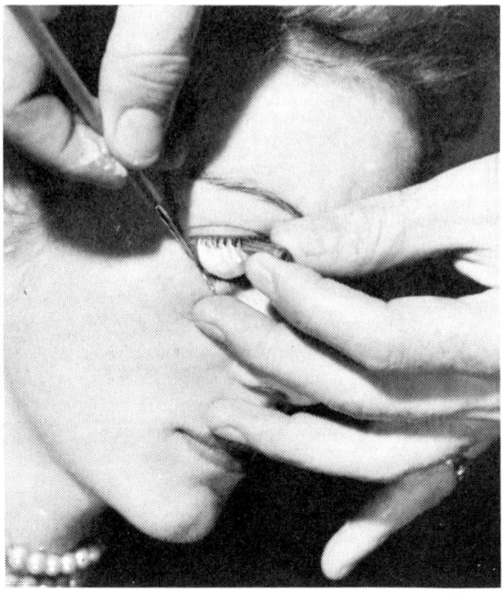

Figure 7–18. Breaking suction of impression to eye by drawing shell handle toward eyebrow and pulling the lower lid with a muscle hook.

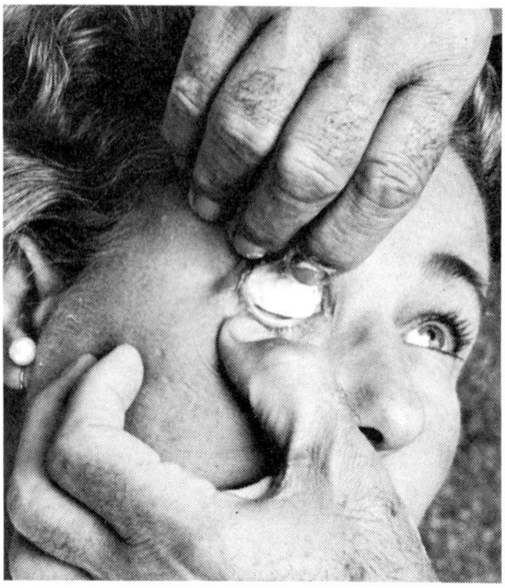

Figure 7–19. Separating shell from lower lid.

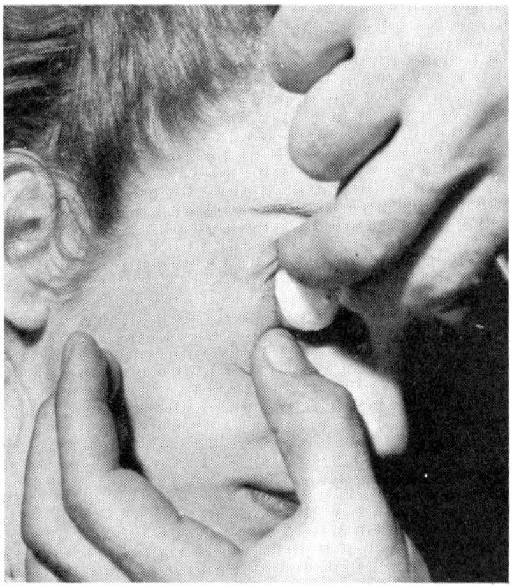

Figure 7–20. Patient looking down while shell is eased out.

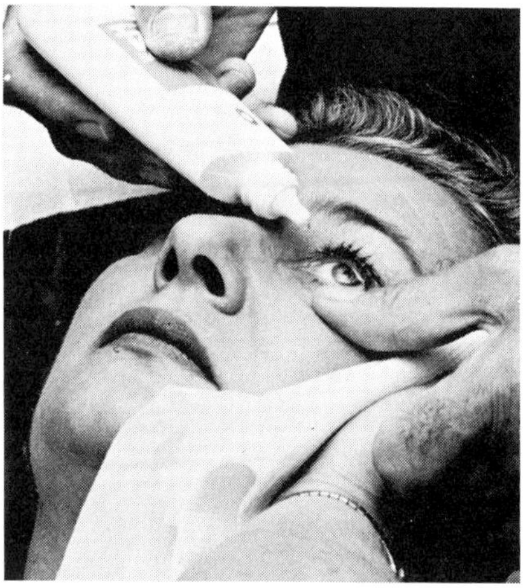

Figure 7–21. Irrigating the eye.

temporally (T) along the 180° line (Fig. 7–23). An *R* is placed at the top of the rear surface of a cast of the right eye and an *L* on a cast of the left eye. The excess dental stone is removed with a knife or razor blade from around the shell, and the cast is then removed from the impression (Fig. 7–24).

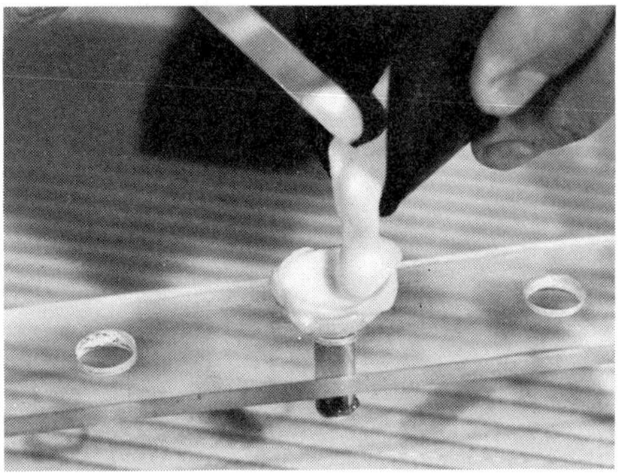

Figure 7–22. Pouring dental stone mixture into impression.

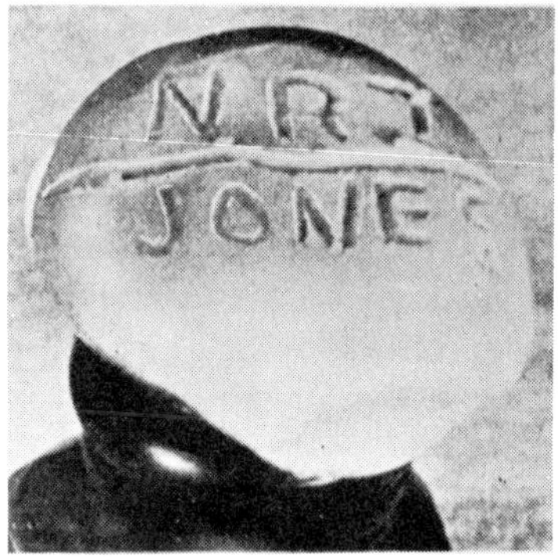

Figure 7–23. Marking cast.

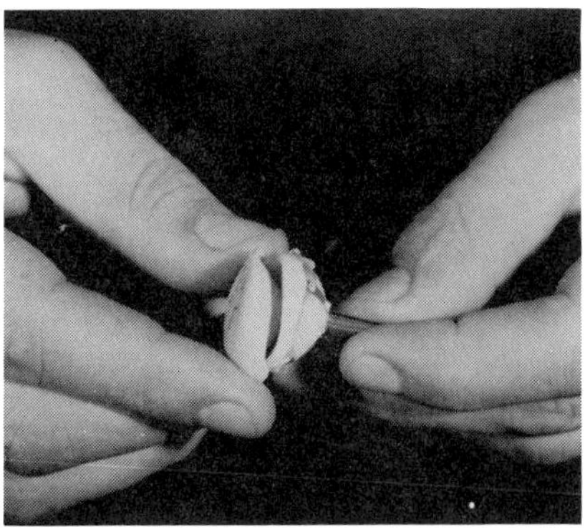

Figure 7–24. Removing the cast from the impression.

LABORATORY PROCEDURES

ORDERING

PREFORMED LENSES. The following specifications are ordered: base curve radius, optic-zone diameter, lens diameter (or diameters if oval, and whether a vertical or horizontal oval is desired), haptic radius (or radii and axis, if toric), optic-zone decentration, back vertex power, and size and location of fenestration (unless this is to be done by the practitioner).[273]

MOLDED LENSES. The appropriately marked cast is sent to the laboratory. The desired lens diameter, the central ophthalmometric readings, the back vertex spectacle power and vertex distance are included. When it is desired, size and position of fenestration may be specified.

VERIFICATION[274]

BASE CURVE. This curve is measured with a radiuscope or an Ophthalmometer. The procedure is similar to that used in verifying corneal contact lenses.

Haptic Radius. This radius may often be measured with a radiuscope or Ophthalmometer. It is important to make certain that the lens is positioned so that the desired area is being measured. Balls of various radii can be matched to the haptic curve.

Corneal and Transitional Zone Diameter. These diameters can be measured with a measuring magnifier, also used in measuring corneal contact lenses.

Lens Diameter. A millimeter ruler is used to measure the lens diameter in a given meridian.

Decentration. The haptic width, measured on each side of the transition along the horizontal meridian of the lens, is determined with a measuring magnifier. Half the difference between these two measurements is the amount of decentration.

Fenestration. Fenestration size is determined by a measuring magnifier. Fenestration quality is evaluated with a stereoscopic microscope.

Refractive Power. Back vertex power is determined on a Lensometer (Vertometer).

Thickness. Gauges are used, as in measuring corneal contact lenses.

Modification[275]

Scleral lens modification is a distinct art. Three basic categories of modification are diameter change, posterior curvature change, and anterior curvature change.

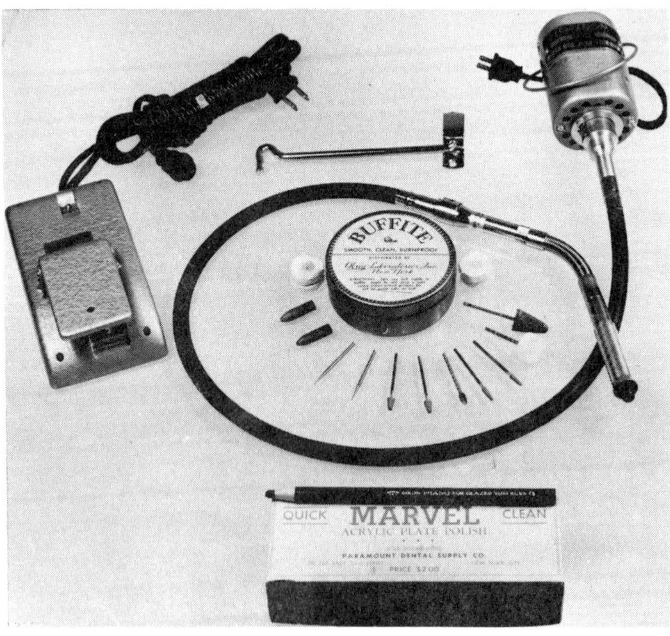

Figure 7–25. Modification equipment, including dental engine and foot rheostat.

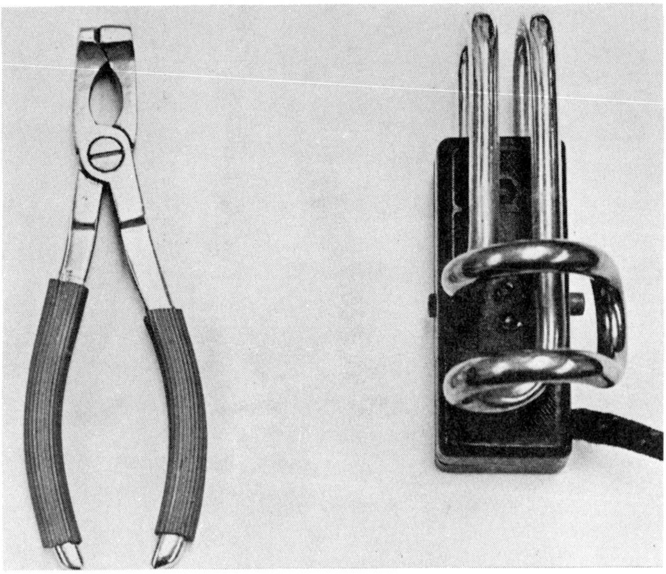

Figure 7–26. Feinbloom forceps and an immersion heater.

Equipment. A motorized unit is needed. This may be a dental engine with a handpiece or a mounted motor-driven spindle, such as is used in corneal contact lens modification (Fig. 7–25). Carborundum balls of various radii, and small grinding disks and points, are needed for plastic removal, and liquid plastic is needed for building up or adding plastic. An immersion heater and forceps may also be used to heat and bend plastic (Fig. 7–26). Felt polishing cones and points and polishing compounds are needed for polishing plastic (Figs. 7–27 and 7–28).

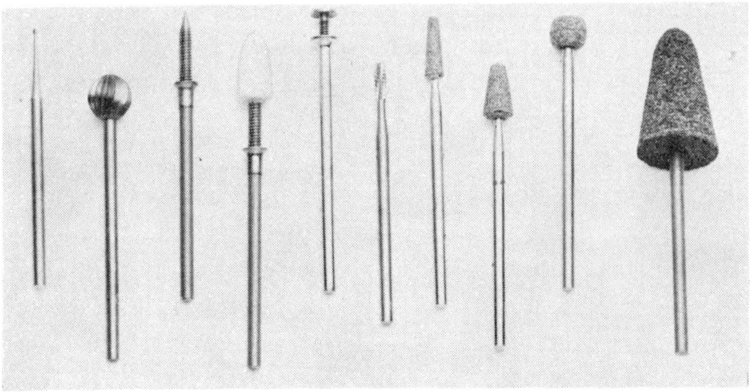

Figure 7–27. Modification tools. Left to right, *dotter, vulcanite burr, pointed mandrel, mandrel and conical buff, flat mandrel, dentate burr, denstone No. 12, denstone No. 13, carborundum stone, and conical carborundum stone.* (Courtesy of Obrig Laboratories, Inc.)

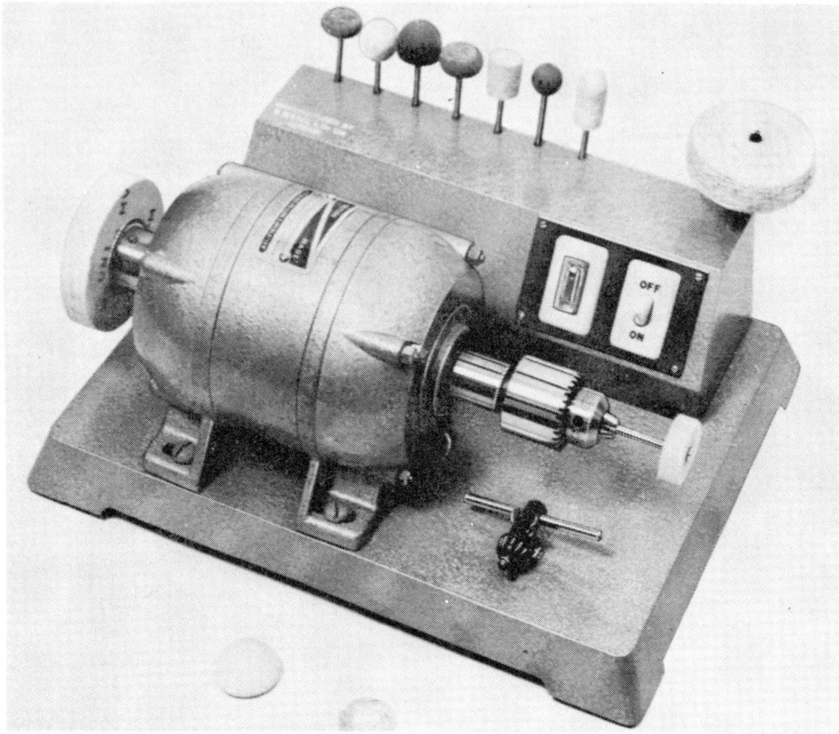

Figure 7–28. Modification unit. (Courtesy of G. Nissel & Co.)

DIAMETER. The area to be cut down is marked with a grease or waterproof marking pencil while the patient wears the lens. After the lens is removed, the marked area is cut away with a conical carborundum stone, and any corners are rounded. Diameter reduction is stopped just before the desired size is reached. A grit-impregnated rubber point is then rolled over the edges. The felt cone or disk is covered with a polishing compound, such as Radoff, and is placed on the dental engine. The cone or disk is rolled over the edge until it is finely polished.

POSTERIOR CURVATURES. Posterior curvatures may be flattened by removing stock from or bending the lens. Removing stock is often termed *grindout* or *easing*. Posterior curvatures may be steepened by adding liquid plastic to or bending the lens. Practitioners should work only on the haptic or transition curvatures. Any alteration of the base curvature is best done by the manufacturer.

The area to be flattened is marked with a grease or waterproof marking pencil while the patient wears the lens. A carborundum stone is placed on the motorized unit. After the lens is removed from the eye, the indicated amount of plastic is ground from the posterior surface under the marked area. The stone should be kept moist with water to avoid marring of the lens surface. The grit-impregnated rubber tool is then placed on the motorized unit and is used to smooth the area. Finally, after the felt cone or disk is placed on the motorized unit, it is covered with a polishing compound, such as Radoff, and the area is polished.

It is possible to flatten part of the haptic area by bending. A pair of forceps is heated 15 to 25 seconds in boiling water in a special immersion heater. The forceps are pressed lightly along the lens area to be flattened. This area is bent slightly toward the front surface of the lens, and the procedure is continued until the desired flattening is established.

The same basic bending procedure may be used for steepening the haptic curvature. In this case, the bending is toward the rear surface. Haptic curvature may also be steepened by the addition of liquid plastic. The loose areas are marked with a grease or waterproof marking pencil while the lens is on the eye. The lens is removed, and a thin coating of liquid plastic is placed on the posterior surface of the lens under the marked area. The coating is then allowed to dry. The procedure is continued until the desired steepening has been accomplished. This area is then polished.

It is possible to move the base curve closer to or further from the cornea by altering haptic thickness. Decreasing the thickness throughout the haptic area moves the base curve closer to the cornea; increasing the thickness moves the base curve further from the cornea. Removing plastic from the haptic is done by grinding. This must be done uniformly throughout the haptic area, and about twice as much is ground out at the transition as at the edge. It is estimated that to decrease corneal clearance 0.1 mm., 0.06 mm. must be ground from the transition edge and 0.03 mm. from the lens edge. There should be a relatively uniform rate of change from transition to edge.

Adding plastic to the haptic area is done in the same manner as in steepening. A thin layer must be applied uniformly throughout the haptic area. After this is dried and polished, the lens is put back on the patient's eye. Successive layers are added until the desired clearance is obtained.

It is possible to change the base curve of a finished lens to alter clearance. This is best done by the manufacturer. Alterations of the transition zone also may accidentally alter the base curve, and it is usually best to leave such changes to the manufacturer.

Anterior Curvatures. The anterior curvature is usually changed to alter refractive power, and such changes are best left to the manufacturer. When there is sufficient center thickness, it is easy for the manufacturer to increase minus power up to 2.50 D. It is more difficult to increase plus power. Often +0.50 D to +0.75 D is the maximum possible change. It is best, therefore, to prescribe maximum plus or minimum minus in all cases.

Education of the Patient

Lens Insertion

The lens is prepared with wetting solution. A right lens is inserted with the right hand and a left lens with the left hand. The thumb holds the temporal side of the lens, the second finger holds the nasal side of the lens, and the index finger is placed against the anterior surface of the optic zone. The patient looks down and pulls back his upper lid with the opposite hand. The lens is placed high on the superior sclera and under the upper lid. As the lens slips up, the upper lid is pulled down over it. The lens is held in this position, and the patient looks up. Then the lower lid is pulled over the lens. A suction cup may be used to hold the lens, with the procedure remaining the same.

Lens Removal

The patient holds his head erect and looks down. To remove the right lens, the index or middle finger of the right hand is placed under the margin of the upper lid near the inner canthus. The upper lid is first pulled away from the lens and then pushed under it. The index or middle finger is moved toward the outer canthus while maintaining pressure against the orbit. The lens will fall into the opposite hand, which is cupped under the eye. Hands are reversed for lens removal from the left eye.

A suction holder may be used for removal. The upper lid is pulled away. The patient looks at the suction holder, and it is attached to the anterior surface of the optic zone of the lens. The patient looks down, and the lens is pulled down and out by the suction holder.

Lens Care

After the lenses are removed, they are cleaned with wetting solution. This is rinsed off with water, and the lenses are then blotted dry with a tissue and usually stored dry.

ARTIFICIAL EYES

An artificial eye is often used after blinding, disfiguring ocular pathologic conditions, or removal of some or all of the orbital contents by accident, enucleation, evisceration, or exenteration.[276–278] An artificial eye is used to improve appearance and to retain the size and shape of the orbit.

Artificial eyes are generally made of polymethyl methacrylate, as are most corneal and scleral contact lenses. This plastic is tolerated well by the tissues, it does not break easily, and it can be modified readily.

An artificial eye has a painted iris, pupil, and sclera to simulate a real eye (Fig. 7–29). When it is in place, an artificial eye should match the appearance of the good eye and palpebral aperture as nearly as possible. It should also provide good movement and comfort, and it should not cause poor sanitation.

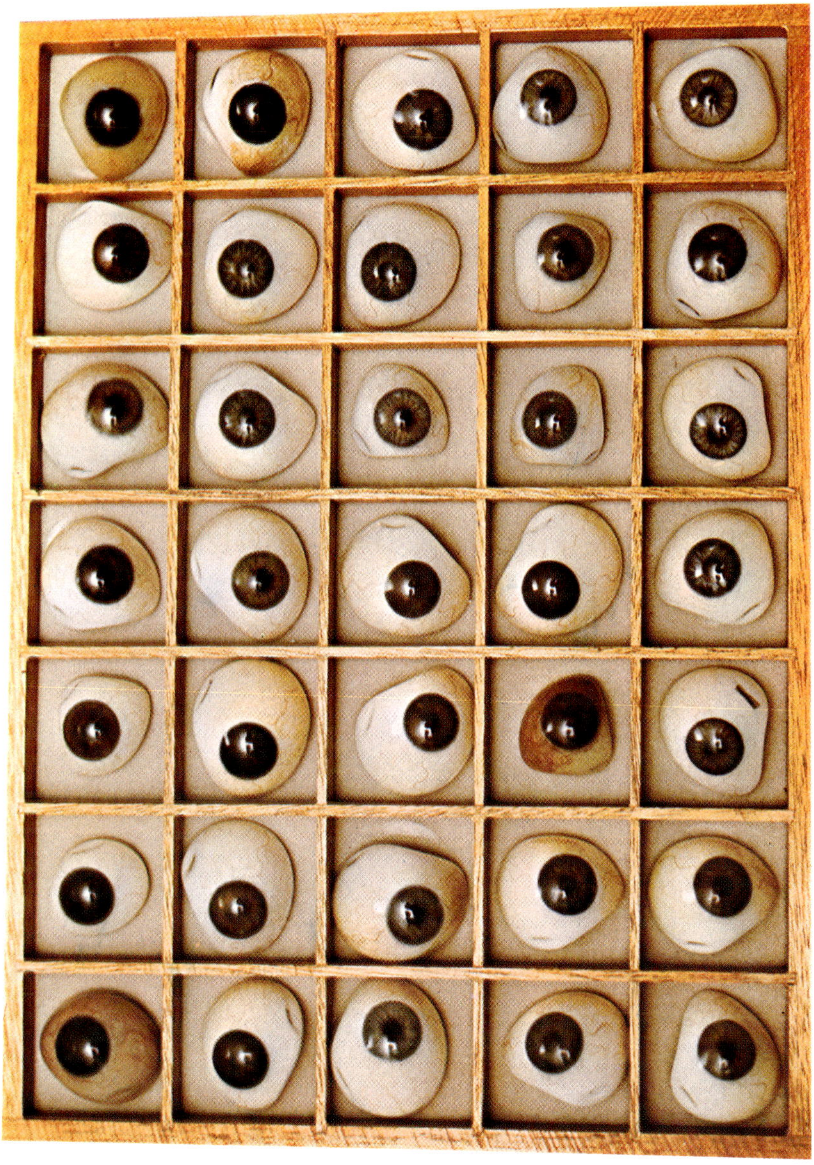

Figure 7–29. Artificial eyes.

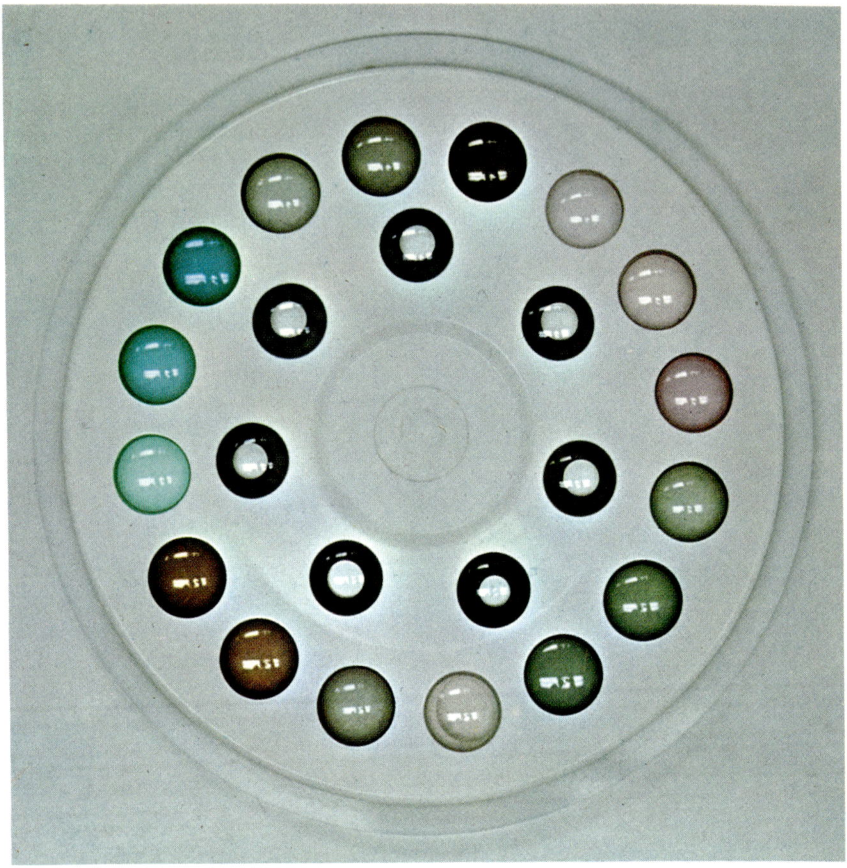

Figure 7–39. Cosmetic corneal contact lenses.

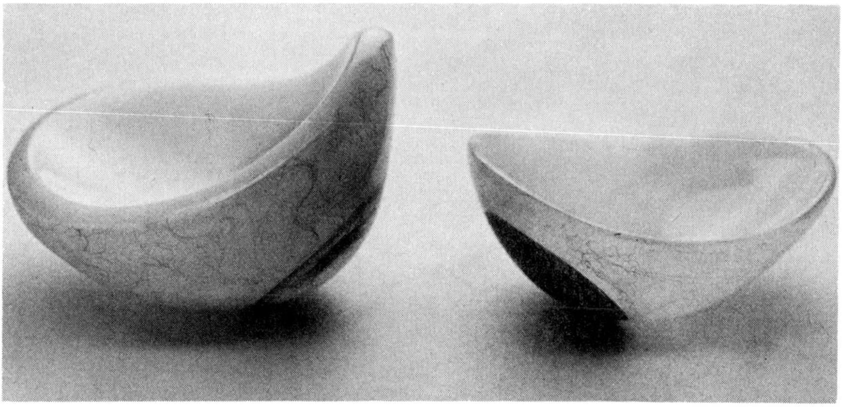

Figure 7–30. Reform and shell eyes. Note the thickness difference.

Types of Artificial Eyes

Based on center thickness, there are two general types of artificial eyes. When the center thickness is about 2 mm. or less, it is termed a *shell eye,* or cosmetic cover lens; when the center thickness is more than 2 mm., it is termed a *reform eye* (Fig. 7–30).

Shell eye and scleral contact lens thickness are similar, and cosmetic scleral contact lenses are often used as shell eyes. Shell eyes are also obtained by direct order or by reduction of the posterior thickness of a reform eye. A shell eye is used when either the natural or artificial orbital contents occupy a considerable amount of space. A shell eye used over scanty orbital contents produces a sunken, enophthalmic appearance with a narrow palpebral aperture. A reform eye is used when either the natural or artificial orbital contents occupy little space. A reform eye used over full orbital contents produces a bulging, exophthalmic appearance with a wide palpebral aperture. The type of artificial eye should be selected to provide a satisfactory appearance by supplementing the thickness of the natural or artificial orbital contents.

Orbital Contents

What is meant by natural or artificial contents of the orbit? Natural contents of the orbit are the orbital and ocular tissues; artificial contents include material surgically implanted.

Implants are often used after enucleation or evisceration to fill the orbital space previously occupied by the removed tissue. The artificial eye is fitted against this implant. Extraocular muscles are attached to the tissue covering the implant or to the implant itself, and this musculature imparts movement as fixation is varied. Movement is also imparted by relationship to and movement of the fornices.

Implants typically are spheres made entirely of plastic, glass, gold, or

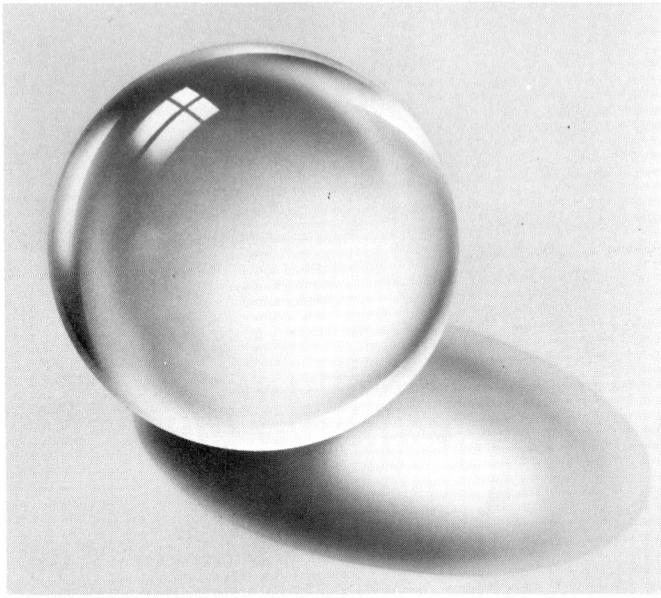

Figure 7–31. Sphere implant. (Courtesy of American Optical Co.)

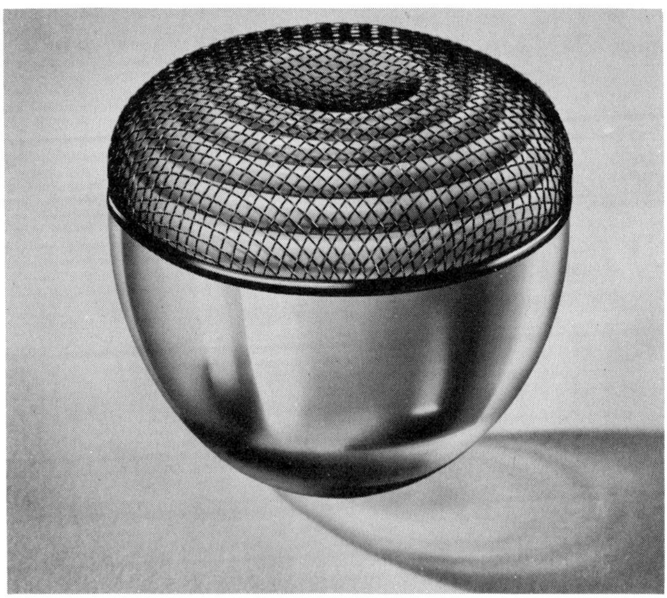

Figure 7–32. Mesh-covered implant. (Courtesy of American Optical Co.)

silicone rubber, or they are made of plastic and a tantalum mesh. Spheres without mesh frequently have grooves or tunnels to which the recti muscles are attached (Fig. 7–31). In spheres with mesh, the recti muscles are usually sutured directly to the mesh (Fig. 7–32).

There are two common procedures related to orbital contents with enucleation. Either the four recti are sutured together as a stump, or an implant is sutured into the cavity formed by the recti muscles, Tenon's capsule, and the conjunctiva. After evisceration, an implant is usually sutured into the scleral cavity (Fig. 7–33).

Implants are either attached or integrated. An *attached implant* is con-

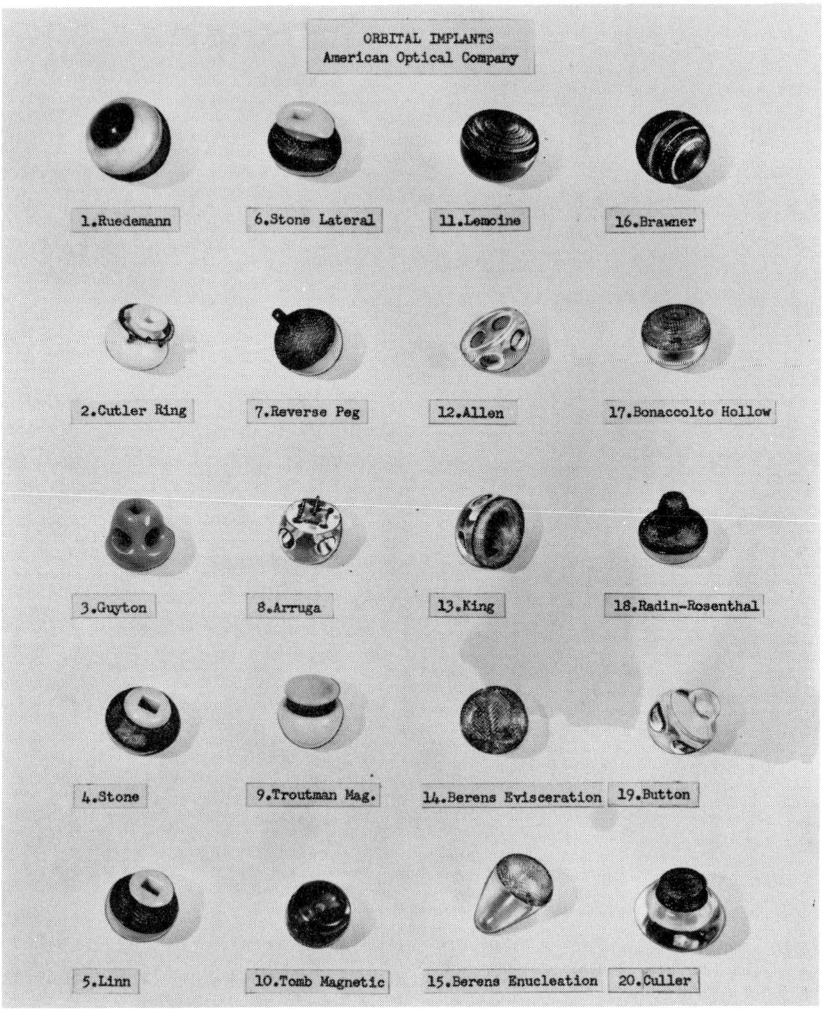

Figure 7–33. Various types of implants. (Courtesy of American Optical Co.)

nected directly to the extraocular muscles, but it is not connected directly to the artificial eye. An *integrated implant* is connected directly to the extraocular muscles and to the artificial eye.

Integration is used to obtain better movement of the artificial eye. Integration is usually done in one of two ways. A peg may be placed on the rear surface of the artificial eye and inserted in an opening on the front surface of the implant, or magnets are placed on the rear surface of the artificial eye and the front surface of the implant (Fig. 7–34).

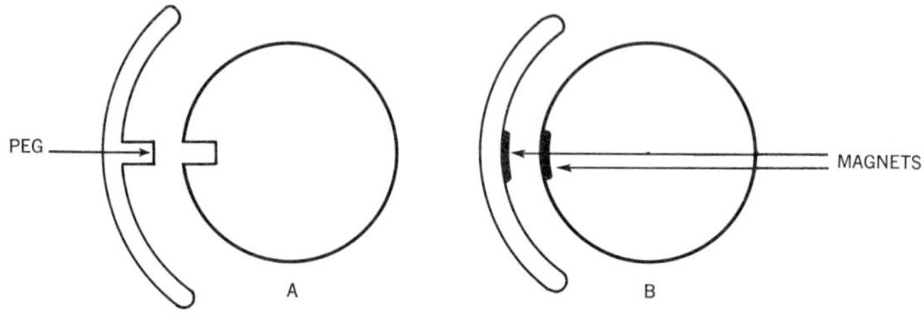

Figure 7–34. A, *Integration of artificial eye and implant by a peg.* B, *Integration of artificial eye and implant by magnets.*

Attached implants and integrated magnetic implants are *buried*—that is, the implant is covered on all surfaces by tissue. Integrated peg implants are *semiburied*—the front surface of the implant is exposed so that the peg can be inserted.

Shell eyes are generally used in a blind, disfigured eye that has not atrophied greatly or an eviscerated eye with an implant (Fig. 7–35). Reform eyes are generally used in an atrophied, blind, disfigured eye or after enucleation or exenteration (Fig. 7–36). A relatively thick reform eye is used when enucleation without an implant, or exenteration, has been performed.

The two most common conditions seen by the fitter of artificial eyes are a blind, disfigured eye or an enucleated eye. Exenteration is a radical procedure used only when there has been a malignant ocular condition. Evisceration is not frequently used owing to the tendency for the implant to be pushed out, or extruded, from the eye.

General Fitting Techniques

There are three general techniques for fitting artificial eyes: the *stock eye technique,* the *customized stock eye technique,* and the *custom eye technique.*

Stock eye technique involves using a set of preformed artificial eyes. The set is designed to include the range of shapes and colors needed by most people. The best shapes and colors for each patient are selected from the preformed eyes and ordered from the manufacturer who stocks these shapes and colors. When the practitioner receives the eye, size and shape may be modified to produce a better fit.

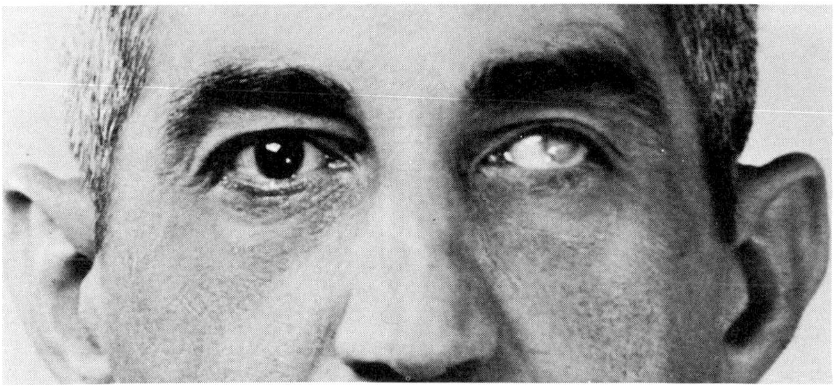

A

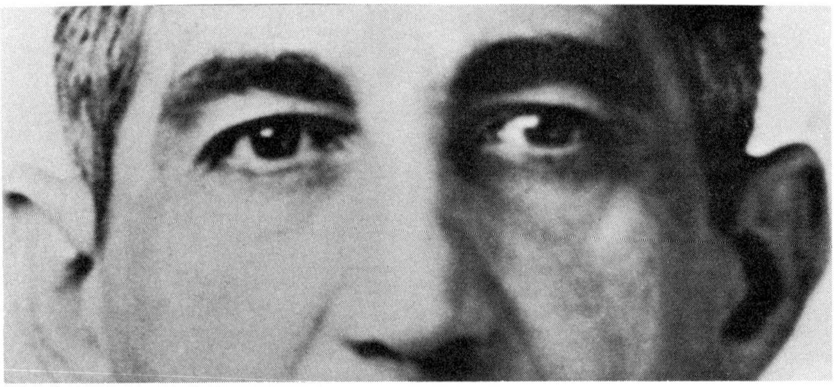

B

Figure 7–35. Fitting a shell artificial eye. A, *Before.* B, *After.*

The customized stock eye technique involves using a stock lens, which is then customized. There are two general types of customization: an impression technique may be used to produce better conformity between the posterior surface of the artificial eye and the anterior surface of the orbital contents, or from direct observation of the patient an artist may paint an uncolored stock eye, which is then annealed.

The custom eye technique involves making a mold and a cast of the anterior area of the orbit and its contents. This cast is used to determine the sizes and shapes of the plastic artificial eye. The iris and sclera are painted from direct observation of the patient by an artist, and the artificial eye is annealed.

Clinical Procedures

After enucleation, a special conformer, or a temporary artificial eye, is used to condition the socket and to aid healing. Only an approximate fit of

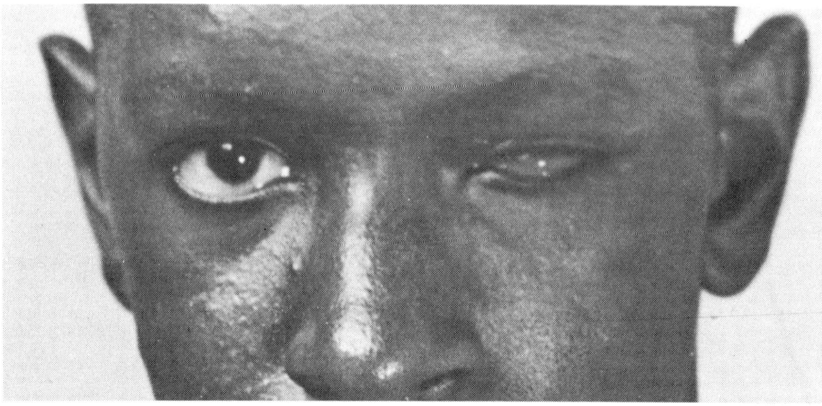

A

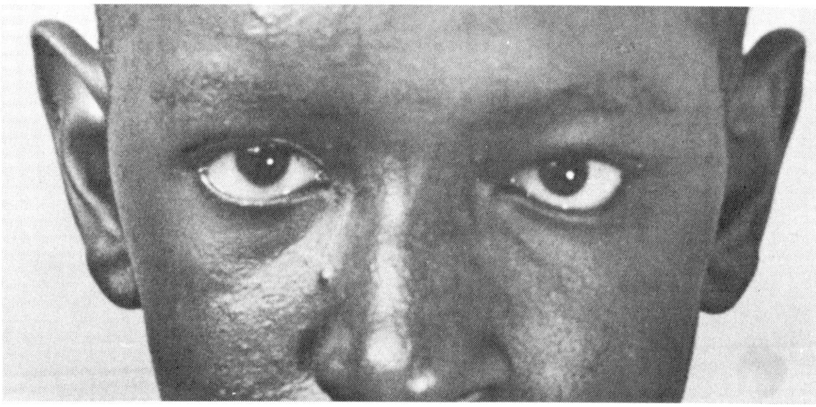

B

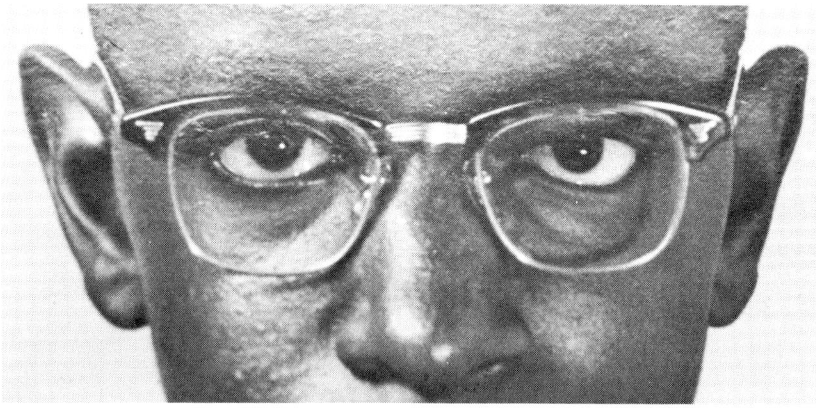

C

Figure 7–36. Fitting a reform artificial eye. A, *Before.* B *and* C, *After.*

size, shape, and color is needed at this point. A prolonged fitting procedure may irritate the semihealed tissues. The temporary eye must be cleaned about once a week.

When the tissues are properly healed, the permanent artificial eye is fitted. It must be fitted to match the appearance of the good eye and palpebral aperture, to move satisfactorily, to be comfortable, and to be sanitary.

Stock Eye Technique

Stock eye techniques vary somewhat with each manufacturer. The technique presented here is a representative technique, and the practitioner is advised to relate this technique to the services and facilities of his manufacturer.

Some manufacturers provide color charts of artificial eyes for the selection of iris and scleral colors. Pupil size, iris size, and position of the good eye, and the orbital size of the other eye are measured. These measurements are sent to the manufacturer, who supplies about two dozen artificial eyes used to determine the fit.

To produce the desired results, the fitter selects the appropriate eye sizes, shapes, and art work from the preformed diagnostic eyes. This procedure is shown in the following schema:

Sizes + shapes + art work = appearance + comfort + movement

Sizes. The first decision is whether to use a shell or a reform eye. When a shell eye is used, the authors prefer to use a fluidless molded cosmetic scleral contact lens. Sizes and shapes are determined as in molded scleral contact lenses (p. 275).

When a reform eye is used, the orbital size is evaluated. Orbits are considered small, medium, or large for purposes of artificial eye fitting. When the horizontal orbital dimension is less than about 24 mm., it is small; when it is 25 to 26 mm., it is medium; and when it is 27 mm. or more, it is large.

Shapes. The shape of the orbit is then evaluated. Various manufacturers use reform eyes of different shapes. There is generally a standard, or round, shape and an oval shape, which are used for the corresponding orbital shape. The practitioner should verify with his manufacturer the specific shapes he maintains in stock.

Art Work. Pupil size, iris color and size, and scleral color of the diagnostic artificial eye are matched as closely as possible with the good eye. Because the pupil size of a human eye varies with illumination, an intermediate pupil size is selected for the artificial eye. Usually, this size is equal to the pupil size measured under ordinary room illumination. The pupils in many preformed artificial eyes are approximately 3.5 mm. in diameter. When a different size is needed, it must be specified.

Initial tentative iris color is selected by comparison of various artificial eyes near the good eye, preferably under natural light. Because of the surrounding skin, eyelashes, and shadows, apparent iris color changes when an artificial eye is placed in the orbit. Final iris color selection should not be made until after the eye has been placed in the orbit. Iris size is determined by measurement of the visible horizontal iris diameter of the good eye. Many preformed artificial eye irises have a diameter of 11.5 mm. When a different size is needed, it must be specified.

Alteration of pupil or iris size from that of the diagnostic preformed eye changes the apparent iris color. Supplementary diagnostic eyes or charts are available from some manufacturers for matching iris color under such conditions.

Evaluation of the Inserted Artificial Eye. The artificial eye is inserted into the orbit. It is advisable to use a contact lens wetting solution on the artificial eye before insertion. Insertion and removal procedures are similar to those used with scleral contact lenses (p. 286).

Aperture size is evaluated to determine two basic and related factors—vertical palpebral aperture size and relation of upper and lower lids to the iris. The vertical palpebral aperture sizes must match reasonably well, although slight variations are not significant. When the vertical aperture is considerably larger when the artificial eye is in place, a staring, exophthalmic appearance is produced; when the aperture is considerably smaller, a squinting, enophthalmic appearance is produced. An excessively wide aperture indicates the need for a smaller or thinner artificial eye; an excessively narrow aperture indicates the need for a larger or thicker artificial eye. The relationship of the upper and lower lids to the irises of the artificial and good eyes must be approximately the same. Appropriate diagnostic eyes are used until aperture size and lid relationship are satisfactory.

Iris color is evaluated. The patient then fixates a distant target, and horizontal and vertical pupil planes of the good and artificial eyes are compared. The artificial eye exhibiting the least horizontal and vertical deviation is best. Because the pupil plane can be altered by modification, moderate initial deviation is acceptable. When the preformed eye of best size and shape displays considerable deviation, compensation should be made in ordering. With the artificial eye in the orbit, the patient assumes primary fixation. A horizontal line and a vertical line are drawn with a grease pencil on the artificial eye to match pupil planes of the good eye. After the artificial eye is removed, a vertical and a horizontal line are drawn through the center of the pupil. The amount of decentration of the iris in each plane is measured. This amount and its direction are specified on the order (Fig. 7-37).

Customized Stock Eye Technique

A stock eye is used and customized as to iris and scleral colors, or to posterior surface. In the former case, an uncolored stock eye is fitted with appropriate size and shape in the usual manner. Then, from direct patient

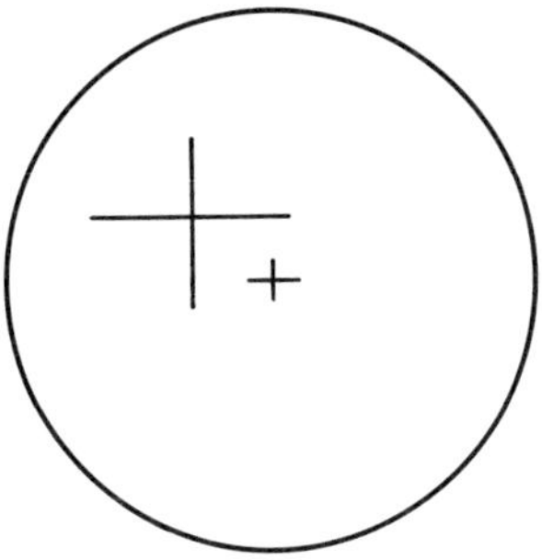

Figure 7–37. Crossed lines help determine the amount of vertical and horizontal iris decentration needed to produce apparent parallelism between artificial and good eyes.

observation or from a matching artificial eye, an artist paints and anneals the iris, pupil, and sclera.

In the latter case, a stock eye is fitted in the usual manner. An impression procedure is then used to produce conformity between the rear surface of the artificial eye and the orbital contents. This operation can be done in the following manner:

A series of small, shallow holes are drilled into the rear of the artificial eye. The rear surface of the eye is filled with impression material, which will adhere to the eye as it fills in the holes. A suction cup is placed toward the center of the front surface of the artificial eye. The patient is seated looking straight ahead with the rear of his head securely held by a headrest. The artificial eye is then inserted.

Using the suction cup, the artificial eye is positioned so that it lines up with the good eye. The artificial eye is gently pressed until it has the same orbital position as the good eye.

The artificial eye is removed, wrapped in cotton, and placed in a jar containing water. The hardening tablet is then used with the impression material. This is mailed to the manufacturer, who will replace the impression material with plastic.

A stock eye can be made into an integrated peg eye. The stock eye technique is followed. A peg is adjusted to fit into the opening on the implant, and is then temporarily attached with wax to the rear surface of the stock eye in approximately the desired position. The artificial eye is tried, using a suction cup to hold it for insertion and removal, and the peg is moved until the proper iris plane is obtained. A scribe is used to trace on the surface of the artificial eye around the base of the peg. The peg is removed, and a depression is cut in the marked area. Plastic cement is used to affix the peg to the artificial eye. Just before the plastic cement is fully set, the eye is tried, and any small adjustments are made.

Modification

Two general categories of artificial eye modification involve removing or cutting away plastic, and adding or building up plastic. Equipment used for scleral contact lens modification can be used for artificial eye modification.

Removal of plastic is accomplished by grinding, followed by polishing. Plastic is added in liquid form, followed by polishing, or the practitioner may build an area with dental wax and send the eye to the laboratory to have the wax replaced with plastic. The removal or addition of plastic should be done gradually. After each alteration the artificial eye is tried, and the procedure is repeated until the desired result is obtained.

Change in Iris Plane

The iris of the artificial eye may be angled so that it produces an apparent tropia. When the iris is angled in this manner, it must be modified. The general procedure is to remove plastic from one side and simultaneously to add it to the opposite side of the eye.

When an esotropic appearance is present, plastic is removed from the temporal posterior surface and edge, and it is added to the nasal posterior surface and edge. When there is an exotropic appearance, plastic is removed from the nasal posterior surface and edge, and it is added to the temporal posterior surface and edge. When the appearance is hypertropic, plastic is removed from the inferior posterior surface and edge, and it is added to the superior posterior surface and edge. When the appearance is hypotropic, plastic is removed from the superior posterior surface and edge, and it is added to the inferior posterior surface and edge.

Change in Iris Position

The iris of the artificial eye may be noticeably higher, lower, or further in or out than that of the normal eye, and in these cases must be modified. This modification differs from a change in iris plane modification because no angling is needed. In general, plastic is removed from the side of the eye corresponding to the desired direction of movement. Plastic is removed uniformly from the anterior surface, edge, and posterior surface. For example, if the iris is to be moved toward the nose, plastic is removed from the nasal side of the eye.

Care must be taken to avoid producing a tropic appearance, which if present, must be eliminated by a change of the iris plane.

Change in Orbital Position

When the artificial eye is positioned so that it produces apparent exophthalmos or enophthalmos, it must be modified. In exophthalmos, plastic is removed uniformly from the posterior surface or from all around the edge. In enophthalmos, plastic is added uniformly to the posterior surface or all around the edge.

Change in Lid Position

If an artificial eye is positioned so that the lids come too far or not far enough over the iris, the eye must be modified. When the lid comes too far onto the iris, plastic should be built up beneath the lid on the anterior scleral surface of the artificial eye. When the lid does not come far enough over the iris, plastic should be removed beneath the lid on the anterior scleral surface of the artificial eye. When blepharoptosis is present, a plastic shelf may be built on the superior sclera of the artificial eye to hold up the lid. A shelf may also be cut into the superior sclera of the artificial eye to hold up a ptotic lid (Fig. 7–38).

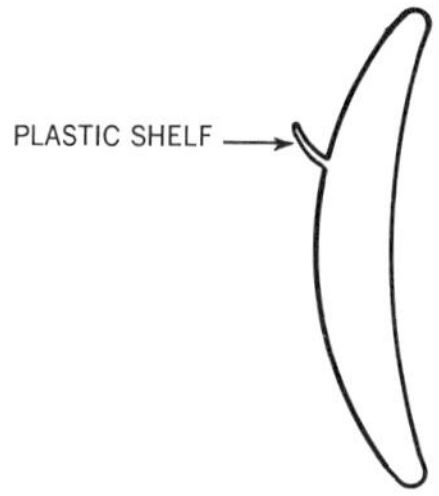

Figure 7–38. A shelf built up on superior sclera of an artificial eye to hold up a ptotic lid.

Change in Apparent Iris Size

Apparent iris size is reduced by thinning of the plastic of the corneal section or by the use of spectacles with a minus lens in front of the artificial eye. Thinning of the corneal section tends to darken the apparent iris color somewhat. Apparent iris size can be increased by the use of spectacles with a plus lens in front of the artificial eye.

Change in Movement

When the artificial eye shows insufficient movement, it must be modified. Insufficient movement is often caused by a poor relationship between the posterior artificial eye and the anterior implant surfaces, by insufficient contact in the fornices, by too large a lens, or by too thick a lens.

When there is insufficient contact between the eye and implant surfaces, an impression customized stock eye technique is used. When there is insufficient contact in the fornices, the superior and inferior edges of the eye are built up to increase contact. When the artificial eye is too large, its size is reduced. When there is too thick an eye, plastic is uniformly removed from the posterior surface.

Responsibility of the Patient

The patient must be taught proper insertion and removal. This is similar to the procedures used with a scleral contact lens (p. 286). A contact lens wetting solution should be used before insertion.

A shell eye should be removed every night, cleaned, and stored in contact lens soaking solution. A reform eye is removed every two to three weeks and cleaned with soap and warm water. After it is rinsed, a soft cloth is used to wipe and polish the eye.

The patient should be checked at least once a year. Modifications to the eye, cleaning, and removal of scratches are done as needed.

COSMETIC CONTACT LENSES

Cosmetic corneal or scleral contact lenses may have one of two forms—transparent tinted, or opaque painted, which is similar to an artificial eye.

Cosmetic contact lenses are used with normal or abnormal eyes. When they are used with normal eyes, their purpose is to change the apparent iris color—a transparent tinted or an opaque painted form is used (Fig. 7–39, p. 286). When they are used with abnormal eyes, their purpose is to mask an unsightly physical defect or to improve vision.[279–282] A totally or partially opaque painted form is used. Examples of masking an unsightly physical defect are the concealing of scar tissue on an eye retaining sight, the concealing of a blind and disfigured eye, or the concealing of a blind and strabismic eye. Improvement of vision may take place when an artificial pupil is provided in aniridia, polycoria, or coloboma of the iris.

Use With Normal Eyes

Tinted contact lenses may change the apparent iris color. Whether they do depends on the original iris color and the type of change desired. There are two basic types of change—a darkening of the same color, and an alteration to another color (Fig. 7–40).

It is usually possible to darken a given iris by the use of a contact lens of the same color. The darker the shade of the contact lens used, the greater the change is. It may or may not be possible to alter iris appearance from one color to another. The lighter the shade of the original iris color, the greater is the possibility of alteration to another color. Table 7–4 is a guide to approximate alteration with medium shades of blue, brown, or gray irises.

Resultant apparent iris color can be determined only by the placement of a lens of the appropriate color on the eye. When a darker lens shade is used, the lens is fitted so that it is relatively large. If it is not, there is a noticeable color difference between the iris area covered by the lens and the surrounding iris area. Because darker shades significantly reduce transmitted visible light, dark lenses should not be used on a full-time basis or during night driving.[283–285] Light transmission should be similar in each eye, otherwise stereoscopic visual performance may be impaired because of the Pulfrich stereo phenomenon. Figure 7–41 is a transmission graph of the more com-

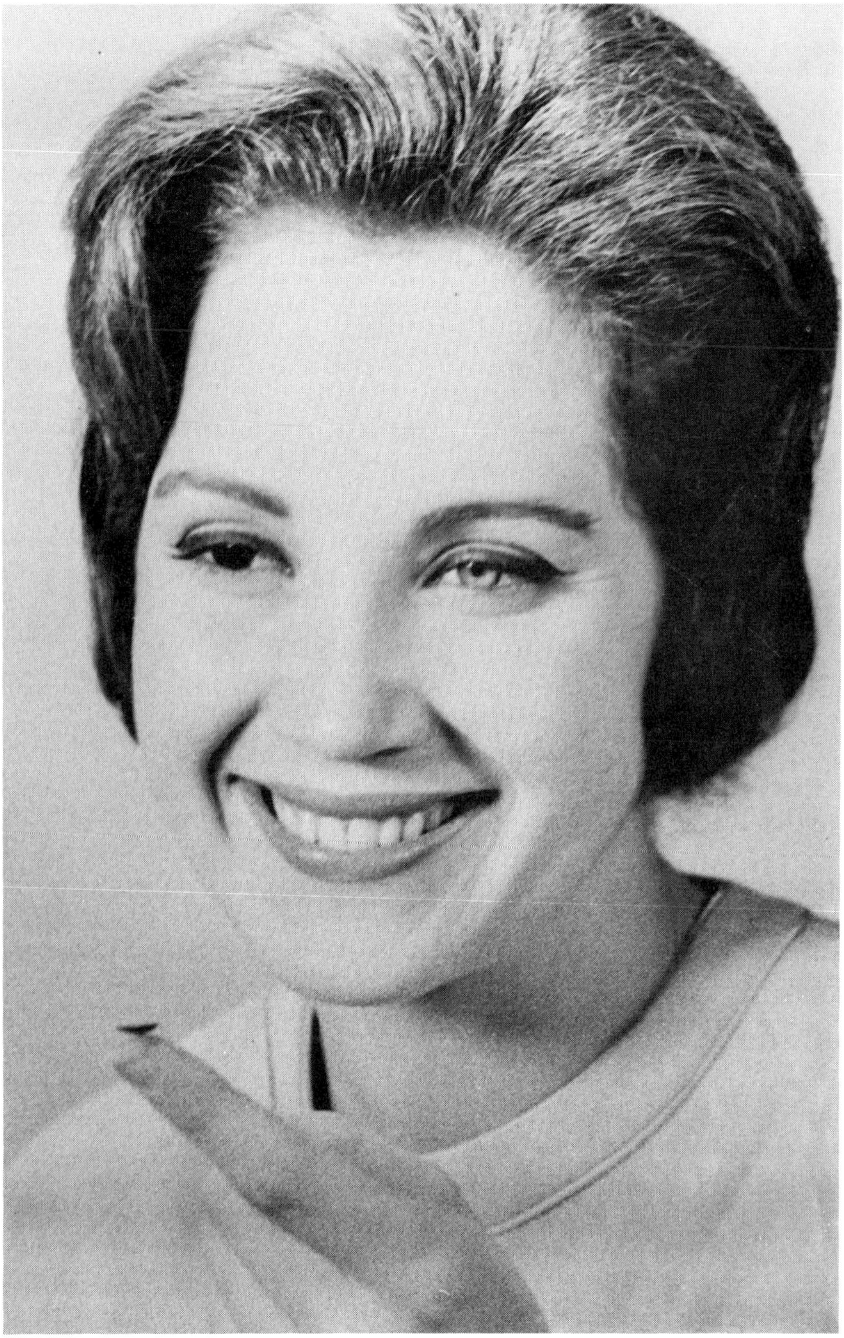

Figure 7–40. Apparent iris color of the right eye is changed by use of a transparent tinted contact lens. (Courtesy of Miss Rita Wilson.)

TABLE 7–4

EFFECT OF TINTED CONTACT LENSES ON APPARENT IRIS COLOR

(Courtesy of Precision–Cosmet Co., Inc.)

Lens Tint	Medium Gray Iris	Medium Brown Iris	Medium Blue Iris
Gray No. 1	Medium gray	Dark brown	Medium blue
Gray No. 2	Dark gray	Black-brown	Black-blue
Gray No. 3	Black	Black	Black
Brown No. 1	Brown-gray	Brown	Brown-blue*
Brown No. 2	Dark brown	Dark brown	Orange-brown*
Brown No. 3	Black	Black	Black-brown
Blue No. 1	Blue-gray	Brown*	Bright blue
Blue No. 2	Blue-gray	Blue-brown*	Dark blue
Blue No. 3	Deep blue	Blue-brown*	Blue-black
Green No. 1	Gray	Brown	Blue
Green No. 2	Yellow-gray*	Brown-green*	Yellow-green
Green No. 3	Dark green	Deep green-black*	Turquoise

* Cosmetically poor except where special effect is desired.

monly used tints. Lenses with a center thickness of approximately 0.20 mm. were used to obtain this graph.

When a desired apparent iris color change cannot be obtained by the use of a transparent tinted contact lens, an opaque painted corneal or scleral contact lens is used. When an opaque painted lens is ultimately to be used, the patient is first fitted with a transparent lens. When a scleral lens is used, a nonfenestrated lens is often cosmetically preferable. The physical fit of the lens and modifications to the posterior lens surface cannot be properly viewed with an opaque painted lens. After the fit is established, the proper opaque painted lens is ordered.

For best cosmetic results, an opaque painted corneal contact lens must be fitted large enough to cover almost the entire visible iris. The lens characteristics must provide this stable coverage while simultaneously maintaining ocular tissue integrity. Because of the very large lenses used, it is difficult to provide comfort and tissue integrity for long wearing periods. The authors prefer opaque painted scleral lenses to opaque painted corneal lenses; better appearance and a much longer wearing time are often obtained.

After the physical fit is established by use of the transparent lens, the iris color and pupil size and position are selected. Iris and scleral colors are selected by the use of trial cosmetic lenses, by the use of a color chart, or by the use of an artificial eye. The pupil size is made equal to the pupil size of the normal eye under ordinary room illumination. To determine pupil position, a dot is placed on the anterior contact lens surface corresponding

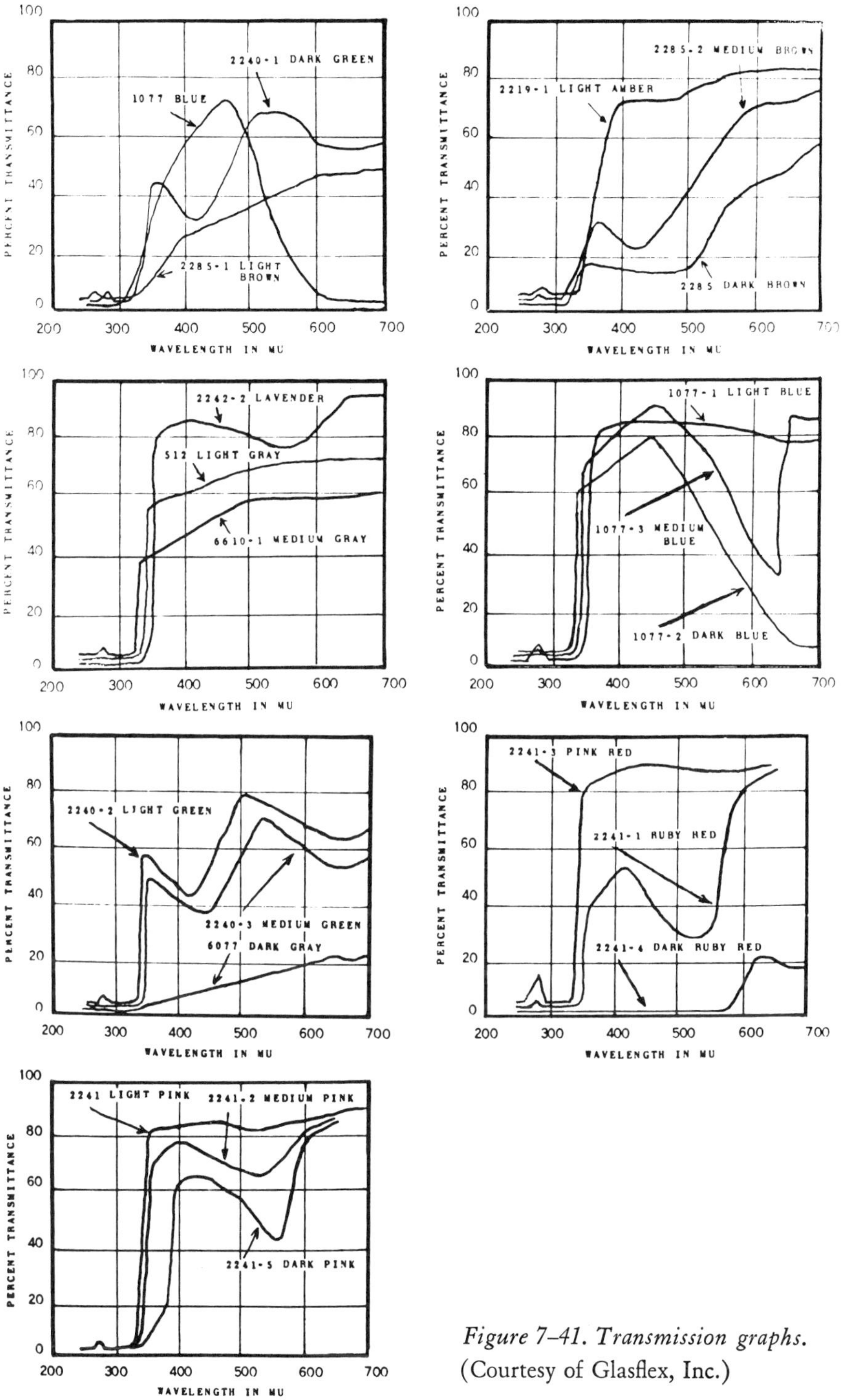

Figure 7–41. Transmission graphs. (Courtesy of Glasflex, Inc.)

to the center of the pupil in primary fixation. This procedure is done with the lens on the eye, and a grease pencil is used. The pupil may be either clear or painted black. Because the eye involved has normal sight, the pupil should be clear to permit vision. The vertical and horizontal iris diameters should be determined.

Use With Abnormal Eyes

Opaque painted scleral lenses are almost always used with abnormal eyes. They are fitted basically the same way any scleral lens is fitted. The chief difference is the art work, which must be made to match the appearance of the good eye.

Molding is frequently the best procedure in fitting cosmetic contact lenses for abnormal eyes because of the abnormal topography of the eye. In the molding of a lens for a strabismic eye, it is essential that proper fixation is maintained with the good eye.

It is possible to have various combinations of painted areas—that is, iris, pupil, and sclera may be either opaque or transparent. Usually, all three areas are appropriately painted when used with blind eyes.

When painted scleral lenses are used in aniridia, polycoria, or coloboma of the iris, an opaque iris and an opaque haptic area are used. The pupil may be completely transparent, or a transparent pinhole area in a black pupil may be used. The pinhole is usually about 1.5 to 2.5 mm. in diameter.

8

Instrumentation, Optics and Manufacture

SLIT-LAMP BIOMICROSCOPE

It is well established that slit-lamp biomicroscopy is an essential aid in four stages of contact lens practice—patient screening, initial design selection, evaluation of adaptation, and lens inspection.[286–292]

Patient Selection. Slit-lamp biomicroscopy is used in the detailed examination of the anterior segment tissues before contact lenses are fitted. When signs of past or present ocular pathologic conditions or abnormalities are detected, contact lenses may be contraindicated completely, or until the condition has been treated and controlled (see pp. 9 and 378).

Initial Design Selection. Slit-lamp biomicroscopy is used in diagnostic lens procedure to aid in the selection of the most logical initial lens design characteristics.

Control and Management of Adaptation. Slit-lamp biomicroscopy is used to evaluate the maintenance of anterior segment tissue integrity after contact lenses have been worn. It also is used to evaluate certain aspects of the fit of the lens and to determine the most logical cause of any undesired signs or symptoms.

Laboratory Procedure. Slit-lamp biomicroscopy is used to inspect certain physical aspects of the contact lens.

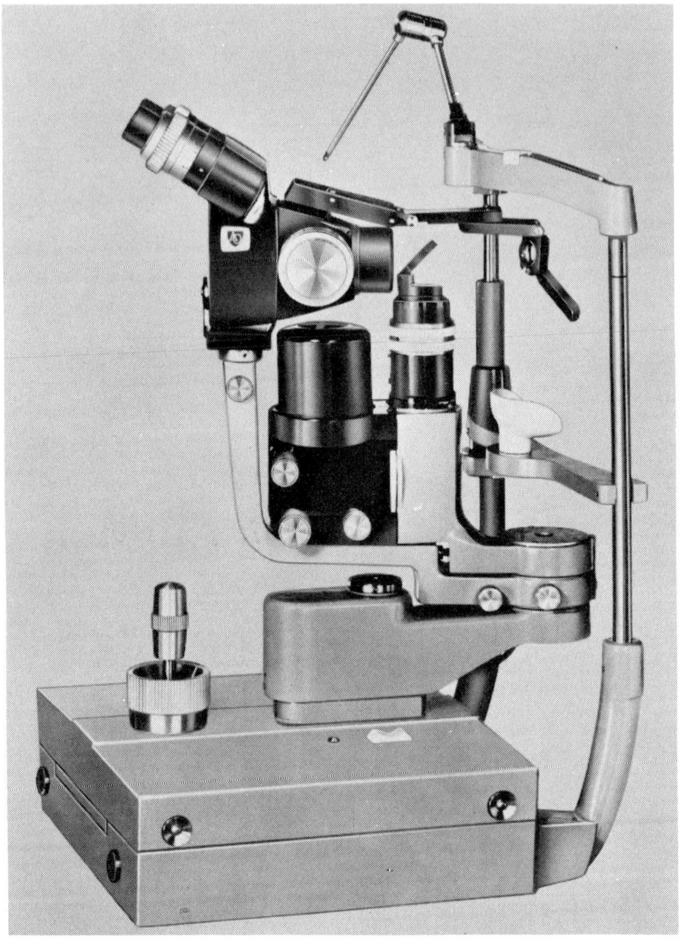

Figure 8–1. A Campbell slit-lamp biomicroscope. (Courtesy of American Optical Co.)

The elements of slit-lamp biomicroscopy related to contact lens practice will be discussed. Readers interested in acquiring a broader background are referred to the textbooks and atlases devoted exclusively to slit-lamp biomicroscopy. Readers interested in learning the mechanics of a specific slit-lamp biomicroscope are referred to the appropriate manufacturer's pamphlet.

Construction

A slit-lamp biomicroscope is used to study ocular tissues in microscopic detail (Fig. 8–1). The instrument has a special type of illumination system (lamp) and a special type of observation system (binocular microscope).

Its function is based partially on a principle known as the Tyndall phenomenon.

Illumination System

To study ocular tissues properly with light, the beam of light should be intense, focused in the proper plane, oblique, and free from shadows. It is not easy to fulfill these criteria. Many years were spent in devising a source of light and a means for concentrating it that would produce desired intensity and focus. Additional time and energy were spent in finding a means for eliminating the shadows that frequently accompany oblique illumination. This was accomplished by using rays of light coming from the image of the light source rather than those coming directly from the light source.

A typical illumination system (Fig. 8–2) works as follows: Light is emitted by an intense *source,* usually a low-voltage nitrogen bulb. The light

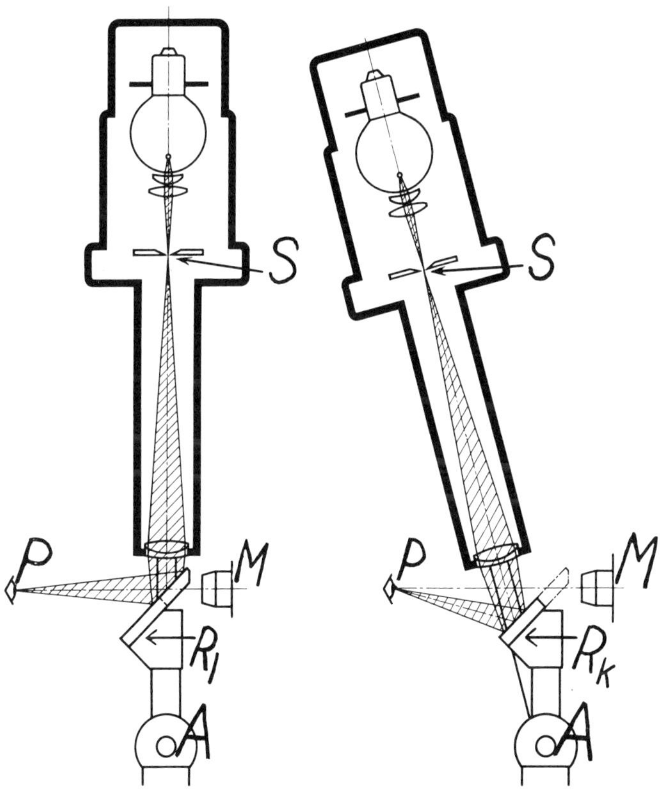

Figure 8–2. Diagram of the illumination system of a Haag-Streit slit-lamp biomicroscope (S, slit; P, slit image; A, axis of inclination; R, long mirror; M, objectives of microscope; and R_K, short mirror). (Courtesy of House of Vision, Inc.)

is then concentrated by a *condensing system,* consisting of two convex lenses with their curved surfaces in apposition. This concentrated light then passes through a *diaphragm* having apertures of various sizes and shapes. Selection of the desired aperture produces the desired shape and size of beam. The apertures and resultant beam are usually either circular or rectangular, and they can be varied from wide to narrow. The narrow rectangular beam is often termed a slit beam.

The resultant beam is collimated by a lens, and an *image* from the light source is focused by the illuminating lens about 7 to 10 cm. from the end of the system.

Observation System

This microscope is binocular and of the Czapski type, consisting of three main parts: the oculars (eyepieces), objectives, and a system of Porro prisms with four reflecting surfaces. The combination of oculars and objectives produces desired levels of magnification, and the Porro prisms positioned between the oculars and objectives aid in producing an erect image. The image seen through such a microscope is of intense luminosity, erect, and magnified. The housing of the eyepieces can be adjusted for the observer's interpupillary distance. This aids in achieving a stereoscopic view.

The most useful magnifications for contact lens work are approximately 12× to 30×. General application for contact lens work is usually done at about 12× to 16×. When it is necessary, study of any small specific detail is done with higher magnification. As magnification is increased, size and brightness of the field are decreased. The field at 15× is usually between 10 and 12 mm., and the field at 30× is usually about half this size.

The illumination and observation systems are on separate arms. Angulation between the two systems is altered by manipulation of the arms. There is usually a plaque calibrated in degrees at the juncture of the two arms to aid in establishing desired angulation (Fig. 8–3).

Tyndall Phenomenon

Slit-lamp biomicroscopy of the anterior segment basically involves properly illuminating an area and then viewing it under desired levels of stereo-

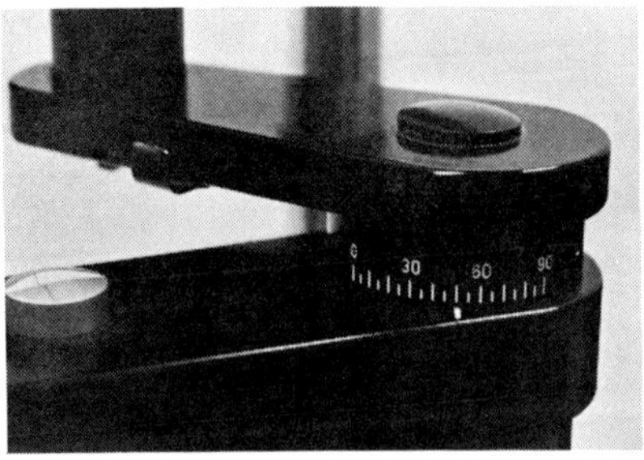

Figure 8–3. A calibrated plaque at the juncture of the arms of illumination and observation systems aids in establishing angulation.

scopic magnification. Another important concept involved in viewing optic media, such as the cornea or a contact lens, is the Tyndall phenomenon.

A beam of light directed through a perfectly transparent and homogeneous optic medium is invisible, whereas nontransparent particles or layers of different refractive indices in an optic medium reflect and scatter light. If the surrounding area is relatively dark, this reflection and scattering produces a contrast between the area through which the light is projected and the surrounding area. The pathway of the beam, the layers of different refractive indices, and the particles become visible. This effect is known as the Tyndall phenomenon.

The Tyndall phenomenon is exemplified by a beam from a searchlight in the sky at night or a beam from a movie projector in a darkened room. The beam and any suspended particles are visible. If the same beam is projected in the sky during daylight or if the movie projector is used in a lighted room, the contrast between the illuminated area and surrounding areas decreases. The beam becomes difficult or impossible to see.

The tissues of the healthy cornea, lens, aqueous, and vitreous are not completely transparent, have different refractive indices for various layers, and have suspended particles. When these tissues become pathologic, there is usually an increase of nontransparent organisms and structures. Because of the Tyndall phenomenon, these structures are made visible by the illumination system of the slit lamp. They are then magnified by and observed through the stereoscopic microscope.

Methods of Illumination

Eight basic illumination methods are used in slit-lamp biomicroscopy of the anterior segment. The various illumination methods are obtained by altering the focal plane of the illumination system relative to that of the observation system, by altering the angle between the illumination and observation systems, and by altering the size and shape of the light beam.

The various methods of illumination are discussed separately in the following paragraphs. In practice, the examiner quickly switches from one method to another by changing the focus, angulation, or aperture of the slit-lamp biomicroscope.

Direct (Focal) Illumination

Focal Plane. The beam and the microscope are both sharply focused at the same area in the same plane (Fig. 8–4). The examiner is therefore looking directly at the illuminated area.

Angle. The microscope is directly in front of the eye being examined, and the angle between the two systems is about 45°.

Aperture and Beam. Either a rectangular or circular beam of varying width is used. When a rectangular beam with a width no greater than

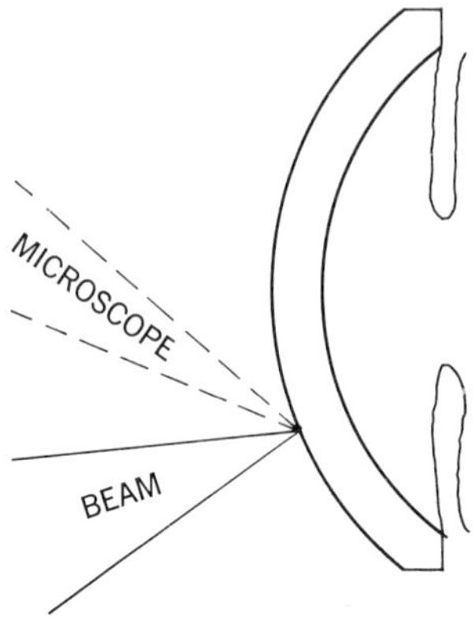

Figure 8–4. For direct illumination, the beam and the microscope are both sharply focused at the same area in the same plane.

the thickness of the structure being examined is projected from an angle of about 45° through an optic medium such as the cornea or a contact lens, an illuminated cross-sectional view is produced. Average central corneal thickness is approximately 0.5 mm. and average peripheral corneal thickness is probably .6 to .75 mm. The shape of the illuminated area is similar to a parallelepiped prism whose outer and inner surfaces are curved due to the curvature of the cornea or the contact lens (Fig. 8–5).

When a parallelepiped is formed on the cornea, it has three general areas: the anterior surface is gray and corresponds to Bowman's membrane, because the epithelium is practically transparent; the posterior surface corresponds to the endothelium; and the thick marble-like area between the two surfaces corresponds to the stroma.

When a parallelepiped is formed on a contact lens, it has three general areas: the anterior surface corresponds to the precorneal fluid on the front of the lens, the posterior surface corresponds to the depth of the precorneal fluid between the lens and the cornea, and the area between the two surfaces corresponds to the body of the contact lens.

When the width of the rectangular beam is narrowed almost to its minimum and projected from an angle of about 45° through the cornea or a contact lens, a sagittal view, or *optic section,* similar to a thin histological section is produced (Fig. 8–6). The widths of the anterior and posterior faces of the section should be about 20 microns.

When an optic section is formed on the cornea, it has five general layers. From anterior to posterior they are: (1) a thin bright layer representing the precorneal fluid, (2) a thin dark layer representing the epithelium, (3) a thin bright layer representing Bowman's membrane, (4) a thick grayish, granular area representing the stroma, (5) a thin bright layer representing the endothelium.

A small circular aperture produces a conical beam. This beam can be projected through the cornea and the aqueous.

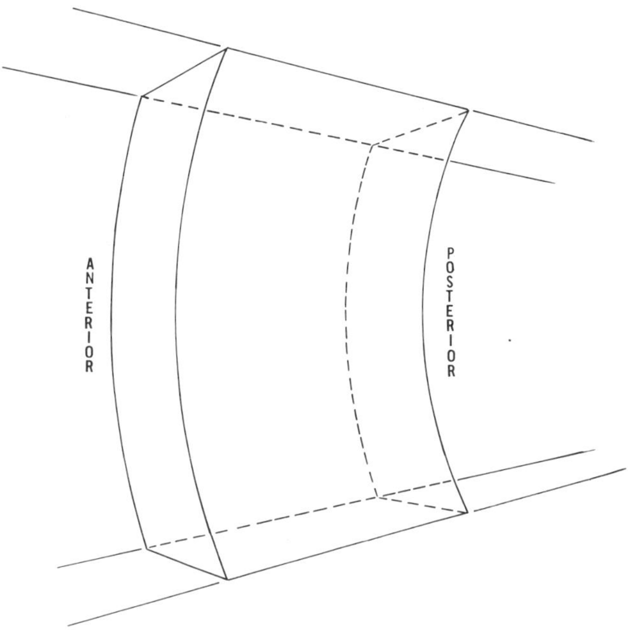

Figure 8–5. A parallelepiped from direct illumination is produced when a rectangular beam .5 to 1.0 mm. wide is projected at about 45° through an optical medium.

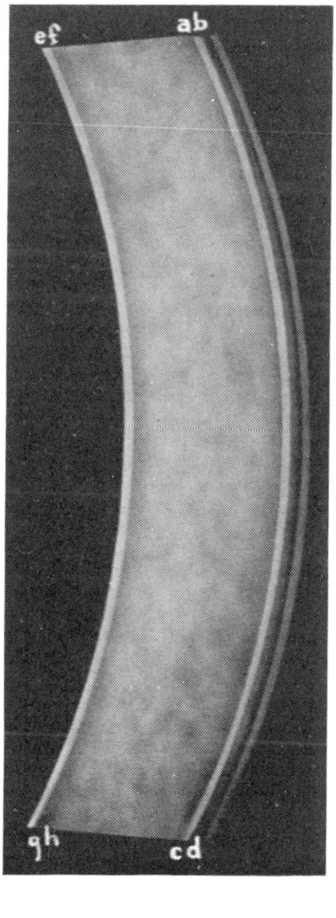

Figure 8–6. Optic section of the cornea. As the beam is narrowed by narrowing the slit the lateral walls of the parallelepiped approach each other, producing a virtual plane or section. The first of the lines on the surface of the cornea is the precorneal tear film line; the dark space between this and the succeeding light line represents the nonrespective epithelium; behind this is the more relucent Bowman's zone; then follows the parenchymal thickness of cornea, the deep edge of which (efgh) *represents the posterior corneal surface* abcd, *anterior surface of the cornea.* (From Berliner, M. L.: *Biomicroscopy of the Eye.* New York, Paul B. Hoeber, Inc.)

TECHNIQUE. The microscope is positioned directly in front of the eye being examined, and the appropriate aperture size is chosen. Both the beam and the microscope are simultaneously focused at the same plane. When a small, conical beam is used, intensity of illumination should be increased, about 25× magnification should be used, and the room should be completely darkened.

USE. Direct focal illumination is used to study any of the tissues of the anterior segment. When a corneal parallelepiped is used, opaque structures, which increase the localized optical density, such as scars, abrasions, corneal nerves, and opacities, appear whiter than the surrounding area. Pigmented areas and precipitates often appear to be reddish brown. Fluid accumulation, which decreases the localized optical density, appears darker than the surrounding area. Edema appears grayish, but it is difficult to see edema clearly with direct focal illumination.

When fluorescein is applied, the precorneal fluid is stained green. Abraded or eroded areas retain a greater amount of fluorescein and appear greener than the surrounding areas. Areas which do not wet properly appear darker than the surrounding areas. Fluorescein evaluation is more apparent when an ultraviolet type of filter is placed in front of the illumination system.

When a contact lens and fluorescein are placed on the eye, a properly focused parallelepiped has three areas: an anterior green surface, which corresponds to the precorneal fluid on the front of the lens; a central clear area when white light is used, and a central black area when ultraviolet light is used, which corresponds to the contact lens; and a posterior green or black surface corresponding to the depth of the precorneal fluid between the lens and cornea in a given area. As the depth of this precorneal fluid is increased, the brightness of the green is increased.

An optic section is used for the same purposes as the parallelepiped. The narrower width permits a more detailed study of a small area and a better appreciation of depth of involvement and degree of thickening or thinning of the structure being viewed. Because a narrow area is viewed, a composite picture of the cornea is obtained by mentally integrating optic sections of all parts of the cornea. In contact lens fitting, a composite fluorescein pattern is obtained by mentally integrating a series of parallelepipeds or optic sections of all parts of the fluorescein pattern. This mental integration is difficult, and a wide beam is preferable for fluorescein pattern evaluation.

A conical beam is used to detect aqueous flare, which indicates pathology. The illumination system should be gently oscillated from side to side. Clumps of fibrin and white blood cells appear grayish white; red blood cells appear reddish-yellow; and pigment granules appear brown.

DIFFUSE ILLUMINATION

FOCAL PLANE. The beam is not sharply focused in the plane of the area being studied. At this plane, the rays of light are either converging or

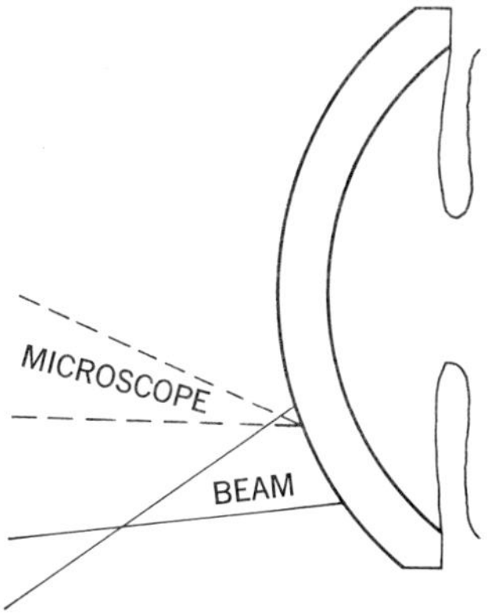

Figure 8–7. For diffuse illumination, the beam is not focused and the microscope is focused in the plane of the area being studied.

diverging. A wide aperture illuminates the entire orbital area, and the microscope is focused in the plane of the area being studied (Fig. 8–7).

ANGLE. The microscope is directly in front of the eye being examined, and the angle between the two systems is usually about 45°.

APERTURE AND BEAM. Any size beam may be used, but it is usually best to have a wide aperture so that a large area is illuminated.

TECHNIQUE. The diaphragm is adjusted to produce a wide rectangular or circular beam. Lack of focus of the beam in the plane of observation and the wide aperture produce a large illuminated area. The microscope is positioned directly in front of the eye being examined, and it is focused for the plane being viewed.

USES. This type of illumination is useful for viewing a large area with relatively intense, uniform illumination under conditions of stereoscopic magnification. A general surface view of the cornea, lids, sclera, conjunctiva, and lacrimal drainage system is obtained. A magnification of about 15× is used.

After application of fluorescein and a contact lens, use of an ultraviolet filter produces a magnified front view of the fluorescein pattern. Evaluation is best done at a magnification of approximately 12 to 15× and a field 10 mm. or more in diameter.

Because prolonged use of a wide beam, especially when no filter is used, produces discomfort, the patient should be given frequent rest periods.

RETROILLUMINATION (TRANSILLUMINATION)

FOCAL PLANE. The beam reflects from a plane posterior to the plane at which the microscope is focused. Light is reflected from the posterior structure, and the structures in the anterior plane at which the microscope is focused are viewed in this reflected light. This type of illumination is most commonly used when the beam reflects from the iris and the microscope is focused on the cornea (Fig. 8–8).

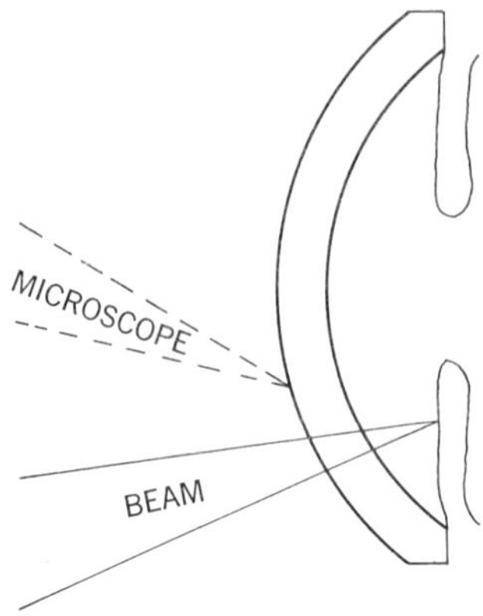

Figure 8–8. For retroillumination, the beam is focused on and reflects from a structure behind the plane being studied. The microscope is focused in the plane being studied.

As a slit beam of light hits the cornea obliquely, some of the light is absorbed and reflected by the corneal tissues, and a corneal block, or parallelepiped, is thus formed. The rest of the light is transmitted; when it strikes the iris, some of the transmitted light is absorbed and the rest is reflected (see Fig. 8–9). If one looks to the side of the parallelepiped, a diffuse, shadowy area of reflected light is observed on the cornea. The color is somewhat affected by the color of the iris, and it is often yellowish when reflected from a brown iris.

Unless some structure in the media obstructs or scatters this reflected light, no special details are observed. The color of structures seen with retroillumination differs from the color of the same structure seen with direct illumination.

Scars, pigment, and vessels containing blood are opaque to light and appear dark on a brighter background when viewed with retroillumination.

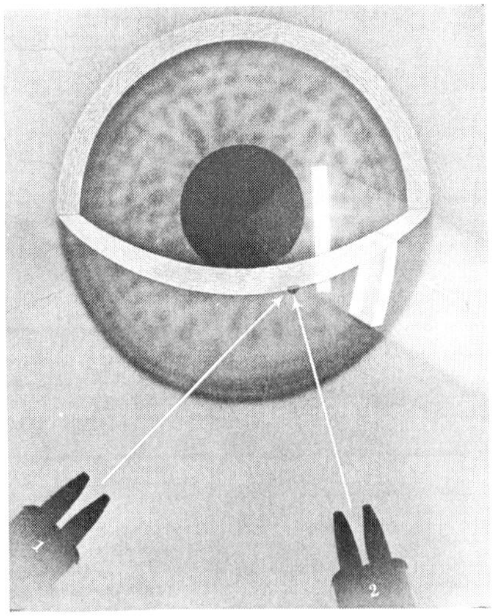

Figure 8–9. Indirect retroillumination. The position of the observer changes from position 1 to position 2 so that the opacity on the surface of the cornea is viewed in the retroreflected light against the black background of the pupil. (Figs. 8–9 to 8–12 from Berliner, M. L.: *Biomicroscopy of the Eye.* New York, Paul B. Hoeber, Inc.)

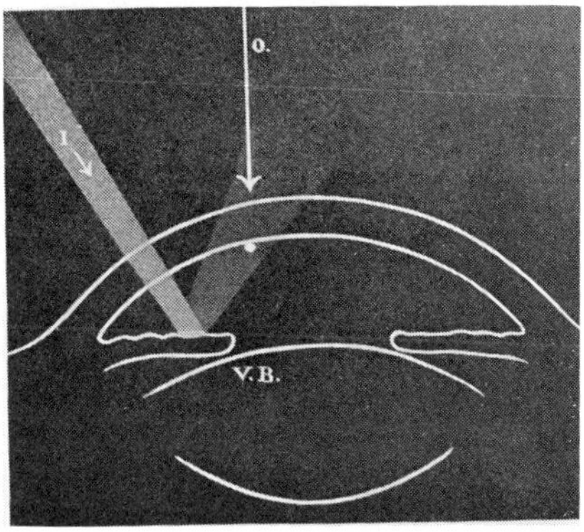

Figure 8–10. Indirect retroillumination. Diagram showing a deposit on the posterior corneal surface as viewed by indirect retroillumination. The angle of observation (O) *does not correspond to the direction of the reflected rays, but is such that the retroilluminated object is viewed against the dark nonilluminated background* (VB) *of the pupil.*

Edema and corneal precipitates scatter light and appear bright on a darker background when viewed with retroillumination.

There are two types of retroillumination—indirect and direct. In indirect retroillumination, the structure, the microscope, and the reflected light do not all lie on the same line (Figs. 8–9 and 8–10). Either the structure is to the side of the path of the reflected light or the microscope is moved away from the path so that the structure is observed against a dark background, such as the pupil or the iris. In direct retroillumination, the structure, the microscope, and the reflected light all lie on the same line (Figs. 8–11 and 8–12). Scars, pigment, and vessels with blood are seen best with direct retroillumination. Edema and precipitates are best seen with indirect retroillumination.

ANGLE. The angle between the two systems is about 45° in indirect retroillumination and 90° in direct retroillumination.

APERTURE AND BEAM. A slit 1 to 2 mm. wide may be used to form the parallelepiped.

TECHNIQUE. The diaphragm is adjusted to produce the desired parallelepiped. For indirect retroillumination, the microscope is directly in front of the eye being examined and the angle between the illumination and observation systems is set at about 45°. For direct retroillumination, both the microscope and the illumination system are set at about 45° to the eye being examined. The angle between the microscope and illumination systems is, therefore, 90°. The systems are moved across the cornea so that all areas are seen in reflected light.

USE. Retroillumination is useful in studying most types of epithelial edema, vacuoles, scars, posterior precipitates, and the channels from blood vessels that have infringed on the cornea.

ILLUMINATION BY SCLEROTIC SCATTER

FOCAL PLANE. The beam is focused at the corneoscleral limbus. The scattering and dispersion of light from the perilimbal sclera produce a halo

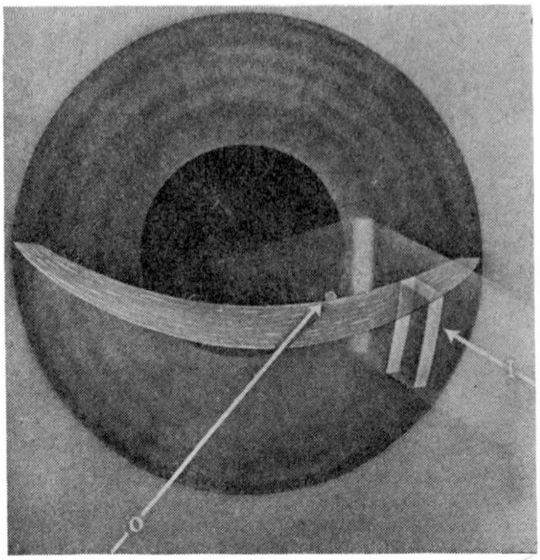

Figure 8–11. Diagram of direct retroillumination (dissected view, upper half of the cornea removed). I, *incident light passing through the cornea forms a parallelepiped and illuminates a sector of the iris surface. The opacity on the posterior corneal surface is viewed by the observer,* O, *in the direction of the retroreflected rays.*

around the cornea. The halo is brightest on the side of the cornea opposite to the focused beam. Internal reflection of the light transversing the cornea illuminates it (Fig. 8–13). Unless there are abnormalities of the cornea which impede or scatter this light, nothing is seen.

The microscope is focused at the plane of the cornea in the area to be examined. In this type of illumination, some things are observed better by the unaided eye of the examiner than by the use of a microscope (p. 230).

ANGLE. The microscope is directly in front of the eye being examined, and the angle between the beam of light and the microscope or unaided eye of the examiner should be at least 45°.

APERTURE AND BEAM. A slit about 1 to 2 mm. wide is used.

TECHNIQUE. The diaphragm is adjusted to produce the desired slit, and the beam is focused at the temporal limbus. The cornea is observed by the unaided eye of the examiner or microscopically with low magnification. The angle between the observation system and the focus of the light is altered until the desired circumcorneal halo appears. If the beam is placed

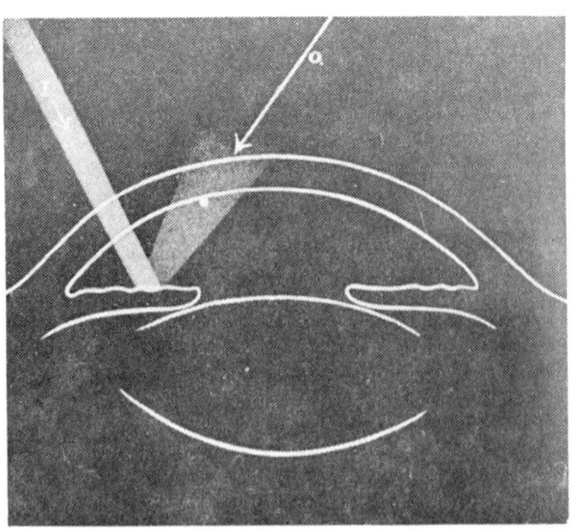

Figure 8–12. Diagram illustrating direct retroillumination of a deposit on the posterior corneal surface. (O, *observer;* I, *incident light.*) *The angle of observation corresponds to the angle of the light reflected from the iris surface.*

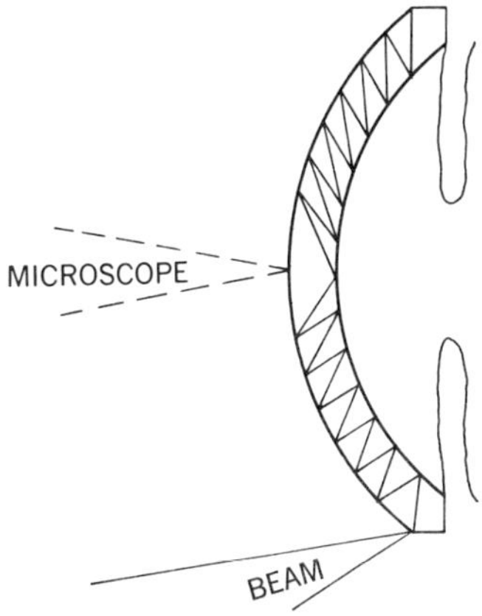

Figure 8–13. For sclerotic scatter illumination, the beam is focused at the limbus and the microscope is focused in the corneal plane being studied.

so that part of it is on the corneoscleral limbus and part on the iris, a combination of sclerotic scatter and retroillumination is produced (split-limbal).

USE. Sclerotic scatter illumination aids in detecting very slight and early changes of the corneal tissue which only mildly obstruct but significantly scatter light. Central circular clouding is probably best determined by this method.

INDIRECT (LATERAL OR PROXIMAL) ILLUMINATION

FOCAL PLANE. A narrow beam is focused on a nontransparent translucent tissue, such as the sclera, iris, or a leukoma of the cornea. The microscope is focused at the same plane slightly to the side of the beam (Fig. 8–14).

ANGLE. The angle between the two systems is 60° or more, thus increasing the amount of internal reflection and the amount of light scatter.

APERTURE AND BEAM. A beam about 1 mm. wide is used.

TECHNIQUE. A narrow slit beam is focused on one of the tissues mentioned. The microscope is focused adjacent to the illuminated area. The light may be oscillated.

USE. This type of illumination is most useful for studying the iris.

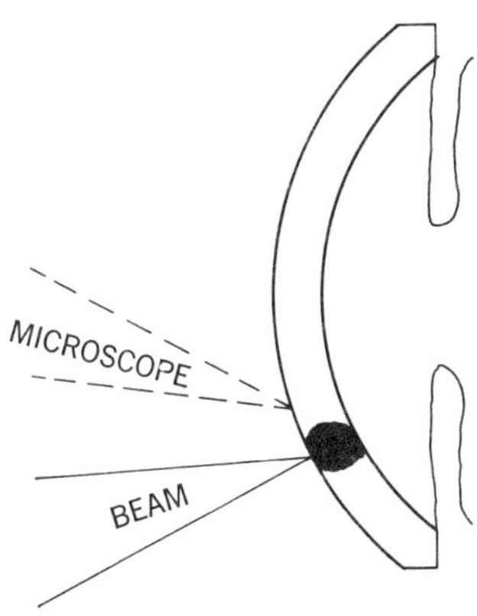

Figure 8–14. For indirect illumination, the beam is focused on a nontransparent area, and the microscope is focused in the same plane slightly to the side of the beam.

Illumination by Specular Reflection

Focal Plane. When a narrow slit beam is focused at the corneal surface, diffuse reflection produces a corneal parallelepiped. There is a significant difference between the indices of air and the precorneal fluid and to a lesser degree between the indices of the aqueous and the endothelium, which produces so-called *zones of discontinuity*. Regular and irregular reflection of light occurs at each zone of discontinuity. As a result of regular (specular) reflection, a catoptric image of the illuminating lens of the slit lamp is formed by the convex mirror-like anterior corneal surface. Because the anterior corneal radius is usually between 7 to 8.2 mm. and because the focus of a convex mirror is at half its radius, the catoptric image of the illuminating lens is about 3.5 to 4.1 mm. in back of the precorneal fluid layer (that is, near the anterior surface of the crystalline lens or on the iris). Because of irregular reflection, details of the reflecting surface itself can be seen, but only when the eye of the observer is in the direct path of the regularly reflected beam. Irregularities on the surface absorb much light and therefore appear as dark spots on the background of the dazzling reflex produced by the regularly reflected light. The microscope is focused on the copper-colored image produced by regular reflection (Fig. 8–15).

Angle. The angle between the two systems is about 60°.

Aperture and Beam. A slit about 1 to 2 mm. wide is used. The vertical height of the slit is reduced to about 4 or 5 mm.

Technique. When the slit beam travels through the cornea, it forms an illuminated corneal area, an illuminated iris area, and the catoptric image of the illuminating lens in the aqueous. The illuminated corneal area is moved in the direction of the catoptric image of the illuminating lens until they lie on the same axis. At this point the angle of incidence equals the angle of reflection, and a dazzle is produced. If the microscope is also on this common axis, the zones of specular reflection come into view.

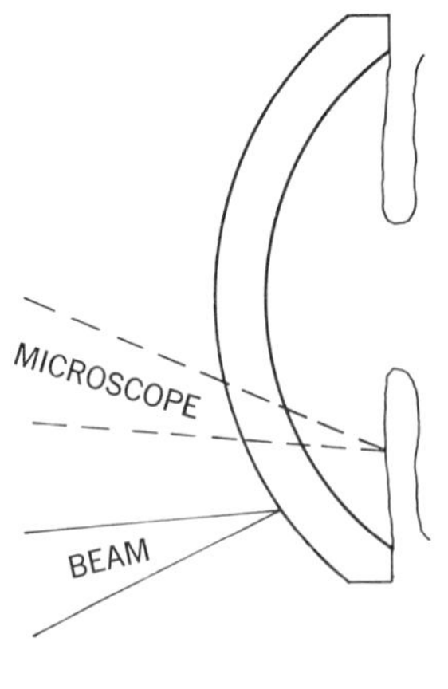

Figure 8–15. For specular reflection illumination, the beam is focused at the corneal surface, and the microscope is focused at the catoptric image of the illuminating lens about 3.5 to 4.1 mm. back of the precorneal fluid.

For placement of the microscope on this common axis, the patient's visual axis must be halfway between the microscope and the illumination system. This can be arranged by having the patient fixate straight ahead and angling both the microscope and the illumination system at 30° to the patient's visual axis. This can also be arranged by placing the microscope directly in front of the eye being examined, angling the illumination system 60° to the microscope, and having the patient fixate halfway between the microscope and the illumination system. Because the tubes of the microscope are separated and usually converge at about a 14° angle, the light reflection and the area of the cornea examined cannot travel through both tubes simultaneously unless the slit is turned horizontally. To see the individual cells, higher levels of magnification, about 20× to 25×, must be used. To see other areas of the cornea, the patient's fixation is altered and the procedure is repeated.

USE. Specular reflection is useful for viewing surface irregularities of the precorneal fluid, corneal epithelium, and corneal endothelium. On the cornea, the front of the zones of specular reflection represents the precorneal fluid, and the rear of the zones represents the smaller, less luminous, golden glow of the endothelium. There is also intrinsic specularity in the stroma from the individual lamellar surfaces, and glistening bronzed striae are seen in it. Mucus, secretions and particles in the precorneal fluid can be seen. Elevations or depressions of the epithelium great enough to disturb the contour of the precorneal fluid can be seen. Blinking helps differentiate between fixed and movable particles. The endothelial mosaic, Hassal-Henle bodies—which appear as dark depressed spots—and endothelial deposits can be seen. Because folds or tears in Descemet's membrane disturb the endothelial contour, they can also be seen.

OSCILLATORY ILLUMINATION

Instead of the beam being kept in focus, it is gently rocked, or oscillated, back and forth, while the microscope is kept in focus. Oscillatory illumination may be used with many of the other types of illumination to change the stimulus and increase the visibility. Details are alternately light and dark.

TANGENTIAL (IRIS-GRAZING) ILLUMINATION

The angle between the two systems is quite wide. The beam grazes the surface of the iris. Freckles, tumors, and the general integrity of the iris may be examined.

GENERAL USE

The mechanics of operation of the slit-lamp biomicroscope are not very complicated. Ability to use the instrument quickly and efficiently and to appreciate and evaluate properly that which is seen does require repeated, consistent use. Slit-lamp biomicroscopy should be part of all patient examinations. It enables a more comprehensive examination for the detection of ocular pathologic conditions, and it concurrently develops a greater facility in use and a better appreciation of normal versus abnormal conditions.

Usually it is best to do a preliminary examination with the unaided eye and with the ophthalmoscope. This facilitates detection of areas needing more detailed inspection. It also helps to reduce the time needed with the intense light of the slit-lamp biomicroscope.

The patient's height and the height of his face are gauged. Chair, table, headrest, and chinrest are positioned in accordance with these patient characteristics to make him as comfortable as possible. The patient is instructed to keep his head firmly against the headrest and to place his chin in the chinrest. His arms may be placed on the table holding the instrument or folded around the base of the instrument when it is mounted on the pole of the ophthalmic unit. Proper stability of the head is necessary to maintain proper focus.

The microscope is then raised or lowered so that it is about level with the patient's eyes. The room illumination is reduced to the lowest point at which the examiner can still see. This allows a proper contrast between the light on the eye and the surrounding area, but at the same time it provides enough general light so that the examiner can see his way around and the patient can see the fixation target. If a method of illumination using very low intensities is employed, it may be necessary almost to completely darken the room so that there is proper contrast.

If the examiner needs spectacles to correct his astigmatism or muscular imbalance, which may interfere with his stereoscopic vision, they should be worn. The separation between the two eyepieces is set for the examiner's interpupillary distance to help ensure stereopsis.

The patient is requested to fixate either into or slightly adjacent to the microscope. If possible, the fixation should be slightly to the side of the microscope and at a somewhat distant target. This helps reduce patient fatigue resulting from prolonged accommodation.

When specular reflection is employed, the patient is usually asked to fixate about halfway between the light and the microscope. When the examiner wishes to study the superior or inferior parts of the anterior segment, the level of the microscope and the illumination system may be altered or the patient may be asked to raise or lower his fixation.

The illumination system is directed toward the temporal limbus and a relatively narrow slit beam with an ultraviolet type of filter is used. This prevents excessive illumination from entering the eye and increases the patient's comfort. With focusing on the temporal side of the eye, most of the light strikes the nasal side of the retina. The fovea is thus not affected as much, and the patient is more comfortable. The light and microscope are focused. The filter is removed, and then the beam is moved onto the cornea. To make certain that the focus is in the proper plane, the patient is asked to blink. If the focus is in the proper plane, the precorneal fluid is seen on the anterior surface of the parallelepiped.

The examiner then begins his survey of the tissues using the various methods of illumination. If examination is to be of long duration, periodic breaks should be taken.

Selection of the Patient

The eyes are examined by routine procedures to detect any pathologic condition. A biomicroscopic study is then done of those areas most directly related to contact lens fitting: cornea, limbus, conjunctiva, lids, and precorneal fluid and drainage system.

Cornea

Sclerotic scatter, focal, and retroillumination are most frequently used in the examination of the cornea. The last two types can be employed almost simultaneously by using a parallelepiped and first examining the area in the direct light of the parallelepiped, and then examining the area in the light reflected from the iris. A magnification of about 15× is used. The conditions listed before under the use of each method of illumination thus may be seen. A more detailed study of specific conditions may be done by an optic section. The beam is moved across the cornea and limbus so that all areas may be examined.

Limbus

As the parallelepiped is moved across the cornea, the limbal area is studied. The examiner looks for limbal loops, pigmented nevi, pterygia or pinguecula infringement, channels from vessels, nerves, and edema. Note that a very mild edema extending about 0.5 mm. on the cornea near the limbus is often physiologic. This edema is probably caused by an imbibition of the nutritive fluids from the neighboring capillary loops.

Conjunctiva

Diffuse illumination is employed, and the exposed bulbar conjunctiva is examined for inflammation, hyperemia, pigmentation, tumors, injection, pinguecula, and pterygia. Any abnormality should be studied in more detail by direct focal illumination.

Lids

The lids are viewed with diffuse illumination to detect the presence of blepharitis, meibomianitis, trichiasis, entropion, ectropion, chalazia, or hordeolum. Details are studied in direct focal illumination. The lids are everted, and the palpebral conjunctiva is studied.

Precorneal Fluid and Drainage System

The precorneal fluid is examined while the cornea is being examined. The presence of excessive debris or dry spots should be noted. This may indicate a diseased cornea and potential wetting problems with contact lens. The inner canthus and drainage system are examined when the conjunctiva is examined to detect any inflammation, blockage of drainage, or an eyelash acting as an irritant. These conditions may interfere with drainage and cause a constant excess of fluid on the eye.

Overall Clinical Procedure

The authors find the following to be an efficient procedure.

A beam about 1 to 2 mm. wide is focused at the temporal limbus, and a combination of sclerotic scatter and indirect retroillumination is obtained. The cornea is studied first with the unaided eye and then with the microscope at a magnification of approximately 15×.

The beam is narrowed to form a parallelepiped which is then moved across the cornea. The corneal tissue and precorneal fluid are studied with direct focal illumination, retroillumination, and specular reflection. An optic section is used when a more detailed study is indicated. The limbus is also studied with direct focal illumination as the parallelepiped is swept across the cornea. When the beam is about halfway across the cornea, the depth of the anterior chamber is approximated. Then the illumination system is angled so that the beam enters the cornea at about a 45° angle from the nasal side, and the parallelepiped is moved toward the nasal limbus. If the beam is not brought in nasally in viewing of the nasal half of the cornea, a distorted beam is produced. A conical beam is used to detect aqueous flare.

Diffuse illumination is then employed, and the exposed bulbar conjunctiva, superficial aspects of the lids, and the inner canthus are examined. Direct focal illumination is used for a more detailed study when necessary.

The lids are everted, and the palpebral conjunctiva is examined with diffuse and direct focal illumination. Fluorescein may be applied, and the procedure may be repeated under conditions of staining.

The crystalline lens and the first third of the vitreous may be studied. Because of the thickness of the crystalline lens, only half of it can be seen in one parallelepiped or optic section. By use of a high minus Hruby lens, the posterior two thirds of the vitreous and the fundus may be examined.

Pathologic structures can be localized by use of an optic section, by focusing the scope, by specular reflection, by parallactic displacement, and by projected shadows. The first four methods should be obvious from previous discussion.

When there is a structure in the cornea, it projects a shadow onto the posterior surface of a parallelepiped or optic section. The posterior surface acts as a screen, and an image of the structure is seen. This *optical reduplication* and the depth of this shadow is helpful in localization.

Initial Lens Design Selection

Slit-lamp biomicroscopy is helpful in diagnostic lens procedure for determining the lens and optic-zone diameters needed to give the desired position, movement, comfort, and vision; the base and secondary curves needed to give the desired relationship between posterior lens and anterior corneal surfaces; and the edge thickness and configuration needed to give the desired comfort.

Lens and Optic-zone Diameters

Position and movement of the lens and its relationship to the lids may be determined. This observation is best made before fluorescein has been placed on the eye, because the use of fluorescein may result in a slightly different fluid composition, which may alter the position and movement of the lens. Light intensity should be reduced somewhat so that excessive lacrimation does not alter the position or movement. The relationship of optic-secondary transition to the pupil may be observed. This evaluation is easier after fluorescein has been used. The possibility of flare should be determined. This technique may be used when determining the positioning of the segments of alternating-vision bifocals. Also the application of a dot to the anterior surface of a lens is of use in evaluating the stability of meridional orientation.

The surfaces of the lens may be inspected, and an evaluation of the wetting may be made. The lens surface should first be viewed without fluorescein because the fluorescein may cause artificial wetting. Dry spots or an excess of sebaceous or mucoid deposits may indicate the poor flow of precorneal fluid over the surface of the lens, or the excessive stimulation of the glands of the lids and conjunctiva. Such stimulation results in the excessive production of sebaceous and oily material.

Lens Curvatures

The static and dynamic fluorescein patterns may be viewed and evaluated by using slit-lamp biomicroscopy. After fluorescein and a diagnostic lens are placed on the eye, the fluorescein pattern is viewed using light from the illumination system, with or without a filter. The light projects enough ultraviolet light to activate the fluorescein, thus making a dull pattern visible. Use of a cobalt type of filter causes the fluorescein to be activated to a much greater degree, enabling better evaluation. It is important that the density of the filter be correct; it should allow sufficient ultraviolet transmission and at the same time not reduce the total light intensity too greatly.

A frontal view of the fluorescein pattern may be obtained by diffuse illumination or by direct illumination with a wide beam. When diffuse illumination or wide-beam direct illumination is used, the magnification should be such that the entire lens may be seen. A magnification of approximately 12 to 15× usually produces a large enough field. This frontal view is the same as that seen with a handheld ultraviolet lamp, but the view is greatly enlarged, which enables a more critical evaluation of the pattern to be made.

A cross-sectional view may be obtained by using a parallelepiped. The outer surface is green if fluorescein is spread over the front surface of the contact lens. The middle section, representing the contact lens, is clear when white light is used and black when ultraviolet light is used. The inner surface is green or black, depending on the depth of the precorneal fluid layer.

Usually, the practitioner tries to match one or, at the most, two base curves and one or two secondary curves to the underlying cornea. The authors find it best to use diffuse illumination or wide-beam direct illumination for fluorescein pattern evaluation. Any areas needing more detailed study are then examined by using a parallelepiped. By the observation of particles and debris, the flow of precorneal fluid between the contact lens and the cornea can be evaluated.

Lens Edges

As the patient blinks, the relationship of the upper lid to the edge of the lens may be observed. The practitioner may determine whether the lid flows smoothly over the edge or is impeded by it, and a decision is made as to which edge thickness and configuration will be satisfactory.

Overall Clinical Procedure

The authors find it best first to make tentative selection of design characteristics by using a stand or handheld ultraviolet lamp. Lens insertion and removal are easier and quicker, and patient comfort is better. Once a tentative selection of design characteristics is made, the characteristics are then refined and verified by using slit-lamp biomicroscopy.

The authors find the following to be an efficient system. Diffuse or wide-beam direct illumination is used. The lens and optic-zone diameters, wetting characteristics, and edge relationships are evaluated, and a parallelepiped is used for more detailed observation. Fluorescein is then instilled, and the relationship of and flow between the posterior surface of the lens to anterior corneal curvatures is evaluated using a cobalt filter and diffuse or wide-beam direct illumination. A parallelepiped is used for more detailed observation.

Control and Management of Adaptation

Certain signs and symptoms may result from or be affected by contact lens wear (p. 229). The signs may result from temporary changes of the anterior segment tissues. There is no substitute for slit-lamp biomicroscopy in the detection of many of these temporary changes. An important possible cause of such changes is the physical fit of the lens. Slit-lamp biomicroscopy is extremely helpful in determining which aspects of the lens design are causing these changes.

Laboratory Procedures

One of the best methods for inspecting the edges and surface quality of a contact lens is by the use of a stereoscopic microscope (p. 149). The slit-lamp stereomicroscope with a magnification of 15 to 20× can be used for this purpose. The illumination system of the slit lamp or an auxiliary lamp can be used for illumination. Often a 100 watt bulb in a gooseneck lamp is satisfactory.

The lens must be held steadily in focus. It may either be held between the thumb and forefinger, or mounted on a holding device such as a suction cup or a stick with double-sided tape.

To inspect the surface quality, the lens is tilted to reflect the light, and it is rotated so various areas can be observed. Surface imperfections will reflect the light irregularly. It is often helpful to have a dark background. Try not to smudge or dirty the lens because smudges or dirt may be misinterpreted as lens flaws.

For inspection of the lens edge, the apex of the edge is directed toward the observer. The lens is rotated and tilted from back to front. This procedure enables evaluation of contour, polish, and thickness to be made.

OPHTHALMOMETRY (KERATOMETRY)

Optics

The Ophthalmometer and Keratometer are designed to determine the radius of curvature of a surface. The function of both instruments is based on laws of reflection applied to convex spherical mirrors (Fig. 8–16).

A target of known size—the mires of the instrument—is placed at a known distance from the mirror-like anterior precorneal fluid surface of the eye. The light is reflected, and the resultant virtual image size is measured by the use of a calibrated doubling device and a short-focus telescope (Fig. 8–17).

It is assumed that the object distance (u) is infinite and that the object (mire) size (O) is small enough so that paraxial rays are reflected. With a convex mirror and paraxial rays, an infinitely distant object has its image in the focal plane—that is, $v = f$. Also the focal length (f) is equal to half the radius (r) of the mirror—that is, $f = (r/2)$.

Thus the following development may be used to determine the radius in terms of the magnification formula:

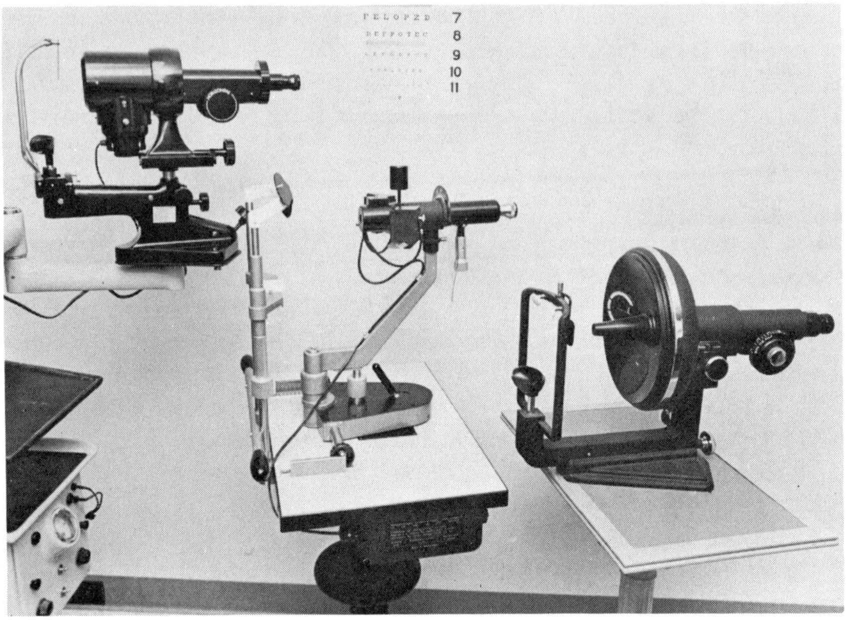

Figure 8–16. Left, *Keratometer* (Bausch & Lomb). Center, *Ophthalmometer* (Haag-Streit). Right, *Ophthalmometer* (American Optical Co.).

$$v = f \text{ (by definition)}$$

$$f = \frac{r}{2} \text{ (by definition)}$$

$$\frac{I}{O} = \frac{v}{u} \text{ (magnification formula)}$$

$$\frac{I}{O} = \frac{f}{u} \text{ (substitute } f \text{ for } v\text{)}$$

$$\frac{I}{O} = \frac{r}{2u} \text{ (substitute } \frac{r}{2} \text{ for } f\text{)}$$

$$rO = 2uI$$

$$r = \frac{2uI}{O} \text{ (approximate formula)}$$

Object size (O) and object distance (u) from the anterior surface are values known from construction of the instrument. Size of the virtual image (I) is measured by the instrument. All values on the right side of the last equation are known, and the radius of the reflecting surface may be determined.

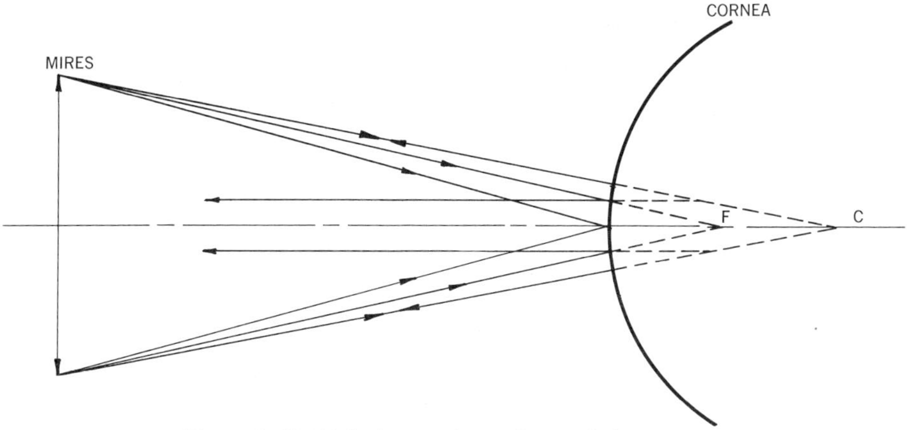

Figure 8–17. Light from mires reflects off the cornea.

Because the assumption of an infinite object distance is incorrect, this equation is only approximate. The equation $r = (2uI/O - I)$ is more accurate (see p. 329).

Areas Measured

There is another factor of clinical importance. The cornea is aspherical, but the Ophthalmometer interprets measurements as spherical reflection. The radius value determined by ophthalmometry is an averaging of the radii of circular curves of two small areas corresponding to the extreme edges of the miral image in a given meridian (Fig. 8–18). The resultant

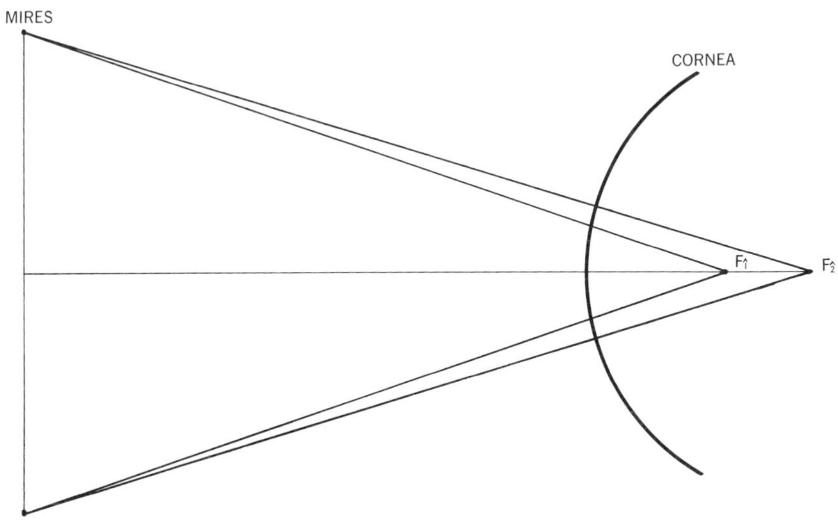

Figure 8–18. As the anterior corneal power increases, the distance between the corneal reflecting areas used in ophthalmometry decreases.

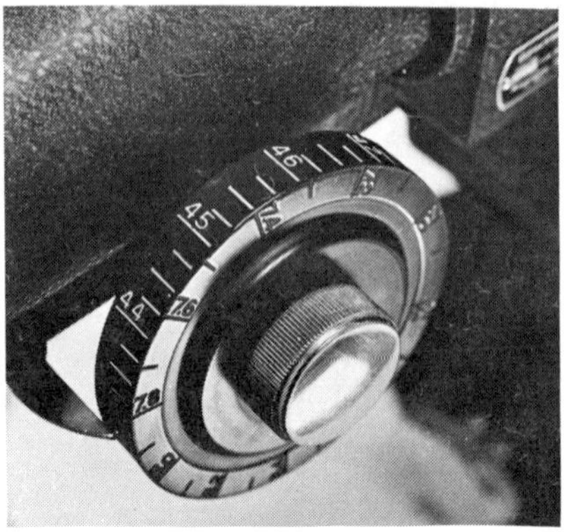

Figure 8–19. Power drum, readings in diopters and radii.

Ophthalmometric radius is similar to the radius of the center of the area being measured.

These two small areas are separated by a distance of approximately 2.3 to 2.7 mm. for the Ophthalmometer and approximately 2.8 to 3.3 mm. for the Keratometer. The smaller distance is for a radius of about 7.10 mm., and the larger distance for a radius of about 8.40 mm.

Conversion Factors

Although the instrument is based on principles of reflection, readings of the surface are on a wheel in terms of diopters of refraction (Fig. 8–19). The reason for this arrangement is that the instrument was originally used in spectacle prescription to determine the amount and axis of the anterior corneal astigmatism, and spectacle power is prescribed in diopters of refraction.

The use of diopters of refraction can lead to confusion and errors in contact lens fitting because there are two types of power produced by a given radius of the anterior precorneal fluid—refracting power and reflecting power.

Assume the measurement of an eye the central anterior surface of which has a true radius of 7.50 mm. spherical. To find the reflecting power:

$$f = \frac{r}{2}$$

$$f = \frac{7.50\text{ mm.}}{2} = 3.75\text{ mm.}$$

$$f = \frac{1000\text{ mm.}}{D} \text{ or } D = \frac{1000\text{ mm.}}{f}$$

$$D = \frac{1000\text{ mm.}}{3.75\text{ mm.}} = 266.67 \text{ (reflecting power)}$$

As can be seen, this mathematical calculation is not affected by the indices involved according to the principles of reflection. The wheel readings of the instrument, however, are in terms of diopters of refraction, and refraction is affected by the indices used. With a constant radius, the power varies in relation to the indices, as shown by the formula:

$$D = \frac{n_2 - n_1}{r} K$$

n_2 = the index of the substance into which light is going

n_1 = the index of the substance from which light is coming

K = the unit factor, 1000 for mm.

With these instruments, light comes from the object (the mires) situated in air, $n = 1.00$ (approximately). It goes into the precorneal fluid, $n_2 = ?$. Some value had to be established for n_2. It is extremely difficult to determine the index of this substance, for the methods used introduce artifacts. Frequently used values are 1.3360 and 1.3375; these are averages, and there may be individual variation. Index 1.3375 establishes a 7.50 mm. radius. It has been suggested that the convenience of these numbers has influenced index acceptance.

The Ophthalmometer calibration is based on an assumed average index of 1.336. The Keratometer calibration is based on an assumed average index of 1.3375. With the use of a known radius of 7.50 mm., it is seen that clinical problems can result:

Ophthalmometer

$$D = \frac{n_2 - n_1}{r} K$$

$$D = \frac{1.336 - 1.00}{7.50} (1000)$$

$$D = 44.80$$

Keratometer

$$D = \frac{n_2 - n_1}{r} K$$

$$D = \frac{1.3375 - 1.00}{7.50} (1000)$$

$$D = 45$$

What problems can result from this discrepancy of having different dioptric powers from the same radius of curvature? If the proper conversion table is used by both practitioner and laboratory, there are no problems. However, if either practitioner or laboratory uses the incorrect table, problems will result.

Assume that the practitioner has used an Ophthalmometer based on an index 1.336 with the proper conversion table for this index. Assume that the laboratory's conversion table is based on the index 1.3375. If the base curve is ordered in diopters rather than radius, an error is introduced by conversion at the laboratory.

Assume that a value of 44.80 D is ordered based on the Ophthalmometer (AO) and its tables and that it is converted by the Bausch & Lomb table:

$$D = \frac{n_2 - n_1}{r} K$$

$$44.80 = \frac{1.3375 - 1.00}{r} (1000)$$

$$r = 7.53 \text{ mm.}$$

This value obviously does not equal the 7.50 mm. radius desired. Both fitting and refractive problems result. These problems also occur when the practitioner uses the incorrect table.

In this way, an error may also be introduced in the clinical calibration of the instrument with the use of a steel ball. Many of these balls have their dioptric power marked on them. It is in relation to this marked dioptric power that the instrument is set. However, the dioptric power has again been computed with the use of an assumed index. Many of these balls have a dioptric power of 42.50 D. They really have a radius of 7.94 mm. determined by the principles of reflection. The balls have two dioptric powers for practical purposes:

Ophthalmometer $$D = \frac{336}{7.94}$$ $$D = 42.32$$

Keratometer $$D = \frac{337.5}{7.94}$$ $$D = 42.50$$

The practitioner should base calibration of his instrument on the radius of the ball only.

Use of the Ophthalmometer (Keratometer)

To obtain accurate readings, the instrument must be properly focused and calibrated before use. Then, proper technique must be employed.

Focusing the Eyepiece

Turn the eyepiece counterclockwise as far as it will go. Turn the light of the instrument on, and hold a piece of firm white paper or cardboard in front of the telescope. Note the out-of-focus black circle (Ophthalmometer) or black cross hairs (Keratometer).

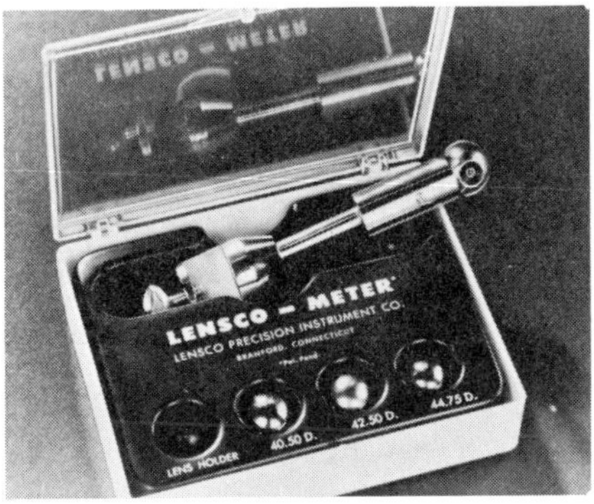

Figure 8–20. Calibration set. (Courtesy of Lensco Precision Instrument Co.)

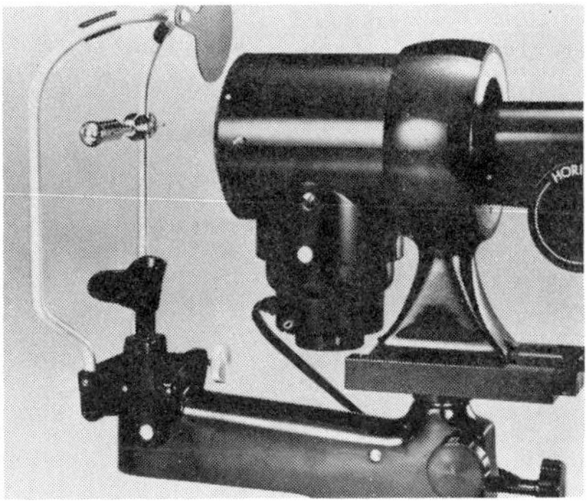

Figure 8–21. Calibration device mounted on a Keratometer. (Courtesy of Lensco Precision Instrument Co.)

Slowly turn the eyepiece clockwise until the cross hairs or circle come into clearest focus. Do not go past this point and return. Undesired accommodation may be introduced. If only one person is to use the instrument, a line may be made from the eyepiece to the telescope for subsequent checking.

Calibration

To verify the accuracy of the instrument, it should be calibrated. This is done by using calibration balls of known *radius*. Several devices can be used to mount the ball on the instrument (Figs. 8–20 and 8–21).

Move the telescope from away toward the ball until it is in focus. Take three readings in each principal meridian. Always stop at the first alignment of the mires so that the effect of lost motion does not introduce an error.

If the three readings vary from one another by more than 0.12 to 0.25 D, the practitioner's technique is inaccurate. If the three readings are within this amount but the mean of the three is 0.25 D more or less than the power of the calibration ball, the instrument should be considered inaccurate.

If the instrument is inaccurate, either a correction factor is considered with each reading, or the set screws of the power drum are loosened, the power drum is set properly, and the screws are tightened. This is done for each principal meridian.

The design of the instrument assumes that the object distance (the mires) is infinite. If it is not, then an instrument calibrated for one radius may not be accurate for other radii. A clinical rule of thumb is that the radius should be shortened by 0.01 mm. for each 0.2 mm. a given reading is shorter than the calibration ball.[293] The radius is lengthened by 0.01 mm. for each 0.2 mm. a given reading is longer than the calibration ball. Assume that calibration was done with an 8.00 mm. ball and that the reading of the radius of a cornea is 7.20 mm. This value would be shortened by 0.03 mm.; the true radius is 7.17 mm. Use may introduce various amounts of play for different radii. This and the preceding factor can cause errors. It is best to use a series of calibration balls of various radii and to establish a calibration chart. A series of calibration balls with radii of 7.10, 7.40, 7.70, 8.00, and 8.30 mm. is often used. The power drum is set for one radius (such as 8.00 mm.), and a compensation chart is established for the other radii.[294]

Technique

Make sure that you and your laboratory are using the proper conversion chart for your instrument, and make sure the eyepiece has retained its focused position. Position the patient so that the outer canthi of his eyes are aligned with the markers (baseline) on each side of the headrest by raising or lowering the chinrest. The patient should be seated with reasonable comfort. To maintain his eye in focus, his forehead should be firmly against the forehead rest and his hands should be folded over the base of the instrument.

Occlude the eye not being measured to make sure that fixation is maintained by the eye under test. If this is not done, a peripheral area of the cornea may be measured by mistake.

Make sure the mires are centered by encircling the primary spokes with the black circle (Ophthalmometer) or by placing the cross hairs in the center of the lower right hand circle (Keratometer) (Fig. 8–22).

Instruct the patient to blink normally, to hold his head steady, and to look in the telescope at the image of his own eye. Keep one hand on the knob that controls the focusing and clarity of the miral images. Keep the other hand on the power drum, which controls the separation of the miral images. Focus the miral images and keep them focused at all times. Overlap the vertical spokes of the Ophthalmometer or the vertical arms of the horizontal plus lines of the Keratometer. Rotate the barrel of the instrument until the horizontal arms of the targets are continuous. This procedure determines the axis.

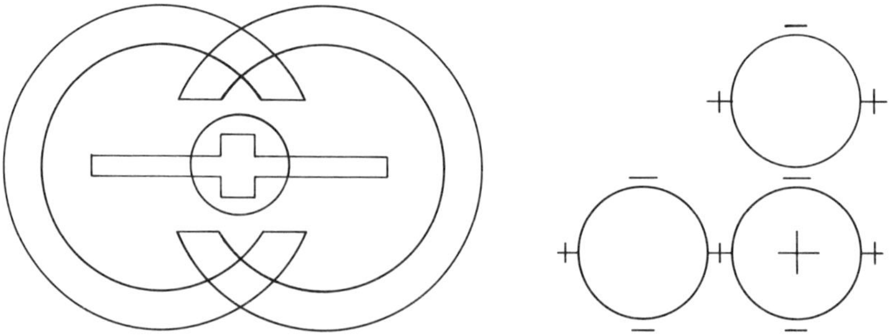

A B

Figure 8–22. Centration, alignment, and superimposition of miral images. A, *Ophthalmometer* (American Optical Co.). B, *Keratometer* (Bausch & Lomb).

Measure the power of the first principal meridian by making the vertical spurs of the Ophthalmometer continuous or by superimposing the vertical arms of the plus signs of the Keratometer. For the second principal meridian, the knob of the Ophthalmometer is rotated to secondary, and the measurement is taken as before. In the Keratometer, the two horizontal dashes are brought together to form a single dash.

Make sure that the mires are focused when the reading is taken. Always take the reading by moving the power wheel in the same direction. If the reading is obtained by going back and forth, a considerable error may be introduced from lost motion.

Three readings should be taken and the mean of the three used. If two of the three are the same, this is the mean. The readings should agree with one another by 0.12 or 0.25 D or less. If they do not, the examiner's technique or the patient's fixation is probably incorrect.

Clinical Considerations

Increasing Accuracy

Certain modifications help produce more accurate and repeatable findings. These modifications change the method of determining alignment from coincident to vernier.[295, 296]

In the Ophthalmometer, a thin wire is placed along one of the spokes. In the Keratometer, part of the mires is covered by black tape (Fig. 8–23).

Increasing the Range

The power range of most instruments is from the middle thirties to the high fifties. To obtain higher readings, a plus lens must be held against the aperture of the telescope. To obtain lower readings, a minus lens must be held against the aperture of the telescope.[297]

Computation has been done when a +1.25 D Bausch & Lomb trial

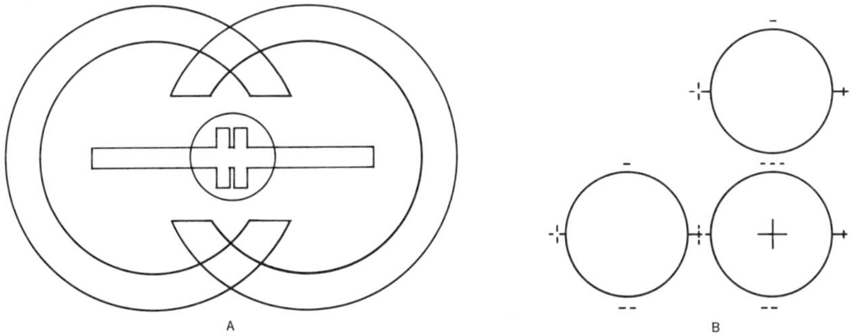

Figure 8–23. Modification of mires to change determination of alignment from coincident to vernier. A, *Ophthalmometer* (American Optical Co.). B, *Keratometer* (Bausch & Lomb).

spectacle lens with a plano back surface and a −1.00 D Bausch & Lomb trial spectacle lens were used (see table in Appendix III).

This table is valid only when these specific lenses are used, because lens shape alters magnification. Because of this and because the calibration characteristics of each Keratometer and Ophthalmometer may differ, the practitioner should make his own calibration chart.

Reading Concave Surfaces

Use of the Ophthalmometer or Keratometer is based on laws of reflection of *convex* mirrors. Conversion tables used to determine the radius of the convex anterior surface of the eye are appropriately computed. These instruments are also used to measure the concave base curve of contact lenses.

The image size from a concave surface of a given radius is smaller than from a convex surface when it is measured by an Ophthalmometer or Keratometer, because the image formed by a convex mirror lies behind it, whereas that formed by a concave mirror lies in front of the mirror. It is this image on which the instrument focuses.

Unless the proper table is used, an error of 0.02 to 0.04 mm. results. The tables most practitioners use are for convex surfaces. Column 2 of the Surface Power Table (Appendix VI) is the column used for concave surfaces.

Peripheral Readings

Peripheral corneal readings are obtained in two ways with the use of an Ophthalmometer or Keratometer. First, the direction of the instrument's optic axis is held constant, and the patient alters his direction of fixation. Fixation targets tabulated in terms of decentration of the patient's visual axis from instrument's optic axis are used. Fixation markings may also be placed directly on the instrument, and decentration can be computed. Second, the patient's fixation is held constant, and the instrument is moved along an arc (Fig. 8–24).

Peripheral corneal readings are sometimes used to select secondary curve radii. However, their validity and accuracy, as currently taken and interpreted, produce questionable practical data.

First, the cornea is aspherical and asymmetrical, a fact which reduces the validity and accuracy of measurements by systems based on spherical, symmetrical reflection. Second, the centers of curvature of the various curves of most contact lenses lie on a common axis. The centers of curvature of the various curves of the cornea do not lie on a common axis. This condition poses a considerable problem in the transferring of data. Third, a contact lens moves and tilts on the cornea, a movement which further complicates selection of secondary curve radii. Finally, any reading, as it is generally performed, measures two areas separated by about 2.5 to 3.5 mm.

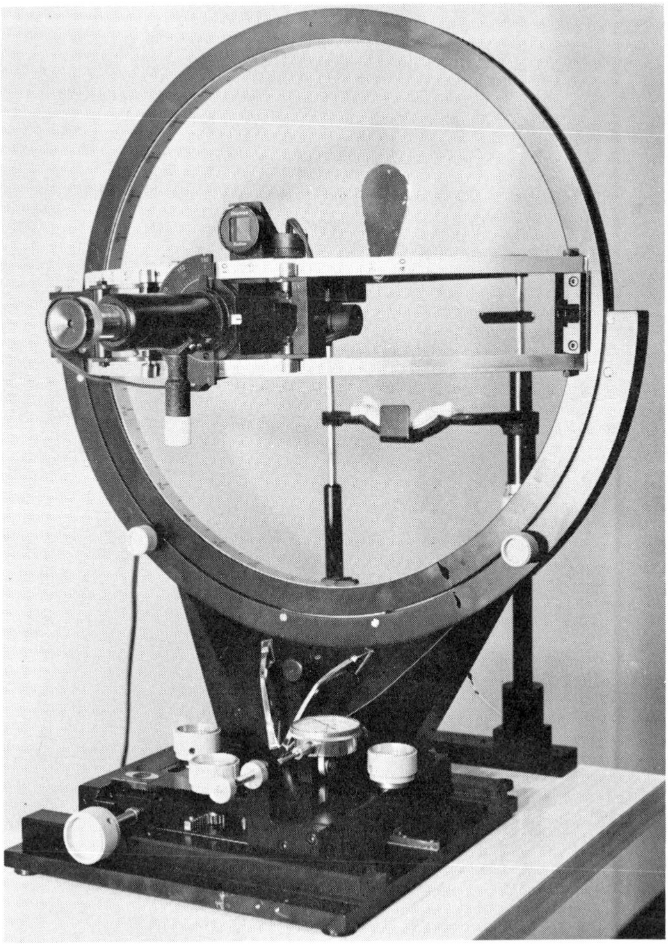

Figure 8–24. The Cornealometer, an ophthalmometer that can be moved along an arc. (Courtesy of Obrig Laboratories, Inc.)

Small-mire Ophthalmometry (Keratometry)

The last problem stated in the previous paragraph is reduced somewhat when an instrument with small mires is used. The separation of the extremities of the miral images may be about 1.0 mm. Too great a reduction of the area measured reduces the accuracy of the measurement.

A small-mire instrument may be used to take central corneal readings. Although there is some disagreement, it seems that central readings taken in this way are the same as those taken with a standard instrument, probably because the instrument interprets the surface it is measuring to be spherical. The resultant reading is not that of the two points, but more nearly that of the area between them.

Central Readings

Central readings give valuable information in contact lens fitting. When possible, they should be used with the diagnostic lens procedure in the selection of the appropriate base curve. The reasons for this are discussed on page 76.

A central ophthalmometric reading is best used with tables of standards or norms based on clinical experience (see Tables 2–7 and 2–8). These tables relate the ophthalmometric reading to the radius necessary in a given optic-zone diameter to establish a desired relationship between the base curve and corneal curves.

The values obtained have two primary uses: they may be a starting guide for diagnostic lens fitting, and they may establish a logical base curve selection when accurate diagnostic lens fitting is impossible.

Central readings are also valuable in the detection of corneal curvature changes arising after lenses have been worn.

TOPOGOMETER

Design and Purpose

The Topogometer consists of a movable point source of light attached to horizontal and vertical scales, and it is usually placed on a Keratometer[298] (Figs. 8–25 and 8–26). It is used simultaneously to control fixation and to measure the decentration of the patient's visual axis from the Keratometer's optical axis.

The purpose of the instrument is to determine the longest and shortest diameters of the cornea's "apical zone," or "corneal cap." This information is used in the selection of contact lens diameters. Usually, lenses with small

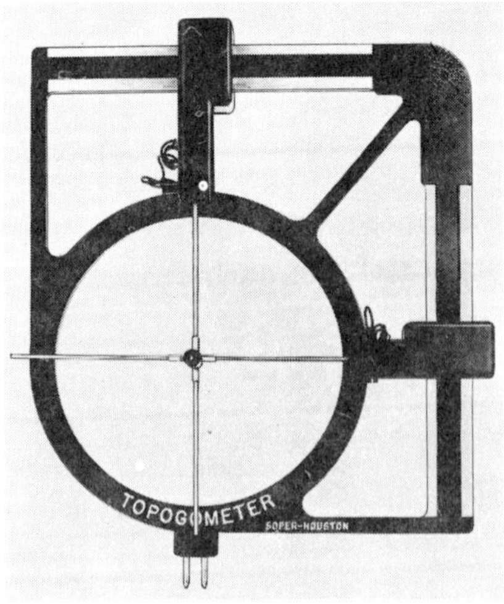

Figure 8–25. Front view of Topogometer. (From Girard, L. J., Soper, J. W., and Sampson, W. G.: *Corneal Contact Lenses.* St. Louis, C. V. Mosby Co., 1964.)

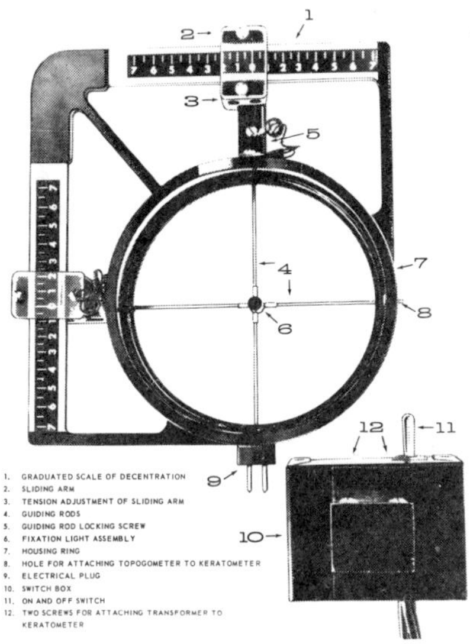

Figure 8–26. Back view of Topogometer. (From Girard, L. J., Soper, J. W., and Sampson, W. G.: *Corneal Contact Lenses.* St. Louis, C. V. Mosby Co., 1964.)

diameters and narrow secondaries result; these lenses are meant to provide considerable exposure of the cornea to its normal environment.

Use

The Keratometer measures two small areas that are separated by a distance related to the radius of the surface. This distance is computed by the use of the formula $r = (2(u)(I)/O)$. In the Keratometer, $u = 75$ mm. and $O = 64$ mm. Table 8–1 gives the resultant chord lengths from various radii.

In this technique, the apical zone is defined as the corneal area with greatest curvature and less than 0.50 D curvature variance, as found by use of a standard Keratometer in a given meridian. As long as the image of both miral extremities lies within this zone, a constant reading results. When one miral extremity lies on the flatter peripheral area, a flatter reading results. This procedure indicates the limit of the apical zone. Serial Keratometry with controlled, measured alteration of fixation is used to determine apical-zone diameters.

Assume that the apical zone is symmetrical with the visual axis. The first keratometric reading is taken with both of the Topogometer scales at zero, so that the visual axis of the eye and the optical axis of the Keratometer coincide. The chord values for these principal meridian readings may be determined from Table 8–1. The light source is then moved nasally one quarter of a scale unit, and a keratometric reading is taken with the patient fixating on the source. This procedure is continued until a reading 0.50 D flatter than the first reading in this meridian is found. When this reading occurs, one extremity of the miral image lies off the apical zone and on the flatter peripheral cornea. The procedure is repeated in temporal fixation.

TABLE 8–1

CHORD LENGTHS

Diopters	Radius (in mm.)	Chord Length (in mm.)
36	9.38	3.8
37	9.12	3.7
38	8.88	3.6
39	8.65	3.5
40	8.44	3.4
41	8.23	3.3
42	8.04	3.2
43	7.85	3.2
44	7.67	3.1
45	7.50	3.0
46	7.34	3.0
47	7.18	2.9
48	7.03	2.8
49	6.89	2.8
50	6.75	2.7
51	6.62	2.7
52	6.49	2.6

Decentration shown on the Topogometer scale from nasal and temporal fixation is added to the chord value of the principal meridian found from the first reading. Each scale unit equals 1.0 mm. of decentration of the patient's visual axis from the optical axis of the Keratometer. The procedure is repeated in superior and inferior fixation, and the decentration is added to the chord value of the principal meridian found from the first reading.

The geometric centers of the corneas and apical zone are determined by the intersection of their greatest and smallest diameters. Decentration of the apical zone is determined by comparison. If the apical zone is not symmetrical with the visual axis, the keratometric reading indicates steepening as the visual axis is decentered from the optical axis.

Determination of Lens Specifications

The lens diameter is 2.0 mm. greater than the longer apical-zone diameter; thus the technique is called *LD* + 2 (lens diameter + 2) or *OC* + 2 (optic cap + 2). Most lens diameters are 7.2 to 8.8 mm. One millimeter is added to the longer apical-zone diameter to compensate for lens movement and to produce adequate pupil coverage. The optic zone is therefore 1.0 mm. greater than the longer apical-zone diameter.

One millimeter is also added to the apical-zone diameter to provide for secondary curves. These are composed of a peripheral curve 0.2 mm. wide with a 13.00 mm. radius, an intermediate curve 0.2 mm. wide with a 9.12

mm. radius, and a blend 0.1 mm. wide with a radius about 0.4 to 0.8 mm. longer than the radius of the base curve.

When the lens diameter is less than 9.0 mm., the base curve radius is the mean of the steepest and flattest apical keratometric readings, or 0.50 D is added, whichever is steeper. When the lens diameter is greater than 9.0 mm., the base curve is equal to the flattest keratometric reading, or one quarter of the corneal keratometric toricity is added to this value.

Thin center thicknesses are used, about one third less than standard. Thickness tables are supplied with the instrument.

Summary

The developers of this technique do not consider it a panacea, and they are aware of the theoretical limitations of topographical keratometry. They believe that it is a practical technique for determining logical initial design characteristics. When the method is integrated into a total contact lens procedure, they believe it is a clinically expedient technique.

RADIUSCOPES

Curvatures of reflecting surfaces having short radii are accurately determined by the use of instrumentation based on the Drysdale technique. Such instruments are called Radiuscopes or optical spherometers.

The instrument is composed of a compound microscope with an aperture in the tube between a 15× ocular and a 5× objective. A special vertical illumination system and a beam splitter are aligned with the aperture. The light source of the illumination system and focal plane of the eyepiece are approximately equidistant from the beam splitter. The beam splitter is placed at 45° to the axis of the microscope (Fig. 8–27).

Light from the vertical illumination system is reflected by the beam splitter to the objective, which focuses it in the anterior focal plane of the microscope. This focused light becomes the object for the reflecting surface being measured. The reflecting surface is positioned facing the microscope in a holder containing fluid, which neutralizes reflection from the other surface and eliminates ghost images. A dial is turned to make the anterior focal plane of the microscope coincident with the vertex of the surface being measured. When an object is placed at the vertex of a mirror, its image lies in the same plane, thus producing a clear surface-image picture of the stellate target. The dial is then set at zero.

A second object position with a mirror makes the image and object planes coincident. This phenomenon occurs when the object is at the center of curvature of the mirror. The distance between the end of the microscope and the surface being measured is altered by use of the dial until the object is at the center of curvature of the reflecting surface. This adjustment produces a clear aerial image of the stellate target. The distance from the vertex

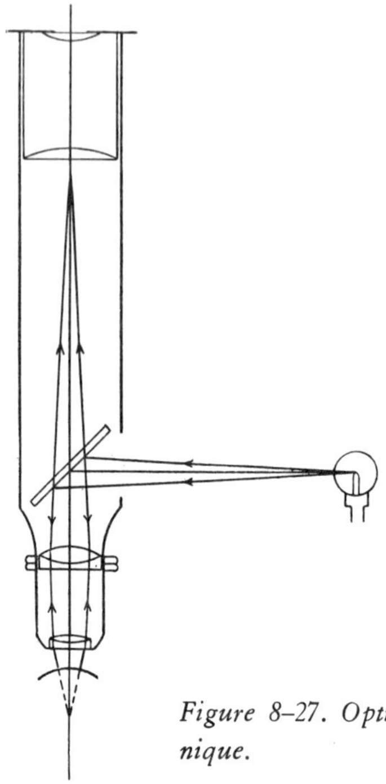

Figure 8–27. Optics of Drysdale technique.

of a surface to its center of curvature is the radius of the surface. Because the instrument has been zeroed at the vertex, the linear distance traversed to bring the object from the vertex to the center of curvature determines its radius. This value is read from a scale. (See p. 153.)

The center of curvature of a concave reflecting surface lies in front of it. To place the object at this point, the distance between the end of the microscope and the surface must be increased. The center of curvature of a convex reflecting surface lies behind it; to place the object at this point, the distance between the end of the microscope and the surface must be decreased.

OPTICS

There are three general areas related to producing satisfactory visual performance in a contact lens wearer: factors related to the selection of contact lens refractive power, factors related to the alteration of visual performance when changing from spectacle to contact lens correction, and factors related to visual performance unique to contact lenses.

Selection of Contact Lens Refractive Powers

There are two basic ways to determine initial refractive power to be incorporated in a contact lens.[299–305] The first involves mathematical computations based on spectacle plane refraction and central ophthalmometric findings. The second involves the refraction over precision diagnostic lenses on the eye. There are advantages and disadvantages to either method.

The following are possible sources of error when one is using only computation: The spectacle refraction may be in error. Vertex distance may be incorrectly measured or neglected. The ophthalmometric findings may be in error. Spherical aberration differs with contact lens and spectacle wear, a factor which may alter the selection of the portion of the bundle of rays that gives optimum focus.

The following are possible sources of error with the use of diagnostic lenses only: Excessive lacrimation may make objective or subjective testing inaccurate. Initial lens positioning may not be the same as final lens positioning. Edema may occur and invalidate the results. The ciliary muscle may spasm, causing an artificial refractive situation. Change of image size from spectacle to contact lenses may cause an initial erroneous subjective acceptance of power. The diagnostic lenses may be switched or altered.

The following are possible sources of error with the use of either computation or diagnostic lens procedure: The tolerance for fabrication and verification of a base curve is 0.02 mm. The tolerance for fabrication and verification of refractive power is 0.12 D. The base curve may be altered by hydration and wear.

To prescribe the refractive power of a contact lens accurately, it is necessary to understand the optics of contact lenses, which is based on certain aspects of geometric, ophthalmic, and physiologic optics. For simplicity, the discussion is limited to paraxial optics related to circular (as opposed to aspherical) curves.

Physical Structure

General. The initial discussion is limited to the optic zone. Three physical characteristics contribute to produce the refractive power of the contact lens: surface radii, index of refraction, and thickness.

Surface Radii. Each surface may be either spherical or toroidal. A spherical surface has the same radius in each meridian, whereas a toroidal surface has a different radius in each meridian of any quadrant. On a toroidal surface, there is a progressive change in each quadrant from longest to shortest radii. The meridians of minimum (shortest) radius and maximum (longest) radius are termed the *principal meridians* and are 90° apart.

If the anterior surface is toroidal and the posterior surface is spherical, the lens is termed an *anterior* or *front surface toric lens.* If the posterior surface is toroidal and the anterior is spherical, the lens is termed a *posterior* or *back surface toric lens.* If both the anterior and posterior surfaces are toroidal, the lens is termed a *bitoric lens.* The axes of the toroidal anterior and posterior surfaces may coincide with, or be oblique to one another. Usually they coincide.

Practically, there are two types of refraction of light: stigmatic and astigmatic. A *stigmatic refraction* of light is one in which light from a point source is brought to a single point focus by a lens or optical system. An *astigmatic refraction* of light is one in which light from a point source is not brought to a single point focus. It is focused as two line images at different distances from the system, generally at right angles to each other.

Single spherical anterior and posterior optic-zone curvatures produce equal refraction of light in all meridians and a resultant point focus. Toroidal anterior or toroidal posterior surfaces produce unequal refraction in the various meridians. The greatest refraction is in the principal meridian of steepest curvature, and the least refraction in the principal meridian of flattest curvature, resulting in the production of two line images.

Temporarily disregarding the effects of center thickness on refraction, assume that the anterior and posterior surfaces of the lens are surrounded by the same medium, and that the optic zone has spherical anterior and posterior surfaces. To produce diverging (negative) refraction, the anterior radius must be longer than the posterior radius. If the radii are fabricated with their centers of curvature on the same axis, there is a progressive increase of thickness from center to edge. To produce converging (positive) refraction, the anterior radius must be shorter than the posterior radius. If the radii are fabricated with their centers of curvature on the same axis, there is a progressive decrease of thickness from center to edge.

Indices. The lens has an index of refraction, and it is surrounded by a medium (or media) that has another index of refraction. The medium surrounding the contact lens is either air or precorneal fluid. The refractive index of the lens plastic is usually 1.49; the index of air is taken to be 1.00; and the index of precorneal fluid is usually given as 1.33 to 1.34.

For each spherical surface, the relationships of the radius and the indicial difference to the refractive power are shown by the following formula:

$$D = \frac{n_2 - n_1 K}{R}$$

where n_2 = Index of substance into which light goes
n_1 = Index of substance from which light comes
K = Unit factor (1,000 for mm.)

Center Thickness. The anterior and posterior surfaces of the lens are separated by the thickness of the lens. Usually the central point, or center thickness, is used for computations.

THIN AND THICK LENSES. When center thickness is less than one per cent of the surface radii, the effect of center thickness on light refraction is negligible—that is, the power of emerging light is relatively the same whether it enters the anterior or posterior surface first. The total power (D_t)

of the lens in any meridian is equal to the algebraic sum of the anterior surface power (D_1) and the posterior surface power (D_2) in that meridian: $D_t = D_1 + D_2$.

Because of the short radii of a contact lens, center thickness is greater than one per cent of surface radii. Although a contact lens is thin physically, it must be considered optically thick. The power of light entering the anterior surface and emerging from the posterior surface is not the same as the power of light entering the posterior surface and emerging from the anterior surface.

Posterior and Anterior Vertex Power. When light enters the anterior (convex) surface and emerges from the posterior (concave) surface, the focal length is measured from the vertex of the posterior surface to the focal point. This measurement is termed the *posterior* (or *back*) *focal length*. The reciprocal of this value is the *posterior* (or *back*) *vertex power.*

When light enters the posterior (concave) surface and emerges from the anterior (convex) surface, focal length is measured from the vertex of the anterior surface to the focal point. This measurement is termed the *anterior* (or front) *focal length,* the reciprocal of which is the *anterior* (or *front*) *vertex power.*

When a spectacle or contact lens is worn, it is positioned with its posterior surface closer to the eye. Light enters the anterior surface and emerges from the posterior surface. The practitioner must determine the necessary posterior vertex power. It is important to remember this factor for prescription and verification purposes.

The posterior vertex power of a minus lens is stronger in minus power than the anterior vertex power. The posterior vertex power of a plus lens is stronger in plus power than the anterior vertex power is. The difference between posterior and anterior vertex powers is greater in plus than in minus lenses, owing to the greater center thickness.

Posterior vertex power of an optically thick lens is determined by the formula:

$$D_P = \frac{D_1}{1 - D_1(t/n)} + D_2$$

where: D_P = Posterior vertex power
D_1 = Power of anterior surface
D_2 = Power of posterior surface
t = Center thickness in *meters*
n = Index of lens material

The anterior vertex power of an optically thick lens is determined by the formula:

$$D_A = \frac{D_2}{1 - D_2(t/n)} + D_1$$

ANTERIOR COMPENSATION. Mathematical computation based on thick lens formulas is somewhat complex and lengthy. When the desired base curve, posterior vertex power, and center thickness are known, the appropriate anterior radius can be determined without thick lens formulas. This is done by treating the lens as a thin lens and compensating for the change of power due to center thickness.[306–308] Compensation involves taking one third the center thickness and adding it to the radius of the anterior surface found by the thin lens formula—that is, $D_t = D_1 + D_2$.

For example, if the base curve of a lens is 8.00 mm. (−60.98 D in air), the desired posterior vertex power is −5 D in air, and a center thickness of 0.15 mm. is desired, then:

$$D_t = D_1 + D_2$$

$$-5 = D_1 + (-60.98)$$

$$+55.98 = D_1$$

$$8.75 = r_1 \text{ (noncompensated)}$$

$$8.75 + \tfrac{1}{3}(.15) = r_1 \text{ (compensated)}$$

$$8.80 = r_1 \text{ (compensated)}$$

Thus, to have a −5 D posterior vertex power in air, the anterior curvature must be 8.80 mm.

POWER OF SINGLE SPHERICAL CURVATURE. The power of a surface depends on the radius of the curvature and the difference between the refractive index of the lens and that of the surrounding medium. Five different indicial relationships are most frequently used in contact lens work. To make calculations simpler and more accurate, powers for various radii with each indicial relationship have been computed (see Appendix VI).

Column 1 lists the various radii of curvature. Column 2 is discussed on page 332.

Column 3 has the power for the corresponding radius in Column 1, based on an n_2 value of 1.3375 and an n_1 value of 1.00. The n_2 value (1.3375) is the assumed refractive index of the precorneal fluid when the Keratometer (Bausch & Lomb) is used, the refractive index of air remaining at 1.00.

Column 4 lists the powers for the corresponding radii in Column 1, based on an n_2 value of 1.336 and an n_1 value of 1.00. The n_2 value (1.336) is the assumed index of the precorneal fluid when the Ophthalmometer (American Optical) is used, and the n_1 value (1.00) is the refractive index of the surrounding air.

Column 5 shows the power for the corresponding radius in Column 1, based on an n_2 value of 1.49 and an n_1 value of 1.00. The n_2 value (1.49) is the refractive index of the lens plastic. The values in this column are positive for the anterior convex surface of the lens and negative for the posterior concave surface of the lens. This column may be used to obtain the true power of a curvature of a contact lens in air.

Column 6 lists the power for the corresponding radius in Column 1 based on an n_2 value of 1.3375 and an n_1 value of 1.49. The n_2 value (1.3375) is the assumed index of the precorneal fluid used with the Keratometer, and the n_1 value (1.49) is the index of plastic. The values in this column, which are negative, indicate the power of a single spherical curvature of a contact lens when it is next to the precorneal fluid—that is, on the eye. Its major use is in relation to the posterior surface of the lens.

Column 7 lists the powers for the corresponding radii in Column 1 based on an n_2 value of 1.336 and an n_1 value of 1.49. The n_2 value (1.336) is the assumed index of the precorneal fluid when the Ophthalmometer is used, and the n_1 value (1.49) is the index of the plastic. The values in this column are negative. This column indicates the power of a single spherical curvature of a contact lens when it is next to the precorneal fluid—that is, on the eye. Its major use is in relation to the back surface of the lens.

Use of Surface Power Table. Consider how Appendix VI is used when measurements are made with an American Optical Ophthalmometer. When a central ophthalmometric measurement is taken, the reading is in diopters, based on a n_2–n_1 relationship of 1.336–1.000. To find the radius corresponding to the power indicated on the instrument scale, refer to Column 4 at the appropriate power. Then refer to the corresponding level in Column 1.

To determine the astigmatic refraction resulting from a toric base curve, look up either the ophthalmometric power of each meridian in Column 4 or its radius in Column 1. Look across on the same line for each power or radius to Column 7 to find the power of each curve on the eye. The difference between the two meridians is the amount of astigmatic refraction.

To determine the radius or true in-air power of a convex curvature of a contact lens measured by an Ophthalmometer, find the ophthalmometric power in Column 4. Read across the same line to Column 1 to find the radius and to Column 5 to find the power. To find the radius of a concave curvature measured on an Ophthalmometer, find the ophthalmometric power in Column 4. Read across the same line to Column 2 to find the corresponding radius. To determine the power in air, find this same radius in Column 1, and read across this line to Column 5.

The same general procedures are used in each instance with the Keratometer. However, Column 3 is used instead of Column 4, and Column 6 instead of Column 7.

Certain relationships between the various columns may be used:

Column 7 is 0.314 of Column 5.
Column 6 is 0.311 of Column 5.
Column 4 is 0.686 of Column 5.
Column 3 is 0.689 of Column 5.
Column 5 is 1.458 of Column 4.
Column 5 is 1.452 of Column 3.
Column 7 is 0.458 of Column 4.
Column 6 is 0.452 of Column 3.
Column 4 is 2.182 of Column 7.
Column 3 is 2.213 of Column 6.

Optical System of the Eye and Its Correction

Two Variables. The eye is an optical system having a dioptric power and an axial length. Refraction of a static eye to determine the needed spectacle lens power indirectly determines the relationship between two distances—the axial length of the eye and the posterior focal length of the dioptric power of the eye. Clinically, neither the axial length nor the total dioptric power and its posterior focal length are determined. Only the relationship, or degree of balance, between these two variables is determined.

In any one meridian of a static eye, there are three possible relationships: the posterior principal focus from entering parallel light falls on the retina, the posterior principal focus from entering parallel light falls in front of the retina, or the posterior principal focus from entering parallel light falls behind the retina.

When the first relationship exists, the meridian is considered to be balanced, or emmetropic. When the second relationship is present, the meridian is considered to be unbalanced, or ametropic, in a myopic direction. When the third relationship exists, the meridian is considered to be unbalanced, or ametropic, in a hyperopic direction. When ametropia is present, a balanced relationship between axial length and posterior focal length must be established, which may be done artificially by the use of lenses of appropriate power placed in an appropriate position in front of the corneal apex.

Spectacle Correction. The far point of a meridian of a static eye is the point in space that is conjugate with the retina. In myopia, this point is a real and finite point in front of the eye. In hyperopia, this point is a virtual point behind the eye (Fig. 8–28).

To establish a balance, a spectacle lens is used to take parallel rays of light and focus them toward the far point. In myopia, through the use of a minus lens, parallel rays are made to diverge, as if coming from the far point. In hyperopia, through the use of a plus lens, parallel rays are made to converge to the far point. To establish a balance, the power of a spectacle

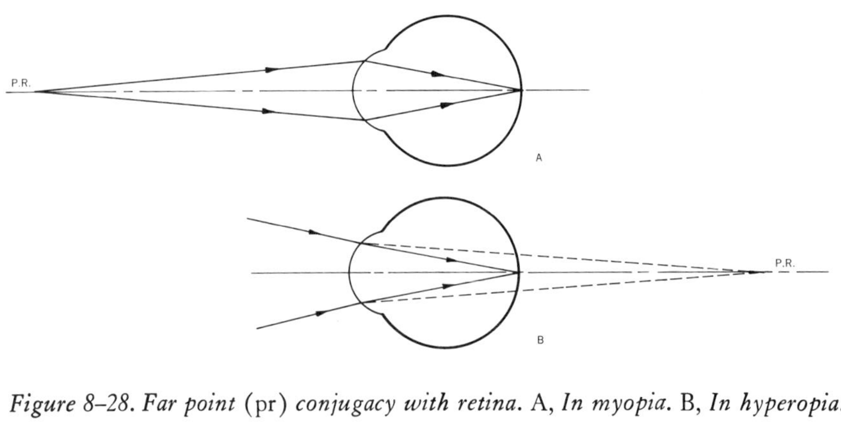

Figure 8–28. Far point (pr) *conjugacy with retina.* A, *In myopia.* B, *In hyperopia.*

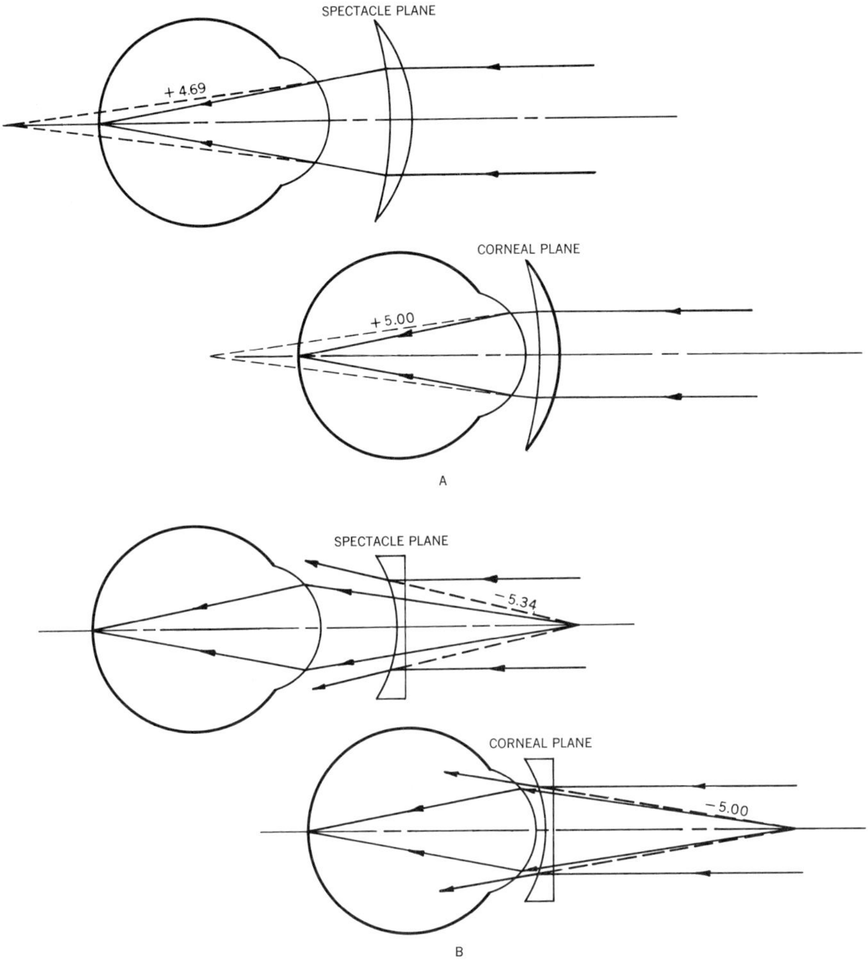

Figure 8–29. A correcting spectacle lens makes the far point of a static eye conjugate with infinity. A, *Because of vertex factors, stronger converging power is needed for corneal plane refraction to produce conjugacy.* B, *Because of vertex factors, weaker diverging power is needed for corneal plane refraction to produce conjugacy.*

lens at a given distance in front of the corneal apex makes the far point conjugate with infinity (Fig. 8–29).

SPECTACLE AND CORNEAL PLANE REFRACTION. The far point of a meridian of a static eye and the focal length of a thin lens for parallel light are constant. The distance between the lens and the far point is variable. The focal length necessary to make the far point conjugate with infinity therefore depends on the distance of the lens from the far point. For any far point, a number of lenses can establish the desired conjugacy. The power needed depends on lens position and is always the reciprocal of the distance between the lens and the far point.

Because it is clinically easier to determine, the distance from the vertex of the posterior surface of the correcting lens to the corneal apex is used. This is termed the *vertex distance*. The vertex distance for a contact lens is taken to be zero, because its posterior surface rests almost on the corneal apex. The vertex distance for a spectacle lens may be any finite number, but it is usually between 12 and 15 mm.

The power needed in a contact lens to achieve conjugacy between the far point and infinity is termed the *corneal plane refraction*. The power needed in a spectacle lens at a specific vertex distance to achieve conjugacy between the far point and infinity is termed the *spectacle plane refraction*. These powers differ as their distances from the far point differ by an amount equal to the vertex distance.

For example, in a spherical myope whose far point is 200 mm. in front of the apex of the cornea, if a lens placed at the corneal apex is 200 mm. from the far point, parallel rays of light striking the lens must receive a divergence of 200 mm. to seem to be coming from the far point. The reciprocal of 200 mm. is -5 D. A lens placed 13 mm. in front of the corneal apex is only 187 mm. from the far point. Parallel rays of light striking the lens must receive a divergence of 187 mm. to seem to be coming from the far point. The reciprocal of 187 mm. is -5.34 D.

In any given myopia, weaker diverging power is needed for corneal plane refraction than for spectacle plane refraction. In any given hyperopia, stronger converging power is needed for corneal plane refraction than for spectacle plane refraction.

This may be visualized by remembering that in myopia the distance from the far point to a spectacle plane is less than the distance from the far point to the corneal plane. The reciprocal of a larger number is less than the reciprocal of a smaller number. In hyperopia, the distance from the far point to a spectacle plane is greater than the distance from the far point to the corneal plane.

Spectacle plane refraction is determined through use of a phoropter or trial frame, which is a certain vertex distance in front of the corneal apex. The spectacle power indicates the total spherical and the total astigmatic imbalance of the eye in terms of a given vertex distance.

To transpose spectacle plane refraction to corneal plane refraction, the equivalent power at the corneal plane must be found. When spectacle plane refraction is less than ± 3 D, this determination need not be made because the difference between spectacle plane refraction and corneal plane refraction is 0.12 D or less (see Appendix V).

The transposition of spectacle plane refraction to equivalent corneal plane refraction may be done by use of the formula:

$$D_{CL} = \frac{D_L}{1 - SD_L},$$ where D_{CL} = Power needed at corneal apex

D_L = Lensometer or phoropter value of spectacle lens

S = Vertex distance in meters spectacles worn at or prescribed for

VERTEX TABLE. It is simpler and often more accurate to do the computation by using Appendix V.

Appendix V is used in the following manner: The spectacle plane refraction is determined in minus cylinder form, and the prescription is placed on an optical cross. The vertex distance of the spectacle plane refraction is then determined. The power of each meridian of the spectacle plane refraction can be found in the left hand column of Appendix V listed under Lensometer reading. Read across to the right on the same line to the appropriate vertex distance to find the total power needed at the corneal plane in each meridian. Powers may be determined from the optical cross to make a spherocylindrical prescription.

For example, a Lensometer reading of -8.00 D $= -3.00 \times 180$ for the spectacle lens is taken, and the spectacles have been worn at a 15 mm. vertex distance. The total powers of this lens are -8.00 D in the 180° meridian and -11.00 D in the 90° meridian.

$$\begin{array}{r} -8 \text{ sph} \\ -3 \text{ cyl} \\ \hline -11 \end{array}$$

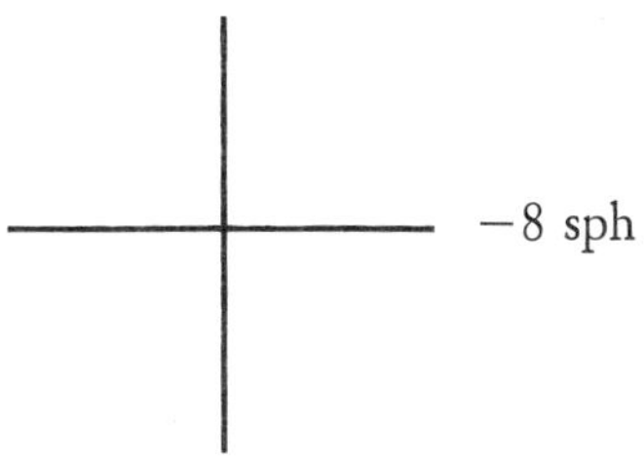

From Appendix V, it may be determined that a Lensometer reading of -8 D on spectacles worn at 15 mm. is equivalent to a power of -7.14 D at the corneal plane; and a Lensometer reading of -11 D on spectacles worn at 15 mm. is equivalent to a power of -9.43 D at the corneal plane. Placing these powers on an optical cross,

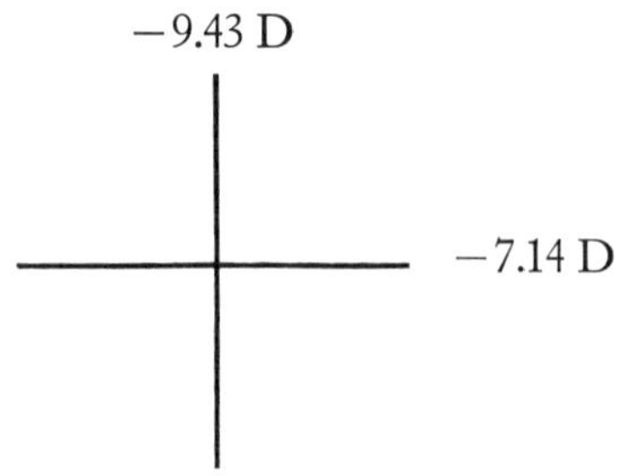

and algebraically combining values,

$$\begin{array}{r} -9.43\ \text{D} \\ -(-7.14\ \text{D}) \\ \hline -2.29\ \text{D} \end{array}$$

result in the power of the cylinder at the corneal plane. The needed refractive power at the corneal plane is $-7.14 = -2.29 \times 180$, or practically $-7.12 = -2.25 \times 180$. The two optical crosses are then compared. In the 180° meridian, there is 0.86 D less corneal plane power, and at the 90° meridian, there is 1.57 D less corneal plane power. The needed corneal plane cylinder power is therefore 0.71 D less than the spectacle plane cylinder power. This procedure must be used and understood. If it is not applied properly, prediction of residual astigmatism and theoretic computation of spherical equivalent power and the power of a toric or bitoric lens will be incorrect (see p. 350).

Contact Lens Correction. Two basic clinical measurements related to contact lens refractive power are usually made. The first is the spectacle refraction at a given vertex distance, which is translated to the equivalent corneal plane refraction. The second is the central ophthalmometric measurement, which indicates the approximate power of the main source of refraction of the eye—the interface between air and the precorneal fluid.

If the ophthalmometric power is combined with the corneal plane power, the eye is made artificially emmetropic. For example, if the central ophthalmometric reading is +45.00 D spherical, and the needed corneal plane power is −5.00 D (which indicates an imbalance between the total power of the eye and its axial length—that is, there is +5.00 D too much power), reducing the ophthalmometric value by 5 D to +40 D would establish artificial emmetropia.

A contact lens on the eye replaces the anterior precorneal fluid as the first and strongest refractive component of the eye's optical system. In the example just given, the contact lens must have a posterior vertex power of +40.00 D *on the eye* to establish artificial emmetropia. The Lensometer reading of this lens will be −5.00 D, representing the amount of imbalance that must be neutralized.

The lens has a −5 D posterior vertex power on the Lensometer but a +40.00 D posterior vertex power on the eye because of the indices of the surrounding media. On the Lensometer, both the anterior and posterior surfaces of the lens are surrounded by air. The power of each surface is, therefore, found in Column 5 of the table in Appendix VI. For simplification, it may be said that the anterior surface of the contact lens on the eye is surrounded by air, but the posterior surface is surrounded by precorneal fluid. The power of the anterior surface is found in Column 5, and the power of the posterior surface in Column 6 or 7 of the table in Appendix VI.

Contact lenses correct ametropia basically by physically changing the power of the eye. Spectacle lenses correct ametropia basically by making the far point of the eye conjugate with infinity. In either case, power is added to or subtracted from the optical system.

Effect of Base Curve—Precorneal Curve Relationship. When a contact lens with a spherical base curve is placed on the eye, the anterior surface of the precorneal fluid assumes the shape of the base curve. If the anterior surface of the precorneal fluid, measured by the Ophthalmometer, is toric, this toricity is eliminated for practical purposes.

Consider this in terms of the flatter ophthalmometric meridian. When a contact lens with a base curve the radius of which is the same as the flatter ophthalmometric meridian is on the eye, the precorneal fluid fills in through all other meridians to form an interface with a single radius. When the base curve does not equal the flatter ophthalmometric radius, the posterior vertex power is altered. This factor must be compensated for.

From Column 7 of Appendix VI, it may be seen that lengthening the base from 7.50 to 7.54 mm. (0.04 mm.) adds +0.11 D to the posterior vertex power of the lens on the eye. It may be seen from Column 5 that the same base curve lengthening adds +0.35 D to the posterior vertex power of the lens in air.

To achieve the same posterior vertex power on the eye, the +0.11 D must be neutralized by lengthening of the anterior curvature so that −0.11 D is added. The indicial difference relating to the anterior surface is, for practical purposes, the same on the eye or in the air; thus, the −0.11 D is the same for both.

In air, therefore, −0.11 D is added to the anterior surface power, and +0.35 D is added to the posterior surface power. The resultant change of posterior vertex power is +0.24 D. On the eye, −0.11 D is added to the anterior surface power, and +0.11 D is added to the posterior surface power. There is no resultant change of posterior vertex power.

Although the numbers vary slightly for different radii, this relationship is valid throughout the range of base curves used. A clinical rule of thumb can be derived. For each 0.04 to 0.05 mm. flatter the base curve is than the flatter central ophthalmometric value, +0.25 D is added to the posterior vertex contact lens power in air; for each 0.04 to 0.05 mm. steeper the base curve is than the flatter ophthalmometric valve, −0.25 D is added. Because of 0.04 to 0.05 mm. radius change equals about 0.25 D of *ophthalmometric or keratometric* change, these values may be interchanged.

Two Components. In contact lens work, the power of the optical system of the eye can be considered to result from two major components. The first component is the interface between air and the anterior surface of the precorneal fluid. This may be measured by the use of an Ophthalmometer or Keratometer. The second major component is that composed of all elements behind, or internal to, the interface between air and the anterior surface of the precorneal fluid.

Astigmatism may in part be caused by the interface between air and the precorneal fluid. This astigmatism is measured by the Ophthalmometer and may be called *ophthalmometric astigmatism* (AO). The remainder of the astigmatism is caused by all the components internal to the interface between air and the precorneal fluid. This portion may be called *internal astigmatism* (AI). The total astigmatism produced by these two components is represented by the astigmatic value of the spectacle refraction referred to the corneal plane. This total may be termed AT, and it may be equated as:

$$AT = AO + AI$$

or

$$AI = AT - AO.$$

Residual Astigmatism. Residual astigmatism is defined as the astigmatism that remains or is residual after the application of a lens having spherical anterior and spherical or toroidal posterior surfaces. This definition indicates that there are two basic residual astigmatism categories: that which occurs when the anterior and posterior surfaces of the lens are spherical, and that which occurs when the anterior surface is spherical and the posterior surface is toroidal.

Central Spherical Anterior and Posterior Lens Curvatures. A contact lens with central spherical anterior and posterior curvatures refracts light stigmatically. Ophthalmometric astigmatism (AO) is eliminated by conformation of the precorneal fluid to the spherical base curve.

A contact lens with central spherical anterior and posterior curvatures does not compensate for the astigmatic refraction caused by internal components of the eye. This astigmatism remains or is residual. The amount of this residual internal astigmatism may be computed by using the formula $AI = AT - AO$.

Residual internal astigmatism may be compensated for in one of two ways by a contact lens. The first involves using a contact lens with a central spherical anterior curvature, producing stigmatic refraction. The spherical equivalent principle is applied, based on the fact that one position between the focal lines of an astigmatic refraction of light produces the best image—the circle of least confusion. By algebraically adding half the needed minus cylinder to the needed sphere, the resultant equivalent sphere places the circle of least confusion on the retina.

To determine the spherical equivalent, the total spectacle power in minus cylinder form is referred back to the corneal plane in each meridian. The formula $AI = AT - AO$ can be used to determine the amount of residual internal astigmatism. Half this cylinder is added to the corneal plane sphere.

For example, spectacle plane refraction at 13 mm. is $-4.00 = -0.75 \times 90$. The ophthalmometric reading is 44.00 D spherical.

Place the spectacle prescription on an optical cross:

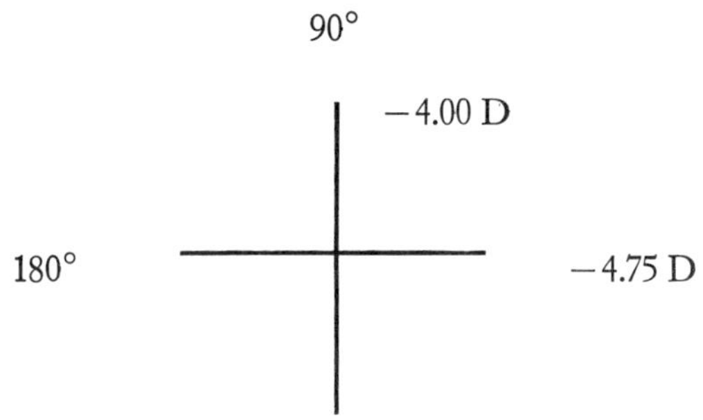

Find the corneal plane power by using the Vertex Distance Tables, Appendix V.

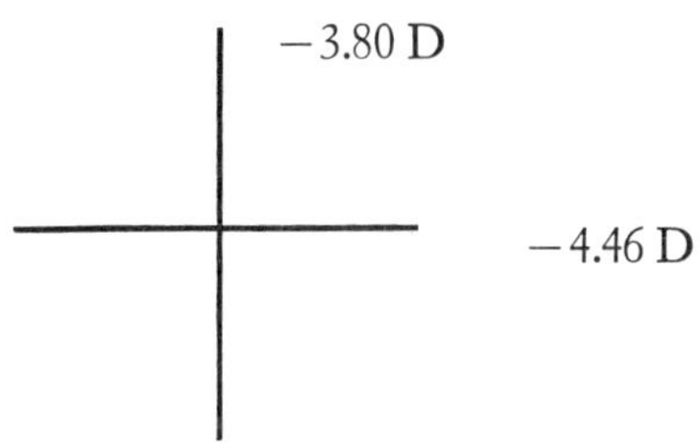

Combine to find the corneal plane spherocylindrical correction: $-3.80 = -0.66 \times 90$.

Use the formula to predict the amount of residual internal astigmatism:

$$AI = AT - AO,$$
$$AI = -0.66 \times 90 - 0 = -0.66 \times 90$$

Add half this cylinder to the sphere to get the equivalent sphere: $-3.80 + (\frac{1}{2})(-0.66) = -4.13$, or practically -4.12.

The second way that a contact lens may correct residual astigmatism involves use of a central toric anterior curvature. The amount of anterior surface cylinder is found by the first four steps of the preceding example. The needed power is $-3.80 = -0.66 \times 90$, or practically $-3.75 = -0.62 \times 90$. Clinical factors may alter the needed power or axis position (see p. 100).

When axes of ophthalmometric astigmatism (*AO*) and total spectacle astigmatism (*AT*) referred to the corneal plane are the same, it may be assumed that the axis of the internal astigmatism is also the same. If the axes of *AT* and *AO* are not the same, it may be assumed that the axis of *AI* is oblique to that of *AO*. To determine the power and axis of *AI*, the formulation for obliquely crossed cylinders is used.

The resultant cylindrical power is found by:

$$C_r^2 = C_1^2 + C_2^2 + 2C_1C_2 \cos 2\,\alpha$$

where C_r = Resultant cylindrical power
C_1 = First cylinder
C_2 = Second cylinder
α = Angle between axes of C_1 and C_2

The resultant cylinder axis is found by:

$$\sin 2\,\phi = \frac{C_2}{C_r} \quad \sin 2\,\alpha$$

where ϕ = Resultant cylinder axis

The resultant sphere is found by:

$$S_r = S_1 + S_2 + \frac{C_1 + C_2 - C_r}{2}$$

where S_r = Resultant sphere
S_1 = First sphere
S_2 = Second sphere

When *AI* and *AO* are oblique to one another by 20° or less, it is usually sufficiently accurate to assume no obliquity for the usual amount of *AI*. It is best clinically to determine the amount and location of residual internal astigmatism by refraction over diagnostic lenses.

Spherical Anterior and Toric Posterior Curvature. A lens having a spherical base curve eliminates *AO*. When a lens having a toric base curve is placed on the eye, the precorneal fluid conforms to the two different radii. There is an astigmatic refraction.[309, 310]

When the lens is in air, the indicial relationship is 1.49 – 1.00 (0.49). When the lens is on the eye, the indicial relationship is either 1.49 – 1.336 (0.154) or 1.49 – 1.3375 (0.1525). Air-to-eye relationships are 0.154/0.490 (31.4 per cent) or 0.1525/0.490 (31.1 per cent). The astigmatic refraction on the eye therefore equals about 31 per cent of the toricity of the base in air. A toric base curve on a lens produces or induces a given amount of astigmatism. This astigmatism is termed *induced astigmatism.*

The amount of induced residual astigmatism is determined by determination of the radius of each principal meridian in Column 1 of Appendix VI. When using the Keratometer, read across to Column 6 on each of these lines. This reading gives the power of each meridian on the eye. The difference between the two is the amount of induced astigmatism. It is always a minus cylinder with its axis corresponding to the meridian of the flatter base curve. The same procedure is used with the Ophthalmometer, but Column 7 is used.

Induced astigmatism is compensated for in one of two ways. First, only the induced astigmatism is corrected, and the internal astigmatism remains uncorrected. This is done when it is felt that the internal astigmatism is insufficient to cause problems in visual acuity or discomfort. Second, the sum of the induced astigmatism and the internal astigmatism is corrected. In either method, compensation is accomplished by the use of a lens having a toric anterior surface.

When only the induced astigmatism is corrected, the anterior cylinder has the same axis as the posterior surface cylinder, and the power in each is equal in amount but opposite in type. For example, if the induced cylinder is −1.50 axis 180, the cylinder placed on the anterior surface is +1.50 axis 180. One cylinder neutralizes the other, and the lens has a spherical power on the eye. Any fluctuation of the meridional orientation of the lens does not cause visual problems from a tilted cylinder. However, the internal astigmatism is uncorrected and may cause problems.

In correcting both the induced astigmatism and internal astigmatism, lens power on the eye is not spherical. Part of the anterior surface cylinder neutralizes the induced astigmatism; the remainder neutralizes the internal astigmatism. The effective residual cylindrical power on the eye equals the internal astigmatism.

At times the axes of the induced astigmatism and internal astigmatism are oblique to one another. Resultant cylindrical power and spherical power may be computed by use of the formula on page 352.

Compensation for fitting a spherical base curve flatter or steeper than the flattest ophthalmometric meridian (see p. 349) is valid for a toric base curve, but compensation must be done for each meridian. For example, if the ophthalmometric readings are 44 at the 180° meridian and 47 at the 90° meridian, and if the ophthalmometric value of the base curve at the 180° meridian is 43.75 (0.25 D flatter) and at the 90° meridian is 46.50 (0.50 D flatter), then +0.25 D must be added to the 180° meridian and +0.50 to the 90° meridian.

Alteration of Visual Performance in Changing from Spectacle to Contact Lenses

Prismatic Effect

The prismatic effect of spectacles and contact lenses is basically the same.

Image Size

There is a difference in image size between spectacle correction and contact lens correction.[311] When this difference is considered in terms of retinal image size—the image (blurred or clear) that falls on the retina—it may be termed *comparative contact lens magnification.*

Disregarding lens shape, at a given vertex distance the image size of a distant object is inversely proportional to lens power. Thus, the retinal image size with a contact lens (*cl*) at corneal plane may be represented as $1/D_{cl}$, and the retinal image size with spectacle at spectacle plane as $1/D_L$.

It has been shown on page 347 that the relationship between corneal plane refraction and spectacle plane refraction can be represented by the equation:

$$D_{cl} = \frac{D_L}{1 - sD_L}$$

A ratio of image size due to power factors when corrected by contact lens and by spectacle lens is used:

$$\frac{\dfrac{1}{D_{cl}}}{\dfrac{1}{D_s}}$$

This may then be equated with needed corneal plane and spectacle plane powers:

$$\frac{\dfrac{1}{D_{cl}}}{\dfrac{1}{D_L}} = \frac{\dfrac{1 - sD_L}{D_L}}{\dfrac{1}{D_L}}$$

The right hand side of the equation simplifies to $1 - sD_s$:

$$\frac{\dfrac{1}{D_{cl}}}{\dfrac{1}{D_L}} = 1 - sD_L$$

The left hand side of the equation is a ratio of contact lens magnification of correction and spectacle lens magnification of correction for a given eye, or the *comparative contact lens magnification:* $CCLM = 1 - sD_L$. If the solution to the equation is a number greater than 1, the difference between the number and 1 indicates an increase of retinal image size of this per cent. The reverse holds when the solution to the equation is a number less than 1.

Comparative contact lens magnification is always greater for a myope and less for a hyperope. That is, a contact lens-corrected myope has a comparatively larger retinal image than a spectacle lens-corrected myope. A contact lens-corrected hyperope has a comparatively smaller retinal image than a spectacle lens-corrected hyperope.

The concept of *relative magnification* may be used to illustrate the effect of contact lens and spectacle lens correction in terms of the aniseikonia (inequality of retinal image size) related to anisometropia. Relative magnification with spectacle correction for an ametropia of solely refractive origin is: $RMR = 1 + dD_L$ where d = distance from spectacle plane to the first principal point.

Relative magnification with spectacle correction for an ametropia of solely axial origin is:

$$RMA = 1 - gD_L$$

where g = distance from anterior focal point of the eye to the spectacle plane.

When a contact lens is on the eye, d is almost zero and RMR is almost unity. A refractive anisometropia results in less aniseikonia when corrected by contact lenses than when corrected by spectacle lenses.

When a contact lens is on the eye, g is greater and the RMA is greater. Axial anisometropia results in more aniseikonia when corrected by a contact lens than when corrected by a spectacle lens.

Accommodation and Convergence

Spectacle lens correction changes the vergence of light from a near object.[312] As a result, a contact lens-corrected myope is required to accommodate more for a given distance than a spectacle-corrected myope. The opposite is true in a hyperope.

To simplify computation, it may be assumed that the corneal apex coincides with the first principal point of the eye and that the second principal point of the correcting lens coincides with the vertex of the posterior surface. Accommodation needed by a spectacle-corrected ametrope for a near object is computed by tracing light from the object to the corneal apex. The amount of accommodation needed by a spectacle-corrected ametrope is the difference between the power of light at the corneal plane and the error of the eye at the corneal plane. This amount of accommodation may be compared with the amount needed by a contact lens-corrected ametrope, which is practically the same as that needed by an emmetrope. The amount of accommodation needed by an emmetrope is practically the reciprocal of the object distance from the corneal apex.

The amount of accommodation needed by a spectacle-corrected ametrope is found more simply by the following formulas:

$$D_c = \frac{1000}{\dfrac{1000}{D_u + D_L} + v},$$

where D_c = Power of light from a near object at corneal plane
D_u = Power of light from a near object at spectacle plane
D_L = Power of spectacle lens
v = Vertex distance (this is $-$ if the sum of $D_u + D_L$ is $+$; and $+$ if the sum of $D_u + D_L$ is $-$)

$$A = D_e - D_c,$$

where A = Accommodation needed
D_e = Corneal plane refractive error (found from Appendix V)
D_c = Power of light from a near object at corneal plane

Take a hyperope corrected by +10 D and a myope corrected by −10 D in spectacle lenses 12 mm. from the corneal apex. The object is 400 mm. (or 1000/400 = −2.5 D) from the spectacle plane.

Hyperope corrected with spectacles:

$$D_c = \frac{1000}{\dfrac{1000}{-2.50 + 10} - 12} = +8.26 \text{ D}$$

$$A = -11.50 + 8.26 = -3.24 \text{ D}$$

Myope corrected with spectacles:

$$D_c = \frac{1000}{\dfrac{1000}{-2.50 - 10} + 12} = -10.87 \text{ D}$$

$$A = +9 - 10.87 = -1.87$$

Emmetrope or contact lens-corrected ametrope:

$$A = \frac{1000}{400 + 12} = -2.43 \text{ D}$$

See Fig. 8–30 for the determination of these values by ray-tracing.

This change of accommodation has clinical significance for two reasons. First, a myopic incipient presbyope able to function reasonably well with

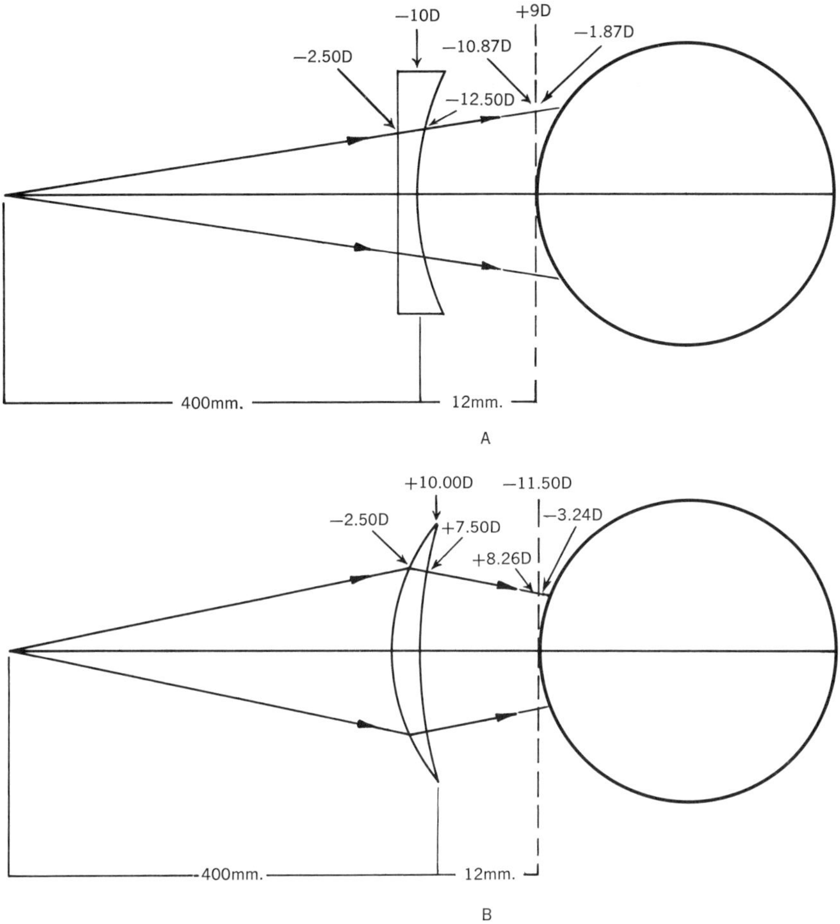

Figure 8–30. An emmetrope must accommodate 2.43 D for an object 412 mm. from the corneal apex. A, *A spectacle-corrected myope must accommodate less than this; for example, 1.87 D in this instance.* B, *A spectacle-corrected hyperope must accommodate more than this; for example, 3.24 D in this instance.*

single-vision spectacle correction may need an addition for near work with contact lenses. The functional onset of presbyopia in a hyperope for the same reason may be retarded slightly by contact lens application. Second, more accommodative convergence is used by a contact lens-corrected myope. It is less for a hyperope corrected with contact lenses than with spectacle lenses. This factor may cause problems related to the balance of the extraocular muscles and excessive demands on fusional reserves.

Because of removal of the base-in effect possessed by a spectacle-corrected myope when fixating at near, a contact lens-corrected myope converges more than a spectacle-corrected myope for a given distance. Because of removal of the base-out effect possessed by a spectacle-corrected hyperope when fixating at near, a contact lens-corrected hyperope converges less than a spectacle-corrected hyperope for a given distance.

Usable Field

The usable field of vision is greater for a contact lens wearer than for a spectacle wearer, owing in part to limitation of the usable field of fixation by the rim of the frame. In plus corrections, the increase of prism with its base opposite to the direction of eccentric fixation further reduces the usable field (see p. 121).

Aberrations

Most contact lenses position and move so that there is a reasonable centration of optic zone with the pupil. The degree of most peripheral aberrations—that is, coma, oblique astigmatism, distortion, and curvature of field—is much less in the use of contact lenses than in spectacle lenses. Chromatic aberration is about the same in contact lens and in spectacle lens correction. Spherical aberration in air is usually worse with contact lenses. The eye, however, eliminates much of this aberration.

Visual Performance Unique to Contact Lenses

Even if a satisfactory initial refractive power has been prescribed, there may be visual problems. Any one of five important conditions may cause poor visual performance: lens coating or hazing, corneal edema or distortion, change of the physical structure of the lens, flare or marginal confusion, and poor lens positioning.

Coating or Hazing of Lenses

Contact lenses are made of polymethyl methacrylate, which is hydrophobic. Thus, lenses may become coated (see also p. 204). Aside from the inherent hydrophobic nature of this plastic, the following factors can contribute to the coating or hazing problem.

Poor hygienic practices may be used by the patient, and body oil or cosmetics may be transferred from the fingers to the lens. The patient may use cold rather than warm water for insertion. Cold water will meet the warmer fluid on the eye, producing vapor.

The patient may use a wetting solution produced by one company and a soaking solution produced by another. Individually, these solutions may function acceptably, but they may not be chemically compatible with one another. The lens surface may be scratched, interfering with proper flow and causing the collection of mucoid material.

The patient may have developed an incomplete or slow blink in an attempt to reduce discomfort from the contact of lid with lens. This type of blink retards the flow of precorneal fluid over the lens. The patient may take a new job or move, with the result that the change in the amount of humidity in the general environment causes lens hazing.

The patient may develop conjunctivitis, with its accompanying increase of mucoid material. The lens edge may be incorrect or marred, resulting in the stimulation of the glands of the lid and the production of a greater amount of sebaceous and mucoid material. The patient may use medication or have a glandular problem, which can cause production of undesired ocular secretions. Finally, the patient may have a cold, sinus trouble, or allergy.

Corneal Edema or Distortion

For light to be refracted properly through the cornea, the tissue must maintain normal transparency and regularity of structure. If the cornea becomes edematous or distorted, light will be refracted improperly.

Change of Physical Structure of the Lens

Because a contact lens is relatively thin and pliable, its physical structure may be altered by hydration or pressure. These factors may cause an undesired spherical or toroidal alteration of the base curve, from which visual problems can result. Proper manufacturing helps to produce a more stable lens. These problems are greater in very thin lenses and in patients having tight lids or a harsh blink action.

Flare or Marginal Confusion

The refraction involved in the secondary area of the lens depends on an optical system of two components. The first is the contact lens, and the second is the lacrimal lens, both producing power and prism. The refractive index of the lens is higher than the index of the precorneal fluid (1.49 to 1.336 or 1.3375). The secondary curve radius is always flatter than the base curve radius. As a result of these two factors, there is more plus power in the secondary area than in the optic zone. There is also a prismatic element with its base toward the center of the lens.

This dual optical system produces two images. The clear one is produced by the optic zone; and the blurred, displaced one is produced by the secondary zone. When the secondary zone covers a considerable area of the pupil, flare or even monocular diplopia is produced. When only the extreme peripheral part of the pupil is covered by the secondary zone, often there is no flare. The direction of the flare or diplopia is opposite to the decentered position of the lens on the eye. At times flare is produced when the anterior curvature of the lens is aberrated.

Poor Lens Positioning

Poor positioning may cause flare or monocular diplopia. Contact lenses also often tilt on the cornea, introducing an undesired spherical and astigmatic component.[313, 314]

MANUFACTURING

General Procedures

Polymethyl methacrylate lenses fabricated under proper manufacturing procedures meet the high tolerances necessary for contact lens application. Contact lenses are manufactured by molding or lathe cutting. The four general types of molding are injection, casting, compression, and sheet forming.

In injection molding, plastic is liquefied by heat and injected at high pressure into a mold having the desired curvatures. Cooling then causes the plastic to solidify, thus forming the lens. Because cooling is accompanied by shrinkage, compensation must be made in the molds or lens warpage may result.

In casting, liquid plastic is freely poured into a mold, and it is chemically or thermally cured. Compensation must be made for possible shrinkage during curing.

In compression molding, plastic powder is put into a mold. Pressure and heat are applied until the mold is filled. Cooling then causes the plastic to solidify into a lens. There is less tendency for shrinkage in this method.

In sheet forming, a softened plastic sheet is pressed against dies of desired curvatures, and heat and pressure are applied. Cooling causes the plastic to solidify. Because of "plastic memory," such lenses often tend to flatten.

Strict manufacturing control can produce good molded contact lenses. Most contact lenses, however, are produced by lathe cutting. Generally, the lathe cutting procedure includes the following steps (Fig. 8–31): (1) A blank is mounted in a holder and placed on a lathe, or radius-turning machine. (2) The base curve is cut—that is, turned or generated. (3) The blank is placed on a polishing machine, and the base curve is polished with convex laps. (4) Secondary curves then may be applied to the resultant semifinished blank. (5) The base curve of the semifinished blank is mounted on a convex arbor, which is placed on a lathe. (6) The properly computed anterior curvature is cut to the proper center thickness. (7) The lens is placed on a polishing machine, and the anterior curvature is polished with concave laps. (8) The resultant uncut lens is reduced to proper lens diameter. (9) If secondary curves were not applied to the semifinished blank, they are now applied. (10) The lens is edged. (11) The lens is inspected and verified.

Equipment

The basic equipment for producing an uncut lens includes plastic blanks, means for mounting the plastic on the machines, lathes to cut the curves, and polishing machines to polish the curves.

Plastic blanks have plano surfaces and are cut from plastic rods (Fig.

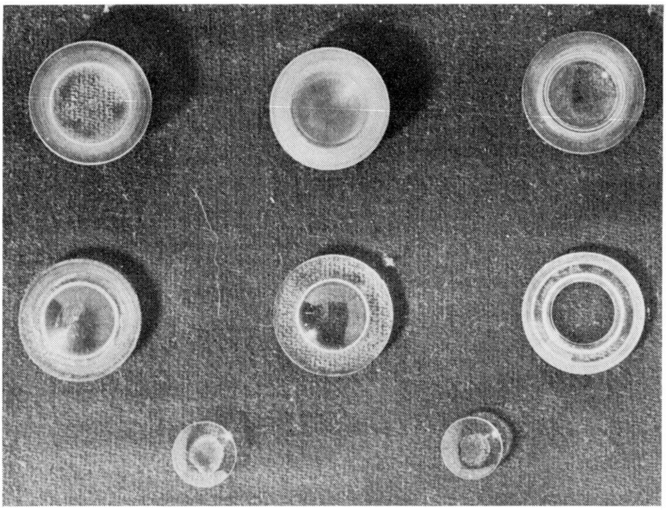

Figure 8–31. Steps in manufacturing procedure. Top row, left to right, *Blank, base curve generated, and base curve polished.* Middle row, *Anterior curve generated, anterior curve polished, and uncut lens punched out.* Bottom row, *uncut lens and finished lens.*

8–32). Blanks are often 11 to 13 mm. in diameter and 3.50 to 5.00 mm. thick. Two commonly used standard diameters are 11.4 and 12.7 mm.

Blanks are mounted in collets or on arbors. Collets may be split and open, or solid and closed. Arbors are steel buttons with flat or convex surfaces (Fig. 8–33). When the base curve is cut, the blank is mounted either in a collet or on a flat arbor. Tightening the collet onto the spindle of the lathe

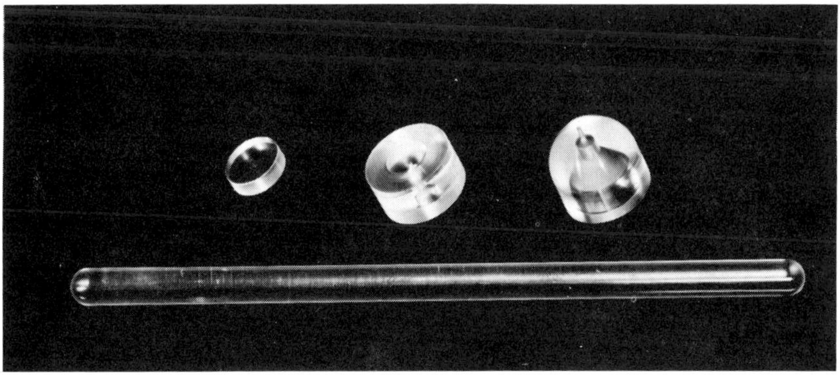

Figure 8–32. Plastic for making lenses. Top row, left to right, *Lens blank, concave mold, and convex mold.* Bottom row, *Centering rod.* (Figs. 8–32 to 8–34 courtesy of Louis Levin & Son, Inc.)

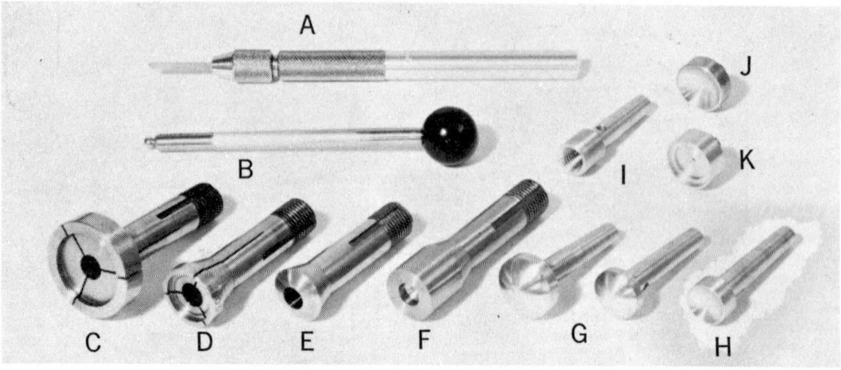

Figure 8–33. Accessories for making lenses. A, *Hand-turning graver and holder.* B, *Ball shank.* C, ¾ *inch collet.* D, ½ *inch collet.* E, *Taper collet.* F, *Flat pad.* G, *Convex lap.* H, *Turning arbor.* I, *Holder for concave laps.* J, *Concave lap.* K, *Cup holder.*

simultaneously secures the blank in the collet head. The blank is secured and centered on a flat arbor with melted wax, which is allowed to cool. When the anterior curve is cut, the base curve of the semifinished blank is mounted with wax or pitch on a convex arbor with the same radius as the base curve.

A contact lens lathe has a diamond cutter and two gauges. One gauge monitors the radius of the cut, and the other monitors the depth of the cut. The lathe also has a variable-speed rotating spindle on which the collet or arbor is placed (Figs. 8–34 and 8–35).

Polishing is done on concave or convex laps the surfaces of which are coated with pitch or made of wax (Fig. 8–33). A pitch lap is curved with the proper concave or convex mold (Fig. 8–32). A wax lap is curved with a lathe or a template.

The following section is an introductory overview of the manufacturing procedure. Each manufacturer, however, develops his own detailed technique in terms of his needs and specific equipment.

Cutting the Base Curve

Before a curvature is cut, the cutter is checked for sharpness and centration. Dull or improperly centered cutters do not generate true surfaces. Surfaces of the spindle and collet or arbor should be checked to make sure they are clean. Small particles between spindle and holder produce misalignment and untrue surfaces.

The radius gauge is appropriately set, and the collet or arbor holding the blank is placed on the spindle. If a collet is tightened too much, stress on the blank may result, possibly producing untrue surfaces. For volume production, a collet closer to control tension is used.

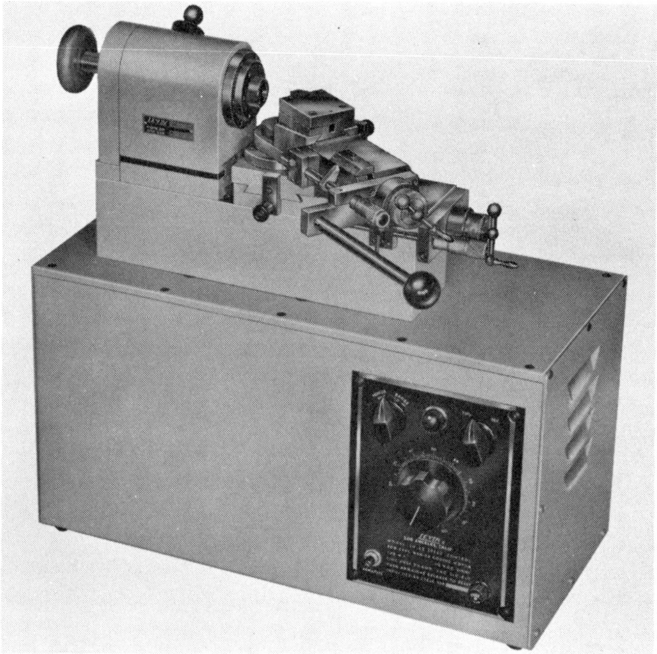

Figure 8–34. Contact lens lathe.

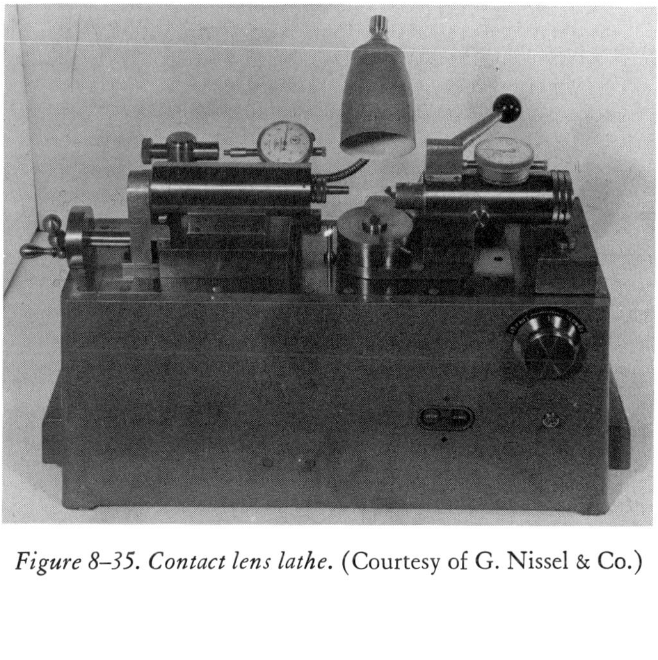

Figure 8–35. Contact lens lathe. (Courtesy of G. Nissel & Co.)

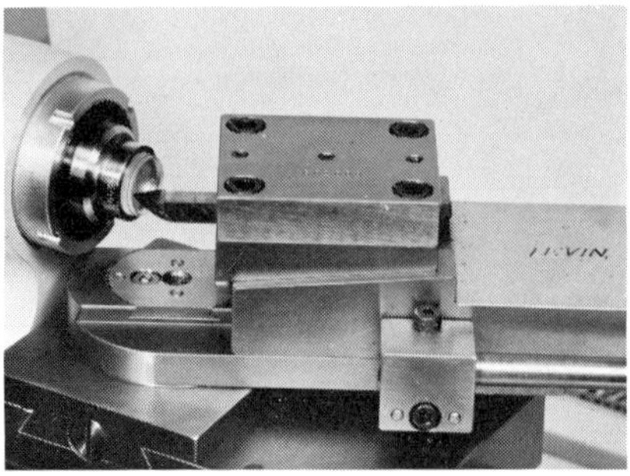

Figure 8–36. Cutting the base curve. (Figs. 8–36 to 8–38 courtesy of Louis Levin & Son, Inc.)

The cutting edge is brought into contact with the blank, and the depth gauge is set at zero. The cutter is withdrawn, the machine is turned on at a high speed, and the cutter is brought into contact with the periphery of the exposed surface of the blank. Light, slow, even strokes about 0.15 mm. deep are taken from one edge of the blank to other. Heavy, uneven, fast, or deep cuts produce excessive heat and poor surfaces. A liquid coolant may be used to prevent excessive surface heat. The final cut is 0.03 to 0.05 mm. deep (Fig. 8–36).

Polishing the Base Curve

Polishing may be done either manually or automatically. A pitch-coated or wax convex lap with a radius equal to the base curve radius is selected and placed on the spindle of the polishing machine. The plano side of the blank is placed in an appropriate holder, or it is left on the steel button or chuck. In manual polishing, a scribe or ball shank holder is inserted into the opening on the back of the blank holder (Fig. 8–33). In automatic pol-

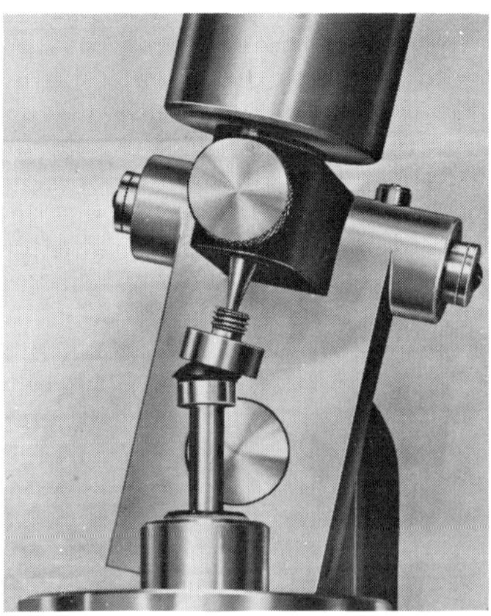

Figure 8–37. Polishing anterior curve automatically.

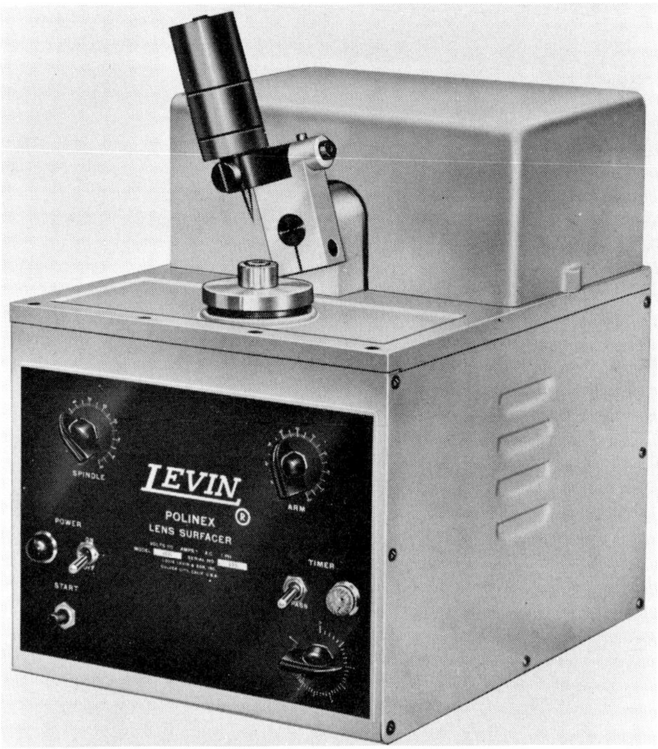

Figure 8–38. Automatic polishing machine.

ishing, the top part of the machine holds the blank holder against the lap (Figs. 8–37 to 8–39). During the polishing procedure, the blank is moved across the lap, and both the lap and blank holder rotate. The lap is continually moistened with polishing compound, and the lens is polished to the proper finish. Polishing takes approximately 2 to 3 minutes.

Manufacturers usually maintain a stock of semifinished lenses with the standard range of base curves. Orders are then more quickly processed.

Secondary Curve Fabrication on Semifinished Blank

Secondary curves may be placed on the relatively thick semifinished blank, which is much less flexible than a thin uncut lens. Unless lens flexibility is slight, secondary curves cannot be fabricated properly. After the curves are cut, they are polished with laps the surfaces of which are covered with tape, pitch, or wax. Pitch or wax polishing produces better surfaces. Secondary curves can be generated by the use of this combination of cutting and polishing or solely by the polishing procedure. Aspherical secondary curves—that is, elliptical, parabolic, or hyperbolic curves—can be generated by the use of special equipment.

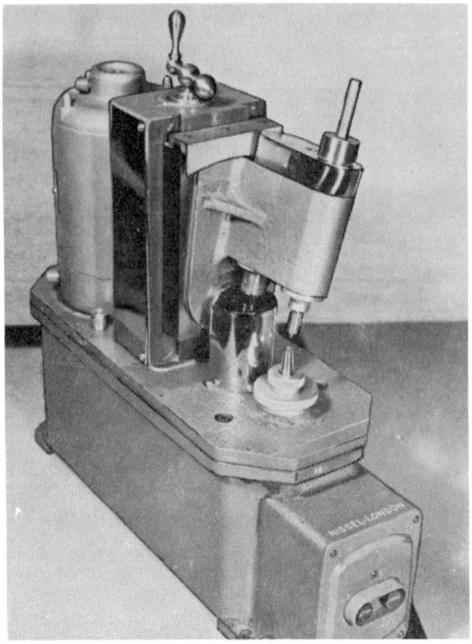

Figure 8–39. Automatic polishing machine. (Courtesy of G. Nissel & Co.)

Cutting Anterior Curve and Center Thickness

The base curve and refractive power are ordered by the practitioner. Center thickness is also ordered by the practitioner, or standard center thickness may be used. The manufacturer must compute the anterior curvature that, combined with the base curve, center thickness, and refractive index, produces the desired posterior vertex refractive power. This computation is done by using the thick lens equations, by using a special slide rule, or by using the anterior surface radius table (Appendix VII).

Center thickness of the semifinished blank is measured, and the desired center thickness is subtracted from this value. The difference is the depth of the plastic that must be removed. The base curve of the semifinished blank is mounted and centered with wax or pitch on a convex arbor with a radius equal to that of the base curve. The arbor is placed on the spindle of the lathe, and it is often held in a taper collet (Fig. 8–33).

The radius gauge is set. The cutting edge is brought into contact with the exposed plano surface of the mounted semifinished blank, and the depth gauge is set at zero. The depth gauge is turned to the depth of plastic that must be removed to produce desired center thickness. Cutting is done as it is in fabricating the base curve.

Polishing the Anterior Curve

The anterior curve is polished in the same manner the base curve is (Fig. 8–37). Concave polishing laps are used (Fig. 8–33).

Additional Procedures

If secondary curvatures are not fabricated on the semifinished blank, they are fabricated on the uncut lens. Lens support and application of pressure must be critically controlled so that the thin uncut lens does not flex. Such flexing would result in improper secondary curves. The sequence of steps in the production of a finished lens from an uncut lens is the same as discussed on page 164. As mentioned, some manufacturers modify lens diameter with a lathe and edge the lens automatically.

Prism is fabricated by inclining the flat front surface of the semifinished blank with the axis of the lathe at an angle equal to the desired amount of prism. Anterior curvature is then fabricated in the usual manner.

Toric surfaces are best produced by the use of toric generators. It is also possible to bend and mount a thin blank over a tool having the desired toricity. A spherical surface is cut and polished. When the lens is removed from the toric arbor, it assumes a toric shape.

Anterior lenticulars are produced by the use of a peripheral anterior curve that differs from the central anterior curve. Thickness at the juncture of these anterior curvatures should be about 0.13–0.15 mm. for plus lenses.

Multiannular bifocal contact lenses are produced with the use of a special lathe (Fig. 8–40).

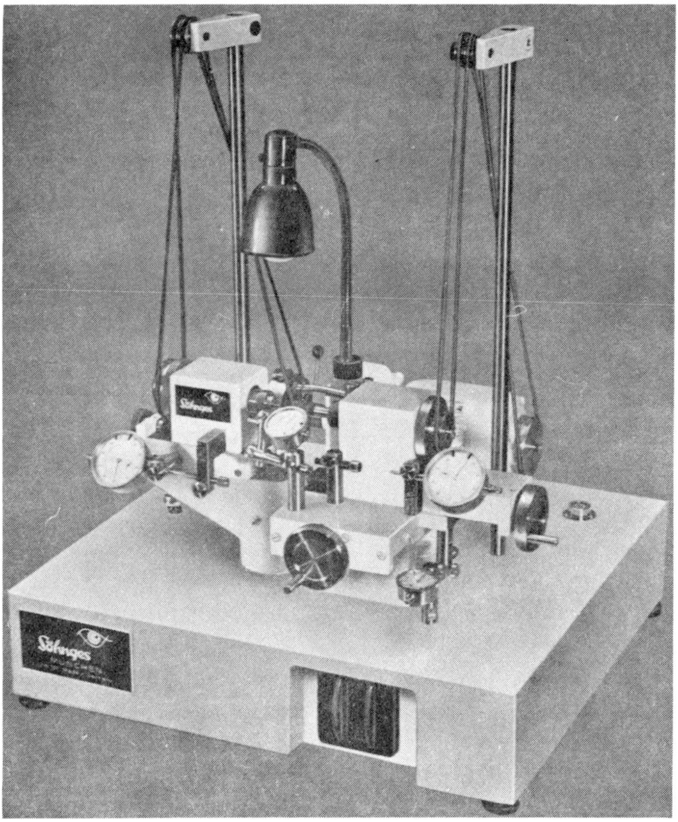

Figure 8–40. Special lathe for cutting multiannular bifocal contact lenses.
(Courtesy of Wilhelm Peter Söhnges)

9

The Cornea and Contact Lenses

Considerable research has been done on the cornea. Owing in part to the interest in fitting contact lenses, the amount of such research is increasing. In spite of this fact, there remains a great deal that is not completely understood.

So much has been written on the cornea that this book cannot possibly include a complete discussion. However, the authors present herein the factors most pertinent to contact lens fitting. The discussion is divided into five general sections: topography, anatomy, physiology, auxiliary mechanisms, and transparency.

CORNEAL TOPOGRAPHY

The following are the only factual generalizations that can be made about corneal topography: It is convex, aspheric, and smooth, and it tends to flatten from center to periphery.[315] There are probably two basic reasons why so little is known about corneal topography. First, the known information is satisfactory for most clinical needs. Unfortunately, it is not entirely satisfactory for contact lens fitting. Second, the measuring procedures used on this complex surface are somewhat inaccurate or invalid.

General methods of determining corneal topography include a direct measurement of the topography, and an indirect measurement with the use of a cast or photograph of the topography.[316] Additional discussion of corneal topography may be found on page 27.

Direct Measurement

Ophthalmometry (Keratometry). This is the most commonly used clinical procedure (p. 323).

Keratoscopy (Use of Placido's Disk). Placido's disk, with alternate white and black concentric circles, is held in front of the examiner's eye so he is able to look through a small central hole in the disk (Fig. 9–1). Light is reflected off the disk into the patient's eye, and images are reflected from the cornea. This is a gross procedure.

Indirect Measurement

Photokeratoscopy. Keratoscopy gives more refined data when the corneal image is photographed and analyzed.[317] This method is called photokeratoscopy. A photokeratoscope consists of a disk with about ten concentric rings cut out. The photokeratoscope measures the curvature only in about ten points on the cornea in a given meridian. These points correspond to the reflection areas of the ten rings. The width of each ring and the separation between the rings is known from construction. A light source behind the disk produces a sufficiently intense image of it to be photographed. The camera is mounted in an opening in the center of the disk (Figs. 9–2 and 9–3).

The corneal image is photographed, and the size or separations of the rings on the photograph are measured. Analysis is based on a principle similar to that used in ophthalmometry. The sizes and separations of the rings of the disk and photograph (object and image) are related by formulas, and the curvature is determined.

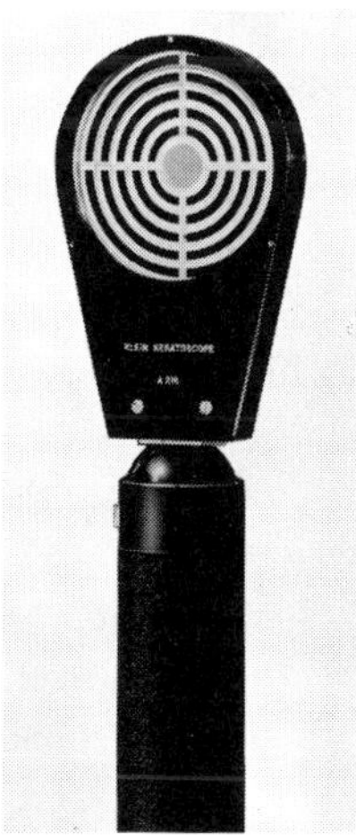

Figure 9–1. A handheld keratoscope. (Courtesy of House of Vision, Inc.)

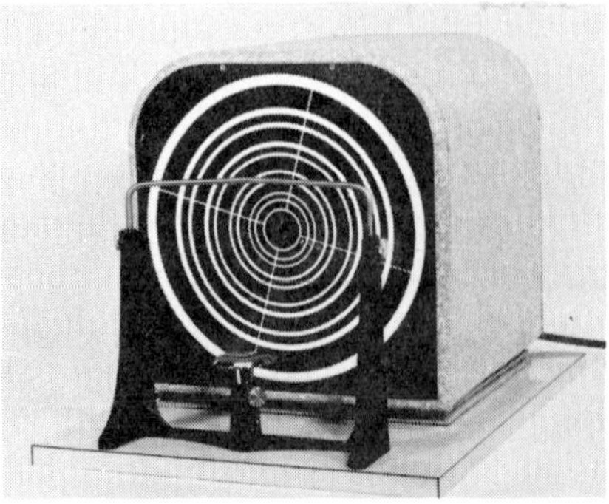

Figure 9–2. Front view of photokeratoscope. (Courtesy of Plastic Contact Lens Co.)

The size or separation of the photograph rings is measured visually or with an electronic scanning device. Visual measurement is inaccurate. When an electronic scanning device is used, the procedure is termed photoelectronic keratoscopy (P.E.K.).[318] Even with a scanning device, accuracy or repeatability of measurement may be less than that obtained with the use of ophthalmometry for central corneal readings.

There are several possible reasons for this. First, camera focus must be critical or blurred borders are produced. The photographic film and development also must meet extremely high standards or blurred borders are produced. Second, most photokeratoscopes have flat disks. Because the cornea is a curved surface, a significant error is introduced beyond the central 6 to 7 mm. of the cornea. Hemispherical or cylindrical disks can be used to

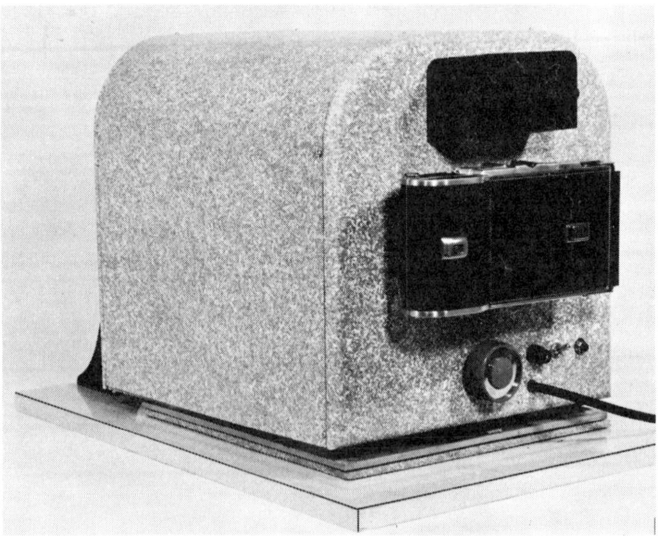

Figure 9–3. Rear view of photokeratoscope showing camera. (Courtesy of Plastic Contact Lens Co.)

eliminate this problem. Third, the corneal principal meridians can be found with the use of the photokeratoscope only by the scanning of all meridians. This is an extremely lengthy procedure. The principal meridians must be known, and they are usually determined by ophthalmometry. Fourth, impractical levels of magnification may be necessary.

Use of Casts. A cast of the cornea may be made, which is then either directly matched to templates of known radii, or a photograph of the cast is matched to templates. There are several significant sources of error in this procedure. An inaccurate cast may be produced owing to corneal compressibility; also the photograph may have blurred borders, or it may be difficult to match curves of small chord values.

Stereophotogrammetry. A stereoscopic photograph is taken of an anesthetized cornea covered with talcum powder. Then the corneal topography is determined by the same stereophotogrammetric methods used in aerial photography of geographic topography.[319, 320]

Diagnostic Lenses

Diagnostic lenses may be used to match curvatures for given chords (p. 76).

ANATOMY

Physical Structure

Classically, the five accepted layers of the cornea from anterior to posterior are stratified squamous epithelium, Bowman's membrane, substantia propria (stroma), Descemet's membrane, and endothelium. It has been suggested that another layer exists in the form of a membrane between the basal layer of the epithelium and Bowman's membrane.[321] It has also been suggested that from a chemical standpoint the cornea may be considered to have only three layers.[322] This suggestion is based on fact that the chemical composition of Bowman's membrane is similar to that of the substantia propria, and that of the endothelium is similar to the epithelium. The basal membrane of the epithelium, the collagen (a gelatin-like protein) and mucoid content of the stroma, and the endothelium are of special interest.

Epithelium. Corneal epithelium is composed of five layers of cells. The basal cells are internal, resting on Bowman's membrane. These basal cells are rich in the glucose and oxygen necessary for normal metabolism.[323] This reserve supply of oxygen and glucose is adequate to maintain proper metabolism for limited periods. When this reserve is consumed, it must be replenished or normal metabolism is disrupted.[324]

Basal cells are also the germinal cells of the epithelium.[325] They provide for normal cellular replacement and cellular replacement for repair. The walls of basal cells differ histologically from the walls of the cells in the other corneal layers, and it has been suggested that they are a separate layer. Most of the oxygen uptake of the cornea is done through the epithelium and endothelium. The stroma has relatively little oxygen uptake.[326] The metabolic rate and activity of the epithelium (and probably also the endothelium) is therefore relatively high compared to that of the stroma.

Much of corneal metabolism occurs in the epithelium.[327] Both the epithelium and the stroma are capable of performing the glycolytic phase of metabolism. However, only the epithelium is capable of performing the respiratory phase.[328] The stroma uses glucose to produce lactic acid, which is transferred to and utilized by the epithelium to complete the metabolic cycle.[329] If the function of the epithelium is hindered, lactic acid accumulates in the stroma and around the basal epithelial cells, thus altering normal metabolism, turgescence, and transparency.

STROMA. The stroma (substantia propria) is composed of interlaced lamellae that run the length of the cornea and the planes of which are nearly parallel to the surface.[330] Each lamella consists of many tiny fibrils. The lamellae are composed principally of collagen surrounded by a mucoid substance. Spaces between the lamellae and fibrils are filled with this mucoid substance, which is similar to aqueous.[331] There appears to be a continuous gradient in the refractive index of each fiber to the surrounding media.[332] The structure of the lattice of the collagen is unusual, and the fibrils are tightly packed, thus enhancing corneal transparency.[333] Any excessive pressure or mechanical irritation that alters the fibril pattern will cause loss of corneal transparency.

The ability of the cornea to absorb fluid is basically due to the collagen and mucoids, which are interrelated.[334] The turgescence, and therefore the transparency, of the cornea is affected by any variation of these substances.

ENDOTHELIUM. This single layer of cells seems to be extremely important. It is known that disease of, or injury to the endothelium results in turgescence and loss of transparency.

CHEMICAL COMPOSITION

The principal constituents of the cornea are water and collagen. One study indicates that the cornea is 81.1 per cent water and 18.9 per cent solids (18.4 per cent collagen and 0.5 per cent inorganic matter, albumin and globulin, water-soluble extractives, lipids, and nucleic acid).[335] These substances have definite relationships to hydration and edema, permeability, metabolic problems, and repair.

The percentage of each substance is critical. It has been suggested that if the water content of the cornea were reduced to that of the sclera (about 65 per cent), the cornea would become opaque.

Each of the layers of the cornea differs somewhat in its chemical composition. For example, the epithelium has a higher content of nucleoproteins, lipids, and ascorbic acid than the substantia propria, but it has less collagen.[336] These differences help account for the unique function of each of the layers.

Innervation and Sensibility

The nonmedullated ciliary nerves from the ophthalmic division of the fifth cranial (trigeminal) nerve richly supply the cornea. After becoming unmyelinated, the free nerve endings extend between the epithelial cells. The resulting extreme sensitivity of the cornea serves to protect it, thus aiding the maintenance of transparency.[337] Interference with the nerve impulses by peripheral stimulation alters corneal metabolism, turgescence, and transparency.[338]

The cornea is extremely sensitive to pain. This sensitivity increases from the periphery to the center in a manner similar to the distribution of the nerve endings.[339] Whether the cornea is truly sensitive of touch has been much discussed. It is now generally felt that it is.[340]

A foreign body produces either a sensation of touch or pain on the cornea, depending on the intensity of the stimulation. A contact lens may be felt on the cornea even if the sensation is not pain. Research indicates that corneal sensitivity decreases with contact lens wear, and that people whose sensitivity is initially lower than average accept contact lenses more readily.[341]

The close association between the nuclei of the fifth cranial nerve and other cranial nerves accounts for reflex weeping, which is often seen during adaptation to contact lenses.[342] Photophobia is related to superficial corneal disturbances. The more superficial the disturbance is, the more intense the photophobia is, owing to the superficial arrangement of the corneal nerves.[343]

PHYSIOLOGY

Nutrition

Nutrition is the process of supplying cells with the food units necessary for their growth, formation, or maintenance. The cornea is nourished by the precorneal fluid, the fluid of the anterior chamber, and the capillary network surrounding the limbus.[344] Although the precise relative importance of each of these pathways is uncertain, the combination brings sufficient nutrients to support adequate metabolism under ordinary circumstances. Research indicates that the lacrimal secretion and fluid of the anterior chamber are more important than the perilimbal plexus in this process.[345–347]

Metabolism

Metabolism is the process in an organism or single cell by which the nutritive material is transformed into living matter (anabolism) and by which it breaks down into simpler substances (katabolism) to perform special functions. It involves all the chemical processes connected with the growth of the tissues, heat production of the tissues, energy supply for the activities of the tissues, and repair of the tissues. In the cornea, metabolism helps to provide for the unique transparency. Corneal metabolism somewhat depends on and is influenced by that of the rest of the body.

Corneal metabolism is probably an intermediate type in which glucose and similar substances are broken down.[348] Two general processes are involved in the breakdown of glucose: glycolysis, in which the molecule is reduced to lactic or pyruvic acids; and respiration, in which lactic acid is oxidized into carbon dioxide and water.

Glycolysis may take place in the presence of oxygen (aerobic glycolysis) or without oxygen (anaerobic glycolysis). Respiration, however, depends on oxygen, which is actively engaged in the reaction. When the oxygen supply to the cornea is insufficient, metabolism is incomplete. The reaction of glucose with oxygen does not result in water, *carbon dioxide,* energy, and heat. It results in water, *lactic acid,* energy, and heat. The energy released is relatively insufficient, unless an excess of glucose is used. If the oxygen supply is insufficient, the excess of lactic acid formed and the glucose used affect basal epithelial cell function. If the reaction is complete, carbon dioxide and heat must be removed from the cornea.

How does the cornea receive its adequate supply of oxygen? It is believed that oxygen is received from the limbal capillaries, the aqueous, and the atmosphere.[349] There has been considerable discussion as to whether atmospheric oxygen is essential. It is believed that corneal metabolism can function normally without atmospheric oxygen for limited periods, such as during sleep. However, metabolism is disrupted if the cornea is almost always cut off from the atmospheric supply of oxygen. This disruption may result in an alteration of the transparency of the cornea. It has even been suggested that, because the cornea is cut off from atmospheric oxygen during sleep, the cornea normally is slightly edematous during sleep.[350]

Permeability

Permeability is the quality or state of the tissues that permits substances (usually fluids or gases) to enter, exit, or spread throughout those tissues. The cornea obviously must have a certain selective permeability to retain its deturgescent state. If this were not so, the aqueous humor, for example, would be able to diffuse through the cornea and evaporate at the surface, producing considerable depletion.

A theory that was long accepted is that the cornea is only unidirectionally permeable to fluids, from exterior to interior.[351] It is now believed that the cornea is permeable to both water and salts (ions) in both directions, but that the epithelium and endothelium are less permeable to salts than is the stroma.[352]

Three general theories have been propounded to account for the permeability of any membrane. The one that seems to apply most adequately to the cornea is the *theory of solubility.*[353, 354] This theory implies that the cornea is a membrane containing a series of solvents that permit passage of only those substances having the necessary solubility in a given layer. Accordingly, the stroma permits passage of substances soluble in water; the epithelium permits passage of substances soluble in fats; and any substance that passes through both the epithelium and stroma must be soluble in both water and fats.[355] Water itself seems to be an exception, for it passes through both the epithelium and stroma.[356] It also should be noted that injuries to a specific tissue apparently alter permeability. For example, injury to the epithelium makes it less permeable to fat-soluble substances and more permeable to water-soluble substances.[357] It has been found that permeability of the epithelium is related to the nervous system. Irritation of the trigeminal nerve seems to increase the water content of the epithelium.[358]

Turgescence

Turgescence is simply a relative swelling of a tissue. The cornea is in a relatively deturgescent state, containing less water than it is capable of accepting from distilled water or salt solutions. This deturgescence is critical to the maintenance of transparency. The cornea tends to absorb water, mainly through the collagen content of the stroma.[359] There must be some means by which this tendency is neutralized to keep the cornea in its relatively deturgescent state. Several theories have been postulated to account for the deturgescence of the cornea. There is no general agreement as to which theory is correct.

It may be advisable at this point, before discussing the first of these theories, to review several elementary definitions. *Osmosis* is the interchange of two fluids of different concentrations through a semipermeable membrane. The fluid flows in the direction of the more concentrated solution, thus equalizing the concentration of the two solutions. *Hypotonic* refers to the less concentrated solution and *hypertonic* to the more concentrated solution. *Isotonic* refers to an equilibrium of the two solutions. The *osmotic pressure* is determined by the rate of flow.

One theory used to explain the deturgescence of the cornea is the *osmotic pump* theory.[360] It states that, because the epithelium and endothelium are impermeable to salts (a point now in question), a difference in osmotic pressure is established between fluids on either side of the cornea and that in the stroma. The hypertonic salt solutions in the case of the cornea, according to this theory, are the tears and the aqueous relative to the stroma. (It is now felt by some that the osmotic pressure of the tears and aqueous is not greater than that of the stroma.)[361] Fluid is thus being drained from the stroma, resulting in an isotonic condition, with the fluid constantly entering the stroma from the limbal capillaries. The equilibrium resulting from these processes keeps the cornea in its state of relative deturgescence, and therefore maintains its transparency. In this theory, it is further propounded that the cornea is transparent because the refractive indices of its elements are approximately the same. Recent work contradicts this contention. Although there may be an osmotic factor involved in maintaining the state of deturgescence, it now is not considered the sole factor.

Another theory is that of the *metabolic* or *physiologic pump*.[362–367] Experiments altering corneal metabolism also alter corneal turgescence, indicating the existence of a metabolic pump. Although the exact nature, structure, and location of this mechanism are unknown, this theory is generally more accepted than that of the osmotic pump. Glycolysis in the presence of air (aerobic glycolysis) and related to the metabolism of the epithelium and endothelium are believed to activate the pump. When oxygen is insufficient (anaerobia), metabolism is incomplete, and the resultant impairment of the metabolic pump increases the turgescence of the cornea. The pump may be located in the endothelium rather than the epithelium, because it has been shown that the epithelium can be destroyed without affecting the pump action.

Maintenance of the cornea in its relatively deturgescent state is necessary for retention of corneal transparency. Clinically, edema as a manifestation of faulty deturgescence is extremely significant. It is possible to have either epithelial, endothelial, or stromal edema, or any combination of these. Epithelial edema is usually the type involved in contact lens fitting.

AUXILIARY MECHANISMS

Regeneration

Superficial corneal lesions heal relatively quickly. A small epithelial abrasion may be completely healed in three hours, moderate ones in about one day, and larger ones in three days.[368]

Epithelial healing takes place in two stages: cells migrate to the abraded area; then the cells undergo mitosis until the area has returned to normal.[369]

Many medications used on the cornea interfere with the healing of the abrasion, either by impeding migration of the cells or, more frequently, by impeding the mitotic activity of the cells.[370] It is believed that natural healing is often best; but care must be taken, of course, to relieve discomfort and to ensure that no infection is setting in.

Vascularization

The cornea is an avascular structure unless there is interference with its normal processes. If corneal vascularization does develop, it apparently is a result of such interference coupled with a need for supplementary oxygen and nutrients supplied by the bloodstream.[371] This additional blood supply is obtained in two ways—through an injection of the normal limbal vessels (pericorneal injection), and through formation of new vessels on the cornea proper (neoformation).[372] It has been suggested that edema is the primary stimulus in these types of vascularization.[373]

TRANSPARENCY

Transparency is the primary requirement of a useful cornea. It results from and is maintained by the unique structure and physiologic processes of the cornea. Anatomic peculiarities of the cornea that contribute to transparency include the regularity and arrangement of the epithelial cells, the uniform size and parallel structure of the lamellae of the stroma, the absence of blood vessels, and the integrity of the endothelium.

It may be said in relation to the metabolic pump theory that if the normal structure of the fibers becomes disarranged or if the refractive indices of the elements are altered, the cornea will lose its transparency. Both fiber arrangement and refractive index depend in part on the corneal deturgescence, which is achieved mainly by a metabolic process dependent on a sufficient supply of atmospheric oxygen.

10

Ocular Pathology and Contact Lenses

For simplicity, ocular disorders may be considered in seven categories: inflammations, degenerative disease, injuries, structural and positional anomalies, neoplasms, general disorders, and symptomatic disorders. The more important disorders in terms of contact lens application are considered under each category.[374–383] A general guide to the relationship of contact lenses and pathologic disorders of the eye may be found on page 10.

INFLAMMATION

Eyelid

Blepharitis, chalazion, dermatitis, hordeolum, and meibomianitis are the most common eyelid inflammations. By direct touch, a contact lens may aggravate these conditions. In addition, the symptoms, signs, temporary tissue changes, and at times the related exudates from these inflammations complicate contact lens fitting. Eyelid inflammations should be cured before the fitting is started. If there is a history of frequent recurrences, the advisability of contact lens application is decreased.

Conjunctiva

Any bacterial, viral, or fungal conjunctivitis should be cured before contact lenses are applied. After trachoma—a viral conjunctivitis—is cured, scleral contact lenses may be indicated to protect the cornea from the abrasive action of the residual scar tissue on the lids.

Allergic conjunctivitis associated with hay fever or vernal conjunctivitis is usually seasonal. Contact lenses should not be fitted during an episode. Because seasonal recurrences are typical, the patient should be informed that during an episode contact lens wear may be less comfortable or may have to be temporarily discontinued.

Chemical conjunctivitis should generally be cured before contact lenses are applied. The exception to this recommendation is related to the fact that some chemically caused cases of conjunctivitis are complicated by an adhesion between the bulbar and palpebral conjunctiva (a symblepharon). At times, a scleral contact lens is used to produce a physical barrier to the development of a symblepharon. Whenever it is possible, the causative agent should be removed from the patient's environment to prevent recurrence. Often the causative agent is related to the patient's occupation and cannot be eliminated. Under such conditions, contact lenses should not be fitted.

Metabolic conjunctivitis (keratoconjunctivitis sicca, Sjögrens syndrome) is a chronic condition marked by reduced lacrimal secretion. Usually, this reduced secretion contraindicates contact lens application. An exception involves the treatment, which is usually by means of periodic introduction of artificial tears and saline irrigations to supplement the reduced natural secretion. At times, a fluid scleral lens may be used to supplement the normal secretion.

Cornea

All suppurative and nonsuppurative keratitis is important in terms of contact lens application. Any keratitis must be cured completely before contact lenses are considered. If contact lenses are fitted, great care and close supervision must be used. Once a person has had keratitis, there is susceptibility to recurrence. The contact lens may act as an exciting agent in the recurrence of keratitis.

Because they are more common or more significant, several types of suppurative keratitis (corneal ulcers, lagophthalmic keratitis, and neuroparalytic keratitis) and several types of nonsuppurative keratitis (interstitial keratitis, pannus or vasculonebulous keratitis, and keratitic precipitates) are discussed separately.

Two excitatory causes of corneal ulcers are trauma and disturbances to corneal nutrition, which may result from the use of contact lenses. Fitting a contact lens to an eye that has had a corneal ulcer should be approached with great caution. Usually, such eyes should be fitted with contact lenses only if visual performance is significantly better with them than with spectacles. Contact lenses may produce superior vision because of the residual scar tissue or irregular astigmatism from the ulcer.

The cause of lagophthalmic keratitis is excessive corneal exposure due to incomplete lid closure. General contact lens fitting should not be tried until proper lid closure is established. However, a fluid scleral lens may be used as a therapeutic measure to retard dehydration.

Neuroparalytic keratitis is due to paralysis of the trigeminal nerve or disease or removal of the Gasserian ganglion. The loss of corneal sensation decreases the patient's ability to appreciate undesired changes in the cornea. Because of this factor and the permanency of the condition, contact lens application is usually not advisable.

Interstitial keratitis must be cured before contact lenses are considered. They then may be considered to replace any resultant irregular anterior corneal surface. It is believed that contact lens application will not cause recurrence of the basic lesion.

After the infiltration of the cornea with new blood vessels in pannus, the channels remain, even though the primary pathologic condition is cured and the blood leaves the channels. A subsequent corneal disorder or irritation can result in the rapid recurrence of pannus through the old channels. Pannus, past or present, thus contraindicates the use of contact lenses. The major exception is in the case of trachoma. Pannus is often a complication of trachoma; use of a scleral lens may be indicated after trachoma to protect the cornea from residual scar tissue on the lid.

The dotlike precipitates on the corneal endothelium (keratic precipitates) may result from exudates from uveitis. Such conditions are discussed on page 381.

Sclera

Contact lenses should not be considered until episcleritis is cured. Then corneal rather than scleral lenses are preferable. Because scleritis is a prolonged disorder and the consequences are serious, contact lenses are usually contraindicated.

Lacrimal System

Dacryocystitis—inflammation of the lacrimal sac—is usually caused by an obstruction in the nasal duct. After the obstruction is cleared, contact lenses may be fitted. Care must be used because corneal ulcers occasionally result from trauma in the presence of pneumococcal dacryocystitis.

Canaliculitis is usually caused by an obstruction. The obstruction should be cleared before contact lenses are applied. Dacryoadenitis—inflammation of a lacrimal gland—is rare, but it should be cured before contact lenses are applied.

Orbit

Orbital cellulitis, orbital periostitis, and cavernous sinus thrombosis are the most frequent orbital inflammations. In general, complications from these inflammations may be severe, and contact lenses are contraindicated.

Uveal Tract

Iritis must be cured for at least three months before contact lenses can be considered. The lens may cause further irritation or trauma, resulting in recurrence of iritis. Great care should be used in contact lens application in a patient who has a history of iritis. If the history indicates more than one episode, contact lens fitting is less advisable.

Cyclitis is frequently associated with iritis (iridocyclitis). This condition affects the use of contact lenses just as iritis does.

If choroiditis exists alone, contact lenses may be applied after the condition has been cured. Frequently, however, choroiditis is accompanied by iritis and cyclitis. This condition of the uveal tract is more like iritis and cyclitis in terms of its effect on contact lens application.

Retina and Optic Nerve

Contact lenses may be applied after retinitis or optic neuritis has been cured or controlled.

DEGENERATIVE DISEASES

Eyelids

Blepharochalasis usually results from aging or after chronic or recurrent edema of the eyelids. When it is a result of aging, contact lens application is not contraindicated. The related loss of tissue tonicity, however, may complicate such application. When blepharochalasis is a result of chronic or recurrent edema, it usually contraindicates contact lens application.

Conjunctiva

Pinguecula and pterygium are conjunctival degenerative disorders. Presence of a pinguecula does not contraindicate contact lens application when the yellowish raised area is away from the limbus. When this area is near the limbus, care must be taken to fit the lens so that it does not touch the pinguecula, or much discomfort may be produced. In addition, excessive irritation may cause a pinguecula to develop into a pterygium.

Pterygia are considered to be caused by prolonged, continued physical irritation, such as exposure to dust and wind. Contact lenses are contraindicated when an active pterygium is present because their use may contribute to such irritation. Furthermore, the growth area of the bulbar conjunctiva on the cornea vastly complicates contact lens fitting. Even after surgical removal, pterygia sometimes recur. The physical irritation of the contact lens may be an excitatory factor in recurrence. When contact lenses are applied after a pterygium has been surgically removed, great care must be taken. Indications of recurrence usually suggest discontinuance of contact lens wear.

Cornea

Corneal degenerative disorders may be considered in three groups for our purposes: keratoconus and keratoglobus, arcus senilis and arcus juvenilis, and others.

Contact lenses application in keratoconus and keratoglobus is discussed on page 105. Contact lens application is not affected by arcus senilis or arcus juvenilis.

Contact lenses are generally contraindicated in any other corneal degenerative disorder. In such cases, the conditions are usually quite serious and progressive. Any tissue insult from a contact lens may complicate the condition considerably. If corneal degeneration progresses sufficiently, use of a corneal transplant may be necessary. Often transplantation results in an irregular corneal surface. Contact lenses may be indicated to provide a regular surface and satisfactory visual acuity.

Sclera

Hyaline degeneration does not contraindicate contact lens application. Corneal rather than scleral contact lenses may be preferable to minimize pressure on the scleral tissues.

Iris

Degenerative diseases of the iris may be considered in three groups for our purposes: those secondary to other ocular or systemic disorders, senile atrophy, and essential (progressive) atrophy.

When iris degeneration is secondary to other pathologic disorders, the primary disorder is usually serious, and tends to contraindicate contact lens application. Senile iris degeneration does not affect contact lens application. Essential atrophy usually leads to absolute glaucoma and complete visual loss. Fortunately, it is usually a unilateral condition, and contact lenses are contraindicated in the affected eye.

Ciliary Body

Senile degeneration or secondary degeneration of the ciliary body affects contact lens fitting the way that degeneration of the iris does.

Choroid

Degeneration of the choroid may be either primary or secondary to other pathologic disorders.

Primary degenerative disorders are usually quite serious. If the macula is affected, visual acuity is lowered considerably. If the peripheral choroid is involved, visual fields are reduced. Such degenerative disorders are often related to myopia and senility. Use of contact lenses probably would not affect the progress of degeneration, nor would the fitting of the contact lenses be complicated by the degenerative process to any great extent. Because visual performance will not be aided better by contact lenses than by spectacle lenses, the use of contact lenses depends on other factors in each case.

Secondary degeneration is often related to glaucoma, diabetes, or nephritis. The use of contact lenses when such conditions exist is discussed on page 387.

Lens

Cataract formation is a common ocular degenerative disorder. Contact lens application is quite valuable in postoperative aphakia (see p. 120).

Retina and Optic Nerve

Contact lenses probably do not affect the progress of retinal degeneration. Contact lens fitting is not complicated very much by retinal degeneration. However, visual performance probably is not aided better by contact lenses than by spectacles. Whether contact lenses should be applied to a person having retinal degeneration depends on the evaluation of other factors.

Optic atrophy may be primary or secondary. Primary atrophy usually results in total or partial amaurosis. Optic atrophy may be secondary to toxicity, glaucoma, retinitis, or circulatory or nutritional disturbances; and the use of contact lenses is related to the primary pathology.

INJURIES

Nonpenetrating Injuries

Nonpenetrating injuries of the eye—those that affect only the external eye—may be classed as abrasions, burns, contusions, or superficial foreign bodies. Such injuries should be properly treated and completely healed before contact lens application is considered. If the injury involves the cornea, great care must be used to detect any recurrence of erosion. Recurrent spontaneous abrasions are frequently related to scratches of the cornea, particularly from fingernails. At times, injuries to the cornea may leave a distorted or irregular surface. Contact lenses may be needed to provide an artificially regular surface so that satisfactory visual acuity is obtained. If the injury is to the sclera, corneal lenses are usually preferable to scleral lenses.

Penetrating Injuries

Penetrating injuries of the eye affect both the external and internal eye. They may be classed as lacerations and injuries involving intraocular foreign bodies. All penetrating injuries should be properly treated and completely healed before contact lenses are considered. Such injuries may be quite serious owing to initial trauma and the introduction of infection. The infection may cause a ring abscess of the cornea, posttraumatic iridocyclitis, or sympathetic ophthalmitis. If one of these secondary inflammations is present, contact lenses are generally contraindicated. If secondary inflammation is not present, great care must be used in contact lens application. If the cornea has been perforated, recurrent corneal erosion is a possibility. If the sclera has been perforated, corneal lenses are usually preferable to scleral lenses.

Postsurgical Injuries

Ocular surgical procedures may have two residual effects concerning contact lens application. Surgery done on or near the cornea may partially desensitize the area because of injury to the sensory nerve supply. This desensitization is common after cataract and corneal transplant operations. Desensitization decreases the patient's ability to appreciate undesired changes of the corneal tissue or the presence of a foreign body. If contact lenses are fitted, there is a need for frequent periodic examinations when desensitization has taken place.

Surgery may also change the topography of the eye by leaving areas of scar tissue or by causing an irregular surface. This change of topography is also common in cataract and corneal transplant operations. It may be somewhat difficult to establish a desired relationship between the posterior surface of a contact lens and the anterior surface of the cornea. Extraocular muscle surgery may leave scar tissue on the bulbar conjunctiva, thus complicating the fitting of a scleral contact lens. If the scar tissue is near the limbus, corneal contact lenses should be fitted so that they do not touch the scar tissue.

STRUCTURAL AND POSITIONAL ANOMALIES

Eyelids

Entropion—the turning inward of the lid margin—often causes irritation to the cornea or conjunctiva. Entropion may be caused by irritation due to keratitis, conjunctivitis, or loose skin (spastic entropion); it may also be caused by disease or injury of the tarsal and conjunctival portions of the lid (cicatricial entropion). Both entropion and its cause should be cured before contact lenses are applied. The advisability of contact lens fitting in light of the cause of the entropion should be carefully considered.

Trichiasis—the inversion of the eyelashes—is often associated with entropion. Trichiasis may also be caused by blepharitis or scars on the lid. The inverted lashes often irritate the eye, and they should be removed before contact lenses are applied.

At times it may be inadvisable to operate or otherwise treat entropion or trichiasis. In these instances, a scleral contact lens may be used to protect the cornea and conjunctiva from irritation by the lids and lashes.

Ectropion—the turning outward of the lid margin—causes epiphora and chronic exposure conjunctivitis, which complicate contact lens fitting. Ectropion should be cured before contact lens application.

Blepharoptosis—the drooping of the upper lid—may complicate corneal contact lens fitting because of narrowing of the palpebral aperture and excessive pressure on the contact lens. Blepharoptosis may be relatively more apparent in contact lens wear than in spectacle wear. Spectacles mask blepharoptosis somewhat, and a ptosis crutch may be incorporated. Because a scleral contact lens tends to widen the palpebral aperture, in blepharoptosis it produces a better cosmetic result than does a corneal contact lens. A special scleral contact lens with a superior ridge to support the upper lid can be used.

Coloboma usually occurs in the upper lid. It may complicate the fitting of a superior-positioned corneal contact lens because of poorer lens retention by the lid. This problem does not occur when aperture-positioning corneal or scleral contact lenses are used.

Epicanthus often gives the impression of a convergent squint. Spectacles tend to conceal this condition more than contact lenses do, and spectacles may thus be cosmetically preferable.

Lagophthalmos is discussed on page 379.

Conjunctiva

The undersurface of the upper lid may be scarred by trachoma, burns, or injuries. In such cases, a contact lens may be applied to protect the cornea from the scarred lid.

Triangular or wedge-shaped white patches on the nasal and temporal bulbar conjunctiva may occur in xerosis. Xerosis may result from a general disease, such as vitamin A deficiency, or be a sequel of a local ocular affection, such as trachoma, burns, pemphigus, or diphtheria. The primary disorder should be treated. Xerosis due to vitamin A deficiency, if not corrected early, can lead to corneal scarring and perforation. The residual effects in each case must be evaluated to determine the advisability of contact lens application. Because diphtheritic conjunctivitis and pemphigus are quite serious, contact lenses are contraindicated.

Cornea

Visual acuity of a patient with an irregular or scarred cornea is often considerably better when contact lenses are applied. Corneal irregularity and scarring often are a result of an ocular pathologic disorder. Advisability of contact lens fitting must be considered in terms of the causative pathologic disorder. Corneal irregularity and scarring may make it somewhat difficult to achieve a desired relationship between the posterior surface of the lens and the anterior corneal surfaces.

Sclera

Anterior scleral staphyloma—a bulging of the anterior sclera—results from a weakening of the scleral structure. Whether congenital or secondary to glaucoma, iridocyclitis, or scleritis, the prognosis is poor. Contact lenses are contraindicated in staphyloma.

Orbit

Extreme abnormal physiologic protrusion of the globe in the orbit (exophthalmos or proptosis) or extreme abnormal physiologic retraction of the globe (enophthalmos) complicates contact lens fitting (see p. 53). Exophthalmos may also be pathologic. Unilateral pathologic exophthalmos may be secondary to orbital cellulitis, tumors of the orbit, or orbital hemorrhages. Bilateral exophthalmos may be secondary to cavernous sinus thrombosis, hyperthyroidism, or symmetrical orbital tumors. If these primary pathologic disorders exist, contact lenses are usually contraindicated.

Iris

Coloboma of the iris or aniridia reduces visual acuity by increasing aberrations and the amount of light entering the eye. Polycoria causes a confused or multiple image. A cosmetic contact lens with an artificial pupil provides a more normal optical system. This improved optical system may help visual performance if amblyopia is not too severe.

The appearance of congenital iridic heterochromia is improved by a cosmetic contact lens. Heterochromia from iritis must be evaluated in terms of the basic pathologic disorder.

Albinism of the iris is usually associated with albinism of the retina and choroid. The amount of light entering the eye is greater than normal, and there is also a greater reflection and scattering of light in the internal eye, which produces veiling and dazzling effects. Visual acuity is decreased, and nystagmus often results. Therapy is aimed at decreasing the amount of light entering the eye. This can be done by cosmetic contact lenses, tinted contact lenses, corneal tattooing, or tinted spectacle lenses. Opinion differs as to whether cosmetic or tinted lenses help (see p. 111). Because so little can be done for such patients, it is worth trying cosmetic contact lenses at an early age. The central pupillary area should be tinted to further reduce the amount of light entering the eye. A noncosmetic, tinted contact lens is less satisfactory than a tinted spectacle lens because less light is absorbed.

In partial albinism, the irises are blue, and the absence of pigment is restricted to the choroid and retina. Use of a darkly tinted contact lens or a tinted spectacle lens may be helpful.

Lens

Contact lens application in aphakia is discussed on page 120.

Retina and Optic Nerve

Coloboma, medullated nerve fibers, and retinal detachment are the most common structural or positional abnormalities. The first two have no special significance relative to contact lens application.

Retinal detachment may be primary or secondary in origin. It may be secondary to the pushing away of the retina due to neoplasms, blood, or exudates. The neoplasm or the primary condition that produces the blood or exudates is usually quite serious, and contact lens application is usually thus contraindicated.

In primary retinal detachment, there is usually a predisposition to recurrence in either eye. Although a contact lens probably does not influence this tendency, it may be best to avoid contact lens application from a legal standpoint. After retinal detachment has occurred in one eye, detachment will take place later in the other eye in about 25 per cent of cases, and a patient may mistakenly believe that the contact lens contributed to the later detachment.

It has been recommended that a contact lens sutured to the conjunctiva be used to maintain corneal clarity during the prolonged surgery required in a retinal detachment operation.

NEOPLASMS

Any malignant growth contraindicates contact lens application. Benign growths of the external eye that are located where they will be touched by a contact lens usually should be excised before contact lens application. If they are not removed, fitting problems and discomfort may be produced.

GENERAL DISORDERS

Many general disorders are related to ocular pathologic disorders and contact lens application.

Vascular Disorders

Vascular disorders of the retina may be associated with local inflammation, but usually they are associated with a serious general disorder. Some of these disorders are arteriosclerosis, diabetes, hypertension, nephritis, syphilis, thrombosis, and toxemia. When it is possible, these pathologic disorders should be cured or controlled before contact lenses are considered. Because diabetes mellitus may result in poor corneal epithelium healing, the advisability of contact lens application, even in a controlled case, is decreased.

Hemorrhages of the internal eye may be quite serious, and they may decrease the advisability of contact lens application. Subconjunctival hemorrhages may not be serious if they are not associated with other pathologic conditions. In such cases, the use of contact lenses may be considered after the hemorrhagic blood is spontaneously absorbed. If contact lenses are fitted before absorption, discomfort or trauma may result, thus aggravating the hematoma. When subconjunctival hemorrhages are associated with other pathologic disorders, the advisability of contact lens application must be considered in terms of this associated condition.

General anemia may decrease the nutritional supply to the cornea and decrease its ability to accept a contact lens.

Endocrine Disorders

During menses, menopause, or pregnancy, instability of endocrine metabolism may exist. This instability can affect corneal sensitivity and turgescence, and the quantity and quality of tear flow. There may also be emotional instability. These factors can complicate contact lens fitting.

Hyperthyroidism and hypothyroidism may change tear flow. The thyroid should be properly regulated before contact lenses are applied.

Adolescent endocrine or metabolic imbalances may produce an excess of sebaceous or mucoid material. When it is possible, these imbalances should be controlled before contact lenses are applied.

Respiratory Disorders

Respiratory disorders, such as asthma, chronic colds, hay fever, nasal infections, and sinusitis, may cause hyperemia and inflammation of conjunctiva. Symptoms such as itching, photophobia, and tearing may be present. Such conditions complicate contact lens fitting, and they should be controlled before contact lenses are applied. Because these conditions are chronic or recur frequently, the patient should be informed that during an episode contact lens wear may become less comfortable or should be temporarily discontinued.

Focal Infections

Focal infections of the teeth, gums, adenoids, or tonsils may cause ocular discomfort. These infections should be cured before contact lenses are fitted.

Medication

Some medication taken in the treatment of general disorders may affect contact lens fitting. Common examples are some medications taken in the treatment of gastrointestinal, weight, or emotional disorders. Such medications may alter corneal turgescence or pupil size. Although the evidence is inconclusive, it seems that contact lens application may be more difficult in some patients using oral contraceptives.

SYMPTOMATIC DISORDERS

Several important conditions are included under this heading and are called "symptomatic" for lack of a better name.

Glaucoma

Opinion differs as to the advisability of contact lens application in cases of glaucoma. Relatively little is known about the effect of contact lenses on intraocular pressure. Scleral lenses may tend to increase intraocular pressure by interfering with the flow through the aqueous veins. It has been hypothesized that corneal contact lenses may decrease intraocular pressure through a massaging action. It has also been hypothesized that corneal contact lenses may increase intraocular pressure by irritating the eye.

Contact lenses are contraindicated in narrow-angle glaucoma. Theoretically, there is the possibility that the lens may cause the anterior chamber of the eye to become more shallow, which in turn may precipitate an acute attack of glaucoma. Open-angle glaucoma should be controlled before contact lenses are considered. It is then probably best to be conservative and to fit contact lenses only when there are significant visual benefits.

Nystagmus

Nystagmus may be aggravated by the poor correction of a refractive error. A contact lens may produce a better image than a spectacle lens because the contact lens causes fewer aberrations, and because there is better coincidence of the optical center of the lens with the visual axis for various directions of fixation. It has been suggested that the improved correction of the refractive error with contact lenses may help to relieve nystagmus. It has also been suggested that the pressure of the contact lens on the eye may reduce nystagmus. The seemingly improved visual performance of some nystagmic patients corrected with contact lenses may be due to these factors, or it may be due to the fact that nystagmus tends to become less severe with age.

If nystagmus is due to albinism or aniridia, a cosmetic contact lens may be helpful. Improvement from the use of contact lenses is hardly certain in nystagmus. However, contact lenses are worth trying because so little else can be done.

Conjunctival Hyperemia

Recurrent or chronic conjunctival hyperemia may be caused by conjunctivitis, exposure to dust or strong light, an improperly corrected error of refraction, gout, hay fever, and other allergic conditions. Contact lenses should not be used until the causative factor is determined and eliminated, or much discomfort may result.

Photophobia

True photophobia is accompanied by pain and is associated with a pathologic condition. The advisability of contact lens application is determined by the primary disorder.

Excessive sensitivity to light with discomfort but no pain is most often found in people having a light complexion. If a patient using spectacles is considerably hypersensitive to light, he will probably be even more light-sensitive with contact lenses because of stimulation of the tissues of the anterior segment by the contact lens.

11

Recent Developments

ASPHERIC SURFACES

The need to aspherize the posterior surface of contact lenses to produce satisfactory relationships with the anterior corneal surface is discussed on page 29. Although aspherization is generally produced by application of spherical secondary curves with longer radii than the base curve, it is also produced in two other ways. First, an optic zone with a spherical base curve surrounded by a secondary zone with true or modified elliptical, parabolic, or hyperbolic curves is used.[384, 385] The proponents of this procedure believe that it produces a better posterior lens–anterior cornea relationship and eliminates transition junctures. Second, a true or modified ellipsoidal, paraboloidal, or hyperboloidal *monocurve* posterior surface is used.[386–389] The proponents of this procedure believe that it produces a better posterior lens–anterior cornea relationship, eliminates transition junctures, and eliminates the flare type of visual problems.

The reason for aspherizing the anterior surface of a contact lens is to aid visual resolution. The proponents of this procedure believe that a properly selected anterior aspheric surface reduces positive, longitudinal spherical aberration, which reduces the size of the retinal disk of confusion.[390]

To understand aspherical conic or modified conic curves and fitting techniques incorporating them, some knowledge of analytic geometry is necessary. Aspherical conic curves have not been used frequently in the ophthalmic field. Because of this fact, pertinent aspects of analytic geometry will be reviewed below.

Selected Aspects of Analytic Geometry

Analytic geometry connects algebra and geometry.[391–393] It uses two aspects of algebra—variables and functions—and two aspects of geometry—graphs and coordinate systems.

In an equation such as $x = 2y$, x and y are unknown quantities, or variables, and 2 is a known quantity, or constant. During a mathematical operation, different values may be assigned to a variable. If in the preceding equation a definite value is assigned to x, the corresponding value of y found is a function of x. That is, the value of y—the dependent variable—depends on the previously selected value of x—the independent variable. For example, values of x from 0 to 10 in increments of 0.5 can be selected and substituted in the preceding equation. After solution of the various equations, each value of x will have a corresponding y value, which is its function. These x and y values can then be placed in a simple table.

It is difficult to visualize the pattern or shape related to this function when it is in a tabular form. Visualization is enhanced when the numbers are placed on a graph. To graph this equation, axes at a right angle are drawn. The horizontal axis is the x axis, or abscissa, and the vertical axis is the y axis, or ordinate. A first-degree equation with positive values of x and y, such as in the preceding equation, produces a linear graph, which may be placed in a single quadrant (Fig. 11–1). The plotting of points is represented by $P(x, y)$, where P stands for point, and the appropriate x and y values are substituted.

When a second-degree equation is used, the graph is a curve with the shape of a circle, ellipse, parabola, or hyperbola. When such curves are about the origin, they cannot be placed in a single quadrant. The abscissa and ordinate are extended, therefore, to produce a Cartesian, or rectangular, co-

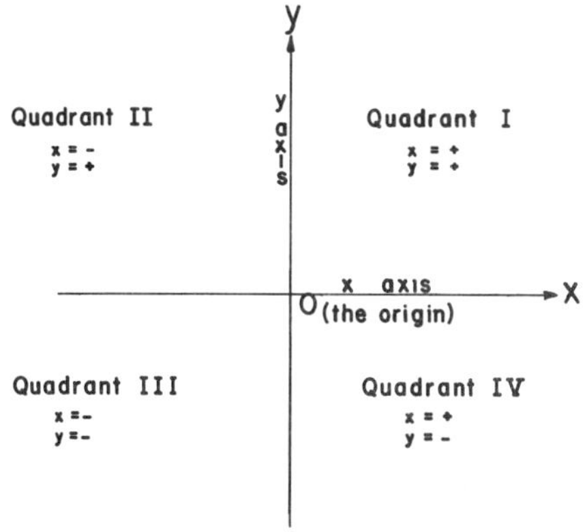

Figure 11–1. Cartesian or rectangular coordinate system.

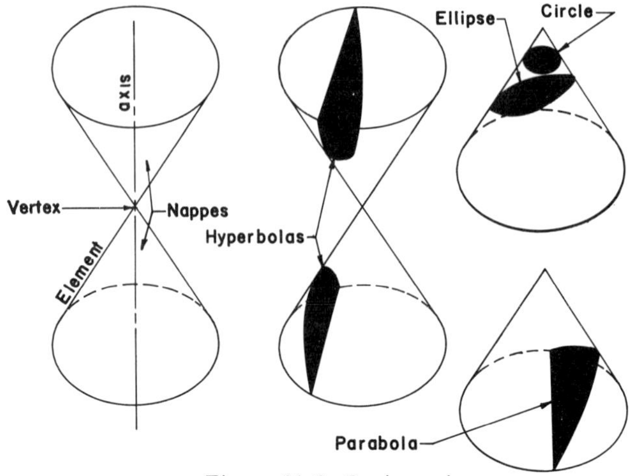

Figure 11–2. Conic sections.

ordinate system with four quadrants (Fig. 11–1). Each point in any quadrant is represented by a value of x and a value of y, which are the coordinates of the point, $P(x, y)$.

Curves of specific geometric form have corresponding algebraic equations. By the use of the algebraic equation for the type of curve under consideration, the coordinates are determined. When these are plotted in a rectangular coordinate system and connected, a graph that is the geometric representation of the curve is produced. If an imaginary point has traced this route, the curve produced is called the locus of the point.

Certain types of curves are produced by the intersection of a plane and a right circular cone, which has an axis, nappes, vertex, and elements (Fig. 11–2). When the cutting plane is perpendicular to the axis of the cone, the section is a circle. When the cutting plane cuts completely across one nappe at an angle oblique to the axis, the curve is an ellipse. When the cutting plane is parallel to an element, the curve is a parabola. When the cutting plane cuts through both nappes of the cone, the curve has two parts and is a hyperbola. Because these curves can be obtained by cutting a cone with a plane, they are often called conic sections, or conics. The circle and ellipse are closed conics, and the parabola and hyperbola are open conics.

Each of these conics may have a common vertex radius, R_v, but each flattens toward the periphery at varying rates (Fig. 11–3). This flattening, or degree of departure from circularity, is called the *eccentricity* (e) of the curve. The eccentricity of a circle is always zero. The eccentricity of an ellipse is between zero and one. The eccentricity of a parabola is always one. The eccentricity of a hyperbola is always more than one. It can be seen that peripheral flattening is zero for a circle, and it increases through an ellipse, to a parabola, to a hyperbola. It can also be seen that there is a central chord over which the various conic curvatures have relative coincidence.

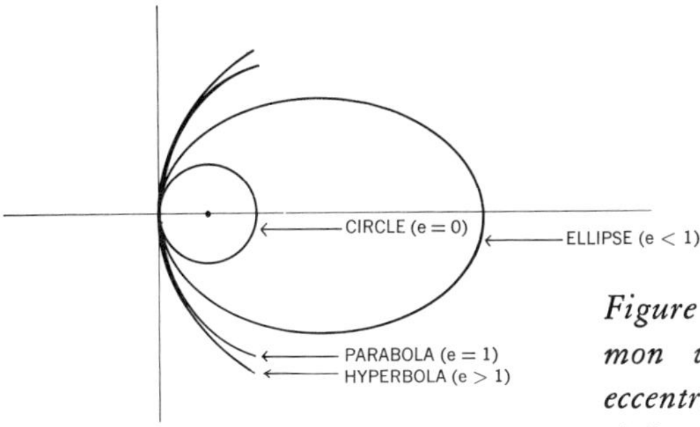

Figure 11–3. Conic curves with common vertex radius (R_v). *Note the eccentricity and relative rates of peripheral flattening.*

In terms of their eccentricities, conics may be defined by their relationship to a fixed line (*directrix*) and fixed point (*focus*). A circle may be defined as the locus of points the ratio of whose undirected distance from the directrix and focus is zero. An ellipse may be defined as the locus of points the ratio of whose undirected distances from the directrix and focus is a constant less than one. A parabola may be defined as the locus of points the ratio of whose undirected distances from the directrix and focus is one. A hyperbola may be defined as the locus of points the ratio of whose undirected distances from the directrix and focus is a constant greater than one.

Conics are a family of curves the equations of which are derived from the standard second-degree equation (Fig. 11–4).

For a circle, this becomes: $x^2 + y^2 = r^2$.

For an ellipse, this becomes: $\frac{x^2}{a^2} + \frac{y^2}{b^2} = 1$.

For a parabola, this becomes: $y^2 = 4Px$.

For a hyperbola, this becomes: $\frac{x^2}{a^2} - \frac{y^2}{b^2} = 1$.

We have discussed some aspects of analytic geometry related to planes. To extend this discussion to surfaces, some aspects of solid analytic geometry must be considered. This factor places things in three-dimensional space, and a three-dimensional rectangular coordinate system is used with a z axis perpendicular to the x and y axes (Fig. 11–5). A conic curve in three dimensions is termed a *quadric surface,* or *conicoid.* Such surfaces of revolution are produced by revolving a conic curve around its principal axis. The conic sections revolved about their principal axis produce conicoids called spheres, ellipsoids, paraboloids, and hyperboloids.

Shape and Size

Each type of unrestricted conic curve has a unique general shape, which may be represented by its eccentricity. Because unrestricted circles and

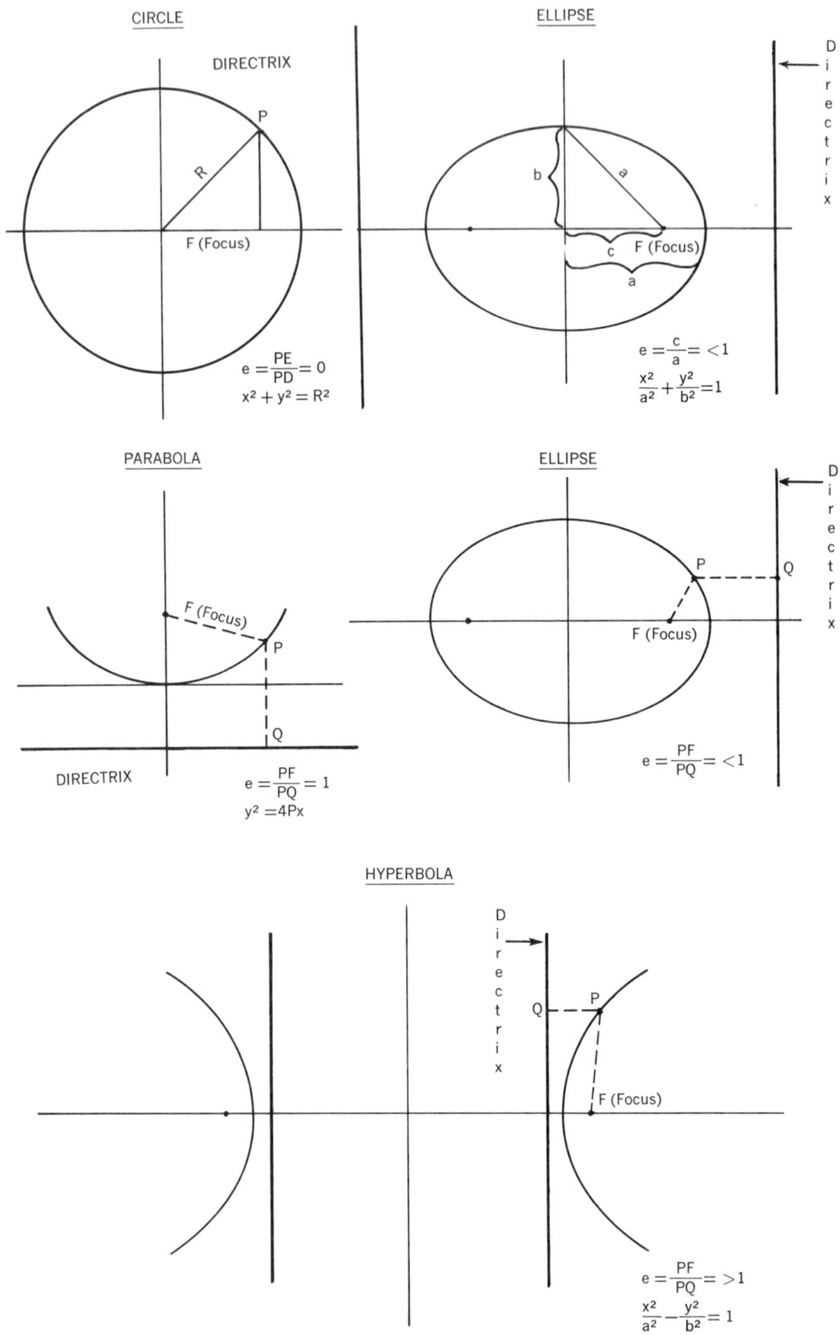

Figure 11–4. Illustration and equations of conics.

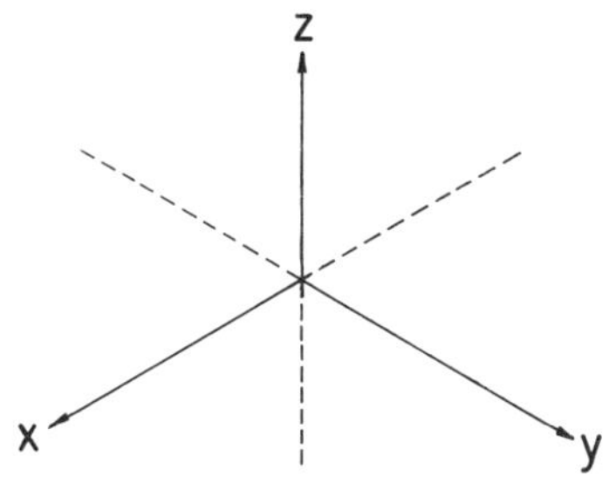

Figure 11–5. Three-dimensional rectangular coordinate system.

parabolas each have one eccentricity—zero and one, respectively—they have constant shapes. Because unrestricted ellipses and hyperbolas have a range of eccentricities, they have a corresponding range of shapes.

With a specified eccentricity and shape, size varies with vertex radius, R_v. Two circles, $e = 0$, with dissimilar radii differ in size but not in shape (Fig. 11–6). Size can also be altered by the use of a different scale. If scale

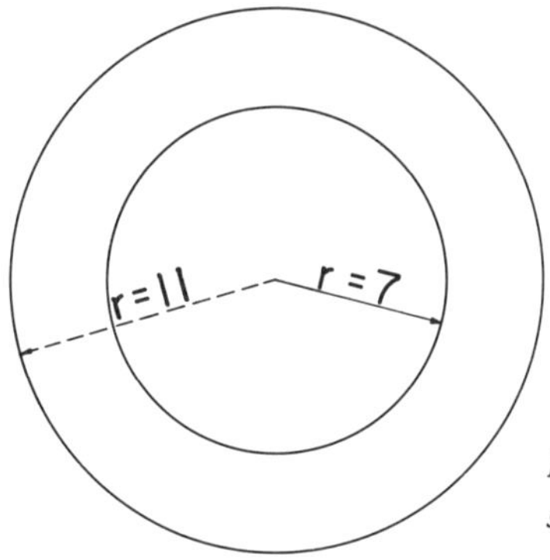

Figure 11–6. With a given eccentricity, size varies with vertex radius (R_v).

and chord or diameter is restricted, a type of apparent comparative shape is produced. For example, two circular curves of differing radii have an apparent comparative shape difference over a 10 mm. diameter—that is, they look different (Fig. 11–7). The terms *flat* or *steep* are used to describe

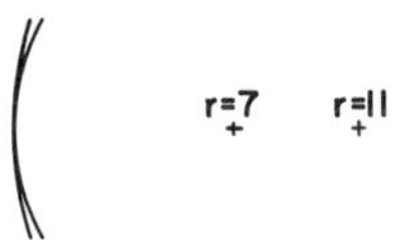

Figure 11–7. When scale and diameter are restricted, a type of comparative shape difference is produced.

apparent comparative shape differences. Flat relates to a long radius, and therefore a larger size; steep relates to a short radius, and therefore a smaller size. Apparent comparative shape differences over a set size are based on rate of change of direction. The curvature of a circle at any point—that is, its rate of change of direction per unit of arc length—equals the reciprocal of the radius. As the radius increases, the rate of change decreases. It should be noted that the reciprocal of the radius is the curvature of a circle only, and other methods must be used to find the curvature of the remaining conics.

Each curve is described by its size and shape. The size is the vertex radius, R_v; and the shape is the eccentricity, e.

With the exception of spheres, it is difficult to manufacture accurate quadric surfaces. Spheres are readily produced by a simple lathe or by using convex and concave surfaces of equal and opposite curvature on a simple rotating machine. Ellipsoidal, paraboloidal, or hyperboloidal surfaces are produced by special, complex generators. Either the mold for casting, the lens surface itself, or the template is generated. There is a new type of lens generator that produces quadric surfaces.[394, 395]

Posterior Aspheric Surfaces

There are two important preliminaries to clinical evaluation or use of lenses with monocurve posterior ellipsoidal, paraboloidal, or hyperboloidal surfaces. First, there must be clinically satisfactory methods to select initial lens design characteristics—lens diameter, size (R_v), shape (e), and refractive power. As with spherical surfaced lenses, the two basic methods for selection of initial lens characteristics are diagnostic lens procedure, and measurements and standards. Second, there must be clinically satisfactory laboratory procedures to order, verify, and modify the lenses. The following discussion indicates the current developmental stage.[389]

Initial Design Selection

Diagnostic Lens Procedure. A recommended initial diagnostic set with 30 lenses has shapes (e) of 0.5, 0.6, and 0.7 combined with sizes (R_v) from 7.30 to 8.10 mm. in 0.1 mm. increments. Lens diameters range from 9.0 to 9.6, with the smaller lens diameters related to shorter vertex radii.

Initial diagnostic lens diameter is 9.0 mm. for an average 11.5 mm. horizontal visible iris diameter. The lens diameter is increased 0.3 mm. for each 0.5 mm. increase of visible iris diameter. The lens diameter is decreased 0.3 mm. for each 0.5 mm. decrease of visible iris diameter.

Initial diagnostic lens size (R_v) is 0.10 mm. shorter than the radius of the longer ophthalmometric principal meridian when there is less than 0.20 mm. of ophthalmometric toricity. R_v is shortened 0.05 mm. for each 0.10 mm. increase of ophthalmometric toricity above 0.20 mm. Initial diagnostic lens shape (e) is 0.6. Subsequent clinical evaluation may indicate that different initial diagnostic lens values of R_v and e are preferable.

Criteria of a satisfactory fit are the same as for any lens design. The desired fluorescein pattern for a cornea with relatively little toricity, however, is thin and uniform throughout. The desired fluorescein pattern for an appreciably toric cornea is thin and uniform along the flatter corneal meridians with relatively more clearance along the steeper meridians. Subsequent clinical evaluation may indicate that other fluorescein patterns are more desirable.

There are two general areas of the fluorescein pattern—central and peripheral—that must be evaluated simultaneously. If there is little corneal asymmetry or toricity, the basic fluorescein patterns and suggested remediations are as shown in Table 11–1.

TABLE 11–1

MONOCURVE ASPHERICAL FLUORESCEIN PATTERN INTERPRETATION

Central	Peripheral	Primary Remediation	Possible Secondary Remediation
Too thin or absent	1. Thin and uniform	Shorten R_v	Increase *e*
	2. Too thin or absent	Shorten R_v and increase *e*	
	3. Thick	Shorten R_v	Decrease *e*
Thick	4. Thin and uniform	Lengthen R_v	Decrease *e*
	5. Too thin or absent	Lengthen R_v	Increase *e*
	6. Thick	Lengthen R_v and decrease *e*	
Thin and uniform	7. Thin and uniform	None	None
	8. Too thin or absent	Increase *e*	Decrease R_v
	9. Thick	Decrease *e*	Increase R_v

A change of either R_v or *e* simultaneously alters both central and peripheral relationships. With the exception of patterns 2 and 6 in Table 11–1, it is probably best to alter either R_v or *e* separately at first. Any residual deficiency of the pattern is corrected with the secondary remediation shown in Table 11–1.

Refractive power is determined by refraction over diagnostic lenses. This is done in the same manner as for lenses with spherical base curves. R_v is used as the base curve radius.

Measurements and Standards. Research has not yet produced a satisfactory means for using the measurements and standards method for selection of initial lens characteristics. Lens diameter can be determined in the same manner used to select initial diagnostic lens diameter. Refractive power can be computed as it is for a spherical base curve lens, and R_v is used as the base curve radius. The problem is to devise a means for selection of R_v and e that produces desired posterior lens–anterior cornea relationships for a satisfactory percentage of patients.[396]

Research may develop satisfactory means for empirically selecting R_v and e based on measurements and standards. This method may involve current or new instrumentation and formulation. If such a means is developed, it also may influence the selection of R_v and e of the initial diagnostic lens.

Laboratory Procedures

Ordering. Lens diameter is ordered to the nearest 0.10 mm., and manufacturing tolerance is plus or minus 0.05 mm. Vertex radius is ordered to the nearest 0.01 mm., and manufacturing tolerance is plus or minus 0.03 mm. Eccentricity is ordered to the nearest 0.10 mm., and manufacturing tolerance is plus or minus 0.05 mm. Refractive power is ordered to the nearest 0.12 D, and manufacturing tolerance is plus or minus 0.12 D. Tint is ordered as desired.

Verification. Lens diameter and thickness are verified in the usual manner. Most contemporary verification equipment for refractive power and vertex radius is based on principles of refraction or reflection from spherical surfaces. Aside from the paraxial regions, these instruments do not verify aspherical quadric surfaces with complete accuracy and validity. An instrument using interference fringes has been developed to measure quadric surfaces.[397] However, until new instrumentation is developed or commonly used, current instrumentation can be used.

Refractive power can be verified with a Lensometer or Vertometer. The aperture is reduced to about 3.0 to 4.0 mm. to eliminate marginal rays, and the lens is centered. If the lens is not centered with the aperture, the Lensometer image quality is poor or an astigmatic refraction is produced.

Vertex radius can be verified with a Radiuscope. The lens is centered on a holder, which is not tilted. If the lens is not centered or the holder is tilted, toricity is read.

Eccentricity can be verified with a Radiuscope or a Toposcope and the use of tables.

Modification. Lens diameter reduction, edging, and power changes are produced in the usual manner. Although it is theoretically unnecessary, secondary curves can be applied.

Research will determine the clinical value of contact lenses with posterior aspherical quadric surfaces.

Anterior Aspherical Surfaces

An aspherical quadric surface has a continuous flattening from center to edge. As a result, the incident angles of paraxial and marginal rays are more uniform than in a spherical surface.[398–400] This factor alters spherical aberration.

In situ, the anterior surface of a contact lens converges light, and its posterior surface diverges light (p. 342). For a given object and image position, an anterior aspherical quadric surface can eliminate positive spherical aberration from a system. However, the other monochromatic aberrations, which relate to extra-axial points and peripheral vision, are not eliminated. Because this discussion is concerned with central vision, chromatic and peripheral aberrations are not considered. A posterior aspherical quadric surface increases positive spherical aberration. The small indicial difference at the interface between the posterior contact lens surface and the precorneal fluid limits this increase, however.

It has been suggested that a paraboloidal anterior surface can be combined with any type of posterior surface to produce a relatively aplanatic system (the eye and contact lens in situ).[390, 401] The single relatively aplanatic focus can be positioned so that a presbyope or prepresbyope will have satisfactory resolution from distance to near fixation.

This theory is based on the belief that visual resolution is limited by retinal element separation and the nature and area of the macular disk of confusion.[402] The area of the disk of confusion depends on the position of the retina along the visual axis (degree of paraxial ametropia) and the amount of spherical aberration. A lens may reduce the size of the macular disk of confusion by moving the paraxial focus toward the retina and by reducing spherical aberration. Satisfactory vision is produced when this retinal disk of confusion is sufficiently small.

In an uncorrected emmetrope, or an ametrope corrected for distance with corrected-curve spectacle lenses or conventional contact lenses, the minimum disk of confusion is near or on the retina and small enough for adequate resolution. It is reasoned that if this disk size could be limited, satisfactory visual resolution should occur at any fixation distance in which the limit could be maintained.

When a relatively aplanatic contact lens is applied to a presbyope, this is accomplished by incorporating an aspheric anterior surface that focuses the marginal and paraxial rays at a point in front of the retina in distant fixation and behind the retina in near fixation. That is, the marginal and paraxial radii combine to produce this single refractive power. The residual macular disk of confusion is reduced by decreasing positive spherical aberration with an anterior paraboloidal surface. It is held that the disk of confusion would then be small enough to be resolved at different levels of fixation without lenticular accommodation.

Because the refractive power is constant throughout the pupil, there is no zonal interference from lens movement, rotation, and translation. Because ballast is not necessary, the associated problems are eliminated. Because visual resolution is satisfactory at any normal fixation distance, it is claimed that there is no restriction within the range of clear vision.

With a relatively aplanatic contact lens for a prepresbyope, the focus for distant fixation is placed on the retina. Because of the reduction of spherical aberration, the smaller macular disk of confusion may heighten visual resolution.

The clinical value of such relatively aplanatic contact lenses will be established by research.

MATERIALS

Materials proposed for contact lens fabrication must be evaluated in terms of weight, mechanical stability, optical characteristics, inertness, ocular tissue compatibility, and ease and accuracy of manufacture.[403–405]

Polymethyl Methacrylate

Early contact lenses made of relatively heavy and breakable glass were unsuccessful. Although experimental work is being done with other materials, almost all contact lenses since the late 1930's have been made of polymethyl methacrylate (PMMA). This plastic is known by the trade names Plexiglas, Lucite, and Perspex, and it has a chemical formula of $CH{=}C(CH_3){-}COOH$.

PMMA lenses weigh about 40 per cent as much as glass lenses of similar size. The specific gravity of this plastic is 1.18 to 1.19.

PMMA lenses have relatively good mechanical stability. With proper care, they can be used for many years without significant undesired alterations to their physical properties. The tensile strength is relatively high (7,000 to 9,000), and they do not break or shatter readily on the eye. The dimensional stability of PMMA lenses is generally good. However, 0.3 to 0.4 per cent of water may be absorbed over a 24-hour period, thus frequently flattening the base curve.

PMMA lenses have good optical clarity and transmission. Because of their dimensional stability, their curvature and refractive power are relatively constant. The refractive index of these lenses is usually between 1.488 and 1.50, with 1.49 used as the standard. Because the refractive index of a plastic stock may vary, a refractive power computation based on a refractive index of 1.49 may be incorrect. Water absorption is too slight to alter the refractive index. Plastic with refractive indices of 1.51, 1.55, and 1.57 have also been used.

PMMA lenses are generally inert, actively and passively. It is highly improbable that chemical constituents, such as methacrylic acid, might leach out of clear PMMA in a high enough concentration to cause ocular irritation. Clinical experience indicates that this is also probably true for colorants added to the basic formulation—through-and-through tints.[406] Colorants added as coatings may not be bound securely to the lens and may migrate to and irritate the ocular tissues. Precorneal fluid and nonmedicated adjunctive solutions do not decompose the lens. Bacteriostatic and fungistatic agents have been polymerized into contact lenses to reduce bacterial contamination. Because it seems that these agents are incorporated so that they do not leach out, their efficacy is doubtful.[407] Lenses from which bacteriostats would leach are considered drugs by the Food and Drug Administration, and they must receive drug approval for ocular application.

PMMA lenses are nontoxic and reasonably compatible with ocular tissues. However, they have several limitations. Because they contain fewer hydrophilic centers (carboxy ester groups) than hydrophobic centers (methyl groups), their surfaces are hydrophobic. These lenses also offer a hard surface for corneal and lid contact, and they hinder the passage of gases between the atmosphere and the eye.

New Materials

Research is being done in an attempt to develop a material that will correct some or all of the problems resulting from use of polymethyl methacrylate. At the same time, however, the good characteristics of polymethyl methacrylate must not be sacrificed.

There are four categories of materials currently being tested or used: cross-linked hydrophilic polymers, organopolysiloxanes, copolymerized resins, and surface treatment materials. These materials are in various stages of development, and research will establish their value.

CROSS-LINKED HYDROPHILIC POLYMERS*

Structure

Contact lenses made of this material have been given various names: hydrophilic contact lenses, gel contact lenses, gel-kontakt flexible lenses, hydrogel contact lenses, hydragel contact lenses, soflenzes, and gelatin contact lenses. We will use the term hydrophilic contact lenses.

Hydrophilic contact lenses are made from a solid colloidal material, which consists of particles, a continuous dispersion medium, and a stabilizing agent. If a liquid colloid (a sol) is to be changed to a solid colloid (a gel), the liquid must be immobilized.

To accomplish immobilization in the material in question, hydrophilic, water-soluble monomers are rapidly polymerized in the presence of water or water-soluble liquids. Starting materials usually include a water-soluble monoester of an olefinic acid from the group of acrylic acid and methacrylic acid, a bifunctional alcohol with an esterifiable hydroxyl group, and at least one additional hydrophilic functional group.[408–412] Typically, glycomonothacrylate is polymerized rapidly in the presence of glycerol so that the

* Dr. Milton M. Kaplan, Research Associate of the Eye-Bank for Sight Restoration, Inc., has generously contributed most of the information on which our discussion of cross-linked hydrophilic polymers is based.

primary particles of the monomer touch in favorable positions and form polymeric chains.[413] These chains are cross-linked in a three-dimensional hydrophilic network.

The resultant plastic is said to be polydioxyethylene methacrylate.[414] Aside from the presence of three oxygen atoms and one OH group in each molecular unit, its formula is the same as that of polymethyl methacrylate. This important chemical difference makes the cross-linked polymer hydrophilic, which results in dehydrated and hydrated states.

Specific Properties

Research is being carried out to establish the specific properties of this material and contact lenses made from it. The following reflects the current state of knowledge.[415–459]

There is no gaseous and questionable fluid interchange through hydrophilic contact lenses. Fluorescein is absorbed, and the lenses glow, often for days. Contaminants from the fingers and antiseptics from contact lens solutions may be absorbed, and subsequent emission may cause ocular tissue irritation. Bacteria and viruses may penetrate the lenses or only cause surface contamination.

In a dehydrated state, hydrophilic contact lenses are hard and brittle. In a hydrated state, hydrophilic contact lenses are soft, gel-like, and flexible. Change from the hard, or dehydrated, to the soft, or hydrated, state may be called *transformation from hydration*. Complete hydration occurs when the lens absorbs approximately 60 per cent of its weight in water. The refractive index and the linear dimensions of hydrophilic contact lenses vary with transformation from hydration.

As the water content increases, the index of refraction decreases. The refractive index in the dehydrated state has been reported to be between 1.525 and 1.54, and the index in the fully hydrated state has been reported to be between 1.425 and 1.432.

As the water content increases, the linear dimensions increase—that is, the lens swells. Linear expansion with full hydration of all diameters, radii, and thicknesses has been reported to be between 15 and 18 per cent. Expansion is inversely related to temperature for the range in which hydrophilic lenses are used, which is contrary to the expansion property of most materials.

Because of flexibility in the soft state, pressures alter the shape of hydrophilic contact lenses. Change of shape from pressure may be called *transformation from bending*.

Transformation from Hydration

Transformation from hydration affects the refractive power and the fitting characteristics of hydrophilic contact lenses. Although hydrophilic contact lenses are worn in the soft state, it may be desirable to order, manufacture, and verify them in the hard state. To do this, a conversion system must be developed that allows prediction of soft characteristics from hard characteristics.[427]

Assuming an 18 per cent expansion of linear dimensions with hydration, the relationship between hard state linear dimensions (L_h) and soft state linear dimensions (L_s) is:

$$\frac{L_h}{L_s} = \frac{1.00}{1.18},$$

$$L_h = 0.8475\ L_s.$$

Assuming an index in the hard state (n'_h) of 1.54 and an index in the soft state (n'_s) of 1.43, the relationship for an optically thin hydrophilic lens between hard state dioptric power (D_h) and soft state dioptric power (D_s) is:

$$\frac{D_h}{D_s} = \frac{\dfrac{n'_h - n}{r_h}}{\dfrac{n'_s - n}{r_s}},$$

$$\frac{D_h}{D_s} = \frac{\dfrac{0.54}{1.00}}{\dfrac{0.43}{1.18}},$$

$$D_h = 1.4818\ D_s.$$

Hydrophilic contact lenses are optically thick, however, as are conventional polymethyl methacrylate lenses. To compensate for the effect of thickness on the power of a hydrophilic contact lens, a precalculated amount of positive power must be added. The amount of positive power compensation varies with thickness in a linear manner within 0.01 D, and it also depends on the base curve radius.[427] Table 11–2 is a simplified approximation of compensation factors. For greater accuracy, more extensive tables can be derived and applied.

TABLE 11–2

COMPENSATION FOR EFFECTS OF THICKNESS ON POWER OF HYDROPHILIC LENSES

Base Curve Radius in Soft State (in mm.)	Add per 1.0 mm. of Soft State Center Thickness
6.00	+0.80 D
6.50	+0.68 D
7.00	+0.59 D
7.50	+0.52 D
8.00	+0.46 D
8.50	+0.41 D
9.00	+0.37 D

Example: A hydrophilic contact lens with the following soft state specification is desired:

Base Curve Radius = 8.00 mm.
Secondary Curve Radius = 8.60 mm.
Lens Diameter = 10.5 mm.
Optic Zone = 7.5 mm.
Secondary Curve Width = 1.5 mm.
Center Thickness = 0.15 mm.
Diopters = −10.00

Find the equivalent hard state characteristics:

Base Curve Radius = 8.00 mm. × 0.8475 = 6.78 mm.
Secondary Curve Radius = 8.60 mm. × 0.8475 = 7.29 mm.
Lens Diameter = 10.5 mm. × 0.8475 = 8.90 mm.
Optic Zone = 7.5 mm. × 0.8475 = 6.36 mm.
Secondary Curve Width = 1.5 mm. × 0.8475 = 1.27 mm.
Center Thickness = 0.15 mm. × 0.8475 = 0.127 mm.
Diopters = −10.00 D × 1.4818 = −14.818 + (0.15)(0.46) = −14.75

Absolute values of refractive index and linear expansion after full hydration are the subject of controversy as of this writing. The stated values are for illustration and may be changed, but the derivation is held to be valid.

When a soft hydrophilic contact lens is placed on the eye, the osmotic balance of the lens is altered. The osmotic balance with the physiologic saline solution, in which the lens is stored, must be changed to osmotic balance with precorneal fluid, in which the lens is worn. It is recommended by some authorities that this adaptation be done by placement of the lens on the sclera for 20 minutes before sliding of the lens onto the cornea.

Transformation from Bending

When a soft hydrophilic contact lens is placed on the cornea, its curvature is transformed by corneal and scleral topography and by lid pressures. Because of its flexibility, the posterior surface of the lens tends to assume the shape of the underlying anterior surface of the cornea and sclera. This change is transmitted to the anterior surface of the lens, which may be altered further by lid pressures.

The transformed anterior surface curvature often has a different central radius and overall shape. That is, a spherical anterior curve of a given radius may be transformed into an aspherical anterior curve of another radius. The quality of the surface may also be altered—a regular surface may be transformed into an irregular surface. Because the anterior surface of a contact lens on the eye is its principal refracting surface, alteration of curvature significantly alters refractive power.

Because the type and amount of refractive power alteration from bending is not yet predictable, refractive power must be determined by refraction over lenses on the eye. Refraction may also be affected by positioning, and internal reflection and dispersion of light. Surface contamination can cause small opacities, which may interfere with vision.

Speculation as to topographic change becomes highly sophisticated.[460] A precise method has been presented to approach the prediction of dimensional change that occurs with bending.[461] This highly complex derivation was determined for programing dioptric change as a consequence of corneal bending in refractive keratoplasty, but the same principles may be said to apply to all flexible lenses.

Clinical Evaluation

Although many types of lens designs have been evaluated clinically, no satisfactory fitting rationale has been developed as of this writing. The only common characteristic to all lens designs has been an almost knifelike edge, which allows merging with the underlying sclera or cornea.

The close adherence of the lens to the cornea limits the thickness of the precorneal fluid layer. Because fluorescein cannot be used, the fit is evaluated by lens movement. There is no gaseous, and questionable fluid, interchange through the lens, and thus movement is necessary for interchange. Insufficient movement has produced significant corneal edema, staining, and associated discomfort. Excessive movement has produced discomfort, poor refraction, and even an opportunity for the lids to fold or eject the lens. It should be noted that optimum movement of hydrophilic contact lenses may differ from that of polymethyl methacrylate lenses.

Hydrophilic contact lenses have been manufactured by a specialized molding procedure or by specialized cutting and polishing procedures. The clinical performance of hydrophilic contact lenses varies with manufacturing procedure.

Molded hydrophilic contact lenses fitted in Czechoslovakia are unmoving on the eye, even with blinking and eye movements. The lens edge merges with the adjacent tissue, and slit-lamp biomicroscopy with wide-beam direct illumination shows normal mucoid layer movement with the blink cycle. Slit-lamp biomicroscopy with a parallelepiped shows the lens as an additional layer, structureless and unmoving, anterior to the cornea. The posterior surface of the contact lens and the anterior corneal surfaces appear as an interface without a precorneal fluid layer between them.

Lathed hydrophilic contact lenses fitted in the United States show dynamic movement with blinking and some lag with eye movements. As the upper lid begins closure at the onset of the blink cycle, it pushes the upper edge of the lens downward. When the upper lid starts to retract, the lens is positioned inferiorly. As the upper lid continues to retract, the lens follows it until the lens regains its primary positioning. The speed of this following movement varies with the fitting relationship of the lens. Research is being undertaken in an attempt to correlate the lens movement, lens parameters, and successful fitting.

Removal of the lens has proved difficult for some people, and there is a greater tendency for damaging lenses by handling. It has been estimated that the average wearer would have to replace lenses three or four times a year. Insertion may be somewhat difficult because of the flexibility of the material, and the lens can easily be turned inside out. Although they are soft, a split lens can cause severe abrasion.

Storage to maintain hydration is recommended to be done in physiologic saline solution. To eliminate surface contamination, nightly boiling in saline solution has been suggested.

Laboratory Procedures

Manufacture. Hydrophilic contact lenses are manufactured by molding in special machines or by specialized cutting and polishing procedures on a lathe.

For molding, the monomer and the solvent are mixed and fed into the refrigerated storage compartment of the machine. Storage temperature is -5° C. During manufacture, the mixture is pumped mechanically through a polyethylene tube into a mold. Each mold has a ground and polished spherical concave surface, which is color keyed for radius. The mold originates at one end of the machine and is manually fed through a glass tube to a turntable. When it reaches the turntable, the mold is automatically pushed onto and linked with a spindle. After linkage, the mold moves to a position where the monomer is poured into it. The mixture is enclosed in carbon dioxide at a temperature of 65° C, which is the most favorable for polymerization. The mold rotates on its spindle as the turntable itself rotates, stopping at each of 60 positions for 5 to 10 seconds. After the turntable completes one revolution, polymerization is complete. The mold is then pushed off the spindle and onto a metal channel, which is enclosed in air at 85° C. Water is pumped onto the lens to replace the glycerol and to hydrate the lens fully. At the end of the channel, each lens is removed manually from its mold and placed in an individual container.

Three factors determine the topography of the posterior surface of the contact lens: dosing, metering, and spinning speed. *Dosing* refers to the percentage of the solvent relative to the monomer. Normal dosing results in a paraboloidal surface, underdosing results in an ellipsoidal surface, and overdosing results in a hyperboloidal surface. *Metering* refers to the amount of pressure used to move the monomer from the refrigeration unit through the tubing to the mold. *Spinning speed* refers to the rotation rate of the mold.

For cutting and polishing, a hard button of polymer is cut from a rod or formed in a mold. The buttons are mounted on tools and chucks with special waxes adapted from dental technology. Cutting and polishing is done on high-speed lathes. Cerium oxide—the polishing compound—is suspended in a mixture of special mineral oil and benzene to prevent hydration of the lens. During the manufacturing procedure, the lens is cleaned periodically by immersion in a test tube filled with hexane in an ultrasonic tank.

Edge Inspection. After a lens in the soft state is pressed flat against the bottom of a water-filled container, a light is projected through the container and onto a screen. Edge contour and smoothness are checked from this shadowgraph.

Power Verification. A special device is used for power verification of a lens in the soft state. The soft contact lens is placed on a hard contact lens of plano power, which is mounted on a hollow brass fitting. A cap with a transparent center is placed over this assembly to protect the soft lens from dust. The assembly is mounted on the arm of a centrifuge. The machine is turned on, and the soft lens is spun against the hard lens. Spinning eliminates surface water and molds the soft lens to a spherical curve. The assembly is removed from the centrifuge, and the power of the soft lens is read from a Lensometer or Vertometer.

Summary

Research must be done to allow better prediction, interpretation, and control of transformation; to allow better means of verifying and selecting lens characteristics; to allow better fluid and gas interchange; to answer the bacteriology questions; and to make the lenses practical for patient handling.

It should be noted that a lens with a hard plastic central area and a soft periphery has been developed.

ORGANOPOLYSILOXANES

Organopolysiloxane elastomers compounded with various types of fillers produce an optically clear silicone rubber material, which is quite permeable to carbon dioxide and oxygen.[462–471] Alteration of the concentration of filler alters the flexibility, pliability, resiliency, and refractive index of this material. Refractive indices from 1.49 to 1.56 have been produced. Dimethyl polysiloxane, with trade names such as Silastic S, or other hydrolyzed hydrocarbon-substituted silanes are used.

Lenses are produced from this silicone rubber by pouring a liquid mixture into a mold and vulcanizing it. Hot pressing may, for example, exert 5 to 20 tons of pressure at a molding temperature of about 300° F. The lens is removed from the mold, and it is cured at a controlled temperature and atmospheric pressure. Changes in the curing conditions alter the softness of the lens. Hardness is directly related to curing time and heat intensity. After the lens is cured, it is cooled, and it can then be cut, ground, and polished. Edges can be formed mechanically or chemically. They are quite thin—almost knifelike. Shrinkage during manufacture is unpredictable at this time, and power and base curves are manufactured by trial and error.

Harder lenses resist change of shape from corneal and lid pressures; softer lenses may have their shape altered in a way similar to that of cross-linked hydrophilic polymers. Adherence between lens and eye, and lid and lens is reduced. As a result, a lens with a given relationship between the posterior surface of the lens and the anterior corneal surface, and a given lens diameter produces different movement when made of transparent silicone rubber from when made of polymethyl methacrylate. Compensation must be made to produce equivalent movement. Posterior lens–anterior cornea relationships can be evaluated with fluorescein.

Much research is yet to be done on this material. Organopolysiloxanes are being used in an attempt to produce a gas-permeable material with a hardness between that of polymethyl methacrylate and that of the cross-linked hydrophilic polymers.

COPOLYMERIZED RESINS

Copolymerized resins are composed of allyldigly colcarbonate (CR 39) (40 to 99 per cent) and of a monomer made from maleic anhydride and glycidyl methacrylate (1 to 60 per cent).[472] Lenses are usually made by casting and curing with heat. They are then placed in an alkaline solution from 1 to 20 per cent of a material from the group of sodium hydroxide, sodium carbonate, potassium hydroxide, sodium acetate, sodium borate, and trisodium phosphate. The alkaline hydrolysis produces hydrophilic surfaces. This material is used in an attempt to produce a lens that is hydrophilic, dimensionally stable, hard, and scratch-resistant.

SURFACE TREATMENT

Two methods of surface treatment have been used to make polymethyl methacrylate surfaces hydrophilic: the surfaces are coated with an inorganic thin film of titanium dioxide or silicon monoxide,[473,474] and the chemical composition of the lens surfaces is changed by placing the lens in a tube and electrically decomposing water, hydrazine, acetic acid, formic acid, and ammonia into free radicals.[475] If such treatments are to be successful, they must be hydrophilically effective for a long time and nonirritating to ocular tissues.

AUXILIARY PROGNOSTIC TESTS

Tests for corneal fragility, corneal sensitivity, lacrimal sufficiency, and lid edema have been suggested for the purpose of gathering auxiliary prognostic data. The tests and conclusions presented here are as reported by their proponents. More research is needed before their validity as prognostic aids can be accepted.

Corneal Epithelium Fragility

The ability of corneal epithelial tissue to withstand pressure apparently varies among individuals. The more fragile the tissues are, the less the probability is that the pressures from a contact lens can be withstood without tissue disturbance. Epithelial fragility is tested by the application of steady pressure to the anesthetized cornea for 4 minutes with the use of a special lens engraved with circles and star-shaped lines fitted on an applanation tonometer.[476,477] Fluorescein is instilled, and the degree of tissue disturbance is shown by staining. There are three categories of patients: negative, slightly positive, and positive. (*Staining from normal lid pressure is important.*)

NEGATIVE ($F = 0$). There is little or no retention of fluorescein or corneal irregularity. About 50 per cent of patients have this response, and from this standpoint they are good contact lens candidates.

SLIGHTLY POSITIVE ($F = +1$). Fine, sinuous, superficial lines or points of staining are scattered over the cornea. About 45 per cent of patients have this response, and they are fair contact lens candidates. Wearing time is increased slowly in this type of patient, and it may have to be restricted to 10 hours or less per day.

POSITIVE ($F = +2$). Large, relatively deep lines, points, or patches of staining are scattered over the cornea. About 5 per cent of patients have this response, and they are poor contact lens candidates.

CORNEAL SENSITIVITY

Corneal sensitivity apparently varies among individuals. The less sensitive the cornea is, the more readily contact lenses are tolerated. Corneal sensitivity is tested with an aesthesiometer that makes use of a nylon thread of known stiffness enclosed in a housing that can regulate the length of exposed thread (Fig. 11–8).[478] The amount of pressure exerted by the thread on the cornea is inversely proportional to the length of exposed thread. Because corneal sensitivity decreases from the center of the cornea to the periphery, a standard area should be established. The limbal area is taken as this standard. When limbal sensitivity is greater than 25 mg., contact lens prognosis is more favorable.

The thread is started at its maximum exposure, and the cornea near the limbus is touched. The length of exposed thread is progressively decreased

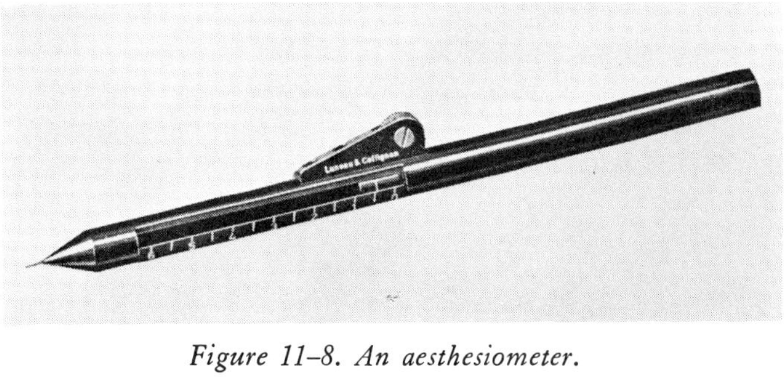

Figure 11–8. An aesthesiometer.

Figure 11–9. A Ronchi ruling.

until the tension is felt by the patient. This length of the exposed thread is read from a scale, and it is converted to milligrams of equivalent pressure by the use of a table.

When hypoesthesia is considerable, the ability of the patient to appreciate symptoms or the presence of a foreign body is reduced. Such patients should be examined more frequently. Hypoesthesia may be caused by surgery for cataracts or by contact lens wear itself.

Lacrimal Sufficiency

Sufficient production of precorneal fluid, which varies among individuals, and proper precorneal wetting are necessary for proper corneal physiologic processes. Lacrimal sufficiency is determined by the Schirmer test.[479] A piece of sterile filter paper is hooked over the nasal part of the lower eyelid. In patients less than 40 years old, at least 15 mm. of paper should be moistened in 5 minutes. In patients more than 40 years old, at least 10 mm. of paper should be moistened in 5 minutes. When lacrimation is insufficient, contact lens prognosis is less favorable. Wetting is evaluated with a slit lamp biomicroscope (see p. 231 and 310).

Lid Edema

The ability of superficial body tissue to withstand pressure without becoming edematous apparently varies among individuals.[480] Pressure applied with a blunt object to the forearm of the patient usually produces a mild redness. In some cases, this redness is followed by a significant swelling—dermographia elevata. When such a swelling is produced, contact lens prognosis is less favorable.

MOIRÉ FRINGES

When two grating sheets of parallel, equispaced lines are superimposed, dark bars called moiré fringes are produced. The gratings, called Ronchi rulings, can have up to 1,000 lines/mm. (Fig. 11–9). If the line frequency and the angulation between the two superimposed sheets are known, the characteristics of the moiré fringes are mathematically predictable.[481–483]

Three factors combine to produce a sensitive, magnified measurement system of reflecting surfaces based on moiré fringes: measurement sensitivity is good when a high frequency grating is used; slight angulation of the superimposed gratings produces a relatively large displacement of the moiré fringes, which is a type of magnification; and image size of a reflecting surface varies linearly with its radius.

Instruments (Toposcopes) for measuring corneal and contact lens parameters based on this system have a variable magnification microscope and two similar gratings (Figs. 11–10 and 11–11).[484, 485] One grating acts as a target

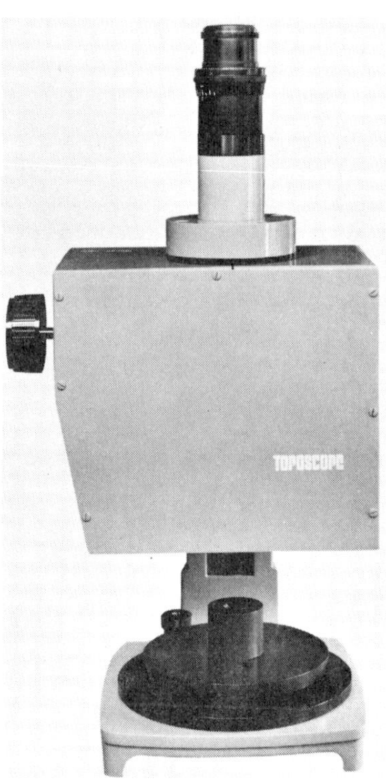

Figure 11–10. Toposcope. (Figs. 11–10 to 11–14 courtesy of Optical Methods, Inc.)

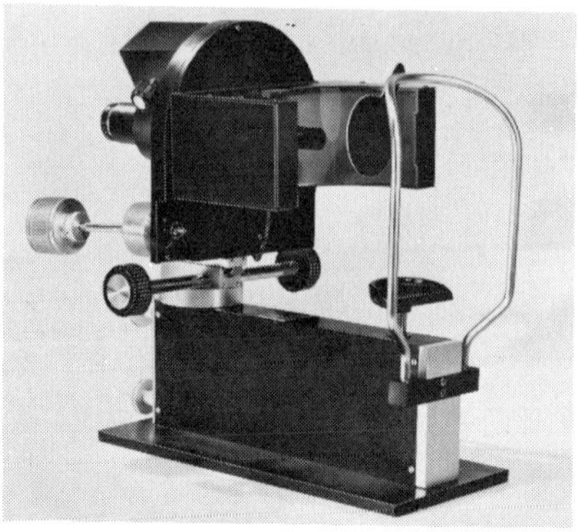

Figure 11–11. Corneal Toposcope.

and reflects off the surface to be measured. The image of this target grating is viewed through the microscope eyepiece, which contains the second grating.

Assume that a surface with a single spherical curvature is being measured. The instrument is designed so that when the magnification of the image of the target grating equals that of the eyepiece grating, fringes parallel to a guideline or index are seen (Fig. 11–12). When the magnification of the image of the target grating differs from that of the eyepiece grating, fringes at an angle to the guideline are produced (Fig. 11–13). Magnification of the image of the target grating and that of the eyepiece grating are equalized by variation of the magnification of the microscope. This adjustment produces parallelism of the fringes and the guideline. It is preferable to evaluate parallelism by concentrating only on the guideline and the adjacent fringe bars.

Magnification variance is produced by turning a dial calibrated in terms of radius of curvature. The final rotation of the dial should be clockwise.

When a surface has more than one spherical curvature in a given meridian, only one radius can be focused at a time. In measuring the posterior surface of the lens, first the fringes in the optic zone and then those in the secondary zone are focused and made parallel to the guideline (Fig. 11–14).

There is a measuring scale in the eyepiece reticle. Optic-zone and lens diameters can be measured by noting the change of curvature between optic and secondary zones and at the edge of the lens, respectively (Fig. 11–14).

Research will establish the clinical significance of instruments based on the use of moiré fringes.

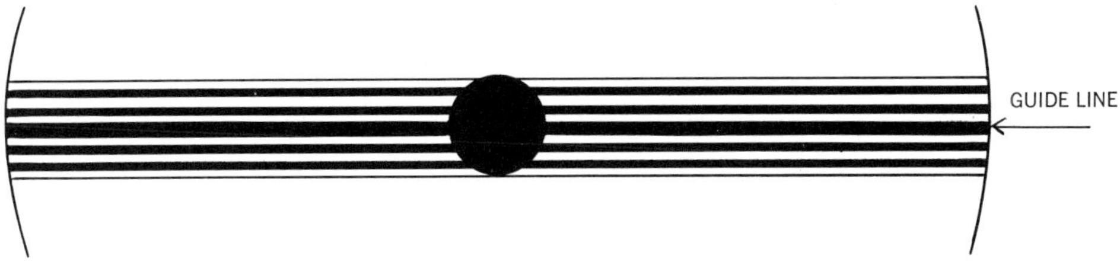

Figure 11–12. Radius is determined by making the fringes parallel to the guide-line.

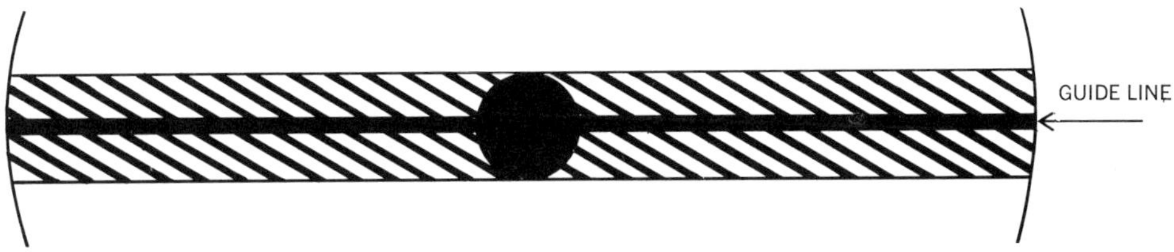

Figure 11–13. Because the fringes are not parallel to the guideline, magnification must be varied to determine the radius.

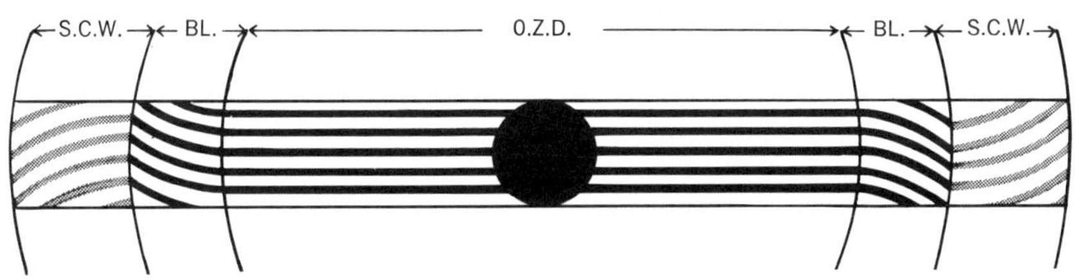

Figure 11–14. Fringes in the optic zone are focused and parallel to the guideline. Fringes in the secondary zone are not focused or parallel to the guideline. (O.Z.D., optic-zone diameter; S.C.W., secondary curve width.)

APPENDICES

Appendix I

HISTORY

Much of the history of contact lenses has been covered in the preceding pages. The contributions of a large number of people, many of whom are listed in the bibliography, constitute the true history of contact lenses. However, a capsule review of the milestones of contact lens history is presented here.

ca. 1508

Leonardo da Vinci outlines the basic optical principle of contact lenses. He conceives and diagrams the idea of neutralizing the anterior corneal power by immersing the eye in water.

ca. 1637

René Descartes first proposes placing lens directly on fluid of eye to correct ametropia. His diagram of this proposal shows a corneal type contact lens separated from the cornea by an extremely deep fluid layer.

ca. 1801

Thomas Young combines da Vinci's neutralizing concept and Descartes' concept of placing lens on the eye. Young uses this combination to determine that cornea is not responsible for accommodation.

ca. 1823 to 1827

Sir John Herschel suggests practical applications of contact lenses. He suggests they can be used with irregular cornea to improve vision and to protect cornea when the eyelids are scarred.

ca. 1887

Adolph Eugen Fick, Friedrich A. Muller, and E. Kalt independently develop the first contact lenses actually worn. Fick's lenses have refractive power; Muller's are more of an artificial eye used to protect cornea from scarred lid. Fick designs scleral lens and corneal lens with diameter equal to corneal diameter. Kalt's lenses are of corneal type. All are made of glass.

ca. 1900 to 1920

The Carl Zeiss Optical Company of Jena produces glass scleral and corneal contact lenses. Because of relatively great weight and possible breakage, these are not successful.

ca. 1929

Josef Dallos makes impressions and casts of eyes. Slightly later, he mentions lenticular, astigmatic, and fenestrated contact lenses.

ca. 1936

William Feinbloom is first American to use plastic for contact lenses. His scleral lenses have plastic haptic and glass corneal portions.

ca. 1938

Istvan Györffy, John Mullen, and Theodore Obrig develop completely plastic scleral contact lenses.

ca. 1938

Josef Dallos suggests fitting scleral contact lenses with minimum corneal clearance.

ca. 1943

Norman Bier develops a fluidless, fenestrated scleral contact lens. It is fitted with minimum corneal clearance, and has transitional curve between corneal and scleral portions to provide limbal clearance. He also discovers importance of bubble in such fitting.

ca. 1947

Kevin Tuohy makes first corneal contact lenses from plastic. Lenses are quite large (11 to 12 mm.) and quite thick. They are monocurve, except for narrow secondary curve.

ca. 1951

Frank Dickinson, John Neill, and Wilhelm Söhnges develop corneal contact lenses that are smaller and thinner than Tuohy lenses. These so-called "micro-lenses" have average diameter of 9.5 mm. and average center thickness of 0.20 mm. The micro-lens is basically a monocurve lens the posterior radius of which is about 0.3 to 0.4 mm. longer than the flatter ophthalmometric principal meridian.

ca. 1956

Norman Bier and Harold Moss develop lenses with relatively small optic zone (6.5 to 7.3 mm.). These lenses are fitted with relative apical alignment or very mild apical clearance. Surrounding the optic zone are secondary curvatures of longer radii than the base curve to allow a slight to moderate secondary clearance relationship. Average lens diameter and thickness are similar to that of micro-lens. Because of conformity to cornea, such lenses are frequently called contour lenses. They usually position superiorly on eye.

ca. 1960 to present

Charles Bayshore, David Ewell, Irving Filderman, Louis Girard, George Jessen, Whitney Sampson, Joseph Soper, and Paul White develop corneal contact lenses to position in palpebral aperture. Such lenses are generally relatively small (8.8 mm. or less).

William Feinbloom and David Volk develop aspheric contact lenses. Walter Becker develops contact lenses made from silicone rubber. Otto Wichterle develops contact lenses made from cross-linked hydrophilic polymers.

Appendix II

PATENTS

Some contact lens history is best summarized by patents currently effective in the United States and Great Britain. The heart of a patent is its claims, which define and limit the exclusive scope of the invention.

The claims and illustrations of selected patents that are currently in effect in the United States and Great Britain and that are related to contact lens constructions are given in the following pages. These patents are listed chronologically to give the reader a historical view of the development of contact lenses.

June 6, 1950; United States Patent 2,510,438; to Kevin M. Tuohy; for Contact Lens.

I CLAIM:

1. A contact lens applicable to the human eye comprising a concavo-convex lens formed of light-transmitting material having a marginal size smaller than the limbus portion of the eye to which it is applicable but larger than the maximum iris opening, said lens having a radius of curvature on its concave side slightly

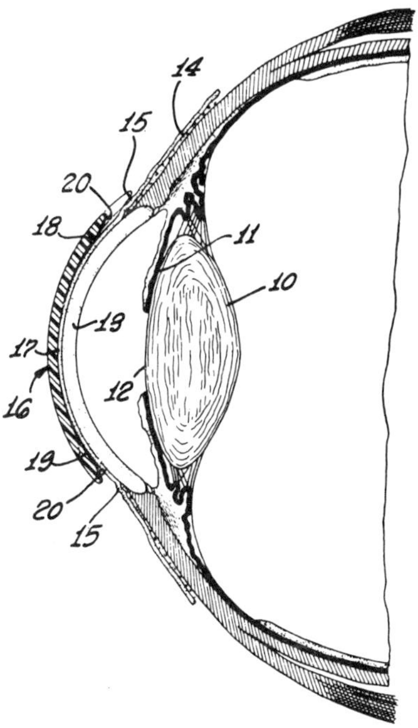

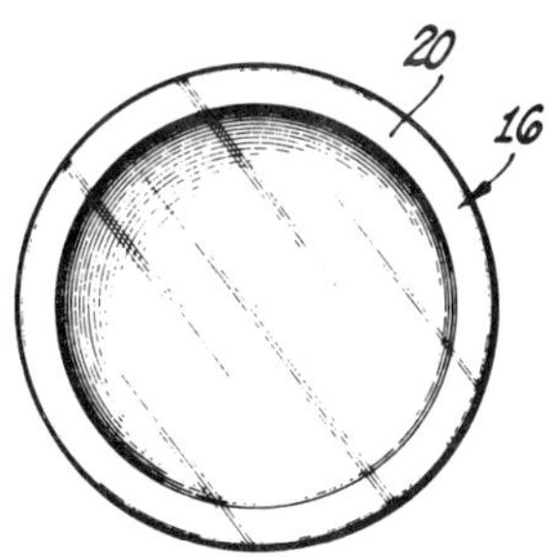

greater than the radius of curvature of the cornea to which it is applied so that radially from the center of the lens there will be a small but gradually increasing clearance for the entry of natural eye fluids between the lens and the cornea, said lens being ground to correct for visual deficiency.

2. A contact lens applicable to the human eye comprising a concavo-convex lens formed of light-transmitting material having a marginal size smaller than the limbus portion of the eye to which it is applicable but larger than the maximum iris opening, said lens having a radius of curvature on its concave side slightly greater than the radius of curvature of the cornea to which it is applied so that radially from the center of the lens there will be a small but gradually increasing clearance for the entry of natural eye fluids between the lens and the cornea, said lens being ground to correct for visual deficiency and having a bevel at its marginal edges on the concave side thereof.

March 6, 1951; United States Patent 2,544,246; to George A. Butterfield; for Corneal Contact Lens.

I CLAIM:

1. A corneal contact lens of concavo-convex form in section and of a size to lie within the area defined by the limbus having an inner central spherical area conforming to the corresponding area of the cornea to which the lens is applied so that undue pressure will not be present at any point, the remainder of said inner surface extending radially outward toward the limbus being formed on a curve different from that of said central area and corresponding in curvature with that portion of the corneal peripheral area to which the lens is applied, whereby space is provided for the natural uninterrupted circulation of lacrimal fluids between said lens and the cornea.

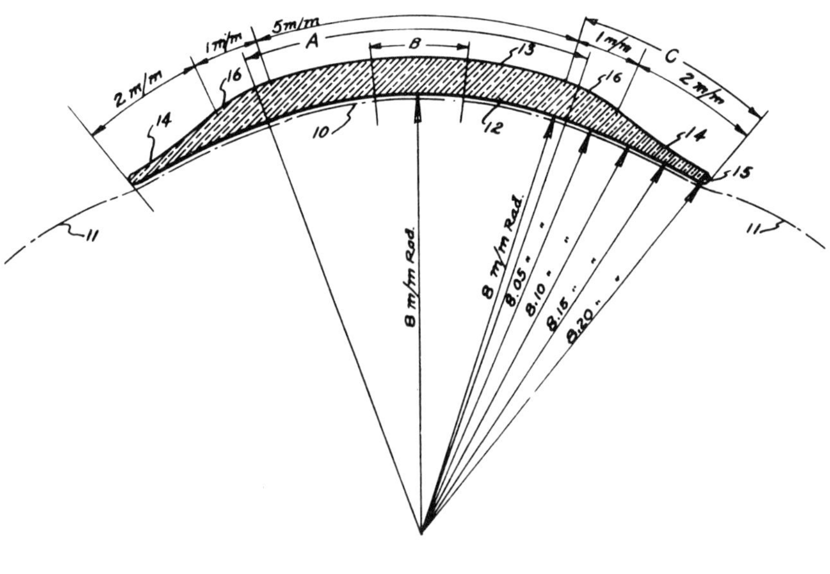

2. A corneal contact lens as in claim 1 wherein the anterior marginal area is gradually reduced in thickness toward the periphery of the lens by an arcuate facing in reverse curvature to the convex surface of the lens, both the junction of said arcuate facing with the remaining central convex portion and the lens edge having a smooth transition whereby the eyelids may pass freely over said edge.

3. A corneal contact lens as in claim 1 wherein the anterior marginal area is gradually reduced in thickness toward the periphery of the lens by a concave facing in reverse curvature to the convex surface of the lens, both the junction of said concave facing with the remaining central convex portion and the lens edge having a smooth transition whereby the eyelids may pass freely over said edge.

June 9, 1953; United States Patent 2,641,161; to Samuel W. Silverstein for Contact Lens.

HAVING DESCRIBED THE INVENTION, WHAT IS CLAIMED AS NEW IS:

1. A contact lens comprising a corneal section of the lens covering a portion of the cornea of the eye and spaced therefrom so as to retain lacrimal fluid between it and the cornea by capillary action, said corneal section being larger than the pupil but smaller in size than the cornea, thus leaving a marginal annular portion of the cornea uncovered, a scleral section of the lens covering a portion of the sclera but leaving an inner substantially annular portion of the sclera uncovered, said scleral section being curved and shaped for contact with the sclera

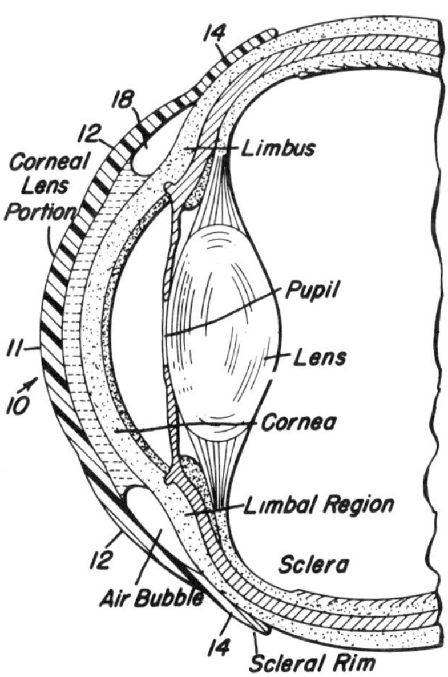

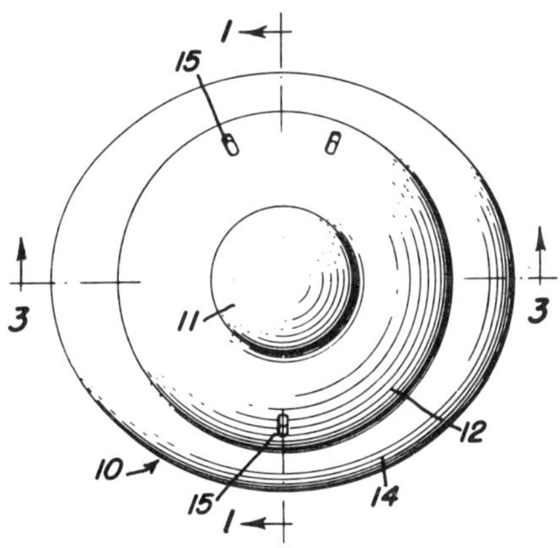

along a limited portion of the same, an intermediate section between said corneal and scleral sections, covering the limbal region of the eye and the adjacent substantially annular corneal and scleral portions, said intermediate section having a curvature of a smaller radius of curvature than the adjacent sections of the eye, so as to produce an enlarged annular space between the contact lens and the eye forming a pocket, bulging outwardly from the eye around the corneal section, the zone of transition joining said intermediate section and the scleral section having a contour shaped in accordance with the shape of the limbal region of the eye, and channels piercing said outwardly bulging intermediate zone for conducting the lacrimal fluid produced on the outside of the contact lens into the pockets on the inside, said pockets being thus filled partly with air and partly by the lacrimal fluid.

2. A contact lens as claimed in claim 1 wherein the curved cross section of the intermediate section has a curvature which is composed of different curves joining each other so as to form a curved line with varying radius of curvature, the resulting combined curve producing the aforesaid outwardly bulging annular section surrounding the corneal section.

3. A contact lens comprising a corneal lens section having an inner surface spaced from the cornea and ground so as to form the outer surface of a fluid meniscus held between the corneal section and the cornea by capillary attraction and adapted to correct a deficiency of vision, said corneal section being larger than the pupil, but smaller than the cornea, so as to leave an outer marginal portion of the cornea uncovered, an intermediary lens section covering the outer marginal portion of the cornea, the limbal region of the eye and the inner marginal portion of the sclera of the eye adjacent to the limbal region, said intermediate section being curved outwardly with an average radius of curvature smaller than the radius of curvature of the region of the eye which is covered, thus forming an outwardly bulging annular pocket of a size wider than the distance between the corneal lens section and cornea around the fluid meniscus held between the corneal lens section and cornea in contact with the sclera and cornea, and a scleral lens section covering a portion of the sclera located around the aforementioned inner marginal portion of the sclera, and having a curvature approximately equal to that of the eye, the contour of the junction line between the scleral lens portion and the outwardly bulging intermediary lens section following approximately the shape of the limbal region of the eye, and channels leading from the outside into the annular outwardly bulging pocket, in order to obtain a free circulation of the lacrimal fluid over the limbal region and through an air filled space over the cornea.

September 29, 1953; United States Patent 2,653,515; to Noel O. Stimson; for Corneal Contact Lens.

WHAT IS CLAIMED IS:

1. A corneal contact lens of approximately the same area as the cornea of a human eye and having a posterior concavity defining a surface predetermined

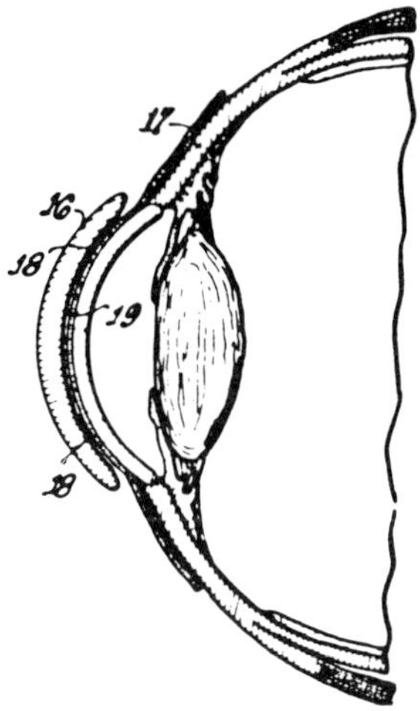

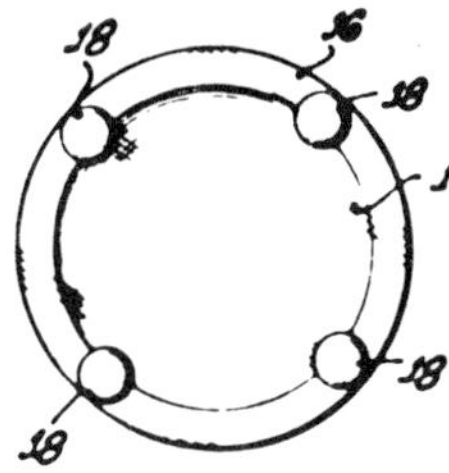

regular curvature extending to the peripheral edges thereof, an even number of circumferentially spaced portions protruding inwardly of said concavity, said protruding portions being symmetrically disposed about the optical axis of said lens and adjacent the periphery thereof in position to simultaneously engage peripheral areas of the corneal surface of an eye to be fitted whereby said lens tends to assume proper orientation on said cornea when rotationally displaced about its optical axis.

2. A lens as defined in claim 1, wherein said concave surface is substantially spherical in shape and wherein there are four of said protruding portions.

3. A corneal contact lens of approximately the same area as the cornea of a human eye and having a concave posterior surface of predetermined regular curvature extending to the peripheral edges thereof, said surface having a predetermined radius of curvature in a first meridian plane and a lesser radius of curvature in a second meridian plane at right angles to said first plane, a pair only of relatively small areas of said lens protruding inwardly from the adjacent areas of said surface adjacent the periphery of said lens and in position to engage peripheral areas of the corneal surface of an eye to be fitted, said protruding portions being positioned at opposite ends of only one of said meridians, the other of said meridians being of such radius of curvature that at least the end portions thereof rest on said corneal surface.

4. A corneal contact lens of approximately the same area as the cornea of a human eye and having a concave posterior surface of predetermined regular curvature extending to the peripheral edges thereof, a plurality of discrete and circumferentially spaced portions of relatively small area protruding inwardly from said surface, said protruding portions being symmetrically disposed about the optical axis of said lens and adjacent the periphery thereof in position to simultaneously engage peripheral areas of the corneal surface of an eye to be fitted, each of said protruding portions defining a substantially flat facet extending chordally of said concave surface.

October 15, 1957; United States Patent 2,809,556; to Joseph J. Hornstein; for Contact Lens.

I CLAIM:

1. A corneal contact lens of concavo-convex form in section and of a size to lie within the area defined by the limbus having an inner central spherical area corresponding in its perimeter to the perimeter of the apical area of the cornea to which the lens is applied and formed on a smaller radius than the radius of said apical area so that a crescent-shaped space is present between said central spherical area and the surface of said apical area, and the remainder of the inner surface of said lens extending radially outwardly toward the limbus being formed on a greater radius than said central area and corresponding in curvature with the corneal peripheral area.

2. A corneal contact lens of concavo-convex form in section and of a size to lie within the area defined by the limbus having an inner central spherical area formed on a radius substantially smaller than the radius of the corresponding area of the cornea to which the lens is applied, so that a crescent-shaped space is present between said central spherical area and said corresponding area of the cornea, whereby pressure on the said corneal area is avoided, and the remainder of the inner surface of said lens extending radially outwardly toward the limbus being formed on a curve different from that of said central area and corresponding in curvature with that portion of the corneal peripheral area to which the lens is applied.

3. A corneal contact lens of concavo-convex form in section and of a size to lie within the area defined by the limbus having an inner central spherical area formed on a radius substantially smaller than the radius of the corresponding

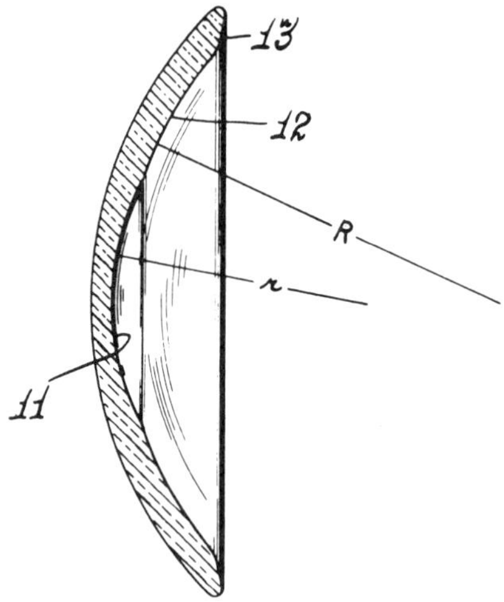

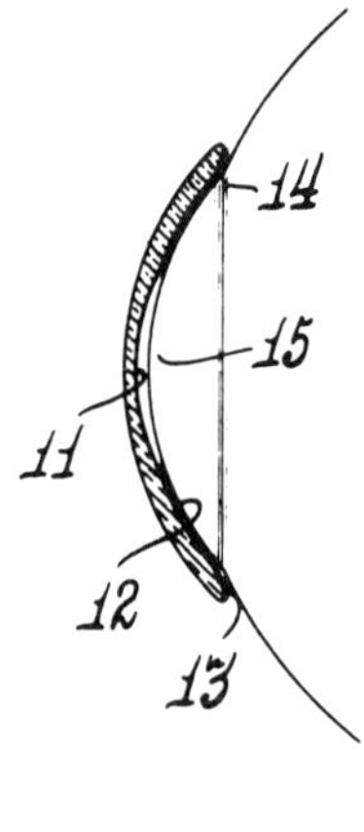

area of the cornea to which the lens is applied, so that a crescent-shaped space is present between said central spherical area and said corresponding area of the cornea, whereby pressure on the said corneal area is avoided, and the remainder of the inner surface of said lens extending radially outwardly toward the limbus being formed on a curve different from that of said central area and corresponding in curvature with that portion of the corneal peripheral area to which the lens is applied, said central spherical area of the lens and the corresponding area of the cornea defining in section a crescent-shaped tear space.

4. A corneal contact lens of concavo-convex form in section having a diameter falling within the area defined by the limbal zone of the cornea to which it is to be fitted, said lens having an inner central spherical area and a wide marginal area, the inside radius of the marginal area being formed on a curve corresponding substantially to the curvature of the peripheral area of the cornea, and the curvature of the central spherical area having a smaller radius than the radius of the corresponding area of the cornea so as to avoid conforming with said corneal area whereby a substantially crescent-shaped space is provided between said central spherical area and the cornea.

June 27, 1961; United States Patent 2,989,894; to Stanley Gordon; for Corneal Contact Lens with Spiral Vent Ducts.

I CLAIM:

A corneal contact lens of generally concavo-convex form having a diameter slightly less than that of the corneal portion of the eye to substantially cover the same without contacting the limbal area or sclera of the eye, the concave surface

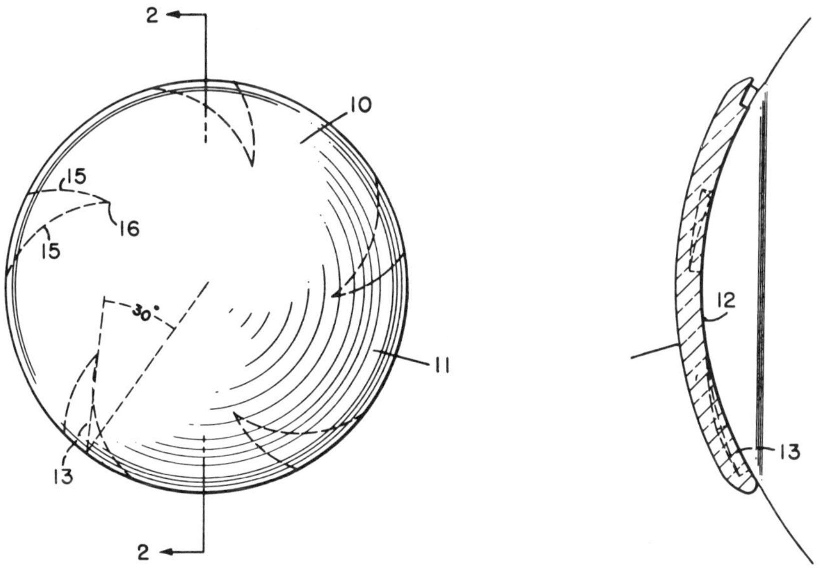

of said lens having a curvature conforming substantially to the natural curvature of the cornea, the inner concave surface of said lens being grooved to form a plurality of equally spaced ducts of generally elongated, spirally curved, tapered configuration extending from the periphery of said lens toward the center thereof, the curvature of said ducts corresponding substantially to the directionality of normal lachrymal flow in said eye whereby said ducts effect accelerated turning moments on said lens thereby to produce continual rotation of said lens at an accelerated rate and in a single direction for a given eye, said ducts being depressed in said concave surface and terminating, in depth, at the lens edge within the body thickness of said lens so as not to impinge on the convex side of said lens, each of said ducts having a relatively wide base adjacent the peripheral edge of said lens defining an arcuate opening substantially conforming to the peripheral edge of said lens for the entry of eye fluid, the arcuate open bases of said plurality of ducts being equally spaced from one another by ungrooved portions of said concave lens surface along the peripheral edge of said lens, the two sides of each said duct being of curved configuration, curved in the same direction relative to one another, and extending from the opposed edges of said arcuate opening in increasing proximity to one another to terminate said duct between the periphery and center of said lens at a location sufficiently distant from the center of said lens so as to avoid interference with vision through the central optical zone of said lens, each of said ducts tapering not only in width but also in depth between said relatively wide base opening and said terminating duct location, each of said ducts being deepest at its base and substantially smoothly merging into said concave surface of said lens at said terminating location, the terminating location of each said duct being angularly displaced from the center point of the duct base in such manner that an acute angle of substantially 30° is described between a lens radius passing through said duct base center point and a line passing from said duct base center point through said terminating duct location, the directionality of curvature for each duct, when each said duct is disposed during rotation adjacent the upper outer portion of an eye, extending generally downward and inwardly from a location adjacent the upper outer corner of the eye toward the inner lower corner of said eye, a pair of said lenses thus having their associated ducts curving in opposing directions in conformity with the opposite directions of normal lachrymal flow in a pair of eyes thereby to effect said continual accelerated rotation of said lenses in a counter-clockwise direction in the right eye, and in a clockwise direction in the left eye, as observed from the outer convex sides of said lenses.

April 3, 1962; United States Patent 3,027,803; to Irving P. Filderman; for Spectacle Lens–Contact Lens System.

I CLAIM AS MY INVENTION:

1. In a spectacle lens-contact system, a spectacle lens having a central objective portion of plus power and a peripheral portion, a corneal contact lens of generally concavo-convex cross-section adapted to be retained on the cornea of the eye by capillary attraction produced by a lacrimal layer between the lens and the cornea,

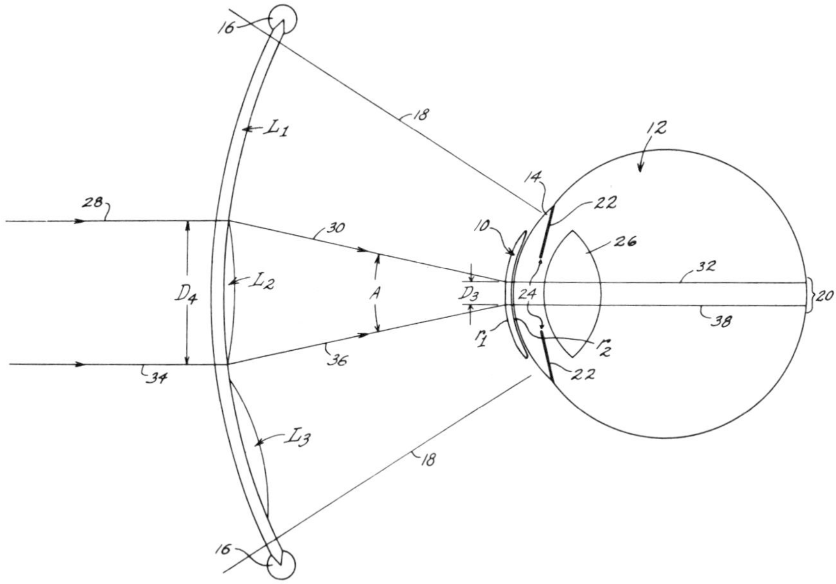

said corneal contact lens having a posterior surface curved to fit the cornea of a patient to which the lens is applied, having an ocular portion of high minus power and a peripheral portion, and having a maximum external dimension smaller than the limbus of eye and greater than the pupil size under normal illumination, said objective portion of said spectacle lens being separated from said ocular portion of said corneal contact lens approximately the normal vertex distance for an eye and a spectacle lens and having a power related to the power of said ocular portion such that the two form a Galilean telescope, said ocular portion of said corneal contact lens defining the exit pupil of said telescope and the diameter of said ocular portion being 2.5 to 3 mm. whereby said telescope involves central vision simultaneously with said peripheral portions of said spectacle and contact lenses involving peripheral vision, said peripheral portions each having dioptic power such that the two of them in conjunction with each other substantially meet the prescription requirements for the peripheral vision of the wearer of the system.

2. The lens system of claim 1 wherein said spectacle lens has a reading add portion off center relative to said objective portion which is optically related to said objective portion which is optically related to and cooperates with said ocular portion of said corneal contact lens.

May 1, 1962; United States Patent 3,031,927; to Newton K. Wesley; for Bifocal Corneal Contact Lens.

I CLAIM AS MY INVENTION:

1. A bifocal corneal contact lens of generally concavo-convex cross-section adapted to be retained on the cornea of the eye by capillary attraction produced by a

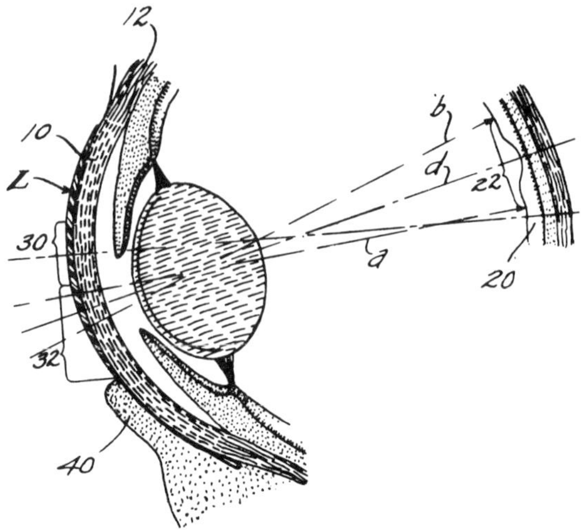

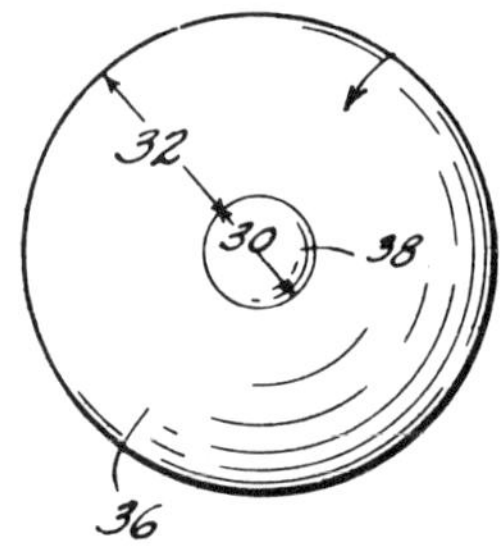

lacrimal layer between the lens and the cornea, said lens having a posterior surface curved to fit the cornea of a patient to which the lens is applied with a tendency to remain centered thereon and having a single base curve in at least the optical area thereof, said lens being of a diameter greater than the normal pupil size and less than the limbal area of the eye, and having its lower peripheral edge normally positioned adjacent the upper edge of the lower eyelid when the lens is centered on the cornea and the patient is looking straight ahead, said posterior surface having its peripheral edge formed to provide clearance between the lens edge and the cornea to facilitate upward shifting movement of the lens whereby, when the eye moves to a downcast position, the lens will be shifted upwardly relative to the cornea by contact of its lower edge with the upper edge of the lower eyelid, said lens having a central zone and a concentric outer zone, said central zone being of substantially circular outline and of a diameter between 3 mm. and 6 mm. whereby central vision may shift therefrom to said outer zone upon engagement of the lower edge of said lens with the upper edge of the lower eyelid, said central zone being powered on the anterior surface for distance vision thereof with respect to the cornea of the patient, said outer zone being powered also on the anterior surface thereof for near vision with respect to such cornea, the anterior surface of said central zone having a radius of curvature flatter than the radius of curvature of the anterior surface of said outer zone to provide the respective distance and near vision powers, said outer zone completely surrounding said central zone so as to be equally effective for near vision in all positions of rotation of said lens with respect to the cornea.

2. A bifocal corneal contact lens of generally concavo-convex cross-section adapted to be retained on the cornea of the eye by capillary attraction produced by a lacrimal layer between the lens and the cornea, said lens having a posterior surface curved to fit the cornea of a patient to which the lens is applied with a tendency to remain centered thereon and having a single base curve in at least the optical area thereof, said lens having a maximum external dimension greater than the normal pupil size and less than the limbal area of the eye and having an

outer lowermost portion normally positioned adjacent the upper edge of the lower eyelid when the lens is centered on the cornea and the patient is looking straight ahead, said posterior surface having its outer peripheral portion formed to provide clearance between the lens edge and the cornea to facilitate upward shifting movement of the lens whereby, when the eye moves to a downcast position the lens will be shifted upwardly relative to the cornea by contact of its lowermost portion with the upper edge of the lower eyelid, said lens having a central zone and an outer zone, said central zone being of substantially circular outline and of a diameter between 3 mm. and 6 mm. whereby central vision may shift therefrom to said outer zone upon engagement of the lowermost portion of said lens with the upper edge of the lower eyelid, said central zone being powered on the anterior surface for distance vision thereof with respect to the cornea of the patient, said outer zone being powered, also on the anterior surface thereof, for near vision with respect to such cornea, the anterior surface of said central zone having a radius of curvature flatter than the radius of curvature of the anterior surface of said outer zone to provide the respective distance and near vision powers.

May 2, 1962; Great Britain Patent 895,334; to Raymonde Jeanne Augustine Koch; for Bifocal Contact Lens.

WHAT I CLAIM IS:

1. A bifocal contact lens having an upper part of one focal length and a lower part of a different focal length, the lower part being of such thickness that the

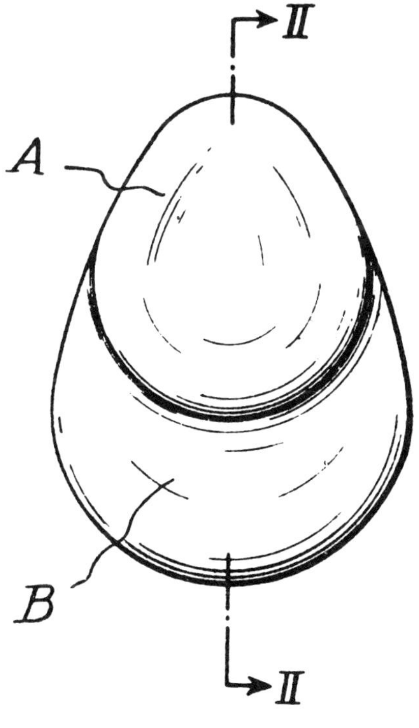

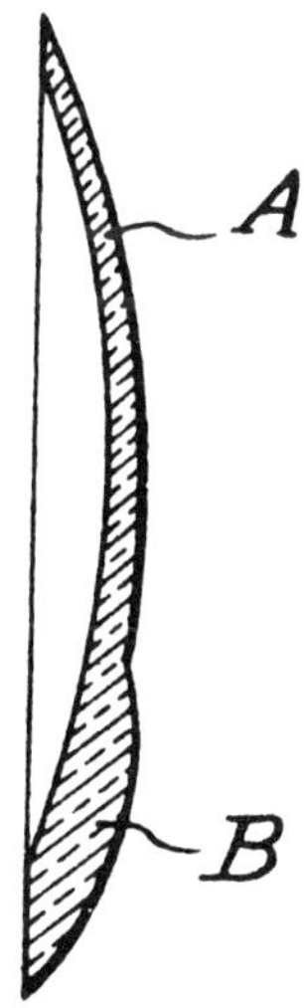

centre of gravity of the lens lies substantially below the centre of the total area of the lens and a gravitational force is thereby set up strongly opposing rotation of the lens on the eyeball.

2. A bifocal contact lens according to Claim 1 wherein the said lower part is of crescent shape.

3. A bifocal contact lens according to Claim 1 or Claim 2 wherein the said two parts of the lens have a common radius of curvature on the concave side of the lens and different radius of curvature on the convex side of the lens, the radius of curvature of the convex lower part being smaller than that of the convex upper part.

4. A bifocal contact lens according to any preceding claim wherein the lens is tapered towards its upper end.

5. A bifocal contact lens according to any preceding claim wherein the lens is of maximum width at a level adjacent the lowermost point of the upper part of the lens.

6. A bifocal contact lens substantially as described herein with reference to the accompanying drawings.

May 15, 1962; United States Patent 3,034,403; to Charles W. Neefe; for Contact Lens of Apparent Variable Light Absorption.

I CLAIM:

A protective contact lens for wear on the eye comprising a transparent concavo-convex lens fitted to the curvature of the eye and having a small, circular, tinted light absorbing area in the center of the lens, the diameter of said area being

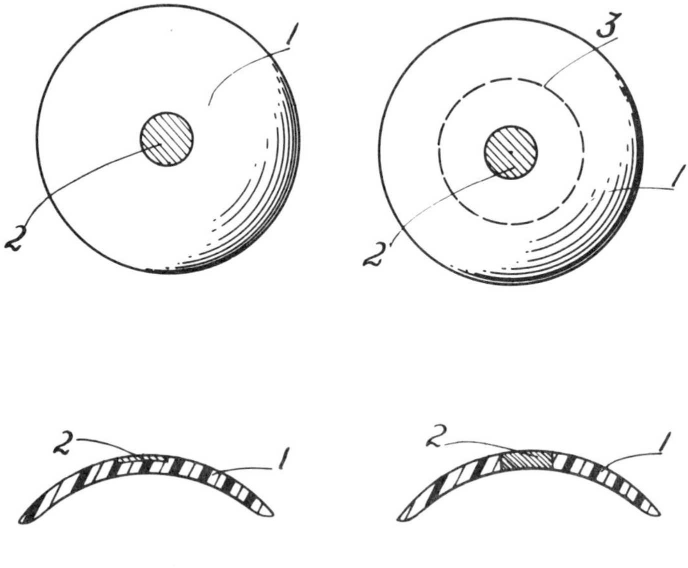

appreciably smaller than the diameter of the eye pupil when dilated in dim light and approximating the diameter of the eye pupil when contracted in bright light, whereby the tinted light absorbing area has a greater effectivity in overall light reduction in bright light and lesser effectivity in dim light.

September 5, 1962; Great Britain Patent 905,289; to the Plastic Contact Lens Company; for Corneal Contact Lens.

WHAT WE CLAIM IS:

1. A polyfocal corneal contact lens adapted to adhere to the cornea by capillary attraction produced by a lacrimal layer having means for preventing rotation of the lens on the cornea.
2. A lens according to Claim 1 wherein rotation of the lens is prevented by constructing the lens so that its centre of gravity is below the lens axis when the lens is in use.
3. A lens according to Claim 1 or Claim 2 divided into two zones of different power.
4. A lens according to Claims 1, 2 or 3 wherein the means for preventing rotation comprises a transparent insert in that part of the lens which is to be lowermost in use.
5. A lens according to Claim 4 in which the insert is of a material having a different refractive index to the material of the lens.
6. A lens according to Claim 4 or Claim 5 in which the insert is of a material of a higher specific gravity than the rest of the lens.
7. A lens according to Claim 3 in which one zone, which is to be the lowermost when the lens is in use, is thicker than the other zone so that the centre of gravity of the lens is spaced from the axis.
8. A lens according to Claim 3 in which one of the zones is circular and is located eccentrically with respect to the other so that it is wholly or partly surrounded by it and so that the centre of gravity of the lens lies to the side of the lens axis remote from the centre of the circular zone.
9. A lens according to Claim 3 wherein both zones have a common posterior curve and different anterior curves in which one anterior curve is generated as a partial surround relative to another curve.

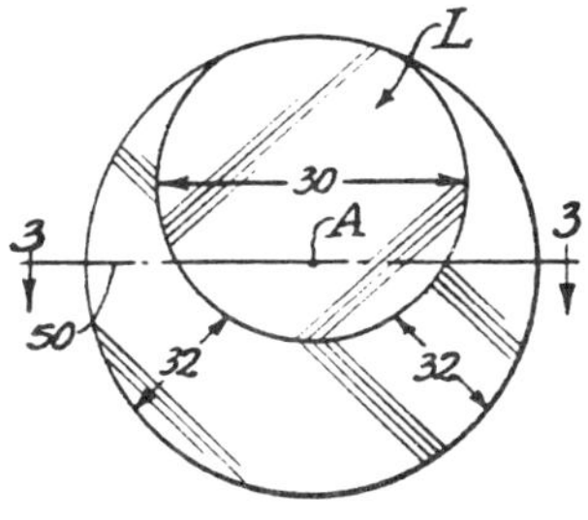

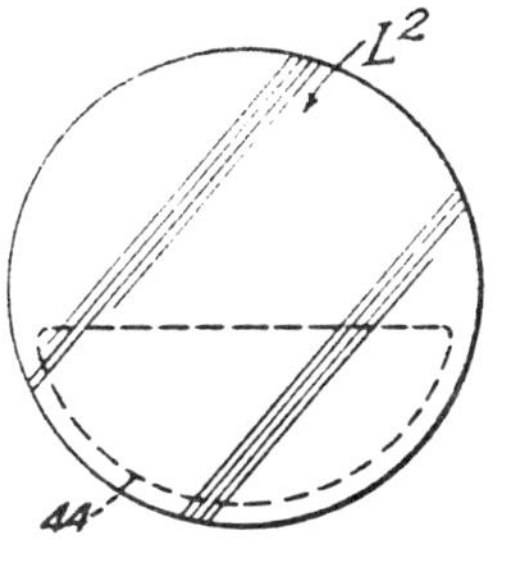

10. A lens according to Claim 9 in which one of the curves undercuts the other so as to reduce the extent of the area of the other said one on the lens.

11. A lens according to any preceding claim wherein the surface to contact the eye is a toric surface.

12. A lens according to any preceding claim in which at least one zone of the lens is of a power and size to accommodate central vision of the retina.

13. A lens according to any preceding claim which is smaller than the limbal area of the eye.

14. A lens according to any preceding claim so shaped as to be capable of movement by the lower eyelid.

15. A polyfocal lens adapted to adhere to the cornea by capillary attraction produced by a lacrimal layer substantially as described herein with reference to Figures 1–4, Figure 5, Figures 6–7, Figure 8, Figure 9, Figure 10, Figures 11–14, and Figures 15–18 of the accompanying drawings.

November 13, 1962; United States Patent Reissue 25,286; to John Trevor de Carle; for Bifocal Corneal Contact Lens.

I CLAIM:

1. A bifocal corneal contact lens of generally concavo-convex form having a maximum external dimension smaller than the limbus of the eye of the patient to whom the lens is applied, said lens including a pair of concentric lens zones having a total area adapted to be only slightly greater than the largest normal area of the pupil of the eye, the central one of said lens zones being circular and having an area approximately half the area of the pupil under average lighting conditions so the patient can see simultaneously through both of said lens zones, the outer one of said lens zones having anterior and posterior curvatures to provide for the patient's prescribed vision at close range, the central lens zone having an anterior surface of the same curvature as said anterior surface of said outer lens zone, the posterior surface of said central lens zone being in the form of a spherical recess of shorter radius of curvature than the radius of curvature of the posterior surface of said outer lens zone and defining, together with the

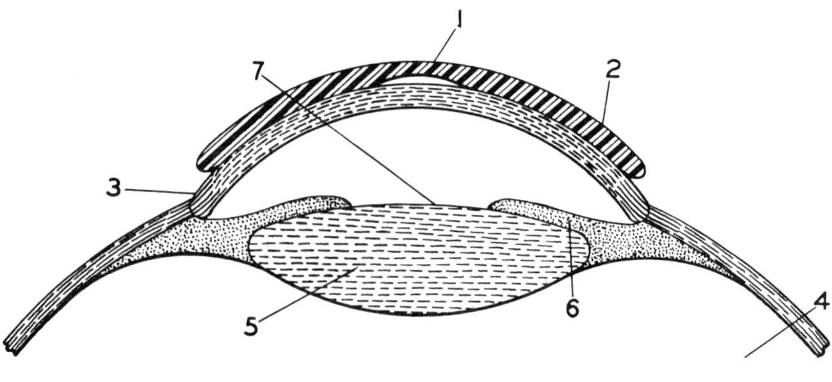

tear fluid filling said recess, the distance prescription for the patient, the curvature of the posterior surface of said outer lens zone substantially conforming to the curvature of the cornea of the eye to provide a relatively tight fit for keeping the lens centered on the eye and for minimal movement so the patient can see simultaneously through both of said lens zones for bifocal vision.

2. A bifocal corneal contact lens of generally concavo-convex form having a maximum external dimension smaller than the limbus of the eye of the patient to whom the lens is applied, said lens including a central lens zone and an outer lens zone which together have a total area adapted to be only slightly greater than the largest normal area of the pupil of the eye, said central lens zone being circular and having an area approximately half the area of the pupil under average lighting conditions so the patient can see simultaneously through both of said lens zones, the outer one of said lens zones having anterior and posterior curvatures to provide for the patient's prescribed vision at close range, the central lens zone having an anterior surface of the same curvature as said anterior surface of said outer lens zone, the posterior surface of said central lens zone being in the form of a spherical recess of shorter radius of curvature than the radius of curvature of the posterior surface of said outer lens zone and defining, together with the tear fluid filling said recess, the distance prescription for the patient, the curvature of the posterior surface of said outer lens zone substantially conforming to the curvature of the cornea of the eye to provide a relatively tight fit for keeping the lens centered on the eye and for minimal movement so the patient can see simultaneously through both of said lens zones for bifocal vision.

November 14, 1962; Great Britain Patent 910,455; to Emanuel Sokel; for Corneal Contact Lens.

WHAT I CLAIM IS:

1. A combination of a corneal lens and a removable additional lens adapted to be located over at least a part of the front surface of the corneal lens and having a rear surface substantially corresponding to that part of the front surface of the corneal lens with which it is to contact.

2. The combination according to Claim 1 in which the additional lens is approximately semicircular and has a front surface such that the focal length of that part of the corneal lens over which the additional lens lies is modified.

3. The combination according to Claim 2 in which the diametrical edge of the additional lens is smoothly curved to obviate sharp corners.

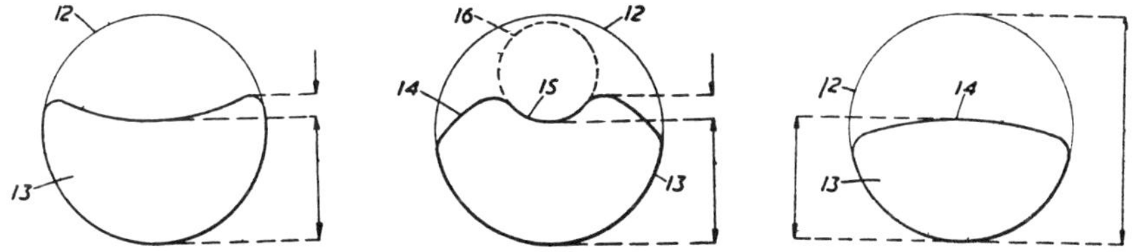

4. The combination according to Claim 2 or Claim 3 in which the diametrical edge of the additional lens is bevelled.

5. The combination according to any of Claims 2 to 4 in which the diametrical edge of the additional lens is centrally and smoothly indented.

6. A removable corneal lens shaped to overlie, as an additional lens, at least part of the front surface of an associated corneal lens and having a concave rear surface adapted to correspond with that part of the front surface of the associated corneal lens over which the additional lens is to lie to form a combination according to any one of the preceding claims.

7. A lens according to Claim 6 shaped to overlie approximately half of the front surface of an associated corneal lens.

8. A removable corneal lens according to Claim 6 and substantially as herein described with reference to any of the figures of the accompanying drawings.

9. The combination of a corneal lens and a removable additional corneal lens according to Claim 1 and substantially as herein described with reference to any of the figures of the accompanying drawings.

August 27, 1963; United States Patent 3,102,157; to Elmer L. Gamber; for Corneal Contact Lens Having Stop Flange Engaged by Eyelid.

WHAT I CLAIM IS:

1. A corneal contact lens comprising a concavo-convex lens formed of light transmitting material having a marginal size smaller than the limbus portion of the

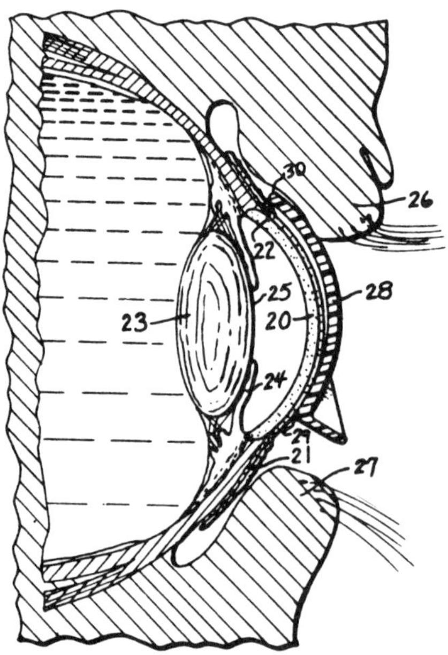

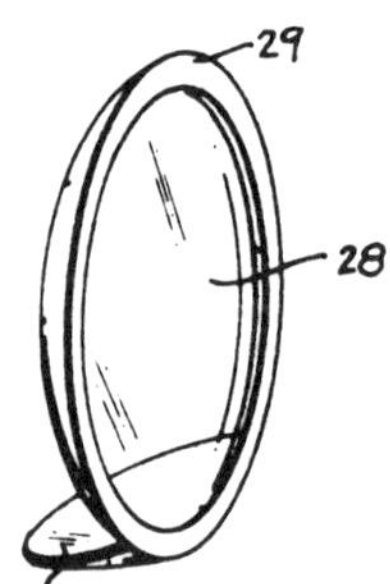

eye and larger than the maximum iris opening thereof, said lens having an elongated downwardly facing stop flange with rounded ends and rounded outer edges projecting substantially normal to the convex side of the lens along the lower edge thereof, said stop flange being downwardly arched to conform to the upper surface of the lower eyelid and projecting forwardly approximately the width of said upper surface to thereby prevent rotation of the lens by engagement of the stop flange with the lower eyelid when urged thereagainst by the upper eyelid.

2. The corneal lens of Claim 1 in which said stop flange is crescent shaped.

3. A bi-focal corneal contact lens comprising a concavo-convex lens formed of light transmitting material having a marginal size smaller than the limbus portion of the eye and larger than the maximum iris opening thereof, said lens having a bottom forwardly projecting stop flange presenting an elongated downwardly facing stop face with rounded ends and rounded outer edges extending substantially normal to the convex side of the lens along the lower edge thereof, said stop face being downwardly arched to conform to the upper surface of the lower eyelid and extending forwardly approximately the width of said upper surface to thereby prevent rotation of the lens by engagement of the stop flange with the lower eyelid when urged thereagainst by the upper eyelid, the portion of said lens immediately above said stop face being thicker than the remainder of said lens and having its front surface formed to provide a bottom near-sight vision area of greater power than said remainder.

October 9, 1963; Great Britain
Patent 939,016; to Wilhelm Peter Söhnges;
for Corneal Contact Lens.

WHAT WE CLAIM IS:

1. A Corneal contact lens comprising concentric zones of different curvatures, characterised by a continuous or substantially continuous change of the lens curvature on the outside of the contact lens.

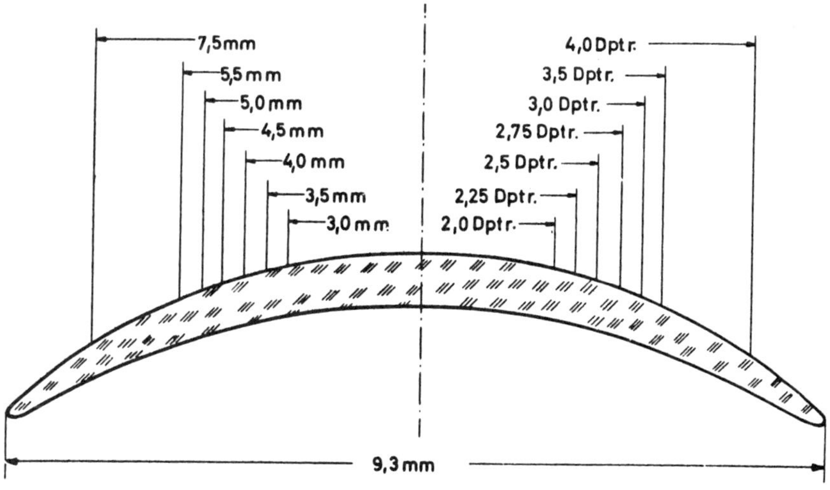

2. A Corneal contact lens as claimed in claim 1, characterised in that the continuous change of the lens curvature extends between the centre point of the lens and its bearing rim.

3. A Corneal contact lens as claimed in either one of claims 1 and 2, characterised in that the annular zones in which the mean variation corresponds to a given diopter value have different widths.

4. A Corneal contact lens substantially as hereinbefore described with reference to and as illustrated in the accompanying drawing.

June 1, 1965; United States Patent 3,187,338; to Charles W. Neefe; for Corneal Contact Lens of Wide Fitting Range with Sine Curve Concave Surface.

I CLAIM:

1. A corneal contact lens of concavo-convex form in section, of a size to lie within the area defined by the limbus and having a concave surface of aspherical form from center to edge composed of a sine curve, the central area having a radius shorter than the cornea to which it is applied and the outer edge having a radius longer than the cornea to which it is applied, whereby the angle of contact between the lens and cornea will remain constant if the radius of the cornea is changed.

2. A corneal contact lens of concavo-convex form in section, of a size to lie within the area defined by the limbus, having a concave, aspheric surface whose curvature is a sine curve, and an outer area having a radius of curvature longer than the cornea to which the lens is applied, whereby a satisfactory fit will result if the cornea or contact lens is of a different radius than the radius designated as correct.

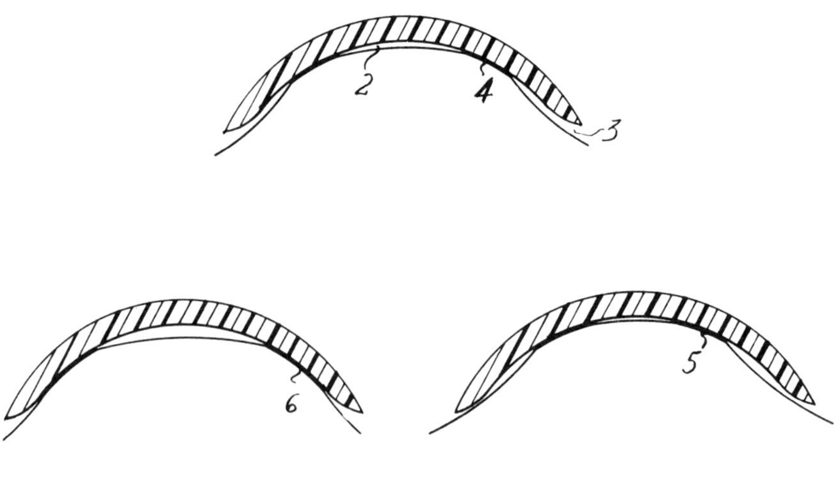

3. A corneal contact lens of concavo-convex form in section, of a size to lie within the area defined by the limbus, having a concave, aspheric surface whose curvature is a sine curve, and a central area having a radius of curvature shorter than the cornea to which the lens is applied, and an outer area having a radius of curvature longer than the cornea to which the lens is applied, whereby a satisfactory fill will result if the cornea or contact lens is of a different radius than the radius designated as correct.

October 12, 1965; United States Patent 3,212,097; to Irving N. Adler; for Truncated Prism Ballast Contact Lens with Indentation and Fluid Drainage Channel at Bottom Edge.

I CLAIM:

In an optical contact lens having a transparent lens body including inner concave and outer convex optical surfaces; there being an interior peripheral reverse undercut tapered continuous bevel formed in said concave surface of decreasing thickness towards its outer edge and transversely rounded to smoothly merge with said outer surface; said body including an off-centered prism ballast of increased thickness in its inferior nasal quadrant adjacent the bottom of the body rendering the lens non-rotatable when applied to the corneal surface of the eye; the improvement comprising:

the peripheral edge of said body at the top thereof having formed therein a radially extending inverted truncation substantially normal to the lens axis, said truncation also extending axially of the lens body for the purpose of gathering tear flow and directing the same toward the center of the eye over which the lens is applied;

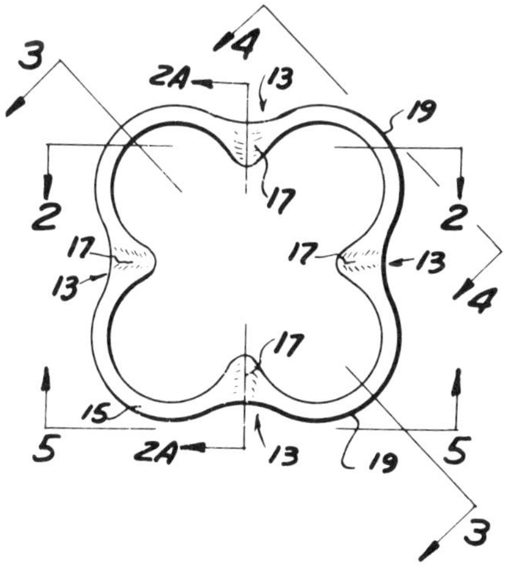

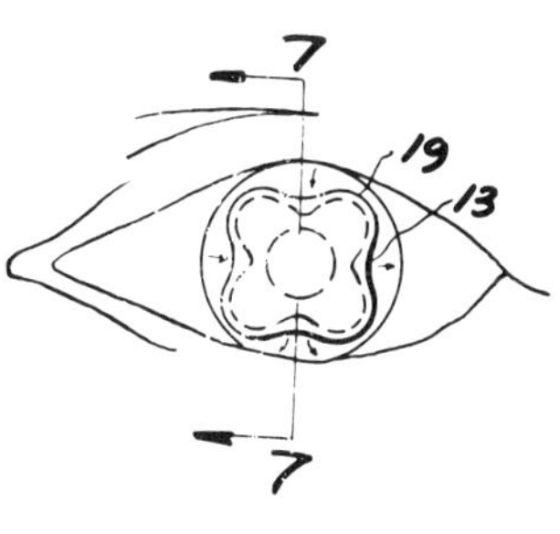

there being an oppositely disposed radial indentation in the peripheral edge of the body extending into said prism ballast at its bottom defining a trough formed at an angle of approximately 90 degrees to the lens axis, said indentation also extending axially of the lens body;

there being a substantially V-shaped radially extending fluid drainage channel formed in the bevel in the bottom edge of the body at said indentation, said channel extending into the concave surface radially inward of said bevel, said channel being defined by converging surfaces in angularly related planes extending radially inward of said body;

said truncation, said indentation and said fluid drainage channel facilitating the flow of precorneal fluid between the lens body and the eye for the purpose of equalizing osmotic pressure and improving in flow and out flow circulation of fluids with accompanying lubrication and improved comfort.

January 4, 1966; United States Patent 3,227,507; to William Feinbloom; for Corneal Contact Lens Having Inner Ellipsoidal Surface.

WHAT IS CLAIMED IS:

1. A corneal contact lens of concavo-convex form and of a size to lie within the area defined by the cornea, having an inner ellipsoidal surface, said ellipsoidal surface having its vertex on the major axis of the ellipsoid wherein in at least a first meridian the ellipse conforms substantially to the equations

$$r_0 = -\frac{b^2}{a} \tag{1}$$

$$r_x = \frac{(a^2x^2 + b^4 - b^2x^2)^{3/3}}{ab^4} \tag{2}$$

where r_0 = the radius of curvature at the apex of the cornea;
r_x = the radius of curvature of the cornea at the point which is a distance x approximately 4.5 mm. from the major axis of the ellipse contained in said meridian;
a = the semi-major axis of the ellipse in said meridian; and
b = the semi-minor axis of said ellipse.

2. A corneal contact lens as defined in claim 1, wherein the central portion of said ellipsoidal surface closely approximates a spherical surface having the radius r_0.

3. A corneal contact lens as defined in claim 1, wherein the meridian at right angles to said first meridian is a circle and said ellipsoidal surface constitutes a toric ellipsoid.

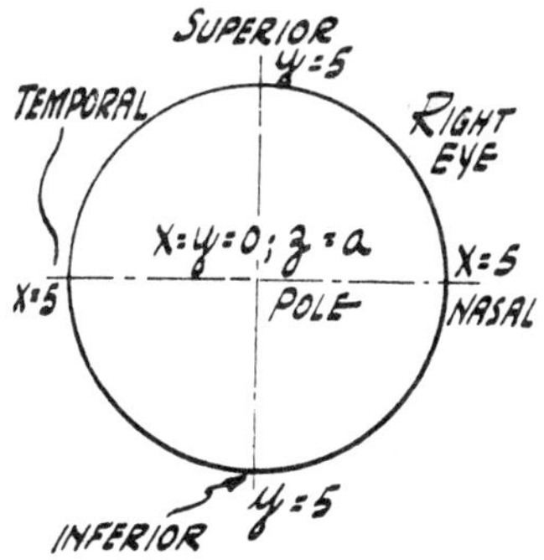

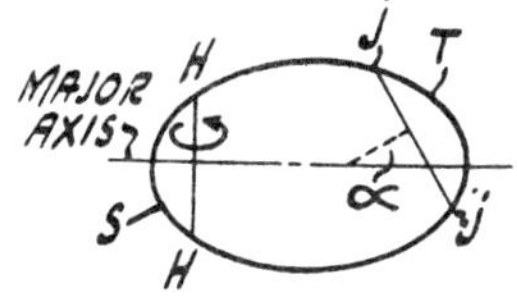

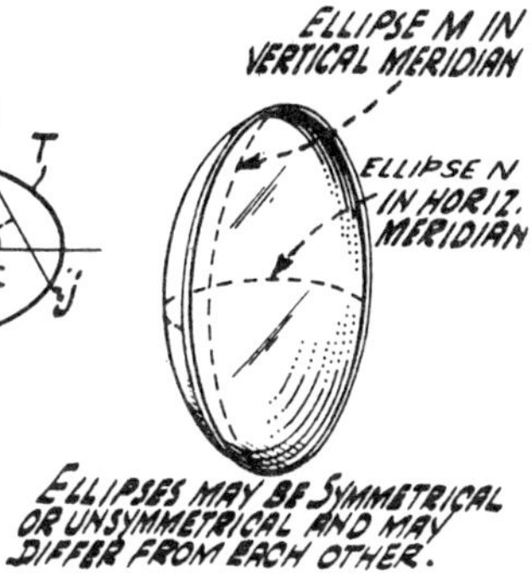

4. A corneal contact lens as defined in claim 1, wherein the meridian at right angles to said first meridian is an ellipse which differs from the ellipse in the first meridian, and said ellipsoidal surface constitutes an elliptical torus.

5. A corneal contact lens as defined in claim 1 having an unfinished outer surface opposite said ellipsoidal surface, and being of sufficient thickness to allow the grinding and polishing of a suitable optical curve on said outer surface to satisfy a desired prescription.

January 11, 1966; United States Patent 3,228,741; to Walter E. Becker; for Corneal Contact Lens Fabricated from Transparent Silicone Rubber.

WHAT IS CLAIMED IS:

1. An improved corneal contact lens of concavo-convex shape adapted to float on and adhere to the cornea, said lens having a concave surface curvature substantially conforming to the cornea, said lens being fabricated from transparent silicone rubber having a softness approximating that of the human cornea, said contact lens being bendable upon itself and capable of returning to its original shape upon release of distorting forces and being substantially unbreakable, said silicone rubber having a gas permeability for oxygen and carbon dioxide of at least about 10,000 cc. per 24-hour period per 100 square inch area per 1 mil thickness at a pressure differential of one atmosphere, thereby providing a contact lens which is substantially non-absorptive of tear fluids in liquid form and whose gas permeability is sufficient to substantially increase its normal safe wearing time.

2. The corneal contact lens of claim 1 wherein said silicone rubber comprises a cured mixture of hydrocarbon substituted polysiloxane and finely divided silica.

3. The corneal contact lens of claim 2 wherein the components of the mixture are selected to provide an index of refraction within the range of from 1.49 to 1.56.

4. The corneal contact lens of claim 1 wherein said silicone rubber comprises a

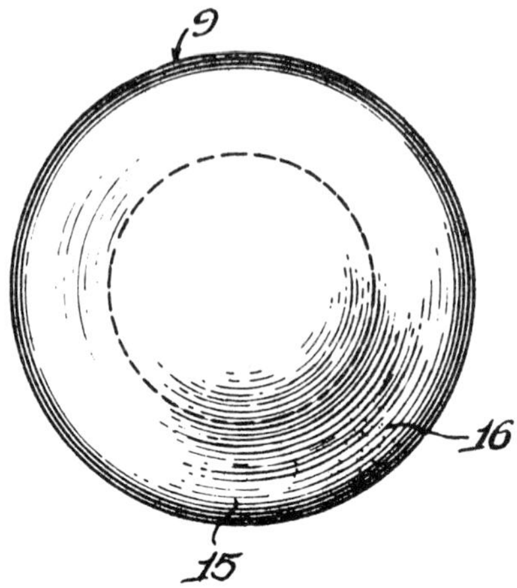

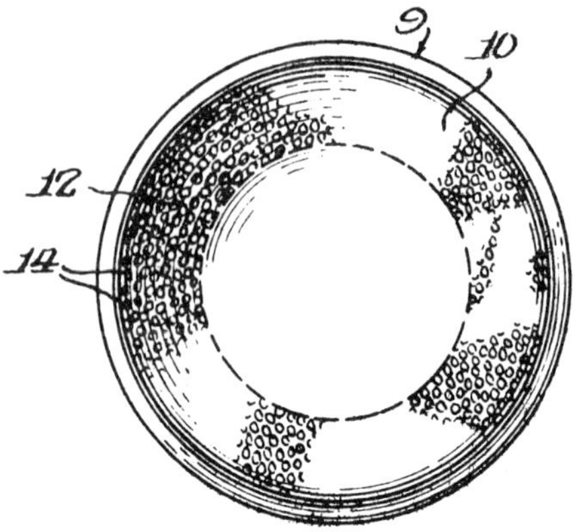

mixture of dimethyl polysiloxane and finely divided silica cured to form a rubbery transparent product.

5. The contact lens of claim 1 wherein said contact lens has fluid channel means in the peripheral portion of the concave surface thereof opening into a substantially smooth pool area in the central portion thereof, whereby tear fluid is readily conductible into the entire area between the contact lens and the cornea when the contact lens is worn.

6. The contact lens of claim 1 wherein the convex surface of said lens has a matte finish which substantially reduces surface tension of tear fluids in contact therewith.

April 14, 1966; Great Britain Patent 1,025,677; to Irving P. Filderman; for Contact Lenses.

WHAT I CLAIM IS:

1. For use upon the human eye, a corneal contact lens having a front convex surface and a rear concave surface curved in accordance with the geometry of the eye of the wearer to enable the lens to be retained upon the cornea of the eye by capillary attraction, the height of said lens being less than the distance between the normally open upper and lower eyelids of the wearer.

2. A corneal contact lens according to claim 1 having a height which is at least one-half millimetre less than the distance between the normally open upper and lower eyelids of the wearer.

3. A corneal contact lens according to claim 1 or 2, wherein the lower peripheral edge of the lens is adapted to be supported upon the lower eyelid of the wearer with the upper peripheral edge of the lens spaced from the upper eyelid.

4. A corneal contact lens according to any one of claims 1 to 3, the height of the lens being substantially equal to the distance between the lower eyelid and the uppermost point of the eye pupil of the wearer.

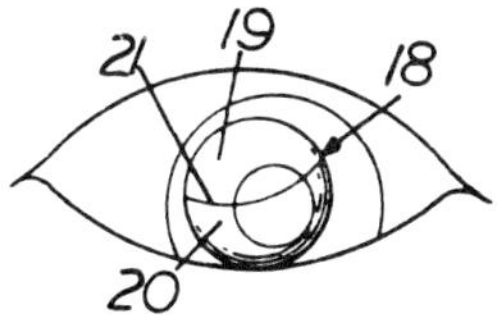

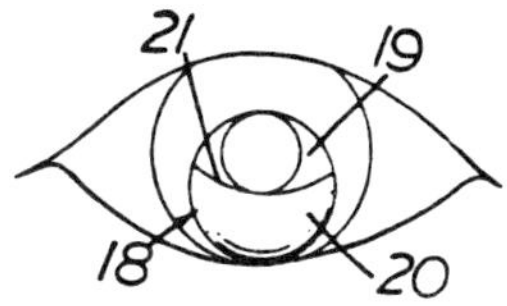

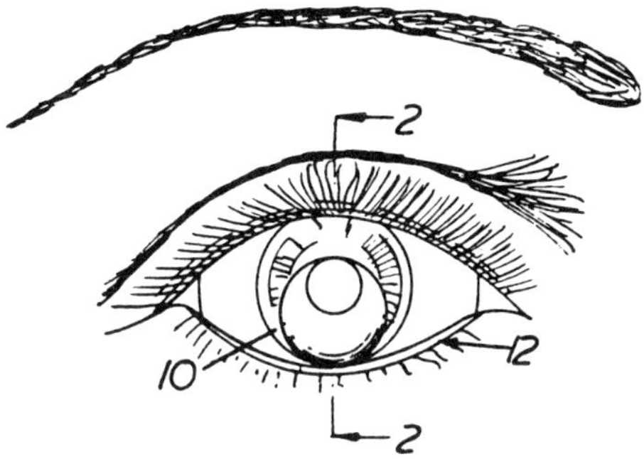

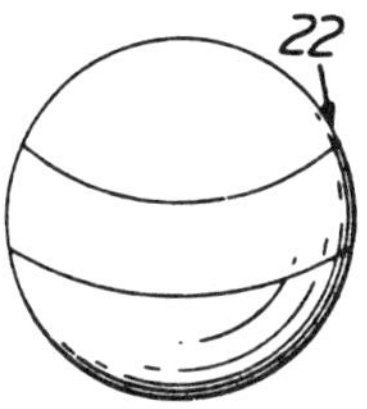

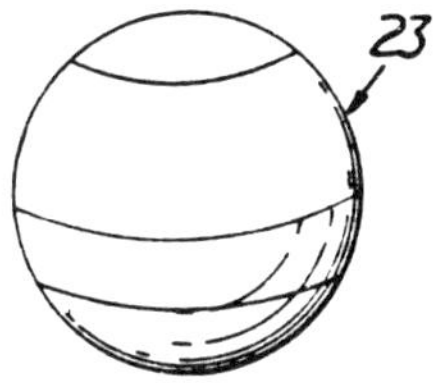

5. A corneal contact lens according to any one of claims 1 to 4, wherein the lens is formed with a plurality of optic zones of different refractive power, with juncture between adjacent zones being demarcated by an upwardly concave line of juncture.

6. A corneal contact lens according to claim 5, wherein the lens is a bifocal contact lens having an upper optic zone, a lower zone and an upwardly concave line of juncture between the said upper and lower optic zones, said line of juncture being spaced from the upper edge of said contact lens a distance substantially equal to the vertical diameter of the human eye pupil of the wearer.

7. A corneal contact lens according to any one of claims 1 to 6, wherein the lower portion of the lens is provided with a ballast.

8. A corneal contact lens according to any one of claims 1 to 7, wherein the diameter of the lens is between 7 and 8 millimetres.

9. A corneal contact lens substantially as hereinbefore described with reference to, and as illustrated in, Figures 1 to 3 of the accompanying drawings.

10. A corneal contact lens substantially as hereinbefore described with reference to, and as shown in, Figures 4 and 5 of the accompanying drawings.

11. A corneal contact lens substantially as hereinbefore described with reference to, and as shown in, Figure 6 or Figure 7 of the accompanying drawings.

April 19, 1966; United States Patent 3,246,941; to Herbert L. Moss; for Contact Lens with Upper Crescent Shaped Scleral Flange and Having Vent Channels and Apertures.

WHAT IS CLAIMED IS:

A contact lens for an eye having a central optic portion, a peripheral portion extending from and about the central portion and having an outer margin within the limbus of the eye and a corneal bearing surfaces conforming to and contacting the peripheral corneal region of the eye, a crescent shaped scleral flange por-

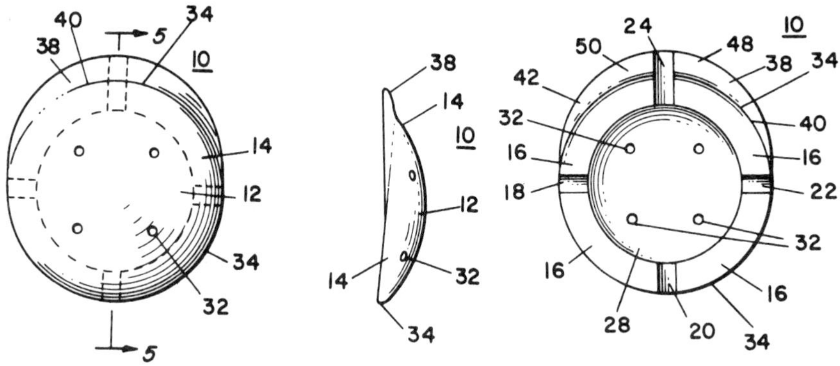

tion extending upwardly from the upper margin of the peripheral portion and having a scleral bearing surface conforming to a contacted superior portion of the sclera, said central portion having a recessed inner surface spaced from the cornea to provide therewith a chamber encompassed by said peripheral portion, and opening means providing for ingress and egress of lacrimal fluid into and out of said chamber, said opening means including a plurality of radial channels provided in the corneal contact surface of said peripheral portion and communicating with said chamber, one of said channels extending to the periphery of said scleral flange and being positioned to bisect said scleral flange, said opening means further including a plurality of apertures extending through said central portion in communication with said chamber, each of said apertures being located between the inner ends of an adjacent pair of channels.

August 30, 1966; United States Patent 3,270,099; to Richard N. Camp; for a Method for Making Multi-focal Length Contact Lenses.

WHAT IS CLAIMED IS:

1. The method of producing a multi-focal lens comprising the steps of, providing a curved optical surface on a cured block of polymerized artificial resinous mate-

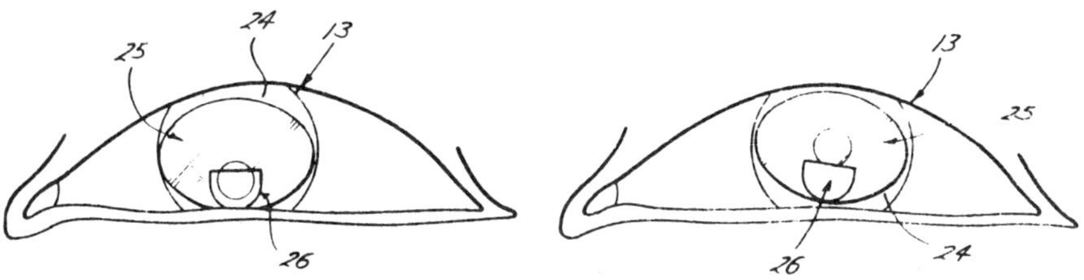

rial having a selected index of refraction, molding a polymerizable mass of artificial resinous material which when cured has a selected different index of refraction from said cured block by polymerization onto the curved optical surface of said cured block to form an integral bond between the resinous materials of the formable mass and the cured block at the curved optical surface, curing the formable mass of resinous material to form a monolithic mass, forming from a portion of said monolithic mass a lens having anterior and posterior optical surfaces of the desired lens optical characteristics having the same general curvature as said cured optical surface with the curved optical surface intersecting at least one of the anterior and posterior surfaces, the portion of the lens containing said three surfaces providing a different focal length than the remainder of the lens.

2. The method of producing a multi-focal lens comprising the steps of, providing a curved optical surface on a cured block of polymerized methyl methacrylate having a selected index of refraction, molding a polymerizable mass comprised of monomers, polymers and mixtures thereof of methyl methacrylate by polymerization onto the curved optical surface of said cured block to form an integral bond between the materials of the formable mass and the cured block at the curved optical surface, said formable mass of polymerizable material when cured having a selected different index of refraction from said cured block, curing the formable mass of material to form a monolithic mass, forming from a portion of said monolithic mass a lens having anterior and posterior optical surfaces of the desired lens optical characteristics having the same general curvature as said curved optical surface with the curved optical surface intersecting at least one of the anterior and posterior surfaces, the portion of the lens containing said three surfaces providing a different focal length than the remainder of the lens.

October 5, 1966; Great Britain Patent 1,045,065; to John Trevor de Carle; for Improvements in Contact Lenses.

WHAT I CLAIM IS:

1. A plastics contact lens assembly which comprises a contact lens having a peripheral skirt which is shaped to conform with the surface of the eyeball and which is constructed from a plastics material which is softer and more flexible from that of the lens.

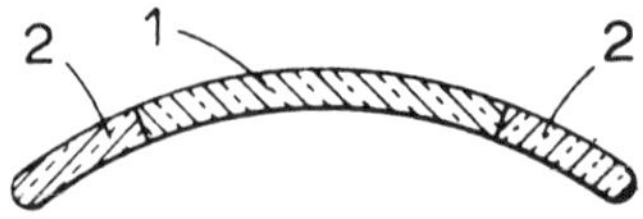

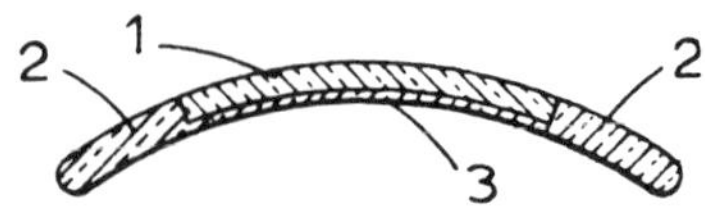

2. An assembly according to claim 1 wherein a layer of plastics material, which is softer and more flexible than that of the lens, extends over the concave back surface of the lens and is integral with the skirt.

3. An assembly according to claim 2 wherein a layer of plastics material, which is softer and more flexible than that of the lens, extends over the convex front surface of the lens and is integral with the skirt so that the lens is totally enclosed within a sheath of plastics material which is softer and more flexible than that of the lens.

4. An assembly according to any one of claims 1 to 3 wherein the skirt is constructed from two or more plastics materials of different degrees of hardness and flexibility so that there is a gradual decrease in the hardness of the assembly coupled with an increase in flexibility from the lens towards the edge of the assembly.

5. An assembly according to any one of the preceding claims wherein the lens and skirt are both constructed from epoxy resins.

6. An assembly according to any one of claims 1 to 4 wherein the lens is constructed from a homopolymer of methyl methacrylate or of ethyl acrylate or from a copolymer of methyl methacrylate with ethyl acrylate.

7. An assembly according to claim 6 wherein the skirt is constructed from a homopolymer of vinyl chloride, a copolymer thereof with vinyl acetate or from a fluorinated copolymer of ethylene and propylene.

8. A method of manufacturing a contact lens assembly as claimed in claim 1 which comprises shaping a cured plastics blank comprising a layer of optical quality plastics material bonded to a layer of softer and more flexible plastics material by cutting a concave cavity into the layer of optical quality plastics material through the layer of softer and more flexible plastic to form the back surface of the assembly and by cutting the opposite face of the blank to form the convex front surface of the assembly.

9. A method according to claim 8 wherein the blank itself has concave and convex outer surfaces, the optical quality plastics material having a convex outer surface, while the softer, more flexible plastics material has a concave outer surface.

10. A method according to claim 8 or 9 wherein the softer and more flexible plastics material is in the form of a plurality of layers of plastics materials having different degrees of hardness and flexibility, the degree of hardness decreasing and the flexibility increasing through the blank in a direction away from the plastics material of optical quality.

11. A method of manufacturing a contact lens assembly according to claim 1 which comprises shaping a blank comprising a cylinder of optical quality plastics material embedded in a flat slab of softer and more flexible plastics material, the axis of the cylinder being at right angles to the plane of the slab.

12. A method of manufacturing a contact lens assembly as claimed in claim 3 which comprises sandwiching the lens between a pair of saucer-shaped members of softer and more flexible plastics material which overlap the edge of the lens and sealing the edges of the saucer-shaped members together to form the skirt.

13. A contact lens assembly substantially as described with reference to Figures 1 to 5 of the accompanying drawings.

14. A method of manufacturing a contact lens assembly substantially as described with reference to Figures 1 to 7 of the accompanying drawings.

October 18, 1966; United States Patent 3,279,878; to William E. Long; for Bi-focal Corneal Contact Lens.

I CLAIM:

1. A bi-focal corneal contact lens of generally concavo-convex cross section adapted to be retained on the cornea of the eye by capillary attraction produced by a lachrymal layer between the lens and the cornea, said lens having a posterior surface curved to fit the cornea of a patient to which the lens is applied with a tendency to remain centered thereon and having a single base curve in at least the optical area thereof, said lens having a maximum external dimension greater than the normal pupil size and less than the limbal area of the eye, said posterior surface having its outer peripheral portion formed to provide clearance between the lens edge and the cornea, said lens having an upper optical zone and a lower optical zone, said upper optical zone being powered on the anterior surface for distance vision thereof with respect to the cornea of the patient, said lower optical zone being powered also on the anterior surface thereof for near vision with respect to such cornea, the anterior surface of said upper optical zone having a radius of curvature flatter than the radius of curvature of the anterior surface of said lower optical zone to provide the respective distance and near vision powers, with the center of curvature of the anterior surface of said upper optical zone being displaced downwardly relative to the axis of the lens and the curvature itself lying within the spherical extension of the anterior surface of said lower optical zone, the line of intersection of the two anterior curves on the

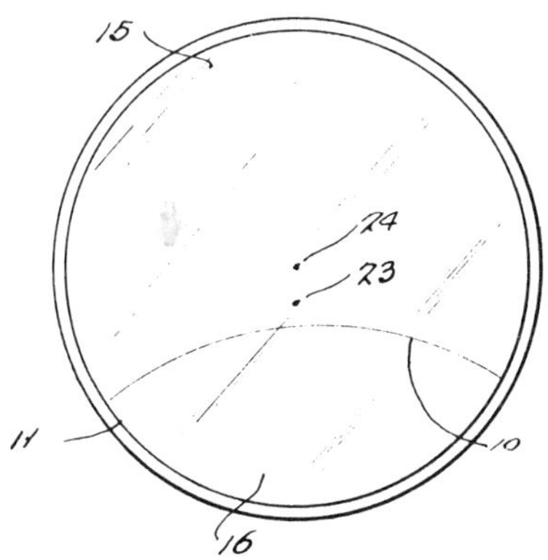

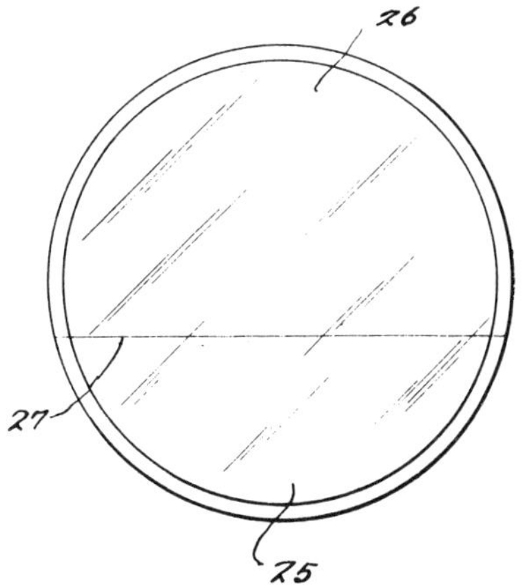

vertical center line of the lens being below the midpoint of said center line, the thickest portion of said lens being below said line of intersection and thereby heavier to restrain the lens from rotating on the cornea and to effect substantially constant positioning of said lower optical zone below said upper optical zone.

2. A bi-focal corneal contact lens of generally concavo-convex cross section adapted to be retained on the cornea of the eye by capillary attraction produced by a lachrymal layer between the lens and the cornea, said lens having a posterior surface curved to fit the cornea of a patient to which the lens is applied with a tendency to remain centered thereon and having a single base curve in at least the optical area thereof, said lens having a maximum external dimension greater than the normal pupil size and less than the limbal area of the eye, said lens having an upper optical zone and a lower optical zone, said upper optical zone being powered on the anterior surface for distance vision thereof with respect to the cornea of the patient, said lower optical zone being powered also on the anterior surface thereof for near vision with respect to such cornea, the anterior surface of said upper optical zone having a radius of curvature flatter than the radius of curvature of the anterior surface of said lower optical zone to provide the respective distance and near vision powers, with the center of curvature of the anterior surface of said upper optical zone being displaced downwardly relative to the axis of the lens and the curvature itself lying within the spherical extension of the anterior surface of said lower optical zone, the line of intersection of the two anterior curves on the vertical center line of the lens being below the midpoint of said center line, the thickest portion of said lens being below said line of intersection and thereby heavier to restrain the lens from rotating on the cornea and to effect substantially constant position of said lower optical zone below said upper optical zone.

3. A bi-focal corneal contact lens of generally concavo-convex cross section adapted to be retained on the cornea of the eye by capillary attraction produced by a lachrymal layer between the lens and the cornea, said lens having a posterior surface curved to fit the cornea of a patient to which the lens is applied with a tendency to remain centered thereon, said lens having a maximum external dimension greater than the normal pupil size and less than the limbal area of the eye, said lens having an upper optical zone and a lower optical zone, said upper optical zone being powered on the anterior surface for distance vision thereof with respect to the cornea of the patient, said lower optical zone being powered also on the anterior surface thereof for near vision with respect to such cornea, the anterior surface of said upper optical zone having a radius of curvature flatter than the radius of curvature of the anterior surface of said lower optical zone to provide the respective distance and near vision powers, with the center of curvature of the anterior surface of said upper optical zone being displaced downwardly relative to the axis of the lens and the curvature itself lying within the spherical extension of the anterior surface of said lower optical zone, the line of intersection of the two anterior curves on the vertical center line of the lens being below the midpoint of said center line, the thickest portion of said lens being below said line of intersection and thereby heavier to restrain the lens from rotating on the cornea and to effect substantially constant positioning of said lower optical zone below said upper optical zone.

Appendix III

Dioptral and mm. Curves for Extended Keratometer Range*

HIGH POWER (+1.25 LENS)

Drum Reading	Corneal Power in Diopters	Radius in mm. Cx	CC
43.000	50.134	6.732	6.759
43.125	50.279	6.712	6.739
43.250	50.425	6.693	6.720
43.375	50.571	6.674	6.701
43.500	50.717	6.655	6.681
43.625	50.862	6.636	6.662
43.750	51.008	6.617	6.643
43.875	51.154	6.598	6.624
44.000	51.299	6.579	6.605
44.125	51.445	6.560	6.587
44.250	51.591	6.542	6.568
44.375	51.737	6.523	6.550
44.500	51.882	6.505	6.531
44.625	52.028	6.487	6.513
44.750	52.174	6.469	6.495
44.875	52.320	6.451	6.477
45.000	52.465	6.433	6.459
45.125	52.611	6.415	6.441
45.250	52.757	6.397	6.423
45.375	52.903	6.380	6.405
45.500	53.048	6.362	6.388
45.625	53.194	6.345	6.370
45.750	53.340	6.327	6.353
45.875	53.486	6.310	6.335
46.000	53.631	6.293	6.318
46.125	53.777	6.276	6.301
46.250	53.923	6.259	6.284
46.375	54.069	6.242	6.267
46.500	54.214	6.225	6.250
46.625	54.360	6.209	6.233
46.750	54.506	6.192	6.217
46.875	54.651	6.175	6.200
47.000	54.797	6.159	6.184
47.125	54.943	6.143	6.167
47.250	55.089	6.126	6.151
47.375	55.234	6.110	6.135
47.500	55.380	6.094	6.119
47.625	55.526	6.078	6.103
47.750	55.672	6.062	6.087
47.875	55.817	6.046	6.071
48.000	55.963	6.031	6.055
48.125	56.109	6.015	6.039
48.250	56.255	5.999	6.024
48.375	56.400	5.984	6.008
48.500	56.546	5.969	5.993
48.625	56.692	5.953	5.977
48.750	56.838	5.938	5.962
48.875	56.983	5.923	5.947
49.000	57.129	5.908	5.931
49.125	57.275	5.893	5.916
49.250	57.421	5.878	5.901
49.375	57.566	5.863	5.886
49.500	57.712	5.848	5.871
49.625	57.858	5.833	5.857
49.750	58.003	5.819	5.842
49.875	58.149	5.804	5.827
50.000	58.295	5.789	5.813
50.125	58.441	5.775	5.798
50.250	58.586	5.761	5.784
50.375	58.732	5.746	5.769
50.500	58.878	5.732	5.755
50.625	59.024	5.718	5.741
50.750	59.169	5.704	5.727
50.875	59.315	5.690	5.713
51.000	59.461	5.676	5.699
51.125	59.607	5.662	5.685
51.250	59.752	5.648	5.671
51.375	59.898	5.635	5.657
51.500	60.044	5.621	5.643
51.625	60.190	5.607	5.630
51.750	60.335	5.594	5.616
51.875	60.481	5.580	5.603
52.000	60.627	5.567	5.589

* Courtesy of Bausch & Lomb, Inc., Rochester, N. Y.

LOW POWER (−1.00 LENS)

Drum Reading	Corneal Power in Diopters	Radius in mm. Cx	CC
36.000	30.874	10.931	10.964
36.125	30.981	10.893	10.926
36.250	31.089	10.856	10.889
36.375	31.196	10.819	10.851
36.500	31.303	10.782	10.814
36.625	31.410	10.745	10.777
36.750	31.518	10.708	10.740
36.875	31.625	10.672	10.704
37.000	31.732	10.636	10.668
37.125	31.839	10.600	10.632
37.250	31.946	10.564	10.596
37.375	32.054	10.529	10.561
37.500	32.161	10.494	10.526
37.625	32.268	10.459	10.491
37.750	32.375	10.425	10.456
37.875	32.482	10.390	10.421
38.000	32.590	10.356	10.387
38.125	32.697	10.322	10.353
38.250	32.804	10.288	10.319
38.375	32.911	10.255	10.286
38.500	33.018	10.221	10.252
38.625	33.126	10.188	10.219
38.750	33.233	10.155	10.186
38.875	33.340	10.123	10.153
39.000	33.447	10.090	10.121
39.125	33.554	10.058	10.088
39.250	33.662	10.026	10.056
39.375	33.769	9.994	10.024
39.500	33.876	9.963	9.993
39.625	33.983	9.931	9.961
39.750	34.090	9.900	9.930
39.875	34.198	9.869	9.899
40.000	34.305	9.838	9.868
40.125	34.412	9.807	9.837
40.250	34.519	9.777	9.806
40.375	34.626	9.747	9.776
40.500	34.734	9.717	9.746
40.625	34.841	9.687	9.716
40.750	34.948	9.657	9.686
40.875	35.055	9.628	9.656
41.000	35.162	9.598	9.627
41.125	35.270	9.569	9.598
41.250	35.377	9.540	9.569
41.375	35.484	9.511	9.540
41.500	35.591	9.483	9.511
41.625	35.698	9.454	9.483
41.750	35.806	9.426	9.454
41.875	35.913	9.398	9.426
42.000	36.020	9.370	9.398

Appendix IV

MEASUREMENTS AND STANDARDS TABLES FOR LENS SPECIFICATIONS

Introduction

There are three methods for determining the most logical initial specifications of corneal contact lenses: (1) Measurements and Standards: Measurements of various factors are taken and related to standards or norms. The commonly used measuring devices are Ophthalmometers or Keratometers and millimeter rulers. (2) Diagnostic Lens Procedure: Lenses with known specifications are systematically observed and tested on the patient's eyes until desired relationships are produced. Sodium fluorescein is added to the precorneal fluid to help determine the relationships between posterior lens and anterior corneal curves. (3) Combination: The information from the measurements and standards method is used to select the initial diagnostic lens. Then diagnostic lens procedure is used. The accuracy and validity of the results from each method are considered, and lens specifications are based on the more accurate and valid method for each patient.

These tables are to be used in the measurements and standards method and in the combination method. Since the combination method provides the most information, it should be used with each patient.

For simplicity, it may be said that there are two categories of corneal contact lenses in terms of positioning on the eye: those that position between the lids with primary fixation, and those that position partially under the upper lid with primary fixation. The former may be called aperture-positioning lenses, and the latter may be called superior-positioning lenses.

The positioning of corneal contact lenses depends on the complex relationships of many factors, and it cannot be predicted accurately from current measurements and standards. However, general guides which relate lens positioning to certain diameters or widths of the anterior segment of the eye and the contact lens can be established. Lenses with smaller diameters (Table 1) tend to position in the palpebral aperture, and lenses with larger diameters (Table 2) tend to position superiorly.

The curvature relationships between the posterior surface of the contact lens and the anterior surface of the cornea cannot be predicted accurately from current measurements and standards. Again, general guides can be established which allow reasonably satisfactory selection of posterior lens curves to produce desired relationships with anterior corneal curves. See Tables 4, 5, and 7. These tables are based on a desire to have relative central alignment or very mild central clearance relationships with superior-positioning contour lenses, and slightly greater central clearance with aperture-positioning Nodema contact lenses. With all lenses, the desired secondary relationship is mild to moderate secondary clearance.

TABLE 1

DIAMETERS AND WIDTHS FOR NODEMA™ CONTACT LENSES

Flat "K"	H.I.D.	V.P.A.	L.D.	O.Z.D.	S.C.W.
Less than 42.00 D	12.5 mm. or more	10.5 mm. or more	8.8 mm.	7.5 mm.	0.65 mm.
42.00 to 42.75 D	12.0 mm.	10.0 mm.	8.5 mm.	7.2 mm.	0.65 mm.
43.00 to 43.75 D	11.5 mm.	9.5 mm.	8.3 mm.	7.0 mm.	0.65 mm.
44.00 to 44.75 D	11.0 mm.	9.0 mm.	8.0 mm.	6.7 mm.	0.65 mm.
45.00 to 46.00 D	10.5 mm.	8.5 mm.	7.8 mm.	6.5 mm.	0.65 mm.
More than 46.00 D	10.0 mm. or less	8.0 mm. or less	7.5 mm.	6.2 mm.	0.65 mm.

H.I.D. = Horizontal iris diameter
V.P.A. = Vertical palpebral aperture
L.D. = Lens diameter
O.Z.D. = Optic-zone diameter
S.C.W. = Secondary curve width
Flat "K" = Ophthalmometric or keratometric power of the flatter principal meridian

TABLE 2

DIAMETERS AND WIDTHS FOR CONTOUR LENSES

Flat "K"	H.I.D.	V.P.A.	L.D.	O.Z.D.	S.C.W.
Less than 42.00 D	12.5 mm. or more	10.5 mm. or more	9.8 mm.	7.8 mm.	1.00 mm.
42.00 to 42.75 D	12.0 mm.	10.0 mm.	9.5 mm.	7.5 mm.	1.00 mm.
43.00 to 43.75 D	11.5 mm.	9.5 mm.	9.3 mm.	7.3 mm.	1.00 mm.
44.00 to 44.75 D	11.0 mm.	9.0 mm.	9.0 mm.	7.0 mm.	1.00 mm.
45.00 to 46.00 D	10.5 mm.	8.5 mm.	8.8 mm.	6.8 mm.	1.00 mm.
More than 46.00 D	10.0 mm. or less	8.0 mm. or less	8.5 mm.	6.5 mm.	1.00 mm.

H.I.D. = Horizontal iris diameter
V.P.A. = Vertical palpebral aperture
L.D. = Lens diameter
O.Z.D. = Optic-zone diameter
S.C.W. = Secondary curve width
Flat "K" = Ophthalmometric or keratometric power of the flatter principal meridian

TABLE 3

SECONDARY CURVE WIDTHS

T.S.C.W.	BL. W.	S.C.W.
0.50 mm.	0.10 mm.	0.40 mm.
0.65 mm.	0.10 mm.	0.55 mm.
0.75 mm.	0.10 mm.	0.65 mm.
1.00 mm.	0.10 mm.	0.90 mm.
1.25 mm.	0.10 mm.	1.15 mm.

T.S.C.W. = Total Secondary Curve Width
S.C.W. = Secondary Curve Width
BL. W. = Blend Width

TABLE 4

B.C.R. WHEN L.D. IS LESS THAN 8.8 MM. AND O.Z.D. IS 6.7 TO 7.2 MM.*

Amount of Ophthalmometric or Keratometric—"K"— Astigmatism	B.C.R.
0.00 to 0.37 D	Flat "K"
0.50 to 1.00 D	Flat "K" +0.25 D
1.12 to 1.50 D	Flat "K" +0.37 D
1.62 to 2.00 D	Flat "K" +0.50 D
2.00 D and over	Flat "K" $+\left(\frac{\text{Steep "K"} - \text{Flat "K"}}{3}\right)$ A toric base curve should also be considered

* When O.Z.D. is 6.2 to 6.6 mm., steepen B.C.R. found in this table by 0.25 D. When O.Z.D. is 7.3 to 7.8 mm., flatten B.C.R. found in this table by 0.25 D. To compensate for lengthening of B.C.R. from hydration, shorten B.C.R. found in this table an empirical average of 0.03 mm. for *all* plus and minus less than 6 D and 0.05 mm. for over minus 6 D.

B.C.R. = Base curve radius
L.D. = Lens diameter
O.Z.D. = Optic-zone diameter
Flat "K" = Power of flatter ophthalmometric or keratometric principal meridian

TABLE 5

B.C.R. WHEN L.D. IS MORE THAN 8.9 MM. AND O.Z.D. IS 6.7 TO 7.2 MM.*

Amount of Ophthalmometric or Keratometric—"K"— Astigmatism	B.C.R.
0.00 to 0.37 D	Flat "K" −0.25 D
0.50 to 1.00 D	Flat "K"
1.12 to 1.50 D	Flat "K" +0.12 D
1.62 to 2.00 D	Flat "K" +0.25 D
2.00 D and over	Flat "K" $+\left(\frac{\text{Steep "K"} - \text{Flat "K"}}{3}\right)$ A toric base curve should also be considered

* When O.Z.D. is 6.2 to 6.6 mm., steepen B.C.R. found in this table by 0.25 D. When O.Z.D. is 7.3 to 7.8 mm., flatten B.C.R. found in this table by 0.25 D. To compensate for lengthening of B.C.R. from hydration, shorten B.C.R. found in this table an empirical average of 0.03 mm. for *all* plus and minus less than 6 D and 0.05 mm. for over minus 6 D.

B.C.R. = Base curve radius
L.D. = Lens diameter
O.Z.D. = Optic-zone diameter
Flat "K" = Power of flatter ophthalmometric or keratometric principal meridian

TABLE 6

CONVERSION TABLE FROM DIOPTERS ($\nabla N = 1.3375 - 1.0000$) TO RADII*

D	R	D	R	D	R	D	R
50.87	6.63	47.87	7.05	44.87	7.52	41.87	8.06
50.75	6.65	47.75	7.07	44.75	7.54	41.75	8.08
50.62	6.67	47.62	7.09	44.62	7.56	41.62	8.11
50.50	6.68	47.50	7.11	44.50	7.58	41.50	8.13
50.37	6.70	47.37	7.12	44.37	7.61	41.37	8.16
50.25	6.72	47.25	7.14	44.25	7.63	41.25	8.18
50.12	6.73	47.12	7.16	44.12	7.65	41.12	8.21
50.00	6.75	47.00	7.18	44.00	7.67	41.00	8.23
49.87	6.77	46.87	7.20	43.87	7.69	40.87	8.26
49.75	6.78	46.75	7.22	43.75	7.72	40.75	8.28
49.62	6.80	46.62	7.24	43.62	7.74	40.62	8.31
49.50	6.82	46.50	7.26	43.50	7.76	40.50	8.33
49.37	6.84	46.37	7.28	43.37	7.78	40.37	8.36
49.25	6.85	46.25	7.30	43.25	7.80	40.25	8.39
49.12	6.87	46.12	7.32	43.12	7.83	40.12	8.41
49.00	6.89	46.00	7.34	43.00	7.85	40.00	8.44
48.87	6.91	45.87	7.36	42.87	7.87	39.87	8.46
48.75	6.92	45.75	7.38	42.75	7.90	39.75	8.49
48.62	6.95	45.62	7.40	42.62	7.92	39.62	8.52
48.50	6.96	45.50	7.42	42.50	7.94	39.50	8.55
48.37	6.98	45.37	7.44	42.37	7.97	39.37	8.57
48.25	7.00	45.25	7.46	42.25	7.99	39.25	8.60
48.12	7.01	45.12	7.48	42.12	8.01	39.12	8.63
48.00	7.03	45.00	7.50	42.00	8.04	39.00	8.65

* This table is accurate to the nearest 0.12 D. It is valid for measuring *convex* surfaces with a Bausch & Lomb Keratometer. For measuring convex surfaces with an American Optical Co. Ophthalmometer, 0.03 mm. is subtracted from the radius determined. For measuring concave surfaces, the following allowances are added to the convex radius:

Radius 7.10 or less add 0.02 mm.
Radius 7.10 to 8.30 add 0.03 mm.
Radius 8.30 or more add 0.04 mm.

TABLE 7

SECONDARY CURVE RADII

S.C.W.	BL. R.	S.C.R.
0.50 mm.	0.60 mm.	1.6 mm.
0.65 mm.	0.60 mm.	1.4 mm.
0.75 mm.	0.60 mm.	1.2 mm.
1.00 mm.	0.60 mm.	1.0 mm.
1.25 mm.	0.60 mm.	0.8 mm.

S.C.W. = Secondary Curve Width on each side of the optic zone
S.C.R. = Secondary Curve Radius. Add this value to B.C.R. and order to nearest 0.1 mm.
BL. R. = Blend Radius. Add this value to B.C.R. and order to nearest 0.1 mm.

TABLE 8

APPROXIMATE STANDARD CENTER THICKNESS FOR MINUS LENSES*

Refractive Power	7.5 to 8.0 mm. L.D.	8.1 to 8.5 mm. L.D.	8.6 to 9.0 mm. L.D.	9.1 to 9.5 mm. L.D.	9.6 to 10.00 mm. L.D.
−1.00 to −1.87 D	0.16 mm.	0.17 mm.	0.18 mm.	0.20 mm.	0.22 mm.
−2.00 to −2.87 D	0.15 mm.	0.16 mm.	0.17 mm.	0.18 mm.	0.19 mm.
−3.00 to −3.87 D	0.14 mm.	0.15 mm.	0.16 mm.	0.16 mm.	0.17 mm.
−4.00 to −4.87 D	0.13 mm.	0.14 mm.	0.15 mm.	0.15 mm.	0.16 mm.
−5.00 to −5.87 D	0.13 mm.	0.13 mm.	0.14 mm.	0.14 mm.	0.15 mm.
−6.00 to −6.87 D	0.12 mm.	0.12 mm.	0.13 mm.	0.13 mm.	0.14 mm.
−7.00 and over	0.11 mm.	0.11 mm.	0.12 mm.	0.12 mm.	0.13 mm.

* If computed center thickness for a standard thickness minus lens is less than 0.13 mm., an anterior lenticular construction with a 0.13 mm. center thickness may be considered. The anterior optic zone is 0.5 mm. larger than the posterior optic zone. If ultrathin lenses are desired, 0.03 mm. is subtracted from the value in the table.

TABLE 9

APPROXIMATE STANDARD CENTER THICKNESS FOR PLUS LENSES

Refractive Power	7.5 to 8.0 mm. L.D.	8.1 to 8.5 mm. L.D.	8.6 to 9.0 mm. L.D.	9.1 to 9.5 mm. L.D.	9.6 to 10.00 mm. L.D.
+1.00 to +1.87 D	0.19 mm.	0.20 mm.	0.22 mm.	0.23 mm.	0.25 mm.
+2.00 to +2.87 D	0.21 mm.	0.22 mm.	0.24 mm.	0.26 mm.	0.28 mm.
+3.00 to +3.87 D	0.22 mm.	0.24 mm.	0.26 mm.	0.28 mm.	0.31 mm.

Appendix V

VERTEX DISTANCE CHARTS*

Minus Chart

Lensometer Reading of Spectacle Lens	10 mm.	11 mm.	12 mm.	13 mm.	14 mm.	15 mm.
3.00	2.91	2.90	2.89	2.88	2.87	2.86
3.25	3.15	3.13	3.12	3.11	3.10	3.09
3.50	3.38	3.37	3.36	3.35	3.34	3.33
3.75	3.62	3.61	3.59	3.58	3.57	3.55
4.00	3.85	3.83	3.82	3.80	3.79	3.77
4.25	4.08	4.07	4.05	4.03	4.02	4.00
4.50	4.31	4.29	4.27	4.26	4.24	4.22
4.75	4.52	4.50	4.48	4.46	4.44	4.42
5.00	4.76	4.74	4.72	4.69	4.67	4.65
5.25	5.00	4.98	4.95	4.93	4.90	4.88
5.50	5.21	5.18	5.15	5.13	5.10	5.08
5.75	5.43	5.41	5.38	5.35	5.32	5.29
6.00	5.65	5.62	5.59	5.56	5.52	5.49
6.25	5.88	5.85	5.81	5.78	5.75	5.71
6.50	6.10	6.06	6.02	5.99	5.95	5.92
6.75	6.33	6.29	6.25	6.21	6.17	6.14
7.00	6.54	6.49	6.45	6.41	6.37	6.33
7.25	6.76	6.71	6.67	6.62	6.58	6.54
7.50	6.99	6.94	6.90	6.85	6.80	6.76
7.75	7.19	7.14	7.09	7.04	6.99	6.94
8.00	7.41	7.35	7.30	7.25	7.19	7.14
8.25	7.63	7.58	7.52	7.46	7.41	7.35
8.50	7.81	7.75	7.69	7.63	7.58	7.52
8.75	8.06	8.00	7.94	7.87	7.81	7.75
9.00	8.26	8.20	8.13	8.06	8.00	7.94
9.25	8.47	8.40	8.33	8.26	8.20	8.13
9.50	8.70	8.62	8.55	8.47	8.40	8.33
9.75	8.85	8.77	8.70	8.62	8.55	8.47
10.00	9.09	9.01	8.93	8.85	8.77	8.70
10.25	9.26	9.17	9.09	9.01	8.93	8.85
10.50	9.52	9.43	9.35	9.26	9.17	9.09
10.75	9.71	9.62	9.52	9.43	9.35	9.26
11.00	9.90	9.80	9.71	9.62	9.52	9.43
11.25	10.10	10.00	9.90	9.80	9.71	9.62
11.50	10.31	10.20	10.10	10.00	9.90	9.80
11.75	10.53	10.42	10.31	10.20	10.10	10.00
12.00	10.75	10.64	10.53	10.42	10.31	10.20
12.25	10.87	10.75	10.64	10.53	10.42	10.31
12.50	11.11	10.99	10.87	10.75	10.64	10.53
12.75	11.36	11.24	11.11	10.99	10.87	10.75
13.00	11.49	11.36	11.24	11.11	10.99	10.87
13.25	11.76	11.63	11.49	11.36	11.24	11.11
13.50	11.90	11.76	11.63	11.49	11.36	11.24
13.75	12.05	11.90	11.76	11.63	11.49	11.36
14.00	12.35	12.20	12.05	11.90	11.76	11.63
14.25	12.50	12.35	12.20	12.05	11.90	11.76
14.50	12.66	12.50	12.35	12.20	12.05	11.90
14.75	12.82	12.66	12.50	12.35	12.20	12.05
15.00	12.99	12.82	12.66	12.50	12.35	12.20

* When ordering, round off to the nearest 0.12 D. For other powers or vertex distances, use the formula:

$$D_c = \frac{D_1}{1 - sD_1},$$

where D_c = Power needed at corneal apex
D_1 = Lensometer or Phoropter value of spectacle lens
s = Vertex distance in meters.

Plus Chart

Lensometer Reading of Spectacle Lens	10 mm.	11 mm.	12 mm.	13 mm.	14 mm.	15 mm.
3.00	3.09	3.10	3.11	3.12	3.13	3.14
3.25	3.36	3.37	3.38	3.39	3.40	3.41
3.50	3.62	3.63	3.64	3.65	3.66	3.67
3.75	3.90	3.92	3.93	3.95	3.97	3.99
4.00	4.17	4.18	4.20	4.22	4.23	4.26
4.25	4.44	4.46	4.48	4.50	4.52	4.55
4.50	4.72	4.74	4.76	4.78	4.81	4.83
4.75	4.98	5.00	5.03	5.05	5.08	5.10
5.00	5.26	5.29	5.32	5.35	5.38	5.41
5.25	5.56	5.59	5.62	5.65	5.68	5.71
5.50	5.81	5.85	5.88	5.92	5.95	5.99
5.75	6.10	6.14	6.17	6.21	6.25	6.29
6.00	6.37	6.41	6.45	6.49	6.54	6.58
6.25	6.67	6.71	6.76	6.80	6.85	6.90
6.50	6.94	6.99	7.04	7.09	7.14	7.19
6.75	7.25	7.30	7.35	7.41	7.46	7.52
7.00	7.52	7.58	7.63	7.69	7.75	7.81
7.25	7.81	7.87	7.94	8.00	8.06	8.13
7.50	8.13	8.20	8.26	8.33	8.40	8.47
7.75	8.40	8.47	8.55	8.62	8.70	8.77
8.00	8.70	8.77	8.85	8.93	9.01	9.09
8.25	9.01	9.09	9.17	9.26	9.35	9.43
8.50	9.26	9.35	9.43	9.52	9.62	9.71
8.75	9.61	9.71	9.80	9.90	10.00	10.10
9.00	9.90	10.00	10.10	10.20	10.31	10.42
9.25	10.20	10.31	10.42	10.53	10.64	10.75
9.50	10.53	10.64	10.75	10.87	10.99	11.11
9.75	10.75	10.87	10.99	11.11	11.24	11.36
10.00	11.11	11.24	11.36	11.49	11.63	11.76
10.25	11.36	11.49	11.63	11.76	11.90	12.05
10.50	11.76	11.90	12.05	12.20	12.35	12.50
10.75	12.05	12.20	12.35	12.50	12.66	12.82
11.00	12.35	12.50	12.66	12.82	12.99	13.16
11.25	12.66	12.82	12.99	13.16	13.33	13.51
11.50	12.99	13.16	13.33	13.51	13.70	13.89
11.75	13.33	13.51	13.70	13.89	14.08	14.29
12.00	13.70	13.89	14.08	14.29	14.49	14.71
12.25	13.89	14.08	14.29	14.49	14.71	14.93
12.50	14.29	14.49	14.71	14.93	15.15	15.38
12.75	14.71	14.93	15.15	15.38	15.63	15.87
13.00	14.93	15.15	15.38	15.63	15.87	16.13
13.25	15.38	15.63	15.87	16.13	16.39	16.67
13.50	15.63	15.87	16.13	16.39	16.67	16.95
13.75	15.87	16.13	16.39	16.67	16.95	17.24
14.00	16.39	16.67	16.95	17.24	17.54	17.86
14.25	16.67	16.95	17.24	17.54	17.86	18.18
14.50	16.95	17.24	17.54	17.86	18.18	18.52
14.75	17.24	17.54	17.86	18.18	18.52	18.87
15.00	17.54	17.86	18.18	18.52	18.87	19.23

Appendix VI

SURFACE POWER TABLE*†

R_{cx}	R_{cc}	Keratometer (Bausch & Lomb) $D = \frac{1.3375 - 1}{R}$	Ophthalmometer (American Optical) $D = \frac{1.336 - 1}{R}$	Plastic $D = \frac{1.49 - 1}{R}$	Posterior Lens–Precorneal Fluid Interface $D = \frac{1.49 - 1.3375}{-R}$	$D = \frac{1.49 - 1.336}{-R}$
5.00	5.02	67.50	67.20	98.00	30.50	30.80
5.01	5.03	67.36	67.06	97.80	30.43	30.73
5.02	5.04	67.23	66.93	97.60	30.37	30.67
5.03	5.05	67.09	66.79	97.41	30.31	30.61
5.04	5.06	66.96	66.66	97.22	30.25	30.55
5.05	5.07	66.83	66.53	97.02	30.19	30.49
5.06	5.08	66.69	66.40	96.83	30.13	30.43
5.07	5.09	66.56	66.27	96.64	30.07	30.37
5.08	5.10	66.43	66.14	96.45	30.01	30.31
5.09	5.11	66.30	66.01	96.26	29.96	30.25
5.10	5.12	66.17	65.88	96.07	29.90	30.19
5.11	5.13	66.04	65.75	95.89	29.84	30.13
5.12	5.14	65.91	65.62	95.70	29.78	30.07
5.13	5.15	65.78	65.49	95.51	29.72	30.01
5.14	5.16	65.66	65.36	95.33	29.66	29.96
5.15	5.17	65.53	65.24	95.14	29.61	29.90
5.16	5.18	65.40	65.11	94.96	29.55	29.84
5.17	5.19	65.28	64.99	94.77	29.49	29.78
5.18	5.20	65.15	64.86	94.59	29.44	29.72
5.19	5.21	65.02	64.73	94.41	29.38	29.67
5.20	5.22	64.90	64.61	94.23	29.32	29.61
5.21	5.23	64.77	64.49	94.04	29.27	29.55
5.22	5.24	64.65	64.36	93.86	29.21	29.50
5.23	5.25	64.53	64.24	93.69	29.15	29.44
5.24	5.26	64.40	64.12	93.51	29.10	29.38
5.25	5.27	64.28	64.00	93.33	29.04	29.33
5.26	5.28	64.16	63.87	93.15	28.99	29.27
5.27	5.29	64.04	63.75	92.97	28.93	29.22
5.28	5.30	63.92	63.63	92.80	28.88	29.16
5.29	5.31	63.79	63.51	92.62	28.82	29.11
5.30	5.32	63.67	63.39	92.45	28.77	29.05
5.31	5.33	63.55	63.27	92.27	28.71	29.00
5.32	5.34	63.43	63.15	92.10	28.66	28.94
5.33	5.35	63.32	63.03	91.93	28.61	28.89
5.34	5.36	63.20	62.92	91.76	28.55	28.83
5.35	5.37	63.08	62.80	91.58	28.50	28.78
5.36	5.38	62.96	62.68	91.41	28.45	28.73
5.37	5.39	62.84	62.56	91.24	28.39	28.67
5.38	5.40	62.73	62.45	91.07	28.34	28.62
5.39	5.41	62.61	62.33	90.90	28.29	28.57
5.40	5.42	62.50	62.22	90.74	28.24	28.51
5.41	5.43	62.38	62.10	90.57	28.18	28.46
5.42	5.44	62.26	61.99	90.40	28.13	28.41
5.43	5.45	62.15	61.87	90.23	28.08	28.36
5.44	5.46	62.04	61.76	90.07	28.03	28.30
5.45	5.47	61.92	61.65	89.90	27.98	28.25
5.46	5.48	61.81	61.53	89.74	27.93	28.20
5.47	5.49	61.70	61.42	89.57	27.87	28.15
5.48	5.50	61.58	61.31	89.41	27.82	28.10
5.49	5.51	61.47	61.20	89.25	27.77	28.05
5.50	5.52	61.36	61.09	89.09	27.72	28.00
5.51	5.53	61.25	60.98	88.92	27.67	27.94

* See discussion on page 342.

† Table prepared by Richard Eckstein.

R_{cs}	R_{oc}	Keratometer (Bausch & Lomb) $D = \frac{1.3375 - 1}{R}$	Ophthalmometer (American Optical) $D = \frac{1.336 - 1}{R}$	Plastic $D = \frac{1.49 - 1}{R}$	Posterior Lens–Precorneal Fluid Interface $D = \frac{1.49 - 1.3375}{-R}$	$D = \frac{1.49 - 1.336}{-R}$
5.52	5.54	61.14	60.86	88.76	27.62	27.89
5.53	5.55	61.03	60.75	88.60	27.57	27.84
5.54	5.56	60.92	60.64	88.44	27.52	27.79
5.55	5.57	60.81	60.54	88.28	27.47	27.74
5.56	5.58	60.70	60.43	88.12	27.42	27.69
5.57	5.59	60.59	60.32	87.97	27.37	27.64
5.58	5.60	60.48	60.21	87.81	27.32	27.59
5.59	5.61	60.37	60.10	87.65	27.28	27.54
5.60	5.62	60.26	60.00	87.50	27.23	27.50
5.61	5.63	60.16	59.89	87.34	27.18	27.45
5.62	5.64	60.05	59.78	87.18	27.13	27.40
5.63	5.65	59.94	59.68	87.03	27.08	27.35
5.64	5.66	59.84	59.57	86.87	27.03	27.30
5.65	5.67	59.73	59.46	86.72	26.99	27.25
5.66	5.68	59.62	59.36	86.57	26.94	27.20
5.67	5.69	59.52	59.25	86.41	26.89	27.16
5.68	5.70	59.41	59.15	86.26	26.84	27.11
5.69	5.71	59.31	59.05	86.11	26.80	27.06
5.70	5.72	59.21	58.94	85.96	26.75	27.01
5.71	5.73	59.10	58.84	85.81	26.70	26.97
5.72	5.74	59.00	58.74	85.66	26.66	26.92
5.73	5.75	58.90	58.63	85.51	26.61	26.87
5.74	5.76	58.79	58.53	85.36	26.56	26.82
5.75	5.77	58.69	58.43	85.21	26.52	26.78
5.76	5.78	58.59	58.33	85.06	26.47	26.73
5.77	5.79	58.49	58.23	84.92	26.42	26.68
5.78	5.80	58.39	58.13	84.77	26.38	26.64
5.79	5.81	58.29	58.03	84.62	26.33	26.59
5.80	5.82	58.18	57.93	84.48	26.29	26.55
5.81	5.83	58.08	57.83	84.33	26.24	26.50
5.82	5.84	57.98	57.73	84.19	26.20	26.46
5.83	5.85	57.89	57.63	84.04	26.15	26.41
5.84	5.86	57.79	57.53	83.90	26.11	26.36
5.85	5.87	57.69	57.43	83.76	26.06	26.32
5.86	5.88	57.59	57.33	83.61	26.02	26.27
5.87	5.89	57.49	57.24	83.47	25.97	26.23
5.88	5.90	57.39	57.14	83.33	25.93	26.19
5.89	5.91	57.30	57.04	83.19	25.89	26.14
5.90	5.92	57.20	56.94	83.05	25.84	26.10
5.91	5.93	57.10	56.85	82.91	25.80	26.05
5.92	5.94	57.01	56.75	82.77	25.76	26.01
5.93	5.95	56.91	56.66	82.63	25.71	25.96
5.94	5.96	56.81	56.56	82.49	25.67	25.92
5.95	5.97	56.72	56.47	82.35	25.63	25.88
5.96	5.98	56.62	56.37	82.21	25.58	25.83
5.97	5.99	56.53	56.28	82.07	25.54	25.79
5.98	6.00	56.43	56.18	81.93	25.50	25.75
5.99	6.01	56.34	56.09	81.80	25.45	25.70
6.00	6.02	56.25	56.00	81.66	25.41	25.66
6.01	6.03	56.15	55.90	81.53	25.37	25.62
6.02	6.04	56.06	55.81	81.39	25.33	25.58
6.03	6.05	55.97	55.72	81.26	25.29	25.53
6.04	6.06	55.87	55.62	81.12	25.24	25.49
6.05	6.07	55.78	55.53	80.99	25.20	25.45
6.06	6.08	55.69	55.44	80.85	25.16	25.41
6.07	6.09	55.60	55.35	80.72	25.12	25.37
6.08	6.10	55.50	55.26	80.59	25.08	25.32
6.09	6.11	55.41	55.17	80.45	25.04	25.28

R_{cx}	R_{cc}	Keratometer (Bausch & Lomb) $D = \frac{1.3375 - 1}{R}$	Ophthalmometer (American Optical) $D = \frac{1.336 - 1}{R}$	Plastic $D = \frac{1.49 - 1}{R}$	Posterior Lens–Precorneal Fluid Interface $D = \frac{1.49 - 1.3375}{-R}$	$D = \frac{1.49 - 1.336}{-R}$
6.10	6.12	55.32	55.08	80.32	25.00	25.24
6.11	6.13	55.23	54.99	80.19	24.95	25.20
6.12	6.14	55.14	54.90	80.06	24.91	25.16
6.13	6.15	55.05	54.81	79.93	24.87	25.12
6.14	6.16	54.96	54.72	79.80	24.83	25.08
6.15	6.17	54.87	54.63	79.67	24.79	25.04
6.16	6.18	54.78	54.54	79.54	24.75	25.00
6.17	6.19	54.70	54.45	79.41	24.71	24.95
6.18	6.20	54.61	54.36	79.28	24.67	24.91
6.19	6.21	54.52	54.28	79.15	24.63	24.87
6.20	6.22	54.43	54.19	79.03	24.59	24.83
6.21	6.23	54.34	54.10	78.90	24.55	24.79
6.22	6.24	54.26	54.01	78.77	24.51	24.75
6.23	6.25	54.17	53.93	78.65	24.47	24.71
6.24	6.26	54.08	53.84	78.52	24.43	24.67
6.25	6.27	54.00	53.76	78.40	24.40	24.64
6.26	6.28	53.91	53.67	78.27	24.36	24.60
6.27	6.29	53.82	53.58	78.14	24.32	24.56
6.28	6.30	53.74	53.50	78.02	24.28	24.52
6.29	6.31	53.65	53.41	77.90	24.24	24.48
6.30	6.32	53.57	53.33	77.77	24.20	24.44
6.31	6.33	53.48	53.24	77.65	24.16	24.40
6.32	6.34	53.40	53.16	77.53	24.12	24.36
6.33	6.35	53.31	53.08	77.40	24.09	24.32
6.34	6.36	53.23	52.99	77.28	24.05	24.29
6.35	6.37	53.14	52.91	77.16	24.01	24.25
6.36	6.38	53.06	52.83	77.04	23.97	24.21
6.37	6.39	52.98	52.74	76.92	23.94	24.17
6.38	6.40	52.89	52.66	76.80	23.90	24.13
6.39	6.41	52.81	52.58	76.68	23.86	24.10
6.40	6.42	52.73	52.50	76.56	23.82	24.06
6.41	6.43	52.65	52.41	76.44	23.79	24.02
6.42	6.44	52.57	52.33	76.32	23.75	23.98
6.43	6.45	52.48	52.25	76.20	23.71	23.95
6.44	6.46	52.40	52.17	76.08	23.68	23.91
6.45	6.47	52.32	52.09	75.96	23.64	23.87
6.46	6.48	52.24	52.01	75.85	23.60	23.83
6.47	6.49	52.16	51.93	75.73	23.57	23.80
6.48	6.50	52.08	51.85	75.61	23.53	23.76
6.49	6.51	52.00	51.77	75.50	23.49	23.72
6.50	6.52	51.92	51.69	75.38	23.46	23.69
6.51	6.53	51.84	51.61	75.26	23.42	23.65
6.52	6.54	51.76	51.53	75.15	23.38	23.61
6.53	6.55	51.68	51.45	75.03	23.35	23.58
6.54	6.56	51.60	51.37	74.92	23.31	23.54
6.55	6.57	51.52	51.29	74.80	23.28	23.51
6.56	6.58	51.44	51.21	74.69	23.24	23.47
6.57	6.59	51.36	51.14	74.58	23.21	23.43
6.58	6.60	51.29	51.06	74.46	23.17	23.40
6.59	6.61	51.21	50.98	74.35	23.14	23.36
6.60	6.62	51.13	50.90	74.24	23.10	23.33
6.61	6.63	51.05	50.83	74.13	23.07	23.29
6.62	6.64	50.98	50.75	74.01	23.03	23.26
6.63	6.65	50.90	50.67	73.90	23.00	23.22
6.64	6.66	50.82	50.60	73.79	22.96	23.19
6.65	6.67	50.75	50.52	73.68	22.93	23.15
6.66	6.68	50.67	50.45	73.57	22.89	23.12
6.67	6.69	50.59	50.37	73.46	22.86	23.08

R_{cs}	R_{cc}	Keratometer (Bausch & Lomb) $D = \frac{1.3375 - 1}{R}$	Ophthalmometer (American Optical) $D = \frac{1.336 - 1}{R}$	Plastic $D = \frac{1.49 - 1}{R}$	Posterior Lens–Precorneal Fluid Interface $D = \frac{1.49 - 1.3375}{-R}$	$D = \frac{1.49 - 1.336}{-R}$
6.68	6.70	50.52	50.29	73.35	22.82	23.05
6.69	6.71	50.44	50.22	73.24	22.79	23.01
6.70	6.72	50.37	50.14	73.13	22.76	22.98
6.71	6.73	50.29	50.07	73.02	22.72	22.95
6.72	6.74	50.22	50.00	72.91	22.69	22.91
6.73	6.75	50.14	49.92	72.80	22.65	22.88
6.74	6.76	50.07	49.85	72.70	22.62	22.84
6.75	6.77	50.00	49.77	72.59	22.59	22.81
6.76	6.78	49.92	49.70	72.48	22.55	22.78
6.77	6.79	49.85	49.63	72.37	22.52	22.74
6.78	6.80	49.77	49.55	72.27	22.49	22.71
6.79	6.81	49.70	49.48	72.16	22.45	22.68
6.80	6.82	49.63	49.41	72.05	22.42	22.64
6.81	6.83	49.55	49.33	71.95	22.39	22.61
6.82	6.84	49.48	49.26	71.84	22.36	22.58
6.83	6.85	49.41	49.19	71.74	22.32	22.54
6.84	6.86	49.34	49.12	71.63	22.29	22.51
6.85	6.87	49.27	49.05	71.53	22.26	22.48
6.86	6.88	49.19	48.97	71.42	22.23	22.44
6.87	6.89	49.12	48.90	71.32	22.19	22.41
6.88	6.90	49.05	48.83	71.22	22.16	22.38
6.89	6.91	48.98	48.76	71.11	22.13	22.35
6.90	6.92	48.91	48.69	71.01	22.10	22.31
6.91	6.93	48.84	48.62	70.91	22.06	22.28
6.92	6.94	48.77	48.55	70.80	22.03	22.25
6.93	6.95	48.70	48.48	70.70	22.00	22.22
6.94	6.96	48.63	48.41	70.60	21.97	22.19
6.95	6.97	48.56	48.34	70.50	21.94	22.15
6.96	6.98	48.49	48.27	70.40	21.91	22.12
6.97	6.99	48.42	48.20	70.30	21.87	22.09
6.98	7.00	48.35	48.13	70.20	21.84	22.06
6.99	7.01	48.28	48.06	70.10	21.81	22.03
7.00	7.02	48.21	48.00	70.00	21.78	22.00
7.01	7.03	48.14	47.93	69.90	21.75	21.96
7.02	7.04	48.07	47.86	69.80	21.72	21.93
7.03	7.05	48.00	47.79	69.70	21.69	21.90
7.04	7.06	47.94	47.72	69.60	21.66	21.87
7.05	7.07	47.87	47.65	69.50	21.63	21.84
7.06	7.08	47.80	47.59	69.40	21.60	21.81
7.07	7.09	47.73	47.52	69.30	21.57	21.78
7.08	7.10	47.66	47.45	69.20	21.53	21.75
7.09	7.11	47.60	47.39	69.11	21.50	21.72
7.10	7.12	47.53	47.32	69.01	21.47	21.69
7.11	7.14	47.46	47.25	68.91	21.44	21.65
7.12	7.15	47.40	47.19	68.82	21.41	21.62
7.13	7.16	47.33	47.12	68.72	21.38	21.59
7.14	7.17	47.26	47.05	68.62	21.35	21.56
7.15	7.18	47.20	46.99	68.53	21.32	21.53
7.16	7.19	47.13	46.92	68.43	21.29	21.50
7.17	7.20	47.07	46.86	68.34	21.26	21.47
7.18	7.21	47.00	46.79	68.24	21.23	21.44
7.19	7.22	46.94	46.73	68.15	21.21	21.41
7.20	7.23	46.87	46.66	68.05	21.18	21.38
7.21	7.24	46.80	46.60	67.96	21.15	21.35
7.22	7.25	46.74	46.53	67.86	21.12	21.32
7.23	7.26	46.68	46.47	67.77	21.09	21.30
7.24	7.27	46.61	46.40	67.67	21.06	21.27
7.25	7.28	46.55	46.34	67.58	21.03	21.24

R_{cx}	R_{cc}	Keratometer (Bausch & Lomb) $D = \frac{1.3375 - 1}{R}$	Ophthalmometer (American Optical) $D = \frac{1.336 - 1}{R}$	Plastic $D = \frac{1.49 - 1}{R}$	Posterior Lens–Precorneal Fluid Interface $D = \frac{1.49 - 1.3375}{-R}$	$D = \frac{1.49 - 1.336}{-R}$
7.26	7.29	46.48	46.28	67.49	21.00	21.21
7.27	7.30	46.42	46.21	67.40	20.97	21.18
7.28	7.31	46.35	46.15	67.30	20.94	21.15
7.29	7.32	46.29	46.09	67.21	20.91	21.12
7.30	7.33	46.23	46.02	67.12	20.89	21.09
7.31	7.34	46.16	45.96	67.03	20.86	21.06
7.32	7.35	46.10	45.90	66.93	20.83	21.03
7.33	7.36	46.04	45.83	66.84	20.80	21.00
7.34	7.37	45.98	45.77	66.75	20.77	20.98
7.35	7.38	45.91	45.71	66.66	20.74	20.95
7.36	7.39	45.85	45.65	66.57	20.72	20.92
7.37	7.40	45.79	45.59	66.48	20.69	20.89
7.38	7.41	45.73	45.52	66.39	20.66	20.86
7.39	7.42	45.66	45.46	66.30	20.63	20.83
7.40	7.43	45.60	45.40	66.21	20.60	20.81
7.41	7.44	45.54	45.34	66.12	20.58	20.78
7.42	7.45	45.48	45.28	66.03	20.55	20.75
7.43	7.46	45.42	45.22	65.94	20.52	20.72
7.44	7.47	45.36	45.16	65.86	20.49	20.69
7.45	7.48	45.30	45.10	65.77	20.46	20.67
7.46	7.49	45.24	45.04	65.68	20.44	20.64
7.47	7.50	45.18	44.97	65.59	20.41	20.61
7.48	7.51	45.12	44.91	65.50	20.38	20.58
7.49	7.52	45.06	44.85	65.42	20.36	20.56
7.50	7.53	45.00	44.80	65.33	20.33	20.53
7.51	7.54	44.94	44.74	65.24	20.30	20.50
7.52	7.55	44.88	44.68	65.15	20.27	20.47
7.53	7.56	44.82	44.62	65.07	20.25	20.45
7.54	7.57	44.76	44.56	64.98	20.22	20.42
7.55	7.58	44.70	44.50	64.90	20.19	20.39
7.56	7.59	44.64	44.44	64.81	20.17	20.37
7.57	7.60	44.58	44.38	64.72	20.14	20.34
7.58	7.61	44.52	44.32	64.64	20.11	20.31
7.59	7.62	44.46	44.26	64.55	20.09	20.28
7.60	7.63	44.40	44.21	64.47	20.06	20.26
7.61	7.64	44.34	44.15	64.38	20.03	20.23
7.62	7.65	44.29	44.09	64.30	20.01	20.20
7.63	7.66	44.23	44.03	64.22	19.98	20.18
7.64	7.67	44.17	43.97	64.13	19.96	20.15
7.65	7.68	44.11	43.92	64.05	19.93	20.13
7.66	7.69	44.06	43.86	63.96	19.90	20.10
7.67	7.70	44.00	43.80	63.88	19.88	20.07
7.68	7.71	43.94	43.75	63.80	19.85	20.05
7.69	7.72	43.88	43.69	63.71	19.83	20.02
7.70	7.73	43.83	43.63	63.63	19.80	20.00
7.71	7.74	43.77	43.57	63.55	19.77	19.97
7.72	7.75	43.71	43.52	63.47	19.75	19.94
7.73	7.76	43.66	43.46	63.38	19.72	19.92
7.74	7.77	43.60	43.41	63.30	19.70	19.89
7.75	7.78	43.54	43.35	63.22	19.67	19.87
7.76	7.79	43.49	43.29	63.14	19.65	19.84
7.77	7.80	43.43	43.24	63.06	19.62	19.81
7.78	7.81	43.38	43.18	62.98	19.60	19.79
7.79	7.82	43.32	43.13	62.90	19.57	19.76
7.80	7.83	43.26	43.07	62.82	19.55	19.74
7.81	7.84	43.21	43.02	62.74	19.52	19.71
7.82	7.85	43.15	42.96	62.65	19.50	19.69
7.83	7.86	43.10	42.91	62.57	19.47	19.66

R_{cx}	R_{cc}	Keratometer (Bausch & Lomb) $D = \frac{1.3375 - 1}{R}$	Ophthalmometer (American Optical) $D = \frac{1.336 - 1}{R}$	Plastic $D = \frac{1.49 - 1}{R}$	Posterior Lens–Precorneal Fluid Interface $D = \frac{1.49 - 1.3375}{-R}$	$D = \frac{1.49 - 1.336}{-R}$
7.84	7.87	43.04	42.85	62.50	19.45	19.64
7.85	7.88	42.99	42.80	62.42	19.42	19.61
7.86	7.89	42.93	42.74	62.34	19.40	19.59
7.87	7.90	42.88	42.69	62.26	19.37	19.56
7.88	7.91	42.82	42.63	62.18	19.35	19.54
7.89	7.92	42.77	42.58	62.10	19.32	19.51
7.90	7.93	42.72	42.53	62.02	19.30	19.49
7.91	7.94	42.66	42.47	61.94	19.27	19.46
7.92	7.95	42.61	42.42	61.86	19.25	19.44
7.93	7.96	42.55	42.37	61.79	19.23	19.41
7.94	7.97	42.50	42.31	61.71	19.20	19.39
7.95	7.98	42.45	42.26	61.63	19.18	19.37
7.96	7.99	42.39	42.21	61.55	19.15	19.34
7.97	8.00	42.34	42.15	61.48	19.13	19.32
7.98	8.01	42.29	42.10	61.40	19.11	19.29
7.99	8.02	42.24	42.05	61.32	19.08	19.27
8.00	8.03	42.18	42.00	61.25	19.06	19.25
8.01	8.04	42.13	41.94	61.17	19.03	19.22
8.02	8.05	42.08	41.89	61.09	19.01	19.20
8.03	8.06	42.02	41.84	61.02	18.99	19.17
8.04	8.07	41.97	41.79	60.94	18.96	19.15
8.05	8.08	41.92	41.73	60.86	18.94	19.13
8.06	8.09	41.87	41.68	60.79	18.92	19.10
8.07	8.10	41.82	41.63	60.71	18.89	19.08
8.08	8.11	41.76	41.58	60.64	18.87	19.05
8.09	8.12	41.71	41.53	60.56	18.85	19.03
8.10	8.13	41.66	41.48	60.49	18.82	19.01
8.11	8.14	41.61	41.43	60.41	18.80	18.98
8.12	8.15	41.56	41.37	60.34	18.78	18.96
8.13	8.16	41.51	41.32	60.27	18.75	18.94
8.14	8.17	41.46	41.27	60.19	18.73	18.91
8.15	8.18	41.41	41.22	60.12	18.71	18.89
8.16	8.19	41.36	41.17	60.04	18.68	18.87
8.17	8.20	41.30	41.12	59.97	18.66	18.84
8.18	8.21	41.25	41.07	59.90	18.64	18.82
8.19	8.22	41.20	41.02	59.82	18.62	18.80
8.20	8.23	41.15	40.97	59.75	18.59	18.78
8.21	8.24	41.10	40.92	59.68	18.57	18.75
8.22	8.25	41.05	40.87	59.61	18.55	18.73
8.23	8.26	41.00	40.82	59.53	18.52	18.71
8.24	8.27	40.95	40.77	59.46	18.50	18.68
8.25	8.28	40.90	40.72	59.39	18.48	18.66
8.26	8.29	40.85	40.67	59.32	18.46	18.64
8.27	8.30	40.81	40.62	59.25	18.44	18.62
8.28	8.31	40.76	40.57	59.17	18.41	18.59
8.29	8.32	40.71	40.53	59.10	18.39	18.57
8.30	8.33	40.66	40.48	59.03	18.37	18.55
8.31	8.35	40.61	40.43	58.96	18.35	18.53
8.32	8.36	40.56	40.38	58.89	18.32	18.50
8.33	8.37	40.51	40.33	58.82	18.30	18.48
8.34	8.38	40.46	40.28	58.75	18.28	18.46
8.35	8.39	40.41	40.23	58.68	18.26	18.44
8.36	8.40	40.37	40.19	58.61	18.24	18.42
8.37	8.41	40.32	40.14	58.54	18.21	18.39
8.38	8.42	40.27	40.09	58.47	18.19	18.37
8.39	8.43	40.22	40.04	58.40	18.17	18.35
8.40	8.44	40.17	40.00	58.33	18.15	18.33
8.41	8.45	40.13	39.95	58.26	18.13	18.31

R_{cx}	R_{cc}	Keratometer (Bausch & Lomb) $D = \frac{1.3375 - 1}{R}$	Ophthalmometer (American Optical) $D = \frac{1.336 - 1}{R}$	Plastic $D = \frac{1.49 - 1}{R}$	Posterior Lens–Precorneal Fluid Interface $D = \frac{1.49 - 1.3375}{-R}$	$D = \frac{1.49 - 1.336}{-R}$
8.42	8.46	40.08	39.90	58.19	18.11	18.28
8.43	8.47	40.03	39.85	58.12	18.09	18.26
8.44	8.48	39.98	39.81	58.05	18.06	18.24
8.45	8.49	39.94	39.76	57.98	18.04	18.22
8.46	8.50	39.89	39.71	57.91	18.02	18.20
8.47	8.51	39.84	39.66	57.85	18.00	18.18
8.48	8.52	39.79	39.62	57.78	17.98	18.16
8.49	8.53	39.75	39.57	57.71	17.96	18.13
8.50	8.54	39.70	39.52	57.64	17.94	18.11
8.51	8.55	39.65	39.48	57.57	17.92	18.09
8.52	8.56	39.61	39.43	57.51	17.89	18.07
8.53	8.57	39.56	39.39	57.44	17.87	18.05
8.54	8.58	39.51	39.34	57.37	17.85	18.03
8.55	8.59	39.47	39.29	57.30	17.83	18.01
8.56	8.60	39.42	39.25	57.24	17.81	17.99
8.57	8.61	39.38	39.20	57.17	17.79	17.96
8.58	8.62	39.33	39.16	57.10	17.77	17.94
8.59	8.63	39.28	39.11	57.04	17.75	17.92
8.60	8.64	39.24	39.06	56.97	17.73	17.90
8.61	8.65	39.19	39.02	56.91	17.71	17.88
8.62	8.66	39.15	38.97	56.84	17.69	17.86
8.63	8.67	39.10	38.93	56.77	17.67	17.84
8.64	8.68	39.06	38.88	56.71	17.65	17.82
8.65	8.69	39.01	38.84	56.64	17.63	17.80
8.66	8.70	38.97	38.79	56.58	17.60	17.78
8.67	8.71	38.92	38.75	56.51	17.58	17.76
8.68	8.72	38.88	38.70	56.45	17.56	17.74
8.69	8.73	38.83	38.66	56.38	17.54	17.72
8.70	8.74	38.79	38.62	56.32	17.52	17.70
8.71	8.75	38.74	38.57	56.25	17.50	17.68
8.72	8.76	38.70	38.53	56.19	17.48	17.66
8.73	8.77	38.65	38.48	56.12	17.46	17.64
8.74	8.78	38.61	38.44	56.06	17.44	17.62
8.75	8.79	38.57	38.40	56.00	17.42	17.60
8.76	8.80	38.52	38.35	55.93	17.40	17.57
8.77	8.81	38.48	38.31	55.87	17.38	17.55
8.78	8.82	38.43	38.26	55.80	17.36	17.53
8.79	8.83	38.39	38.22	55.74	17.34	17.51
8.80	8.84	38.35	38.18	55.68	17.32	17.50
8.81	8.85	38.30	38.13	55.61	17.30	17.48
8.82	8.86	38.26	38.09	55.55	17.29	17.46
8.83	8.87	38.22	38.05	55.49	17.27	17.44
8.84	8.88	38.17	38.00	55.42	17.25	17.42
8.85	8.89	38.13	37.96	55.36	17.23	17.40
8.86	8.90	38.09	37.92	55.30	17.21	17.38
8.87	8.91	38.04	37.88	55.24	17.19	17.36
8.88	8.92	38.00	37.83	55.18	17.17	17.34
8.89	8.93	37.96	37.79	55.11	17.15	17.32
8.90	8.94	37.92	37.75	55.05	17.13	17.30
8.91	8.95	37.87	37.71	54.99	17.11	17.28
8.92	8.96	37.83	37.66	54.93	17.09	17.26
8.93	8.97	37.79	37.62	54.87	17.07	17.24
8.94	8.98	37.75	37.58	54.80	17.05	17.22
8.95	8.99	37.70	37.54	54.74	17.03	17.20
8.96	9.00	37.66	37.50	54.68	17.02	17.18
8.97	9.01	37.62	37.45	54.62	17.00	17.16
8.98	9.02	37.58	37.41	54.56	16.98	17.14
8.99	9.03	37.54	37.37	54.50	16.96	17.13

R_{cs}	R_{cc}	Keratometer (Bausch & Lomb) $D = \frac{1.3375 - 1}{R}$	Ophthalmometer (American Optical) $D = \frac{1.336 - 1}{R}$	Plastic $D = \frac{1.49 - 1}{R}$	Posterior Lens–Precorneal Fluid Interface $D = \frac{1.49 - 1.3375}{-R}$	$D = \frac{1.49 - 1.336}{-R}$
9.00	9.04	37.50	37.33	54.44	16.94	17.11
9.01	9.05	37.45	37.29	54.38	16.92	17.09
9.02	9.06	37.41	37.25	54.32	16.90	17.07
9.03	9.07	37.37	37.20	54.26	16.88	17.05
9.04	9.08	37.33	37.16	54.20	16.86	17.03
9.05	9.09	37.29	37.12	54.14	16.85	17.01
9.06	9.10	37.25	37.08	54.08	16.83	16.99
9.07	9.11	37.21	37.04	54.02	16.81	16.97
9.08	9.12	37.16	37.00	53.96	16.79	16.96
9.09	9.13	37.12	36.96	53.90	16.77	16.94
9.10	9.14	37.08	36.92	53.84	16.75	16.92
9.11	9.15	37.04	36.88	53.78	16.73	16.90
9.12	9.16	37.00	36.84	53.72	16.72	16.88
9.13	9.17	36.96	36.80	53.66	16.70	16.86
9.14	9.18	36.92	36.76	53.61	16.68	16.84
9.15	9.19	36.88	36.72	53.55	16.66	16.83
9.16	9.20	36.84	36.68	53.49	16.64	16.81
9.17	9.21	36.80	36.64	53.43	16.63	16.79
9.18	9.22	36.76	36.60	53.37	16.61	16.77
9.19	9.23	36.72	36.56	53.31	16.59	16.75
9.20	9.24	36.68	36.52	53.26	16.57	16.73
9.21	9.25	36.64	36.48	53.20	16.55	16.72
9.22	9.26	36.60	36.44	53.14	16.54	16.70
9.23	9.27	36.56	36.40	53.08	16.52	16.68
9.24	9.28	36.52	36.36	53.03	16.50	16.66
9.25	9.29	36.48	36.32	52.97	16.48	16.64
9.26	9.30	36.44	36.28	52.91	16.46	16.63
9.27	9.31	36.40	36.24	52.85	16.45	16.61
9.28	9.32	36.36	36.20	52.80	16.43	16.59
9.29	9.33	36.32	36.16	52.74	16.41	16.57
9.30	9.34	36.29	36.12	52.68	16.39	16.55
9.31	9.35	36.25	36.09	52.63	16.38	16.54
9.32	9.36	36.21	36.05	52.57	16.36	16.52
9.33	9.37	36.17	36.01	52.51	16.34	16.50
9.34	9.38	36.13	35.97	52.46	16.32	16.48
9.35	9.39	36.09	35.93	52.40	16.31	16.47
9.36	9.40	36.05	35.89	52.35	16.29	16.45
9.37	9.41	36.01	35.85	52.29	16.27	16.43
9.38	9.42	35.98	35.82	52.23	16.25	16.41
9.39	9.43	35.94	35.78	52.18	16.24	16.40
9.40	9.44	35.90	35.74	52.12	16.22	16.38
9.41	9.45	35.86	35.70	52.07	16.20	16.36
9.42	9.46	35.82	35.66	52.01	16.18	16.34
9.43	9.47	35.79	35.63	51.96	16.17	16.33
9.44	9.48	35.75	35.59	51.90	16.15	16.31
9.45	9.49	35.71	35.55	51.85	16.13	16.29
9.46	9.50	35.67	35.51	51.79	16.12	16.27
9.47	9.51	35.63	35.48	51.74	16.10	16.26
9.48	9.52	35.60	35.44	51.68	16.08	16.24
9.49	9.53	35.56	35.40	51.63	16.06	16.22
9.50	9.54	35.52	35.36	51.57	16.05	16.21
9.51	9.55	35.48	35.33	51.52	16.03	16.19
9.52	9.56	35.45	35.29	51.47	16.01	16.17
9.53	9.57	35.41	35.25	51.41	16.00	16.15
9.54	9.58	35.37	35.22	51.36	15.98	16.14
9.55	9.59	35.34	35.18	51.30	15.96	16.12
9.56	9.60	35.30	35.14	51.25	15.95	16.10
9.57	9.61	35.26	35.10	51.20	15.93	16.09

R_{cx}	R_{cc}	Keratometer (Bausch & Lomb) $D = \frac{1.3375 - 1}{R}$	Ophthalmometer (American Optical) $D = \frac{1.336 - 1}{R}$	Plastic $D = \frac{1.49 - 1}{R}$	Posterior Lens–Precorneal Fluid Interface $D = \frac{1.49 - 1.3375}{-R}$	$D = \frac{1.49 - 1.336}{-R}$
9.58	9.62	35.22	35.07	51.14	15.91	16.07
9.59	9.63	35.19	35.03	51.09	15.90	16.05
9.60	9.64	35.15	35.00	51.04	15.88	16.04
9.61	9.65	35.11	34.96	50.98	15.86	16.02
9.62	9.66	35.08	34.92	50.93	15.85	16.00
9.63	9.67	35.04	34.89	50.88	15.83	15.99
9.64	9.68	35.01	34.85	50.82	15.81	15.97
9.65	9.69	34.97	34.81	50.77	15.80	15.95
9.66	9.70	34.93	34.78	50.72	15.78	15.94
9.67	9.71	34.90	34.74	50.67	15.77	15.92
9.68	9.72	34.86	34.71	50.61	15.75	15.90
9.69	9.73	34.82	34.67	50.56	15.73	15.89
9.70	9.74	34.79	34.63	50.51	15.72	15.87
9.71	9.75	34.75	34.60	50.46	15.70	15.85
9.72	9.76	34.72	34.56	50.41	15.68	15.84
9.73	9.77	34.68	34.53	50.35	15.67	15.82
9.74	9.78	34.65	34.49	50.30	15.65	15.81
9.75	9.79	34.61	34.46	50.25	15.64	15.79
9.76	9.80	34.57	34.42	50.20	15.62	15.77
9.77	9.81	34.54	34.39	50.15	15.60	15.76
9.78	9.82	34.50	34.35	50.10	15.59	15.74
9.79	9.83	34.47	34.32	50.05	15.57	15.73
9.80	9.84	34.43	34.28	50.00	15.56	15.71
9.81	9.85	34.40	34.25	49.94	15.54	15.69
9.82	9.86	34.36	34.21	49.89	15.52	15.68
9.83	9.87	34.33	34.18	49.84	15.51	15.66
9.84	9.88	34.29	34.14	49.79	15.49	15.65
9.85	9.89	34.26	34.11	49.74	15.48	15.63
9.86	9.90	34.22	34.07	49.69	15.46	15.61
9.87	9.91	34.19	34.04	49.64	15.45	15.60
9.88	9.92	34.15	34.00	49.59	15.43	15.58
9.89	9.93	34.12	33.97	49.54	15.41	15.57
9.90	9.94	34.09	33.93	49.49	15.40	15.55
9.91	9.95	34.05	33.90	49.44	15.38	15.53
9.92	9.96	34.02	33.87	49.39	15.37	15.52
9.93	9.97	33.98	33.83	49.34	15.35	15.50
9.94	9.98	33.95	33.80	49.29	15.34	15.49
9.95	9.99	33.91	33.76	49.24	15.32	15.47
9.96	10.00	33.88	33.73	49.19	15.31	15.46
9.97	10.01	33.85	33.70	49.14	15.29	15.44
9.98	10.02	33.81	33.66	49.09	15.28	15.43
9.99	10.03	33.78	33.63	49.04	15.26	15.41
10.00	10.04	33.75	33.60	49.00	15.25	15.40
10.01	10.05	33.71	33.56	48.95	15.23	15.38
10.02	10.06	33.68	33.53	48.90	15.21	15.36
10.03	10.07	33.64	33.49	48.85	15.20	15.35
10.04	10.08	33.61	33.46	48.80	15.18	15.33
10.05	10.09	33.58	33.43	48.75	15.17	15.32
10.06	10.10	33.54	33.39	48.70	15.15	15.30
10.07	10.11	33.51	33.36	48.65	15.14	15.29
10.08	10.12	33.48	33.33	48.61	15.12	15.27
10.09	10.13	33.44	33.30	48.56	15.11	15.26
10.10	10.14	33.41	33.26	48.51	15.09	15.24
10.11	10.15	33.38	33.23	48.46	15.08	15.23
10.12	10.16	33.34	33.20	48.41	15.06	15.21
10.13	10.17	33.31	33.16	48.37	15.05	15.20
10.14	10.18	33.28	33.13	48.32	15.03	15.18
10.15	10.19	33.25	33.10	48.27	15.02	15.17

R_{cs}	R_{cc}	Keratometer (Bausch & Lomb) $D = \frac{1.3375 - 1}{R}$	Ophthalmometer (American Optical) $D = \frac{1.336 - 1}{R}$	Plastic $D = \frac{1.49 - 1}{R}$	Posterior Lens–Precorneal Fluid Interface $D = \frac{1.49 - 1.3375}{-R}$	$D = \frac{1.49 - 1.336}{-R}$
10.16	10.20	33.21	33.07	48.22	15.00	15.15
10.17	10.21	33.18	33.03	48.18	14.99	15.14
10.18	10.22	33.15	33.00	48.13	14.98	15.12
10.19	10.23	33.12	32.97	48.08	14.96	15.11
10.20	10.24	33.08	32.94	48.03	14.95	15.09
10.21	10.25	33.05	32.90	47.99	14.93	15.08
10.22	10.26	33.02	32.87	47.94	14.92	15.06
10.23	10.27	32.99	32.84	47.89	14.90	15.05
10.24	10.28	32.95	32.81	47.85	14.89	15.03
10.25	10.29	32.92	32.78	47.80	14.87	15.02
10.26	10.30	32.89	32.74	47.75	14.86	15.00
10.27	10.31	32.86	32.71	47.71	14.84	14.99
10.28	10.32	32.83	32.68	47.66	14.83	14.98
10.29	10.33	32.79	32.65	47.61	14.82	14.96
10.30	10.34	32.76	32.62	47.57	14.80	14.95
10.31	10.35	32.73	32.58	47.52	14.79	14.93
10.32	10.36	32.70	32.55	47.48	14.77	14.92
10.33	10.37	32.67	32.52	47.43	14.76	14.90
10.34	10.38	32.64	32.49	47.38	14.74	14.89
10.35	10.39	32.60	32.46	47.34	14.73	14.87
10.36	10.40	32.57	32.43	47.29	14.72	14.86
10.37	10.41	32.54	32.40	47.25	14.70	14.85
10.38	10.42	32.51	32.36	47.20	14.69	14.83
10.39	10.43	32.48	32.33	47.16	14.67	14.82
10.40	10.44	32.45	32.30	47.11	14.66	14.80
10.41	10.45	32.42	32.27	47.07	14.64	14.79
10.42	10.46	32.38	32.24	47.02	14.63	14.77
10.43	10.47	32.35	32.21	46.97	14.62	14.76
10.44	10.48	32.32	32.18	46.93	14.60	14.75
10.45	10.49	32.29	32.15	46.88	14.59	14.73
10.46	10.50	32.26	32.12	46.84	14.57	14.72
10.47	10.51	32.23	32.09	46.80	14.56	14.70
10.48	10.52	32.20	32.06	46.75	14.55	14.69
10.49	10.53	32.17	32.03	46.71	14.53	14.68
10.50	10.54	32.14	32.00	46.66	14.52	14.66
10.51	10.55	32.11	31.96	46.62	14.50	14.65
10.52	10.56	32.08	31.93	46.57	14.49	14.63
10.53	10.57	32.05	31.90	46.53	14.48	14.62
10.54	10.58	32.02	31.87	46.48	14.46	14.61
10.55	10.59	31.99	31.84	46.44	14.45	14.59
10.56	10.60	31.96	31.81	46.40	14.44	14.58
10.57	10.61	31.92	31.78	46.35	14.42	14.56
10.58	10.62	31.89	31.75	46.31	14.41	14.55
10.59	10.63	31.86	31.72	46.27	14.40	14.54
10.60	10.64	31.83	31.69	46.22	14.38	14.52
10.61	10.65	31.80	31.66	46.18	14.37	14.51
10.62	10.66	31.77	31.63	46.13	14.35	14.50
10.63	10.67	31.74	31.60	46.09	14.34	14.48
10.64	10.68	31.71	31.57	46.05	14.33	14.47
10.65	10.69	31.69	31.54	46.00	14.31	14.46
10.66	10.70	31.66	31.51	45.96	14.30	14.44
10.67	10.71	31.63	31.49	45.92	14.29	14.43
10.68	10.72	31.60	31.46	45.88	14.27	14.41
10.69	10.73	31.57	31.43	45.83	14.26	14.40
10.70	10.74	31.54	31.40	45.79	14.25	14.39
10.71	10.75	31.51	31.37	45.75	14.23	14.37
10.72	10.76	31.48	31.34	45.70	14.22	14.36
10.73	10.77	31.45	31.31	45.66	14.21	14.35

R_{cs}	R_{co}	Keratometer (Bausch & Lomb) $D = \frac{1.3375 - 1}{R}$	Ophthalmometer (American Optical) $D = \frac{1.336 - 1}{R}$	Plastic $D = \frac{1.49 - 1}{R}$	Posterior Lens–Precorneal Fluid Interface $D = \frac{1.49 - 1.3375}{-R}$	$D = \frac{1.49 - 1.336}{-R}$
10.74	10.78	31.42	31.28	45.62	14.19	14.33
10.75	10.79	31.39	31.25	45.58	14.18	14.32
10.76	10.80	31.36	31.22	45.53	14.17	14.31
10.77	10.81	31.33	31.19	45.49	14.15	14.29
10.78	10.82	31.30	31.16	45.45	14.14	14.28
10.79	10.83	31.27	31.13	45.41	14.13	14.27
10.80	10.84	31.25	31.11	45.37	14.12	14.25
10.81	10.85	31.22	31.08	45.32	14.10	14.24
10.82	10.86	31.19	31.05	45.28	14.09	14.23
10.83	10.87	31.16	31.02	45.24	14.08	14.21
10.84	10.88	31.13	30.99	45.20	14.06	14.20
10.85	10.89	31.10	30.96	45.16	14.05	14.19
10.86	10.90	31.07	30.93	45.11	14.04	14.18
10.87	10.91	31.04	30.91	45.07	14.02	14.16
10.88	10.92	31.02	30.88	45.03	14.01	14.15
10.89	10.93	30.99	30.85	44.99	14.00	14.14
10.90	10.94	30.96	30.82	44.95	13.99	14.12
10.91	10.95	30.93	30.79	44.91	13.97	14.11
10.92	10.96	30.90	30.76	44.87	13.96	14.10
10.93	10.97	30.87	30.74	44.83	13.95	14.08
10.94	10.98	30.85	30.71	44.78	13.93	14.07
10.95	10.99	30.82	30.68	44.74	13.92	14.06
10.96	11.00	30.79	30.65	44.70	13.91	14.05
10.97	11.01	30.76	30.62	44.66	13.90	14.03
10.98	11.02	30.73	30.60	44.62	13.88	14.02
10.99	11.03	30.70	30.57	44.58	13.87	14.01
11.00	11.04	30.68	30.54	44.54	13.86	14.00

Appendix VII

ANTERIOR SURFACE RADIUS TABLE*

This table is used to determine the required anterior surface radius. The desired base curve radius is looked up in the left hand column, and the desired posterior vertex power is looked up in the top column.

The coordinate of these two columns gives the noncompensated anterior surface radius. Compensation for power introduced by thickness is made by adding ⅓ of the center thickness to the noncompensated anterior surface radius. For example, desired base curve radius is 7.50 mm. and desired posterior vertex power is −5.00 D. Noncompensated anterior surface radius is 8.11 mm. If a 0.15 mm. center thickness is to be used, compensated anterior surface radius is 8.11 + ⅓(.15) = 8.16 mm. If a base curve radius which is not listed is used, interpolation is used with this table.

* Courtesy of Quality Optics, Inc.

	-725	-700	-675	-650	-625	-600	-575	-550	-525	-500	-475	-450	-425	-400	-375	-350	-325	-300	-275	-250	-225	-200	-175	-150	-125	-100	-75	-50	-25	-0
696=4850																														696
699=4825	780	776	773	770	767	764	761	758	755	753	750	747	744	741	738	736	733	730	728	725	722	720	717	714	712	709	706	704	701	699
703=4800	784	781	778	775	772	769	766	763	760	757	754	751	748	745	742	740	737	734	732	729	726	724	721	718	715	713	710	707	705	703
707=4775	789	786	783	780	777	774	771	768	765	762	759	756	753	750	747	744	741	739	736	733	731	728	725	722	719	717	715	712	709	707
711=4750	793	790	787	784	781	778	775	772	769	766	763	760	757	754	751	748	745	742	739	737	734	731	729	726	723	721	718	715	713	711
714=4725	798	795	791	788	785	782	779	776	773	770	767	764	761	758	755	752	749	746	743	741	738	735	733	730	727	725	722	719	716	714
718=4700	803	800	796	793	790	787	784	780	777	774	771	768	765	762	759	756	753	750	747	745	742	739	737	734	731	729	726	723	720	718
722=4675	808	805	802	799	795	792	789	785	782	779	776	773	770	767	764	761	758	755	752	749	746	744	741	738	736	733	730	727	724	722
726=4650	813	810	807	803	800	797	793	790	787	783	780	777	774	771	768	765	762	759	756	753	750	748	745	742	740	737	734	731	728	726
730=4625	818	815	812	808	805	802	798	795	792	788	785	782	779	776	773	770	767	764	761	758	755	752	749	747	744	741	738	735	732	730
734=4600	823	820	816	813	810	806	803	800	796	793	790	786	783	780	777	774	771	768	765	762	759	756	753	750	748	745	742	739	736	734
738=4575	828	825	821	818	815	811	808	805	801	798	795	791	788	785	782	779	776	773	770	767	764	761	758	755	752	749	746	743	741	738
742=4550	833	830	826	823	819	816	813	809	805	802	799	796	793	789	786	783	780	777	774	771	768	765	762	759	756	753	750	747	745	742
746=4525	838	834	831	828	824	821	818	814	810	807	804	801	798	794	791	788	785	782	779	775	772	769	766	763	760	757	754	752	749	746
750=4500	843	839	836	832	829	826	822	818	815	811	808	805	802	798	795	792	789	786	783	780	777	774	771	768	765	762	759	756	753	750
754=4475	848	844	841	837	834	831	827	823	820	816	813	810	806	803	800	797	794	791	787	784	781	778	775	772	769	766	763	760	757	754
758=4450	854	850	846	842	839	836	832	828	825	821	818	815	811	808	805	802	799	795	792	789	785	782	779	776	773	770	767	764	761	758
763=4425	860	856	852	848	845	841	837	834	830	827	824	820	817	814	810	807	804	800	797	794	790	787	784	781	778	775	772	769	766	763
767=4400	865	861	857	853	850	846	842	839	835	832	828	824	821	818	814	811	808	804	801	798	794	791	788	785	782	779	776	773	770	767
771=4375	870	864	862	859	855	851	848	844	840	837	833	829	826	822	819	816	812	809	806	802	799	796	792	789	786	783	780	777	774	771
776=4350	876	872	868	864	860	856	853	849	845	842	838	834	831	827	824	821	817	814	810	807	804	800	797	794	791	788	785	782	779	776
780=4325	882	878	874	870	866	862	858	854	851	847	843	840	836	833	830	826	822	819	815	812	809	805	802	799	795	792	789	786	783	780
785=4300	887	883	879	875	871	867	863	859	855	851	848	845	841	837	833	830	827	824	820	817	813	810	807	803	800	797	794	791	788	785
789=4275	893	889	885	881	877	873	869	866	862	858	854	850	846	843	839	836	833	829	825	822	818	815	812	808	805	802	798	795	792	789
794=4250	899	895	891	887	883	879	875	871	867	863	859	855	851	848	844	841	837	833	830	826	823	820	816	813	810	806	803	800	797	794
799=4225	905	900	896	892	888	884	880	876	872	869	865	861	857	853	849	846	842	838	835	831	828	825	821	818	815	811	808	805	802	799
804=4200	911	907	903	899	895	891	887	883	879	875	871	867	863	859	855	851	848	844	840	837	833	830	826	823	820	816	813	810	807	804
808=4175	917	913	909	905	901	897	893	889	885	881	877	873	869	865	861	857	853	850	846	842	839	835	832	829	825	821	818	814	811	808
813=4150	924	919	915	911	907	903	899	895	891	887	883	879	875	871	867	863	859	855	851	847	844	841	837	833	830	826	822	819	816	813
818=4125	930	926	921	917	913	909	905	901	896	892	888	884	880	877	873	869	865	861	857	853	849	846	843	839	835	832	828	824	821	818
823=4100	937	932	927	923	919	915	910	906	902	898	894	890	886	882	878	874	870	866	862	858	854	851	848	844	840	837	833	829	826	823
828=4075	944	939	934	930	925	921	917	912	908	904	900	896	892	888	884	880	876	872	868	864	860	857	853	849	846	842	838	835	831	828
833=4050	951	946	941	937	932	928	923	919	915	910	906	902	898	894	890	886	882	878	874	870	866	862	859	855	851	848	844	840	837	833
839=4025	958	953	949	944	939	935	930	926	922	917	913	909	905	901	897	892	888	884	880	876	873	869	865	861	857	853	850	846	842	839
844=4000	964	959	955	950	945	941	936	931	927	923	919	914	910	906	902	898	894	890	886	882	878	874	870	866	862	858	855	851	847	844
849=3975	971	966	961	956	952	947	942	938	933	929	925	920	916	912	908	904	900	895	891	887	883	879	876	872	868	864	860	856	853	849
854=3950	978	973	968	963	959	954	949	944	940	936	931	927	922	918	914	910	905	901	897	893	889	885	881	877	873	869	866	862	858	854
860=3925	985	980	975	971	966	961	956	951	947	943	938	933	929	924	920	916	911	907	903	899	895	891	887	883	879	875	871	868	864	860

FRONT RADIUS = CHART POWER = 1/3 CENTER THICKNESS
THICKNESS (mm) = CORRECTION FACTOR

	-1475	-1450	-1425	-1400	-1375	-1350	-1325	-1300	-1275	-1250	-1225	-1200	-1175	-1150	-1125	-1100	-1075	-1050	-1025	-1000	-975	-950	-925	-900	-875	-850	-825	-800	-775	-750
696=4850																														
699=4825	885	881	877	873	869	865	862	858	854	851	847	843	840	836	832	829	825	822	819	815	812	809	805	802	799	795	792	789	786	783
703=4800	892	888	884	880	876	872	868	864	860	856	853	849	845	842	838	834	830	827	824	820	817	814	810	806	803	800	797	794	791	788
707=4775	898	894	890	886	882	878	874	870	866	862	858	855	851	847	844	840	836	833	829	826	823	819	815	812	808	805	802	799	796	793
711=4750	904	899	895	891	887	883	879	875	871	867	863	860	856	852	849	845	841	837	834	831	827	823	820	816	813	810	806	803	800	797
714=4725	910	905	901	897	893	889	885	881	877	873	869	865	861	858	854	850	847	843	839	836	832	828	825	821	818	815	811	808	805	801
718=4700	916	911	907	903	899	895	891	887	883	879	875	871	867	863	859	856	852	849	845	841	837	833	830	826	823	820	816	813	809	806
722=4675	922	918	914	910	905	901	897	893	889	885	881	877	873	869	865	862	858	854	851	847	843	839	835	832	829	825	821	818	814	811
726=4650	929	924	920	916	912	907	903	899	895	891	887	883	879	875	871	867	863	859	856	852	848	844	840	837	834	830	824	822	819	816
730=4625	936	931	927	922	918	914	909	905	901	897	893	889	885	881	877	873	869	865	861	857	854	850	846	843	839	835	832	828	825	822
734=4600	942	937	933	928	924	920	916	911	907	903	899	894	890	886	882	878	874	870	866	862	858	854	851	848	844	840	837	833	830	826
738=4575	949	944	939	935	931	926	922	918	913	909	905	900	896	892	888	884	880	876	872	869	865	861	857	853	849	846	842	838	835	831
742=4550	955	950	946	941	937	932	928	924	919	915	911	907	902	898	894	890	886	882	878	874	870	866	862	859	855	851	847	843	840	836
746=4525	962	957	952	948	943	939	935	930	925	921	917	913	909	904	900	896	892	888	884	880	876	872	868	864	861	857	853	849	845	841
750=4500	968	964	959	954	950	945	941	936	931	927	923	919	914	910	906	902	898	894	890	886	882	878	874	870	866	862	858	854	850	846
754=4475	975	970	966	961	956	952	947	942	938	933	929	925	920	916	912	907	903	899	895	891	887	883	879	875	871	867	864	860	856	852
758=4450	983	978	973	968	963	959	954	949	945	940	936	931	927	922	918	914	909	905	901	897	893	889	885	881	877	873	869	866	862	858
763=4425	991	986	981	976	971	966	961	957	952	947	943	938	933	929	924	920	916	912	908	904	899	895	891	887	883	879	875	871	868	864
767=4400	997	992	987	982	977	972	967	963	958	953	949	944	939	934	930	926	921	917	913	909	905	901	897	893	889	885	881	877	873	869
771=4375	1004	999	994	989	984	979	974	969	964	960	955	950	946	941	936	932	927	923	919	914	910	906	902	898	894	890	886	882	870	874
776=4350	1011	1006	1001	996	991	986	981	976	971	967	961	957	952	947	943	938	933	928	924	920	916	912	908	904	900	896	892	888	883	880
780=4325	1019	1014	1009	1004	999	994	989	984	979	974	969	964	959	954	950	945	940	936	931	927	923	918	914	910	906	902	898	894	890	886
785=4300	1027	1021	1016	1011	1006	1001	996	991	986	981	976	971	996	961	956	951	947	942	937	932	928	924	920	916	912	908	903	899	895	891
789=4275	1035	1029	1023	1018	1013	1008	1003	998	993	988	983	978	973	968	963	958	954	949	944	940	935	931	927	922	918	914	909	905	901	897
794=4250	1043	1037	1031	1025	1020	1015	1010	1005	1000	995	990	985	980	975	970	965	960	955	951	946	942	938	933	928	924	920	915	911	907	903
799=4225	1052	1046	1040	1034	1028	1023	1018	1012	1007	1002	997	992	987	982	977	972	967	962	958	953	949	945	940	935	931	926	922	918	913	909
804=4200	1060	1054	1048	1041	1036	1031	1025	1020	1015	1010	1005	1000	995	990	985	980	975	970	965	960	955	951	947	942	937	933	928	924	920	915
808=4175	1068	1062	1056	1050	1044	1039	1033	1028	1023	1017	1012	1007	1002	997	992	987	982	977	972	967	963	958	953	949	944	939	935	930	926	922
813=4150	1076	1070	1064	1058	1053	1047	1041	1036	1031	1025	1020	1015	1010	1005	1000	995	990	985	980	975	970	965	960	955	951	946	941	937	932	928
818=4125	1085	1079	1073	1067	1062	1056	1050	1045	1039	1033	1028	1022	1017	1012	1007	1002	997	992	987	982	977	972	967	962	957	953	948	944	940	935
823=4100	1094	1088	1082	1076	1070	1064	1058	1053	1047	1041	1036	1030	1025	1020	1015	1009	1004	999	994	989	984	979	974	969	964	960	955	950	946	942
828=4075	1103	1096	1090	1084	1078	1072	1067	1061	1055	1050	1044	1038	1033	1027	1022	1017	1011	1006	1001	996	991	986	981	976	972	967	962	957	952	948
833=4050	1112	1106	1100	1094	1088	1082	1076	1070	1064	1058	1053	1047	1041	1035	1030	1025	1019	1014	1009	1004	999	994	989	984	979	974	969	964	960	955
839=4025	1122	1116	1110	1103	1097	1091	1085	1079	1073	1067	1061	1056	1050	1044	1039	1033	1028	1023	1017	1012	1007	1002	997	992	987	982	977	972	967	963
844=4000	1132	1125	1118	1112	1106	1100	1094	1088	1082	1076	1070	1064	1058	1052	1046	1040	1035	1030	1025	1019	1014	1009	1004	999	994	989	984	979	974	969
849=3975	1142	1134	1127	1121	1115	1108	1102	1096	1090	1084	1078	1072	1066	1060	1054	1048	1043	1037	1032	1027	1021	1016	1011	1006	1001	996	991	986	981	976
854=3950	1151	1144	1137	1130	1124	1117	1111	1105	1099	1093	1087	1081	1075	1069	1063	1057	1051	1046	1040	1035	1029	1024	1018	1013	1008	1003	998	993	988	983
860=3925	1160	1153	1146	1140	1133	1126	1120	1114	1108	1102	1095	1089	1083	1077	1071	1066	1060	1054	1049	1043	1037	1032	1026	1021	1016	1010	1005	1000	995	990

FRONT RADIUS = CHART POWER + 1/3 CENTER THICKNESS
THICKNESS (mm) = CORRECTION FACTOR

	+25	+50	+75	+100	+125	+150	+175	+200	+225	+250	+275	+300	+325	+350	+375	+400	+425	+450	+475	+500	+525	+550	+575	+600	+625	+650	+675	+700	+725	+750
696=4850	693	691	688	686	683	681	679	677	674	672	670	668	665	663	661	659	656	654	652	650	648	646	643	641	639	637	635	633	631	629
699=4825	696	693	691	689	687	684	682	679	677	674	672	670	668	665	663	661	659	656	654	652	650	647	645	643	641	639	637	635	633	631
703=4800	700	697	695	692	690	688	686	683	681	678	676	673	671	669	667	664	662	660	658	655	652	650	648	686	644	642	640	638	636	634
707=4775	704	701	699	696	694	692	690	687	685	682	680	677	675	673	671	668	666	664	662	659	657	655	653	650	648	646	644	642	640	638
711=4750	708	705	702	700	697	695	693	690	688	685	683	680	678	676	674	671	669	666	664	662	660	658	655	653	651	649	647	645	643	641
714=4725	711	709	706	704	701	699	696	694	691	689	686	684	681	679	677	674	672	670	667	665	663	661	658	656	654	652	650	648	646	644
718=4700	715	712	710	707	705	702	700	697	695	692	690	687	685	682	680	678	676	674	672	669	666	664	661	659	657	655	653	651	649	647
722=4675	719	716	714	711	709	706	704	701	699	696	694	691	689	686	684	681	679	676	674	672	670	667	665	663	661	658	656	654	652	650
726=4650	723	720	718	715	713	710	708	705	702	700	697	694	692	690	687	685	682	680	678	675	673	671	668	666	664	662	659	657	655	653
730=4625	727	724	722	719	717	714	712	709	706	703	701	698	696	693	691	688	686	684	682	679	677	674	672	669	667	665	663	660	658	656
734=4600	731	728	725	723	720	718	715	712	710	707	704	702	700	697	695	692	690	687	685	682	680	677	675	673	671	668	666	663	661	659
738=4575	735	732	729	727	724	722	719	716	713	711	708	706	703	701	698	696	693	691	688	686	683	681	679	676	674	672	669	667	665	663
742=4550	739	736	733	731	728	726	723	720	717	714	712	709	707	704	702	699	696	694	692	689	687	684	682	679	677	675	673	670	668	666
746=4525	743	740	737	735	732	730	727	724	721	718	716	713	711	708	706	703	701	698	696	693	691	688	686	683	681	678	676	674	672	669
750=4500	747	744	741	739	736	734	730	728	725	722	719	716	714	711	708	706	704	702	699	697	694	691	689	686	684	681	679	677	675	672
754=4475	751	748	745	743	740	738	734	732	729	726	723	720	718	715	713	710	708	705	703	700	698	695	693	690	688	685	683	680	678	676
758=4450	755	752	749	747	744	742	739	736	733	730	727	724	722	719	717	714	711	709	706	704	701	699	696	694	691	689	686	684	681	679
763=4425	760	757	754	751	748	746	743	740	737	734	731	729	726	724	721	718	715	713	710	708	705	703	700	698	695	693	690	688	685	683
767=4400	764	761	758	755	752	750	747	744	741	738	735	732	730	728	725	722	719	716	714	711	708	706	704	701	698	690	693	691	688	686
771=4375	768	765	762	759	756	754	751	748	745	742	739	736	734	731	728	725	723	720	717	714	712	709	707	704	702	699	697	694	692	689
776=4350	773	770	767	764	761	758	755	752	749	746	743	740	737	734	731	729	727	724	721	718	716	713	711	708	705	702	700	697	695	692
780=4325	777	774	771	768	765	762	759	756	753	750	746	743	741	738	736	733	731	728	725	722	720	717	715	712	709	706	704	701	699	696
785=4300	782	778	775	772	769	766	763	760	758	754	751	748	746	743	740	738	735	732	729	726	724	721	718	716	713	710	708	705	702	700
789=4275	786	783	779	776	773	770	767	764	761	758	755	752	750	747	744	741	739	736	733	730	728	725	722	719	716	714	712	709	706	704
794=4250	791	788	785	781	777	774	772	769	766	763	760	757	754	752	749	746	743	740	738	735	732	729	726	723	720	718	715	712	710	707
799=4225	796	792	789	786	783	779	777	774	771	768	765	762	759	757	753	750	747	744	741	738	736	733	730	727	725	722	719	716	714	711
804=4200	800	797	794	790	787	784	781	778	775	772	769	766	763	760	757	754	751	748	745	742	740	737	734	731	729	726	723	720	718	715
808=4175	804	801	798	794	791	788	785	782	779	776	773	770	767	764	761	758	755	752	749	746	744	741	738	735	733	730	727	724	722	719
813=4150	809	806	803	799	796	793	790	786	783	780	777	774	771	768	765	762	759	756	753	750	748	745	742	739	737	734	731	728	726	723
818=4125	814	811	808	804	801	798	795	791	788	785	782	779	776	773	770	767	764	761	758	755	752	749	746	743	741	738	735	732	730	727
823=4100	819	816	813	810	808	803	800	796	793	790	786	783	780	777	774	771	768	765	762	759	756	753	751	748	745	742	740	737	734	731
828=4075	824	821	818	814	811	808	805	801	798	794	791	788	785	782	779	776	773	770	767	763	760	757	754	751	749	747	745	741	738	735
833=4050	829	826	823	819	816	813	810	806	803	799	796	793	789	786	783	780	777	774	771	768	765	762	759	756	753	751	748	745	742	739
839=4025	835	832	828	824	821	818	815	811	808	804	801	798	794	791	788	785	782	779	776	773	770	767	764	761	758	755	752	749	746	743
844=4000	840	837	833	829	826	823	819	816	813	809	806	803	799	796	792	789	786	783	780	777	774	771	768	765	762	759	756	753	750	747
849=3975	845	842	838	834	831	828	824	821	818	814	810	807	803	800	797	794	791	788	784	781	778	775	772	769	766	763	760	757	754	751
854=3950	850	847	843	839	836	832	828	825	822	819	815	811	808	804	801	798	795	792	788	785	782	779	776	773	770	767	764	761	758	755
860=3925	856	852	848	844	841	837	834	830	827	823	820	816	813	809	806	803	800	797	793	790	787	784	781	778	775	772	769	766	763	760

FRONT RADIUS = CHART POWER + 1/3 CENTER THICKNESS
THICKNESS (mm) = CORRECTION FACTOR

	+775	+800	+825	+850	+875	+900	+925	+950	+975	+1000	+1025	+1050	+1075	+1100	+1125	+1150	+1175	+1200	+1225	+1250	+1275	+1300	+1325	+1350	+1375	+1400	+1425	+1450	+1475	+1500
696=4850	627	625	623	621	619	617	615	613	611	609	607	606	604	602	600	598	596	595	593	591	589	588	586	584	582	581	579	577	575	574
699=4825	629	627	625	623	621	619	618	616	614	612	610	608	606	604	602	600	598	596	595	593	591	589	588	586	584	582	581	579	577	575
703=4800	632	630	628	626	624	622	621	619	617	615	613	611	609	607	605	603	601	599	597	595	594	592	590	588	586	585	583	581	580	578
707=4775	636	634	632	630	628	626	624	622	620	618	616	614	612	610	608	606	604	602	600	598	597	595	593	591	590	588	586	584	583	581
711=4750	639	637	635	633	631	629	627	625	623	621	619	617	615	613	611	609	607	605	603	601	599	597	596	594	592	590	588	586	584	583
714=4725	642	640	638	635	633	631	629	627	625	623	621	619	617	615	613	612	610	608	606	604	602	600	599	597	595	593	591	589	588	586
718=4700	645	643	641	638	636	634	632	630	628	626	623	622	620	618	616	614	612	610	609	608	606	604	602	600	598	596	594	592	590	588
722=4675	648	646	644	641	639	637	635	633	631	629	627	625	623	621	619	617	615	613	612	610	608	606	604	502	600	598	597	595	593	591
726=4650	651	649	647	644	642	640	638	636	634	632	630	628	626	624	622	620	618	616	614	612	610	608	606	605	603	601	599	597	595	593
730=4625	654	652	650	648	646	643	641	639	637	635	633	631	629	627	625	623	621	619	617	615	613	611	609	608	606	604	602	600	598	596
734=4600	657	655	653	650	648	646	644	642	640	638	636	634	632	630	628	626	624	622	620	618	616	614	612	610	608	606	605	603	600	598
738=4575	660	658	656	654	651	649	647	645	643	641	639	637	635	633	631	629	627	625	623	621	619	617	615	613	611	609	607	606	603	601
742=4550	664	661	659	657	654	652	650	648	646	644	642	640	638	636	634	632	630	628	626	624	622	620	618	616	614	612	610	608	606	604
746=4525	667	665	663	660	658	656	654	651	649	647	645	643	641	639	637	635	633	631	629	627	625	623	621	619	617	615	613	611	609	607
750=4500	670	668	666	664	661	659	657	654	652	650	648	646	644	642	640	638	635	633	631	629	627	625	623	621	619	617	615	613	611	609
754=4475	674	671	669	667	665	662	660	658	656	653	651	649	647	645	643	641	638	636	634	632	630	627	625	623	621	619	617	615	614	612
758=4450	677	674	672	670	668	665	663	661	659	656	654	652	650	648	646	644	641	639	637	635	633	630	628	626	624	622	620	618	617	615
763=4425	680	678	676	674	671	669	667	665	662	660	658	656	653	651	649	647	645	643	641	639	636	634	632	630	628	626	624	622	620	618
767=4400	684	681	679	677	675	671	669	667	665	663	661	658	656	654	652	649	647	645	643	641	639	637	635	633	631	629	627	625	623	621
771=4375	687	684	682	680	678	675	673	670	668	666	664	661	659	657	655	652	650	648	646	644	642	640	638	636	634	632	630	628	626	624
776=4350	690	688	686	684	681	678	676	673	671	669	667	665	662	659	657	655	653	651	649	647	645	643	641	639	637	635	633	631	629	627
780=4325	694	691	689	687	685	682	680	677	675	672	670	668	666	663	661	659	657	654	652	650	648	646	644	642	640	638	636	634	632	630
785=4300	697	695	693	690	688	685	683	680	677	675	673	671	669	667	665	662	660	657	654	652	650	648	646	644	642	640	638	636	634	633
789=4275	701	699	696	694	692	689	687	684	681	679	677	675	672	670	668	666	663	661	659	657	653	650	648	646	644	642	640	639	637	636
794=4250	705	702	700	697	695	692	690	687	685	683	681	678	676	673	671	669	667	664	662	659	657	654	652	650	648	646	644	642	640	638
799=4225	709	706	704	701	699	696	694	691	689	687	685	682	680	677	675	672	670	668	666	663	661	659	657	654	652	650	648	646	644	642
804=4200	712	709	707	705	702	699	697	694	692	690	688	685	683	680	678	675	673	671	669	666	664	662	660	658	656	653	651	649	647	645
808=4175	716	713	711	708	706	703	701	698	696	693	691	688	686	684	681	679	677	674	672	670	668	665	663	661	659	656	654	652	650	648
813=4150	720	717	715	712	710	707	704	702	699	697	694	692	689	686	684	682	680	678	676	673	670	668	666	664	662	659	657	655	653	651
818=4125	724	721	719	716	714	711	708	706	703	701	698	696	693	691	688	686	683	681	679	677	674	672	670	668	665	663	661	659	656	654
823=4100	728	725	723	720	718	715	712	709	707	704	702	699	697	694	692	689	686	684	682	680	677	675	673	671	669	666	664	661	659	657
828=4075	732	729	727	724	722	719	716	713	711	708	706	703	701	698	696	693	691	688	686	683	681	678	676	673	671	669	667	664	662	660
833=4050	736	733	730	728	726	723	720	717	715	712	710	707	705	702	700	697	695	692	690	687	685	682	680	678	675	672	669	666	664	663
839=4025	741	738	735	732	730	727	724	721	719	716	714	711	709	706	704	701	699	696	694	691	689	686	684	681	679	676	674	671	669	666
844=4000	745	742	739	736	733	730	728	725	722	719	717	714	712	709	707	704	702	699	697	694	692	689	687	684	682	679	677	674	672	669
849=3975	749	746	743	740	737	734	732	729	726	723	721	718	715	713	711	708	706	703	701	698	696	693	691	688	686	683	681	678	676	673
854=3950	753	750	747	744	741	738	736	733	730	727	725	722	719	716	714	711	709	706	704	701	699	696	694	691	689	686	684	681	679	676
860=3925	757	754	751	748	745	742	740	737	734	731	729	726	723	720	718	715	713	710	708	705	703	700	698	695	693	690	688	685	683	680

FRONT RADIUS = CHART POWER + 1/3 CENTER THICKNESS
THICKNESS (mm) = CORRECTION FACTOR

	+1525	+1550	+1575	+1600	+1625	+1650	+1675	+1700	+1725	+1750	+1775	+1800	+1825	+1850	+1875	+1900	+1925	+1950	+1975	+2000
696=4850																				
699=4825	574	572	570	568	567	566	564	562	561	559	558	556	555	553	551	549	548	546	545	544
703=4800	576	574	573	571	569	568	566	564	563	561	560	558	557	555	553	551	550	548	547	546
707=4775	579	577	576	574	572	570	569	567	566	564	563	561	559	557	556	554	553	551	550	548
711=4750	581	579	578	576	574	573	571	569	568	566	565	563	561	559	558	556	555	553	552	550
714=4725	584	582	580	579	577	576	574	572	570	569	567	565	563	562	560	559	557	556	554	553
718=4700	586	584	582	581	579	578	576	574	572	571	569	567	565	564	562	561	559	558	556	555
722=4675	589	587	585	583	582	580	579	577	576	574	572	570	569	567	565	563	562	560	558	557
726=4650	591	589	588	586	584	582	581	579	578	576	574	573	571	569	567	565	564	562	560	559
730=4625	594	592	591	589	587	585	584	582	580	578	577	575	573	571	570	568	566	564	563	561
734=4600	596	595	593	591	589	588	586	584	582	581	579	577	575	574	572	570	568	566	565	563
738=4575	599	598	596	594	592	591	589	587	585	584	582	580	578	577	575	573	571	570	568	566
742=4540	602	600	598	596	595	593	591	589	588	586	584	582	581	579	577	575	574	572	570	569
746=4525	605	603	601	599	598	596	594	592	591	589	587	585	584	582	580	578	577	575	573	572
750=4500	608	606	604	602	600	598	596	594	593	591	589	587	586	584	582	580	579	577	575	574
754=4475	610	608	607	605	603	601	599	597	595	593	592	590	588	586	585	583	581	579	578	576
758=4450	613	611	610	608	606	604	602	600	598	596	594	592	590	588	587	585	583	582	580	578
763=4425	617	615	613	611	609	607	605	603	601	600	598	596	594	592	590	588	586	585	583	581
767=4400	619	617	615	613	611	609	607	605	603	602	600	598	596	594	592	590	589	587	585	584
771=4375	622	620	618	616	614	612	610	608	606	604	602	600	599	597	595	593	592	590	588	587
776=4350	625	623	621	619	617	615	613	611	609	607	605	603	601	599	598	596	594	592	590	589
780=4325	628	626	624	622	620	618	616	614	612	610	608	606	604	602	601	599	597	595	593	591
785=4300	630	628	626	624	622	620	618	616	614	612	610	609	607	605	603	601	599	597	595	593
789=4275	633	631	629	627	625	623	621	619	617	615	613	611	609	608	606	604	602	600	598	596
794=4250	636	634	632	630	628	626	624	622	620	618	617	615	613	611	609	607	605	603	601	599
799=4225	640	638	636	634	632	630	628	626	624	622	620	618	616	614	612	610	608	606	604	602
804=4200	642	640	638	636	634	632	630	628	626	624	622	620	618	616	614	612	610	609	607	605
808=4175	645	643	641	639	637	635	633	631	629	627	625	623	621	619	617	615	613	611	610	608
813=4150	648	646	644	642	640	638	636	634	632	630	628	626	624	622	620	618	616	614	612	610
818=4125	652	650	647	645	643	641	639	637	635	633	631	629	627	625	623	621	619	617	615	613
823=4100	655	653	650	648	646	644	642	640	638	636	634	632	630	628	626	624	622	620	618	616
828=4075	658	656	654	652	650	647	645	643	641	639	637	635	633	631	629	627	625	623	621	619
833=4050	662	660	658	656	653	650	648	646	644	642	640	638	636	634	632	630	628	626	624	622
839=4025	665	663	661	658	656	654	652	649	647	645	643	641	639	637	635	633	631	629	627	625
844=4000	668	666	663	661	659	657	654	652	650	648	646	644	642	640	638	636	634	632	630	628
849=3975	671	669	666	664	662	660	657	655	653	651	649	647	645	643	641	639	637	635	633	631
854=3950	674	672	669	667	665	663	660	658	656	654	652	650	648	646	644	642	640	638	636	634
860=3925	678	675	673	671	669	666	664	662	660	657	655	653	651	649	647	645	643	641	639	637

FRONT RADIUS = CHART POWER + 1/3 CENTER THICKNESS
THICKNESS (mm) = CORRECTION FACTOR

Appendix VIII

EDGE THICKNESS DETERMINATION BY MEANS OF SAGITTAL DEPTH TABLE

EDGE THICKNESS DETERMINATION

Formulas

The change of thickness (ΔT) between the center and edge of a finished but unedged contact lens is the difference between the posterior surface sagittal depth (S_P) and the anterior surface sagittal depth (S_A), or $\Delta T = S_P - S_A$.

Edge thickness of a *finished but unedged lens* is the algebraic sum of center thickness and ΔT, or $E.T. = C.T. + \Delta T$.

Standard edge thickness for a finished but unedged lens is 0.13 ± 0.02 mm., and ultrathin edge thickness for a finished but unedged lens is 0.10 ± 0.02 mm.

Tables

Sagittal depth for a curve of a given radius (r) over a given diameter (d) is found by the formula

$$s = \sqrt{r - r^2 - \left(\frac{d}{2}\right)^2}.$$

It is quicker and often more accurate to find sagittal depths by using the sagittal depth table on page 476. The radius of the curve is listed in the lefthand column and its diameter in the top column.

Before S_A can be found, the anterior surface radius must be determined. This can be done by compensation of the thin lens formula ($D_t = D_1 + D_2$). Using Column 5 of Appendix VI, the negative power in air of the base curve D_2 is determined. The desired posterior vertex power (D_t) is combined with this value. Then the radius of this resultant power (D_1) is found, and the result is the noncompensated anterior surface radius. The compensated radius is found by adding one third the center thickness to the noncompensated radius (see example on p. 342).

It is quicker to find the anterior surface radius by using the anterior surface radius table (Appendix VII).

During computations, a center thickness must be assumed. The thickness listed in the tables on page 63 may be used.

Surface Sagittal Depths

S_P is the sum of the sagittal depths of all posterior curvatures. The base curve sagittal depth (S_B) is found by looking up the base curve radius and the optic-zone diameter. The sagittal depth of each secondary curve is found by looking up its radius and subtracting the sagittal depth of its inner diameter from that of its outer diameter. For a bicurve lens, $S_P = S_B + S_1$. For a tricurve lens, $S_P = S_B + S_1 + S_2$.

Unless a lenticular construction is used, S_A is found by looking up the compensated anterior surface radius and the lens diameter.

Bicurve Lens Example

Known:	*B.C.R.*	*O.Z.D.*	*S.C.R.*	*L.D.*	D_P
	7.70 mm.	7.0 mm.	8.80 mm.	8.6 mm.	−3.00 D

Find: The center thickness that produces a 0.13 mm. edge thickness when this lens is finished but unedged.

1. $\Delta T = S_P - S_A$

2. Find S_P

$S_P = S_B + S_1$

S_B (7.70 rad. and 7.0 diam.)	=	+0.841
S_1 outside (8.80 rad. and 8.6 diam.)	=	+1.122
S_1 inside (8.80 rad. and 7.0 diam.)	=	−0.726
S_P		+1.237

3. Find S_A

From Appendix VII, 7.70 base curve and −3.00 posterior vertex power gives noncompensated anterior radius 8.09. From Tables 2–11, assume *C.T.* = 0.16 mm. Compensated anterior radius = 8.09 + ⅓ (.16) = 8.15 mm.

S_A = (8.15 rad. and 8.6 diam.) = 1.227

4. $\Delta T = S_P - S_A$

$\Delta T = +1.237 - 1.227 = +.010$

5. $E.T. = C.T. + \Delta T$

$0.13 = C.T. + 0.01$

$C.T. = .12$

Tricurve Lens Example

Known:	*B.C.R.*	*O.Z.D.*	*I.C.R.*	*I.C.W.*	*P.C.R.*	*P.C.W.*
	7.70 mm.	7.0 mm.	8.80 mm.	0.6 mm.	11.00 mm.	0.2 mm.
	L.D.	D_P				
	8.6 mm.	−3.00				

Find: The center thickness that produces a 0.13 mm. edge when this lens is finished but unedged.

1. $\Delta T = S_P - S_A$

2. Find S_P

   $S_P = S_B + S_1 + S_2$

S_B (7.70 rad. and 7.0 diam.)	=	+0.841
S_1 outside (11 rad. and 8.6 diam.)	=	+0.876
S_1 inside (11 rad. and 8.2 diam.)	=	−0.793
S_2 outside (8.80 rad. and 8.2 diam.)	=	+1.013
S_2 inside (8.80 rad. and 7.0 diam.)	=	−0.726
S_P		+1.211

3. Find S_A

   From Appendix VII, 7.70 base curve and −3.00 posterior vertex power gives noncompensated anterior radius 8.09. From Tables 2–11, assume $C.T. = 0.16$ mm. Compensated anterior radius = 8.09 + ⅓ (0.16) = 8.15 mm.

   S_A = (8.15 rad. and 8.6 diam.) = 1.227

4. $\Delta T = S_P - S_A$

   $\Delta T = +1.211 - 1.227 = -0.016$

5. $E.T. = C.T. + \Delta T$

   $0.13 = C.T. - 0.016$

   $C.T. = 0.146$ or practically 0.15 mm.

Appendix IX

BAUBLITZ SAGITTA TABLE*

RAD. MM	R²	5.00	5.50	5.60	5.80	6.00	6.20	6.40	6.50	6.60	6.80	7.00	7.20	7.40	7.50	7.60	7.80	8.00	8.20
		DIAMETER IN MILLIMETERS																	
6.00	36.00	.546	.667	.693	.747	.804	.863	.925	.956	.989	1.056	1.127	1.200	1.277	1.316	1.357	1.440	1.528	1.619
6.05	36.60	.541	.661	.687	.741	.796	.855	.916	.947	.980	1.046	1.115	1.188	1.264	1.302	1.343	1.425	1.511	1.601
6.10	37.21	.536	.655	.681	.733	.789	.846	.907	.938	.970	1.035	1.104	1.176	1.250	1.289	1.328	1.410	1.495	1.583
6.15	37.82	.531	.649	.675	.727	.782	.839	.898	.929	.961	1.026	1.093	1.164	1.238	1.276	1.315	1.395	1.479	1.566
6.20	38.44	**.526**	**.643**	**.668**	**.720**	.774	**.831**	**.890**	**.920**	**.951**	1.015	**1.082**	**1.152**	**1.225**	1.262	1.301	**1.380**	**1.463**	**1.549**
6.25	39.06	.522	.638	.662	.714	.767	.823	.882	.911	.942	1.006	1.072	1.141	1.213	1.250	1.288	1.366	1.448	1.533
6.30	39.69	.517	.632	.656	.707	.760	.815	.873	.903	.933	.996	1.062	1.130	1.201	1.237	1.275	1.352	1.433	1.517
6.35	40.32	.513	.626	.651	.701	.754	.808	.865	.895	.925	.987	1.052	1.119	1.190	1.225	1.263	1.339	1.418	1.501
6.40	40.96	.508	.621	.645	.695	.747	.801	.857	.886	.916	.978	1.042	1.109	1.178	1.213	1.250	1.326	1.404	1.486
6.45	41.60	**.504**	**.616**	**.640**	**.689**	.740	**.794**	**.850**	**.879**	**.908**	.969	**1.032**	**1.098**	**1.167**	1.202	1.238	**1.313**	**1.390**	**1.471**
6.50	42.25	.500	.610	.634	.693	.734	.787	.842	.870	.900	.960	1.023	1.088	1.156	1.191	1.226	1.300	1.377	1.496
6.55	42.90	.496	.605	.629	.677	.728	.780	.835	.865	.892	.952	1.014	1.078	1.145	1.180	1.215	1.288	1.363	1.442
6.60	43.56	.492	.600	.623	.671	.721	.773	.827	.856	.884	.943	1.004	1.068	1.135	1.169	1.204	1.276	1.350	1.428
6.65	44.22	.488	.595	.619	.666	.715	.767	.821	.848	.877	.935	.996	1.059	1.125	1.158	1.193	1.264	1.338	1.415
6.70	44.89	**.484**	**.590**	**.613**	**.660**	.709	**.760**	**.814**	**.842**	**.869**	.927	.987	**1.049**	**1.114**	1.147	1.182	**1.252**	**1.325**	**1.401**
6.75	45.56	.480	.586	.608	.655	.703	.754	.807	.834	.862	.919	.978	1.040	1.105	1.137	1.171	1.241	1.313	1.389
6.80	46.24	.476	.580	.603	.649	.698	.748	.800	.827	.854	.911	.970	1.031	1.095	1.127	1.161	1.230	1.301	1.375
6.85	46.92	.473	.576	.599	.644	.692	.742	.794	.820	.847	.904	.962	1.022	1.085	1.118	1.151	1.219	1.289	1.363
6.90	47.61	.469	.571	.594	.639	.686	.736	.787	.813	.840	.896	.954	1.014	1.076	1.108	1.141	1.208	1.278	1.350
6.95	48.30	**.465**	**.567**	**.589**	**.633**	.681	**.730**	**.781**	**.807**	**.834**	.889	**.946**	**1.005**	**1.067**	1.098	1.131	**1.198**	**1.267**	**1.338**
7.00	49.00	.462	.563	.584	.629	.675	.724	.774	.800	.827	.881	.938	.997	1.058	1.089	1.121	1.187	1.256	1.326
7.05	49.70	.458	.558	.580	.624	.670	.718	.768	.794	.820	.874	.930	.989	1.049	1.080	1.112	1.177	1.245	1.315
7.10	50.41	.455	.554	.575	.619	.665	.713	.762	.787	.813	.867	.923	.980	1.040	1.071	1.103	1.167	1.234	1.303
7.15	51.12	.451	.550	.571	.615	.660	.707	.756	.781	.807	.860	.915	.972	1.032	1.062	1.094	1.157	1.224	1.293
7.20	51.84	**.448**	**.546**	**.567**	**.610**	.655	**.702**	**.750**	**.775**	**.801**	.853	**.908**	**.965**	**1.023**	1.053	1.085	**1.148**	**1.213**	**1.281**
7.25	52.56	.445	.542	.563	.605	.650	.696	.745	.769	.795	.847	.901	.957	1.015	1.045	1.076	1.139	1.203	1.271
7.30	53.29	.441	.538	.558	.601	.645	.691	.739	.763	.788	.840	.894	.949	1.007	1.037	1.067	1.129	1.193	1.260
7.35	54.02	.438	.534	.554	.596	.640	.686	.733	.757	.783	.834	.887	.942	.999	1.029	1.059	1.120	1.184	1.250
7.40	54.76	.435	.530	.550	.592	.635	.681	.728	.752	.777	.827	.880	.935	.991	1.020	1.050	1.111	1.174	1.240
7.45	55.50	**.432**	**.526**	**.546**	**.588**	.631	**.676**	**.722**	**.746**	**.771**	.821	**.873**	**.928**	**.984**	1.012	1.042	**1.103**	**1.165**	**1.230**
7.50	56.25	.429	.522	.542	.584	.626	.671	.717	.741	.765	.815	.867	.921	.976	1.005	1.034	1.094	1.156	1.220
7.55	57.00	.426	.519	.539	.579	.622	.666	.712	.735	.759	.809	.860	.914	.969	.997	1.026	1.085	1.147	1.210
7.60	57.76	.423	.515	.535	.575	.617	.661	.707	.730	.754	.803	.854	.907	.961	.989	1.018	1.077	1.138	1.201
7.65	58.52	.420	.511	.531	.571	.613	.656	.702	.725	.749	.797	.848	.900	.954	.982	1.011	1.069	1.129	1.192
7.70	59.29	**.417**	**.508**	**.527**	**.567**	.608	**.652**	**.696**	**.719**	**.743**	.791	**.841**	**.893**	**.947**	.975	1.003	**1.061**	**1.120**	**1.182**
7.75	60.06	.414	.504	.524	.563	.604	.647	.692	.714	.738	.786	.835	.887	.940	.968	.996	1.053	1.112	1.174
7.80	60.84	.411	.501	.520	.559	.600	.642	.687	.709	.732	.780	.829	.880	.933	.961	.988	1.045	1.104	1.164
7.85	61.62	.409	.497	.517	.555	.596	.638	.682	.704	.727	.775	.824	.874	.927	.954	.981	1.037	1.096	1.156
7.90	62.41	.406	.494	.513	.552	.592	.634	.677	.699	.722	.769	.818	.868	.920	.947	.974	1.030	1.088	1.147
7.95	63.20	**.403**	**.491**	**.510**	**.548**	.588	**.629**	**.673**	**.695**	**.717**	.764	**.812**	**.862**	**.914**	.940	.967	**1.023**	**1.080**	**1.139**
8.00	64.00	.401	487	.506	.544	.584	.625	.668	.690	.712	.758	.806	.856	.907	.933	.960	1.015	1.072	1.130
8.05	64.80	.398	.484	.503	.541	.580	.621	.664	.685	.708	.753	.801	.850	.901	.927	.954	1.008	1.064	1.123
8.10	65.61	.395	.481	.499	.537	.576	.617	.659	.680	.703	.748	.795	.844	.894	.920	.947	1.001	1.056	1.114
8.15	66.42	.393	.478	.496	.534	.572	.613	.655	.676	.698	.743	.790	.838	.888	.914	.940	.994	1.049	1.107
8.20	67.24	**.390**	**.475**	**.493**	**.530**	.568	**.609**	**.650**	**.671**	**.693**	.738	**.784**	**.832**	**.882**	.907	.934	**.987**	**1.042**	**1.099**
8.25	68.06	.388	.472	.490	.527	.565	.605	.646	.666	.689	.733	.779	.827	.876	.901	.927	.980	1.035	1.091
8.30	68.89	.385	.469	.487	.523	.561	.601	.642	.662	.684	.728	.774	.821	.870	.895	.921	.973	1.027	1.083
8.35	69.72	.383	.466	.484	.520	.558	.597	.638	.658	.680	.724	.769	.816	.865	.889	.915	.967	1.020	1.076
8.40	70.56	.381	.463	.480	.516	.554	.593	.634	.654	.675	.719	.764	.810	.859	.883	.909	.761	1.013	1.069
8.45	71.40	**.378**	**.460**	**.477**	**.513**	.551	**.589**	**.630**	**.650**	**.671**	.714	**.759**	**.805**	**.853**	.878	.903	**.954**	**1.007**	**1.061**
8.50	72.25	.376	.457	.474	.510	.547	.585	.625	.646	.667	.710	.754	.800	.848	.872	.897	.947	1.000	1.054
8.55	73.10	.374	.454	.472	.507	.544	.582	.622	.642	.663	.705	.749	.795	.842	.866	.891	.941	.994	1.047
8.60	73.96	.371	.451	.469	.504	.540	.578	.618	.638	.658	.701	.744	.790	.837	.860	.885	.935	.987	1.040
8.65	74.82	.369	.449	.466	.501	.537	.575	.614	.634	.654	.696	.740	.785	.831	.855	.880	.929	.981	1.034
8.70	75.69	**.367**	**.446**	**.463**	**.498**	.534	**.571**	**.609**	**.630**	**.650**	.692	**.735**	**.780**	**.826**	.849	874	**.923**	**.974**	**1.027**
8.75	76.56	.365	.44[illegible]	.460	.495	.531	.568	.606	.626	.646	.688	.731	.775	.821	.844	.868	.917	.968	1.020
8.80	77.44	.363	.441	.457	.492	.527	.564	.602	.622	.642	.683	.726	.770	.816	.839	.863	.911	.962	1.013
8.85	78.32	.361	.438	.455	.489	.524	.561	.599	.618	.638	.679	.722	.765	.811	.834	.857	.906	.956	1.007
8.90	79.21	.358	.436	.452	.486	.521	.557	.595	.614	.634	.675	.717	.761	.806	.828	.852	.900	.950	1.001
	$\left(\frac{D}{2}\right)^2$	6.25	7.56	7.84	8.41	9.00	9.61	10.24	10.56	10.89	11.56	12.25	12.96	13.69	14.06	14.44	15.21	16.00	16.81

* Courtesy Frederick U. Baublitz.

RAD. MM	R²	8.40	8.50	8.60	8.80	9.00	9.20	9.40	9.50	9.60	9.80	10.00	10.20	10.40	10.60	10.80	11.00	11.20	11.40
6.00	36.00	1.715	1.764	1.816	1.921	2.031	2.148	2.270	2.334	2.400	2.537	2.683	2.842						
6.05	36.60	1.696	1.744	1.794	1.898	2.006	2.121	2.241	2.303	2.368	2.502	2.644	2.796						
6.10	37.21	1.676	1.724	1.773	1.875	1.982	2.094	2.212	2.272	2.336	2.467	2.606	2.753						
6.15	37.82	1.658	1.705	1.753	1.853	1.958	2.068	2.184	2.244	2.306	2.434	2.570	2.713						
6.20	38.44	1.639	1.686	1.733	1.832	1.935	2.043	2.158	2.215	2.276	2.401	2.534	2.674						
6.25	39.06	1.622	1.667	1.715	1.812	1.913	2.019	2.131	2.188	2.248	2.371	2.500	2.638						
6.30	39.69	1.604	1.649	1.696	1.791	1.891	1.995	2.105	2.161	2.220	2.340	2.467	2.601						
6.35	40.32	1.588	1.632	1.678	1.772	1.870	1.973	2.080	2.136	2.193	2.311	2.436	2.567						
6.40	40.96	1.571	1.615	1.660	1.752	1.849	1.950	2.056	2.110	2.167	2.283	2.405	2.533						
6.45	41.60	1.555	1.598	1.643	1.734	1.829	1.928	2.033	2.087	2.142	2.256	2.376	2.502						
6.50	42.25	1.540	1.582	1.626	1.716	1.810	1.908	2.010	2.063	2.117	2.229	2.347	2.470	2.600					
6.55	42.90	1.524	1.566	1.609	1.698	1.791	1.887	1.988	2.040	2.094	2.204	2.319	2.440	2.568					
6.60	43.56	1.509	1.550	1.593	1.681	1.772	1.867	1.967	2.018	2.070	2.179	2.292	2.411	2.536					
6.65	44.22	1.494	1.535	1.578	1.664	1.754	1.848	1.946	1.996	2.048	2.155	2.264	2.383	2.505					
6.70	44.89	1.480	1.520	1.562	1.647	1.736	1.829	1.925	1.975	2.026	2.131	2.230	2.355	2.475					
6.75	45.56	1.466	1.506	1.547	1.632	1.719	1.810	1.906	1.954	2.005	2.108	2.216	2.333	2.452					
6.80	46.24	1.452	1.492	1.532	1.616	1.702	1.792	1.886	1.934	1.983	2.085	2.191	2.302	2.418					
6.85	46.92	1.439	1.478	1.518	1.600	1.686	1.775	1.867	1.915	1.963	2.064	2.168	2.277	2.391					
6.90	47.61	1.426	1.464	1.504	1.585	1.669	1.757	1.848	1.895	1.943	2.042	2.145	2.252	2.365					
6.95	48.30	1.413	1.451	1.490	1.570	1.654	1.740	1.831	1.877	1.924	2.022	2.123	2.229	2.339					
7.00	49.00	1.400	1.438	1.476	1.556	1.638	1.724	1.813	1.858	1.905	2.001	2.101	2.205	2.314	2.427	2.546	2.670	2.800	2.937
7.05	49.70	1.388	1.425	1.463	1.542	1.632	1.708	1.796	1.840	1.887	1.982	2.080	2.183	2.290	2.401	2.518	2.640	2.767	2.902
7.10	50.41	1.375	1.412	1.450	1.528	1.608	1.692	1.778	1.823	1.868	1.962	2.059	2.160	2.266	2.376	2.490	2.610	2.735	2.867
7.15	51.12	1.364	1.400	1.438	1.514	1.594	1.677	1.762	1.806	1.851	1.943	2.039	2.139	2.243	2.351	2.464	2.582	2.705	2.834
7.20	51.84	1.352	1.388	1.425	1.501	1.580	1.661	1.746	1.789	1.834	1.925	2.019	2.118	2.220	2.327	2.438	2.554	2.675	2.801
7.25	52.56	1.341	1.376	1.413	1.488	1.566	1.647	1.730	1.773	1.817	1.907	2.000	2.097	2.198	2.303	2.413	2.527	2.646	2.770
7.30	53.29	1.330	1.365	1.401	1.475	1.552	1.632	1.714	1.753	1.800	1.889	1.981	2.077	2.177	2.280	2.388	2.500	2.617	2.739
7.35	54.02	1.318	1.353	1.389	1.463	1.539	1.618	1.699	1.741	1.784	1.872	1.963	2.058	2.156	2.258	2.364	2.475	2.590	2.710
7.40	54.76	1.308	1.342	1.378	1.450	1.526	1.604	1.681	1.726	1.768	1.855	1.945	2.038	2.135	2.236	2.340	2.449	2.563	2.681
7.45	55.50	1.297	1.331	1.367	1.438	1.513	1.590	1.670	1.711	1.753	1.838	1.927	2.020	2.115	2.215	2.318	2.425	2.537	2.653
7.50	56.25	1.286	1.320	1.355	1.426	1.500	1.576	1.655	1.696	1.737	1.822	1.910	2.001	2.095	2.193	2.295	2.401	2.511	2.626
7.55	57.00	1.276	1.310	1.344	1.416	1.488	1.563	1.642	1.682	1.723	1.806	1.893	1.983	2.076	2.173	2.274	2.378	2.486	2.599
7.60	57.76	1.266	1.300	1.334	1.403	1.476	1.550	1.628	1.667	1.708	1.791	1.876	1.965	2.057	2.153	2.252	2.355	2.462	2.573
7.65	58.52	1.256	1.289	1.323	1.392	1.464	1.538	1.615	1.653	1.695	1.776	1.860	1.948	2.039	2.134	2.232	2.333	2.438	2.548
7.70	59.29	1.246	1.279	1.313	1.381	1.452	1.525	1.601	1.640	1.679	1.760	1.844	1.931	2.021	2.114	2.211	2.311	2.415	2.523
7.75	60.06	1.237	1.269	1.303	1.370	1.441	1.513	1.588	1.629	1.666	1.746	1.829	1.915	2.004	2.096	2.191	2.290	2.393	2.499
7.80	60.84	1.227	1.259	1.292	1.360	1.429	1.501	1.575	1.613	1.652	1.731	1.813	1.898	1.986	2.077	2.172	2.269	2.370	2.476
7.85	61.62	1.218	1.250	1.283	1.349	1.418	1.489	1.563	1.600	1.640	1.717	1.799	1.883	1.970	2.059	2.153	2.249	2.349	2.453
7.90	62.41	1.209	1.240	1.273	1.339	1.407	1.477	1.550	1.587	1.626	1.703	1.784	1.867	1.953	2.042	2.134	2.229	2.328	2.430
7.95	63.20	1.200	1.231	1.264	1.329	1.396	1.466	1.538	1.575	1.613	1.690	1.769	1.852	1.937	2.025	2.116	2.210	2.307	2.408
8.00	64.00	1.191	1.222	1.254	1.319	1.386	1.455	1.526	1.563	1.600	1.676	1.755	1.836	1.921	2.008	2.097	2.191	2.387	2.387
8.05	64.80	1.183	1.213	1.245	1.309	1.376	1.444	1.515	1.551	1.588	1.663	1.741	1.822	1.905	1.991	2.080	2.172	2.267	2.366
8.10	65.61	1.174	1.204	1.236	1.300	1.365	1.433	1.503	1.539	1.576	1.650	1.727	1.807	1.890	1.975	2.063	2.154	2.248	2.345
8.15	66.42	1.166	1.196	1.227	1.290	1.355	1.423	1.492	1.527	1.564	1.638	1.714	1.793	1.875	1.964	2.046	2.136	2.229	2.325
8.20	67.24	1.157	1.189	1.218	1.281	1.345	1.412	1.481	1.516	1.552	1.625	1.701	1.779	1.860	1.943	2.029	2.118	2.210	2.305
8.25	68.06	1.150	1.179	1.209	1.272	1.336	1.402	1.470	1.505	1.540	1.613	1.688	1.765	1.845	1.928	2.013	2.101	2.192	2.286
8.30	68.89	1.141	1.170	1.201	1.262	1.326	1.391	1.459	1.493	1.529	1.601	1.675	1.752	1.831	1.913	1.997	2.084	2.174	2.267
8.35	69.72	1.133	1.163	1.193	1.254	1.317	1.382	1.449	1.483	1.518	1.589	1.663	1.739	1.817	1.898	1.981	2.067	2.156	2.248
8.40	70.56	1.125	1.154	1.184	1.245	1.307	1.372	1.438	1.472	1.507	1.577	1.650	1.725	1.803	1.883	1.966	2.051	2.139	2.230
8.45	71.40	1.118	1.147	1.176	1.236	1.298	1.362	1.428	1.462	1.496	1.566	1.638	1.713	1.790	1.869	1.951	2.035	2.122	2.212
8.50	72.25	1.110	1.139	1.168	1.228	1.289	1.353	1.418	1.451	1.485	1.555	1.626	1.700	1.776	1.855	1.936	2.019	2.105	2.194
8.55	73.10	1.103	1.131	1.160	1.219	1.280	1.343	1.408	1.441	1.475	1.544	1.615	1.688	1.763	1.841	1.921	2.004	2.089	2.177
8.60	73.96	1.095	1.123	1.152	1.211	1.271	1.334	1.398	1.431	1.464	1.533	1.603	1.675	1.750	1.827	1.907	1.989	2.073	2.160
8.65	74.82	1.088	1.116	1.145	1.203	1.263	1.325	1.389	1.421	1.454	1.522	1.592	1.664	1.738	1.814	1.893	1.974	2.058	2.144
8.70	75.69	1.081	1.109	1.137	1.195	1.254	1.316	1.379	1.411	1.444	1.511	1.580	1.652	1.725	1.801	1.871	1.959	2.042	2.127
8.75	76.56	1.074	1.101	1.130	1.187	1.246	1.307	1.370	1.402	1.434	1.501	1.570	1.640	1.713	1.788	1.865	1.945	2.027	2.111
8.80	77.44	1.067	1.094	1.122	1.179	1.238	1.298	1.362	1.392	1.424	1.491	1.559	1.629	1.701	1.775	1.852	1.931	2.012	2.096
8.85	78.32	1.060	1.087	1.115	1.172	1.230	1.290	1.351	1.383	1.415	1.481	1.548	1.617	1.689	1.763	1.839	1.917	1.997	2.080
8.90	79.21	1.053	1.080	1.108	1.164	1.222	1.281	1.342	1.373	1.405	1.470	1.537	1.606	1.677	1.750	1.825	1.903	1.983	2.065
		17.64	18.00	18.49	19.36	20.25	21.16	22.09	22.56	23.04	24.01	25.00	26.01	27.04	28.09	29.16	30.25	31.36	32.49

RAD. MM	R²	DIAMETER IN MILLIMETERS 5.00	5.50	5.60	5.80	6.00	6.20	6.40	6.50	6.60	6.80	7.00	7.20	7.40	7.50	7.60	7.80	8.00	8.20
8.95	80.10	.356	.433	.449	.483	.518	.554	.592	.610	.631	.671	.713	.756	.801	.823	.847	.895	.944	.994
9.00	81.00	.354	.430	.447	.480	.515	.551	.588	.607	.627	.667	.708	.751	.796	.818	.842	.889	.938	.989
9.05	81.90	.352	.428	.444	.477	.512	.548	.585	.604	.623	.663	.704	.747	.791	.813	.837	.884	.932	.982
9.10	82.81	.350	.425	.441	.474	.509	.544	.581	.600	.619	.659	.700	.742	.786	.808	.831	.878	.926	.976
9.15	83.72	.348	.423	.439	.472	.506	.541	.578	.597	.616	.655	.696	.738	.782	.804	.826	.873	.921	.970
9.20	84.64	.346	.420	.436	.469	.503	.538	.574	.593	.612	.655	.692	.734	.777	.799	.821	.868	.915	.964
9.25	85.56	.344	.418	.434	.466	.500	.535	.571	.590	.609	.648	.688	.729	.772	.794	.817	.862	.910	.958
9.30	86.49	.342	.416	.432	.464	.497	.532	.568	.586	.605	.644	.684	.725	.768	.789	.812	.857	.904	.953
9.35	87.42	.341	.414	.429	.461	.494	.529	.565	.583	.602	.640	.680	.721	.763	.785	.807	.852	.899	.947
9.40	88.36	.339	.411	.427	.459	.492	.526	.561	.580	.598	.636	.676	.717	.759	.780	.802	.847	.894	.941
9.45	89.30	.337	.409	.424	.456	.489	.523	.558	.576	.595	.633	.672	.713	.755	.776	.798	.842	.888	.936
9.50	90.25			.422	.453	.486	.520	.556	.573	.592	.629	.668	.709	.750	.771	.793	.837	.883	.930
9.55	91.20			.420	.451	.484	.517	.552	.570	.588	.626	.665	.705	.746	.767	.789	.833	.878	.925
9.60	92.16			.417	.448	.481	.514	.549	.567	.585	.622	.661	.701	.742	.763	.784	.828	.873	.920
9.65	93.12			.415	.446	.478	.512	.546	.564	.582	.619	.657	.697	.738	.758	.780	.823	.868	.914
9.70	94.09			.412	.444	.476	.509	.543	.561	.579	.615	.653	.693	.733	.754	.775	.819	.863	.909
9.75	95.06			.411	.441	.473	.506	.540	.558	.576	.612	.650	.689	.729	.750	.771	.814	.858	.904
9.80	96.04			.409	.439	.470	.503	.537	.554	.572	.609	.646	.685	.725	.746	.767	.809	.853	.899
9.85	97.02			.406	.437	.468	.501	.534	.552	.569	.606	.643	.682	.721	.742	.763	.805	.849	.894
9.90	98.01			.404	.434	.465	.498	.531	.549	.566	.602	.639	.678	.717	.738	.758	.801	.844	.889
9.95	99.00			.402	.432	.463	.495	.529	.546	.563	.599	.636	.674	.714	.734	.754	.796	.840	.884
10.00	100.00			.400	.430	.461	.493	.526	.543	.560	.596	.632	.670	.710	.730	.750	.792	.835	.879
10.05	101.00			.398	.428	.458	.490	.523	.540	.557	.593	.629	.667	.706	.726	.746	.788	.830	.874
10.10	102.01			.396	.426	.456	.488	.520	.537	.554	.590	.626	.663	.702	.722	.742	.783	.826	.870
10.15	103.02			.394	.423	.453	.485	.518	.534	.552	.587	.623	.660	.699	.718	.738	.779	.822	.865
10.20	104.04			.392	.421	.451	.482	.515	.531	.549	.583	.619	.656	.695	.714	.734	.775	.817	.860
10.25	105.06			.390	.419	.449	.480	.512	.529	.546	.580	.616	.653	.691	.711	.731	.771	.813	.856
10.30	106.09			.388	.417	.447	.478	.510	.526	.543	.577	.613	.650	.687	.707	.727	.767	.808	.851
10.35	107.12			.386	.415	.444	.475	.507	.523	.540	.574	.610	.646	.684	.703	.723	.763	.804	.847
10.40	108.16			.384	.413	.442	.473	.505	.521	.537	.571	.607	.643	.680	.699	.719	.759	.800	.842
10.45	109.20			.382	.411	.440	.471	.502	.518	.535	.569	.604	.640	.677	.696	.715	.755	.796	.838
10.50	110.25			.380	.408	.438	.469	.500	.515	.532	.566	.601	.636	.673	.692	.712	.751	.792	.834
10.55	111.30			.378	.407	.436	.467	.498	.513	.530	.563	.598	.633	.670	.689	.708	.747	.788	.829
10.60	112.36			.376	.405	.434	.464	.495	.511	.527	.560	.595	.630	.667	.685	.705	.743	.784	.825
10.65	113.42			.375	.403	.432	.462	.493	.508	.524	.557	.592	.627	.663	.682	.701	.740	.780	.821
10.70	114.49			.373	.401	.430	.460	.490	.505	.522	.554	.589	.624	.660	.679	.698	.736	.776	.817
10.75	115.56			.371	.399	.428	.458	.487	.503	.519	.552	.586	.621	.657	.675	.694	.732	.772	.813
10.80	116.64			.369	.397	.425	.456	.485	.500	.517	.549	.583	.618	.654	.672	.691	.729	.768	.808
10.85	117.72			.367	.395	.423	.453	.483	.498	.514	.547	.580	.615	.650	.669	.687	.725	.764	.805
10.90	118.81			.366	.393	.421	.450	.481	.496	.512	.544	.577	.612	.647	.665	.684	.722	.760	.801
10.95	119.90			.364	.391	.419	.448	.479	.493	.509	.541	.575	.609	.644	.662	.681	.718	.757	.798
11.00	121.00			.362	.389	.417	.446	.476	.491	.507	.539	.572	.606	.641	.659	.677	.715	.753	.793
11.05	122.10			.361	.387	.415	.444	.474	.489	.504	.536	.569	.603	.638	.656	.674	.711	.750	.789
11.10	123.21			.359	.385	.413	.442	.472	.486	.502	.534	.566	.600	.635	.653	.671	.708	.746	.785
11.20	125.44			.356	.382	.409	.438	.467	.482	.497	.529	.561	.594	.629	.646	.664	.701	.739	.778
11.30	127.69			.353	.378	.406	.433	.463	.477	.493	.524	.556	.589	.623	.640	.658	.694	.732	.770
11.40	129.96			.349	.375	.402	.430	.459	.473	.488	.519	.551	.583	.617	.634	.652	.688	.725	.763
11.50	132.25			.347	.371	.398	.425	.455	.469	.484	.514	.546	.578	.611	.628	.646	.681	.718	.756
11.60	134.56			.343	.369	.394	.422	.451	.464	.479	.509	.541	.573	.606	.623	.640	.675	.711	.750
11.70	136.89			.340	.365	.391	.419	.446	.460	.475	.505	.536	.568	.600	.617	.634	.669	.705	.742
11.80	139.24			.337	.362	.387	.415	.442	.456	.471	.500	.531	.563	.595	.612	.629	.663	.699	.734
11.90	141.61			.334	.359	.384	.411	.438	.452	.467	.496	.526	.558	.590	.606	.623	.657	.692	.724
12.00	144.00			.331	.356	.381	.408	.435	.448	.463	.492	.522	.553	.585	.601	.618	.651	.686	.721
12.10	146.41			.329	.353	.378	.404	.431	.445	.459	.487	.517	.548	.580	.596	.612	.646	.680	.716
12.20	148.84			.326	.350	.375	.401	.427	.441	.455	.483	.513	.543	.575	.591	.607	.640	.674	.710
12.25	150.06			.325	.348	.374	.399	.425	.439	.453	.481	.511	.541	.572	.588	.604	.637	.671	.707
12.50	156.25			.318	.341	.365	.390	.417	.430	.443	.471	.500	.530	.560	.576	.592	.624	.657	.693
14.00	196.00											.445	.471	.498	.512	.526	.555	.584	.614
17.00	289.00											.364	.386	.408	.419	.433	.453	.477	.502
	$\left(\frac{D}{2}\right)^2$	6.25	7.56	7.84	8.41	9.00	9.61	10.24	10.56	10.89	11.56	12.25	12.96	13.69	14.06	14.44	15.21	16.00	16.81

RAD. MM	R²	8.40	8.50	8.60	8.80	9.00	9.20	9.40	9.50	9.60	9.80	10.00	10.20	10.40	10.60	10.80	11.00	11.20	11.40
8.95	80.10	1.047	1.073	1.101	1.157	1.214	1.273	1.334	1.365	1.396	1.461	1.527	1.595	1.666	1.738	1.813	1.890	1.969	2.050
9.00	81.00	1.040	1.067	1.094	1.149	1.206	1.263	1.325	1.356	1.387	1.451	1.517	1.584	1.654	1.726	1.800	1.876	1.954	2.035
9.05	81.90	1.034	1.060	1.087	1.142	1.198	1.257	1.316	1.347	1.378	1.442	1.507	1.574	1.643	1.714	1.788	1.863	1.941	2.021
9.10	82.81	1.027	1.053	1.080	1.135	1.191	1.248	1.308	1.338	1.369	1.432	1.497	1.563	1.632	1.703	1.775	1.850	1.927	2.006
9.15	83.72	1.021	1.047	1.074	1.128	1.183	1.240	1.300	1.330	1.360	1.423	1.487	1.553	1.621	1.691	1.764	1.838	1.914	1.992
9.20	84.64	1.015	1.040	1.067	1.120	1.176	1.233	1.291	1.321	1.352	1.414	1.477	1.543	1.614	1.680	1.752	1.825	1.901	1.979
9.25	85.56	1.009	1.034	1.060	1.114	1.169	1.225	1.283	1.313	1.343	1.405	1.468	1.533	1.600	1.669	1.740	1.813	1.888	1.965
9.30	86.49	1.002	1.028	1.054	1.107	1.161	1.217	1.275	1.304	1.335	1.396	1.459	1.523	1.590	1.658	1.728	1.807	1.875	1.952
9.35	87.42	.997	1.022	1.048	1.100	1.154	1.210	1.267	1.296	1.326	1.387	1.449	1.514	1.580	1.647	1.717	1.789	1.863	1.939
9.40	88.36	.991	1.015	1.041	1.093	1.147	1.202	1.259	1.288	1.318	1.378	1.440	1.504	1.569	1.637	1.706	1.777	1.850	1.925
9.45	89.30	.985	1.010	1.035	1.087	1.140	1.195	1.252	1.281	1.310	1.370	1.431	1.495	1.560	1.626	1.696	1.766	1.838	1.913
9.50	90.25	.979	1.004	1.029	1.080	1.133	1.188	1.244	1.273	1.302	1.361	1.422	1.485	1.550	1.616	1.684	1.754	1.826	1.900
9.55	91.20	.973	.998	1.023	1.074	1.127	1.181	1.237	1.265	1.293	1.353	1.414	1.476	1.540	1.606	1.673	1.743	1.814	1.888
9.60	92.16	.967	.992	1.017	1.068	1.120	1.174	1.229	1.257	1.286	1.345	1.405	1.467	1.530	1.596	1.663	1.732	1.803	1.875
9.65	93.12	.962	.986	1.011	1.062	1.114	1.167	1.222	1.250	1.279	1.337	1.397	1.458	1.521	1.586	1.653	1.721	1.791	1.863
9.70	94.09	.956	.980	1.005	1.055	1.107	1.160	1.215	1.243	1.271	1.329	1.388	1.449	1.512	1.576	1.642	1.710	1.780	1.851
9.75	95.06	.951	.975	1.000	1.049	1.101	1.154	1.208	1.235	1.264	1.321	1.380	1.440	1.503	1.566	1.632	1.700	1.769	1.840
9.80	96.04	.946	.969	.994	1.043	1.094	1.147	1.201	1.228	1.256	1.313	1.372	1.432	1.493	1.557	1.622	1.689	1.758	1.828
9.85	97.02	.940	.964	.988	1.038	1.088	1.140	1.194	1.221	1.249	1.306	1.364	1.423	1.485	1.548	1.612	1.679	1.747	1.817
9.90	98.01	.935	.959	.983	1.032	1.082	1.134	1.187	1.214	1.242	1.298	1.355	1.415	1.476	1.538	1.602	1.668	1.736	1.806
9.95	99.00	.931	.953	.977	1.026	1.076	1.127	1.180	1.207	1.235	1.290	1.348	1.407	1.467	1.529	1.593	1.658	1.726	1.795
10.00	100.00	.925	.948	.972	1.020	1.070	1.121	1.173	1.200	1.227	1.283	1.340	1.398	1.458	1.520	1.583	1.648	1.715	1.784
10.05	101.00	.920	.943	.967	1.015	1.064	1.115	1.167	1.193	1.221	1.276	1.332	1.390	1.450	1.511	1.574	1.639	1.705	1.773
10.10	102.01	.915	.938	.961	1.009	1.058	1.108	1.160	1.187	1.213	1.268	1.324	1.382	1.441	1.502	1.565	1.629	1.695	1.762
10.15	103.02	.910	.933	.956	1.004	1.052	1.102	1.154	1.180	1.207	1.261	1.317	1.374	1.433	1.494	1.556	1.619	1.685	1.752
10.20	104.04	.905	.928	.951	.998	1.046	1.096	1.147	1.173	1.200	1.254	1.310	1.367	1.425	1.485	1.547	1.610	1.675	1.741
10.25	105.06	.900	.923	.946	.993	1.041	1.090	1.141	1.167	1.194	1.247	1.302	1.359	1.417	1.477	1.538	1.601	1.665	1.731
10.30	106.09	.895	.918	.941	.987	1.035	1.084	1.135	1.161	1.187	1.240	1.295	1.351	1.409	1.468	1.529	1.591	1.655	1.721
10.35	107.12	.891	.913	.936	.982	1.030	1.079	1.129	1.154	1.180	1.234	1.288	1.344	1.401	1.460	1.521	1.582	1.646	1.711
10.40	108.16	.886	.908	.931	.977	1.024	1.073	1.123	1.148	1.174	1.227	1.281	1.336	1.393	1.452	1.512	1.573	1.636	1.701
10.45	109.20	.881	.903	.926	.972	1.019	1.067	1.117	1.142	1.168	1.220	1.274	1.329	1.386	1.444	1.503	1.565	1.627	1.692
10.50	110.25	.877	.899	.921	.966	1.013	1.061	1.111	1.136	1.161	1.213	1.267	1.322	1.378	1.436	1.495	1.556	1.618	1.682
10.55	111.30	.872	.894	.916	.961	1.008	1.056	1.105	1.130	1.155	1.207	1.260	1.315	1.371	1.427	1.487	1.547	1.609	1.673
10.60	112.36	.868	.889	.911	.956	1.003	1.050	1.099	1.124	1.149	1.201	1.253	1.308	1.363	1.420	1.479	1.539	1.600	1.663
10.65	113.42	.863	.885	.907	.952	.998	1.045	1.093	1.118	1.143	1.194	1.247	1.301	1.356	1.413	1.471	1.530	1.591	1.654
10.70	114.49	.859	.880	.902	.947	.992	1.039	1.088	1.112	1.137	1.188	1.240	1.294	1.349	1.405	1.463	1.522	1.582	1.645
10.75	115.56	.855	.876	.898	.942	.987	1.034	1.082	1.106	1.131	1.182	1.234	1.287	1.341	1.397	1.455	1.514	1.574	1.636
10.80	116.64	.850	.871	.893	.937	.982	1.029	1.076	1.101	1.125	1.176	1.227	1.280	1.334	1.390	1.447	1.505	1.565	1.627
10.85	117.72	.846	.868	.889	.932	.977	1.024	1.071	1.095	1.120	1.170	1.221	1.273	1.327	1.383	1.439	1.497	1.557	1.618
10.90	118.81	.842	.863	.884	.928	.972	1.018	1.065	1.089	1.114	1.163	1.214	1.267	1.320	1.375	1.432	1.489	1.549	1.609
10.95	119.90	.838	.859	.880	.923	.967	1.013	1.060	1.084	1.108	1.158	1.208	1.260	1.314	1.368	1.424	1.482	1.540	1.601
11.00	121.00	.833	.854	.876	.918	.963	1.008	1.055	1.078	1.103	1.152	1.202	1.254	1.307	1.361	1.417	1.474	1.532	1.592
11.05	122.10	.829	.850	.872	.914	.957	1.003	1.050	1.073	1.097	1.146	1.196	1.247	1.300	1.354	1.409	1.466	1.524	1.584
11.10	123.21	.825	.846	.867	.910	.952	.999	1.044	1.068	1.092	1.140	1.190	1.241	1.293	1.347	1.402	1.458	1.517	1.575
11.20	125.44	.818	.837	.859	.901	.944	.989	1.034	1.057	1.081	1.129	1.179	1.229	1.280	1.333	1.388	1.443	1.501	1.559
11.30	127.69	.810	.830	.850	.892	.935	.979	1.024	1.047	1.071	1.118	1.167	1.216	1.268	1.320	1.374	1.429	1.485	1.543
11.40	129.96	.802	.822	.842	.883	.926	.969	1.016	1.037	1.060	1.107	1.155	1.205	1.255	1.307	1.360	1.415	1.470	1.527
11.50	132.25	.794	.814	.835	.876	.917	.960	1.006	1.027	1.050	1.096	1.144	1.193	1.243	1.294	1.347	1.401	1.456	1.512
11.60	134.56	.787	.807	.827	.868	.909	.951	.996	1.017	1.040	1.086	1.133	1.182	1.231	1.282	1.334	1.387	1.441	1.497
11.70	136.89	.780	.800	.819	.859	.901	.942	.986	1.008	1.030	1.075	1.122	1.170	1.219	1.269	1.321	1.373	1.428	1.482
11.80	139.24	.773	.793	.812	.850	.892	.932	.976	.998	1.020	1.067	1.112	1.150	1.208	1.257	1.309	1.360	1.413	1.468
11.90	141.61	.766	.785	.804	.844	.886	.925	.966	.989	1.011	1.056	1.102	1.148	1.195	1.245	1.296	1.347	1.400	1.454
12.00	144.00	.759	.777	.797	.835	.875	.916	.958	.980	1.003	1.046	1.091	1.138	1.186	1.234	1.284	1.335	1.387	1.441
12.10	146.41	.752	.771	.790	.829	.868	.909	.950	.972	.993	1.037	1.082	1.127	1.175	1.222	1.272	1.322	1.374	1.427
12.20	148.84	.747	.764	.783	.821	.860	.901	.942	.963	.986	1.028	1.071	1.117	1.164	1.212	1.261	1.310	1.361	1.414
12.25	150.06	.744	.761	.781	.818	.857	.897	.938	.959	.981	1.023	1.067	1.112	1.159	1.206	1.255	1.305	1.355	1.407
12.50	156.25	.727	.744	.764	.801	.838	.877	.917	938	.959	1.000	1.044	1.087	1.133	1.181	1.227	1.275	1.325	1.375
14.00	196.00	.646	.658	.677	.710	.743	.778	.809	.831	.849	.885	.933	.962	1.002					
17.00	289.00	.527	.538	.553	.579	.606	.634	.663	.677	.692	.721	.752	.783	.814					
		17.64	**18.00**	**18.49**	**19.36**	**20.25**	**21.16**	**22.09**	**22.56**	**23.04**	**24.01**	**25.00**	**26.01**	**27.04**	**28.09**	**29.16**	**30.25**	**31.36**	**32.49**

Appendix X

PATIENT RECORD FORM

NAME | PARENT OR SPOUSE | DATE

ADDRESS | HOME PH.

BUS. PH.

BIRTHDAY | AGE

REFERRED BY | OCCUPATION

	SPH.	CYL.	AXIS	TINT	DEC. IN.	DEC. OUT	FRAME #1
R							
L							
	ADD	BIFOCAL OR TRIFOCAL	SEG. HT.	INSET	TOT. DEC.		
R							
L							

PRISM | TEMPROSS | INDUSTRIAL T. | PLASTIC | P.D.

CURVES

	SPH.	CYL.	AXIS	TINT	DEC. IN.	DEC. OUT	FRAME #2
R							
L							
	ADD	BIFOCAL OR TRIFOCAL	SEG. HT.	INSET	TOT. DEC.		
R							
L							

	SPH.	CYL.	AXIS	TINT	DEC. IN	DEC. OUT	FRAME #3
R							
L							
	ADD	BIFOCAL OR TRIFOCAL	SEG. HT.	INSET	TOT. DEC.		
R							
L							

SERVICES | FEE

PAYMENT PLAN

DELIVERY DATE | M T W T F S | 8 9 10 11 12 1 2 3 4 5 6 7 8

CALL | WILL CALL | MAIL

RECALL

PROGRESS ANALYSIS

DATE	MISCELLANEOUS	FEE	DATE	MISCELLANEOUS	FEE

CASE HISTORY

I. VISION	II. COMFORT	III. APPEARANCE	IV. OCULAR HEALTH		VII. ENVIRONMENTAL DEMANDS
blur dist.	photophobia	redness	disease	sinus	vocation
blur near	burn	water	injury	diabetes	avocation
blur const.	itch	lumps	other	heart	general
diplopia	sting	granulation	correction	blood p.	safety
rainbows	ache	swelling	spectacles	stomach	lighting
spots	tire	squint	V. GENERAL HEALTH	kidneys	
lt. flashes	pain	close one eye	last physical	child dis.	
shifting	draw	cover one eye	last dental	pregnancy	
	headaches		medication	emotions	
	dizziness		treatment	VI. FAMILY	
	nausea		allergies	oc. prob.	
				spectacles	
				gen. dis.	

		SPH.	CYL.	AXIS	TINT	DEC.	ADD	SEG. HT.	BI. OR TRI.	OTHER
OLD RX #1	R.									
	L.									
OLD RX #2	R.									
	L.									

EXTERNAL: TENSION R. L. | PUPILLARY REFLEXES

	LIDS	CONJ.	LAC.	CORNEA	DIRECT	CONSEN.	NEAR
R.							
L.							

ACUITY AIDED	DISTANT	NEAR	UNAIDED	DISTANT	NEAR
R.	/		R.	/	
L.	/		L.	/	

SLIT: R. L. | MEDIA: R. L.

COVER TEST | ROTATIONS | FUSION

PP. CONV. | VERSIONS | DOM. EYE | DOM. HAND

FUNDI: R.

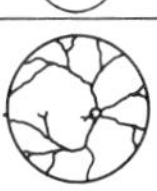

L.

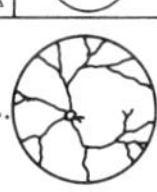

		DISTANCE				NEAR	
KERATOMETRY	R.	/	@		DYNAMIC ADD	R.	
	L.	/	@			L.	
STATIC REFRACTION	R.	=	x	20/	CROSS CYLS MON.	R.	L.
	L.	=	x	20/	BIN.		
SUBJ. REFRACTION	R.	=	x	20/	L. PHORIA		
	L.	=	x	20/	A.C./A. RATIO		
	BIN. ADD			20/	ADDUCTION	/ /	
LATERAL PHORIAS	HAB.				ABDUCTION	/ /	
	IND.				V. PHORIA		
ADDUCTION		/ /			V. DUCTION	R. /	L. /
ABDUCTION		/			ACC. AMP.	R.	L.
V. PHORIA					PRA		NRA
V. DUCTION	R. /	L. /			NEAR ADD	R.	L.
					NEAR V.A.	R.	L.

RECOMMEND:	DIST. WEAR	SUN	REFERRED TO:
CONST. WEAR	BIFOCAL	VIS. TRAINING	
NEAR WEAR	TRIFOCAL	C.L.	

ADDITONAL INFORMATION

CAMPIMETRY: L.

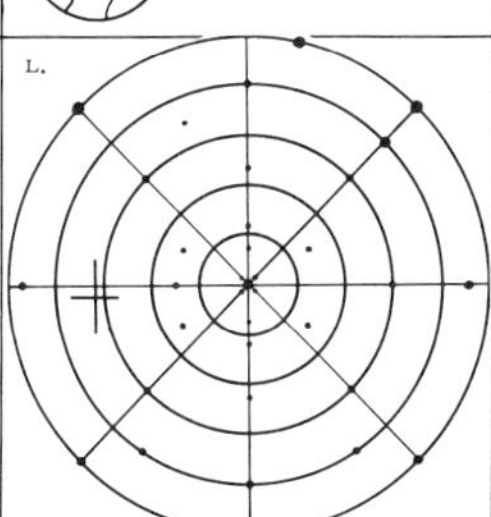

R.

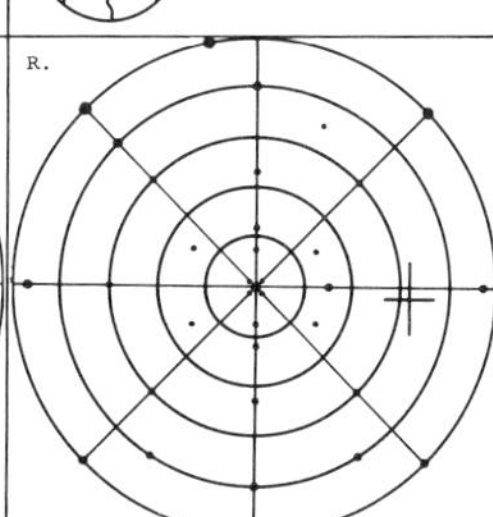

PERIMETRY

		S.	I.	N.	T.	S.N.	I.N.	S.T.	I.T.		S.	I.	N.	T.	S.N.	I.N.	S.T.	I.T.
WHITE	R.									L.								
BLUE																		
RED																		
GREEN																		

PATIENT SELECTION

PSYCHOLOGICAL FACTORS	VISUAL NEED			
MOTIVATION				
MATURITY	TENTATIVE LENS DESIGN CATEGORY			
CONCEPTIONS				
PATHOLOGICAL FACTORS				
PRESENT OCULAR PATHOLOGY				
PAST OCULAR PATHOLOGY				

ACUITY		D.	N.		D.	N.
AIDED	R.	/		UNAIDED R.	/	
	L.	/		L.	/	

NEEDED SPECTACLE POWER: R. / L.

TENTATIVE LENS DESIGN CATEGORY:

1. SPHERICAL SINGLE VISION
2. POSTERIOR TORIC
3. ANTERIOR TORIC
4. PRESBYOPIC
5. APHAKIC
6. SUBNORMAL VISION

ADDITIONAL FACTORS

	R.	L.		
LID POSITION U.			LID TENSION	
LID POSITION L.			BLINK ACTION	
VERTICAL APERTURE			GLOBAL POSITION	
IRIS DIAMETER			PHYSIOL. FACTORS	
IRIS COLOR			ENVIRON-MENT	
PUPIL SIZE				

INITIAL DESIGN SELECTION

MEASUREMENTS AND STANDARDS

	R.	L.
LENS DIAMETER (L.D.)		
OPTIC ZONE (O.Z.)		

BASE CURVE (B.C.)

CENTRAL OPHTHALMOMETRIC OR KERATOMETRIC READINGS

R.	L.
/ @	/ @
/ @	/ @
/ @	/ @
MEAN VALUES	MEAN VALUES
DIOPTERS	DIOPTERS
RADII	RADII
COMPENSATE FOR O.Z.	COMPENSATE FOR O.Z.
COMPENSATE FOR TORICITY	COMPENSATE FOR TORICITY
COMPENSATE FOR HYDRATION	COMPENSATE FOR HYDRATION
FINAL RADIUS	FINAL RADIUS

SECONDARY CURVE WIDTH (S.C.W.) & SECONDARY CURVE RADIUS (S.C.R.)

R.	L.
#1	#1
#2	#2
#3	#3
#4	#4

REFRACTIVE POWER

R.	L.
SPECTACLE POWER	SPECTACLE POWER
VERTEX COMPENSATION	VERTEX COMPENSATION
AI=AT-AO	AI=AT-AO
SPH. + 1/2 AI (SPH. EQ.)	SPH. + 1/2 AI (SPH. EQ.)
B.C. COMPENSATION	B.C. COMPENSATION
TOTAL	TOTAL

COMMENTS

USE COLUMN ON RIGHT FOR C.T. (CENTER THICKNESS) COMPUTATION

DIAGNOSTIC LENS PROCEDURE

	B.C.	S.C.	POWER	L.D.	O.Z.	T.	AUX. POWER	V.A.
#1								
R.								/
L.								/
COMMENTS								
#2								
R.								/
L.								/
COMMENTS								
#3								
R.								/
L.								/
COMMENTS								
#4								
R.								/
L.								/

REFRACTIVE POWER

R.	L.
DIAGNOSTIC LENS POWER	DIAGNOSTIC LENS POWER
AUXILIARY POWER	AUXILIARY POWER
VERTEX COMPENSATION	VERTEX COMPENSATION
B.C. COMPENSATION	B.C. COMPENSATION
TOTAL	TOTAL

C.T. COMPUTATION

R.

L.

ADDITIONAL COMMENTS

ORDER	B.C.	S.C.	S.C.	BL.	POWER	L.D.	O.Z.	TINT	OTHER	C.T.
R.										
L.										

CONTROL AND MANAGEMENT OF ADAPTATION

	Date:	Date:	Date:
Clinician			
Instructor			
	Average wear:	Average wear:	Average wear:

AND EXAMINER QUESTIONING				
GENERAL EXTERNAL EXAMINATION	R.	Appearance: good( ) fair( ) poor( )	Appearance: good( ) fair( ) poor( )	Appearance: good( ) fair( ) poor( )
		Blink: full( ) incomplete( )	Blink: full( ) incomplete( )	Blink: full( ) incomplete( )
		fast( ) normal( ) slow( )	fast( ) normal( ) slow( )	fast( ) normal( ) slow( )
		Position: sl-s-c-i-il tl-t-c-n-nl	Position: sl-s-c-i-il tl-t-c-n-nl	Position: sl-s-c-i-il tl-t-c-n-nl
		Movement: tight( ) normal( ) loose( )	Movement: tight( ) normal( ) loose( )	Movement: tight( ) normal( ) loose( )
	L.	Appearance: good( ) fair( ) poor( )	Appearance: good( ) fair( ) poor( )	Appearance: good( ) fair( ) poor( )
		Blink: full( ) incomplete( )	Blink: full( ) incomplete( )	Blink: full( ) incomplete( )
		fast( ) normal( ) slow( )	fast( ) normal( ) slow( )	fast( ) normal( ) slow( )
		Position: sl-s-c-i-il tl-t-c-n-nl	Position: sl-s-c-i-il tl-t-c-n-nl	Position: sl-s-c-i-il tl-t-c-n-nl
		Movement: tight( ) normal( ) loose( )	Movement: tight( ) normal( ) loose( )	Movement: tight( ) normal( ) loose( )

VISUAL ANALYSIS			v.a.	sph.	cyl.	axis	v.a.	flare		v.a.	sph.	cyl.	axis	v.a.	flare		v.a.	sph.	cyl.	axis	v.a.	flare
	R.	cls.							cls.							cls.						
		specs.							specs.							specs.						
	L.	cls.							cls.							cls.						
		specs.							specs.							specs.						

FLUORESCEIN PATTERN EVALUATION	R.	flow: good( ) fair( ) poor( )	flow: good( ) fair( ) poor( )	flow: good( ) fair( ) poor( )
		wetting: good( ) fair( )	wetting: good( ) fair( )	wetting: good( ) fair( )
		poor( )	poor( )	poor( )
	L.	flow: good( ) fair( ) poor( )	flow: good( ) fair( ) poor( )	flow: good( ) fair( ) poor( )
		wetting: good( ) fair( )	wetting: good( ) fair( )	wetting: good( ) fair( )
		poor( )	poor( )	poor( )
TISSUE INTEGRITY EVALUATION	R.	"K" ▼K R D	"K" ▼K R D	"K" ▼K R D
		slit lamp	slit lamp	slit lamp
		flow: good( ) fair( ) poor( )	flow: good( ) fair( ) poor( )	flow: good( ) fair( ) poor( )
	L.	"K" ▼K R D	"K" ▼K R D	▼K R D
		slit lamp	slit lamp	slit lamp
		flow: good( ) fair( ) poor( )	flow: good( ) fair( ) poor( )	flow: good( ) fair( ) poor( )
PHYSICAL STRUCTURE EVALUATION				
PATIENT RESPONSIBILITY EVALUATION				
REMEDIATION AND INSTRUCTION				

LABORATORY PROCEDURES

	R.											L.										
	DATE	B.C.	S.C.	S.C.	BL.	POWER	L.D.	O.Z.	TINT	OTHER	C.T.	DATE	B.C.	S.C.	S.C.	BL.	POWER	L.D.	O.Z.	TINT	OTHER	C.T.
ORDERED																						
VERIFIED																						
MODIFIED		SURFACE POLISH	SECONDARY CURVES			POWER	L.D.	O.Z.	EDGES	OTHER			SURFACE POLISH	SECONDARY CURVES			POWER	L.D.	O.Z.	EDGES	OTHER	
		B.C.	S.C.	S.C.	BL.	POWER	L.D.	O.Z.	TINT	OTHER	C.T.		B.C.	S.C.	S.C.	BL.	POWER	L.D.	O.Z.	TINT	OTHER	C.T.
ORDERED																						
VERIFIED																						
MODIFIED		SURFACE POLISH	SECONDARY CURVES			POWER	L.D.	O.Z.	EDGES	OTHER			SURFACE POLISH	SECONDARY CURVES			POWER	L.D.	O.Z.	EDGES	OTHER	
		B.C.	S.C.	S.C.	BL.	POWER	L.D.	O.Z.	TINT	OTHER	C.T.		B.C.	S.C.	S.C.	BL.	POWER	L.D.	O.Z.	TINT	OTHER	C.T.
ORDERED																						
VERIFIED																						
MODIFIED																						
ORDERED																						
VERIFIED																						
MODIFIED																						
ORDERED																						
VERIFIED																						
MODIFIED																						
ORDERED																						
VERIFIED																						
MODIFIED																						

PATIENT EDUCATION

LOSS REPLACEMENT PROGRAM		DATE	LENS(ES) LOST	PROMISED	FEE	DATE	LENS(ES) LOST	PROMISED	FEE

LITERATURE		REMOVAL		STORAGE		SOAKING SOL.		WEARING SCHEDULE
INSERTION		CENTRATION		WETTING SOL.		CLEANING SOL.		

Appendix XI

DIAGNOSTIC LENS UNITS

In accordance with his fitting philosophy, the practitioner can use the following outline to develop diagnostic lens sets of *bicurve, unblended tricurve,* or *blended tricurve* lenses. Lens diameters, optic-zone diameters, refractive powers, and thicknesses are the same for any of these three lens constructions. Except for the keratoconic lenses, base curves range from 7.10 to 8.40 mm. in 0.10 mm. increments. Secondary curve widths and radii are determined from the following tables. All blends should be fabricated with a soft pad, such as velveteen. The secondary curves of all bicurve lenses and the intermediate and peripheral curves of all tricurve lenses should be ground on and then polished with a hard pad. However, the intermediate curves of lenses with total secondary width of 0.50 mm. on each side of the optic zone should be fabricated with a soft pad, to act as a blend. When lenticular lenses are ordered, the bowl, or anterior optic zone, should be about 0.30 to 0.50 mm. larger than the posterior optic zone. The transition between the bowl and the carrier should be smooth and its thickness should be about 0.13 mm. for plus lenses. Lenticular plus lenses have minus carriers.

Bicurve Lenses

S.C.W.	S.C.R.
0.50 mm.	1.6 mm.
0.65 mm.	1.4 mm.
0.75 mm.	1.2 mm.
1.00 mm.	1.0 mm.
1.25 mm.	0.8 mm.

S.C.W. = Secondary Curve Width
S.C.R. = Secondary Curve Radius. Add this value to the base curve radius and order to the nearest 0.10 mm.

Unblended Tricurve Lenses

S.C.W.	I.C.W.	P.C.W.
0.50 mm.	0.20 mm.	0.30 mm.
0.65 mm.	0.35 mm.	0.30 mm.
0.75 mm.	0.45 mm.	0.30 mm.
1.00 mm.	0.70 mm.	0.30 mm.
1.25 mm.	0.95 mm.	0.30 mm.

S.C.W.	I.C.R.	P.C.R.
0.50 mm.	1.6 mm.	12.50 mm.
0.65 mm.	1.4 mm.	12.00 mm.
0.75 mm.	1.2 mm.	11.00 mm.
1.00 mm.	1.0 mm.	10.50 mm.
1.25 mm.	0.8 mm.	10.50 mm.

S.C.W. = Secondary Curve Width
I.C.W. = Intermediate Curve Width
P.C.W. = Peripheral Curve Width
I.C.R. = Intermediate Curve Radius. Add this value to the base curve radius and order to the nearest 0.10 mm.
P.C.R. = Peripheral Curve Radius. Order as shown in table.

Blended Tricurve Lenses

S.C.W.	B.L.W.	I.C.W.	P.C.W.
0.50 mm.	0.10 mm.	0.10 mm.	0.30 mm.
0.65 mm.	0.15 mm.	0.20 mm.	0.30 mm.
0.75 mm.	0.15 mm.	0.30 mm.	0.30 mm.
1.00 mm.	0.15 mm.	0.55 mm.	0.30 mm.
1.25 mm.	0.15 mm.	0.80 mm.	0.30 mm.

S.C.W.	B.L.R.	I.C.R.	P.C.R.
0.50 mm.	0.60 mm.	1.6 mm.	12.50 mm.
0.65 mm.	0.60 mm.	1.4 mm.	12.00 mm.
0.75 mm.	0.60 mm.	1.2 mm.	11.00 mm.
1.00 mm.	0.60 mm.	1.0 mm.	10.50 mm.
1.25 mm.	0.60 mm.	0.8 mm.	10.50 mm.

S.C.W. = Secondary Curve Width
B.L.W. = Blend Width
I.C.W. = Intermediate Curve Width
B.L.R. = Blend Radius. Add this value to the base curve radius and order to the nearest 0.10 mm.
I.C.R. = Intermediate Curve Radius. Add this value to the base curve radius and order to the nearest 0.10 mm.
P.C.R. = Peripheral Curve Radius. Order as shown in table.

UNIT I

−3.25 D Single Cut Anterior Surfaces

L.D.	S.C.W.	O.Z.D.	C.T.
7.0 mm.	0.50 mm.	6.0 mm.	0.14 mm.
7.5 mm.	0.75 mm.	6.0 mm.	0.14 mm.
7.5 mm.	0.50 mm.	6.5 mm.	0.14 mm.
8.0 mm.	0.75 mm.	6.5 mm.	0.14 mm.
8.0 mm.	0.50 mm.	7.0 mm.	0.14 mm.
8.5 mm.	0.75 mm.	7.0 mm.	0.15 mm.
8.5 mm.	0.50 mm.	7.5 mm.	0.15 mm.
9.0 mm.	1.00 mm.	7.0 mm.	0.16 mm.
9.0 mm.	0.75 mm.	7.5 mm.	0.16 mm.
9.0 mm.	0.50 mm.	8.0 mm.	0.16 mm.
9.5 mm.	1.25 mm.	7.0 mm.	0.16 mm.
9.5 mm.	1.00 mm.	7.5 mm.	0.16 mm.
9.5 mm.	0.75 mm.	8.0 mm.	0.16 mm.
10.0 mm.	1.25 mm.	7.5 mm.	0.17 mm.
10.0 mm.	1.00 mm.	8.0 mm.	0.17 mm.

UNIT II

−3.25 D Lenticular Cut Anterior Surface
(one set −6 D carrier and one set −9 D carrier)

L.D.	S.C.W.	O.Z.D.	C.T.
7.5 mm.	0.75 mm.	6.0 mm.	0.10 mm.
8.0 mm.	0.75 mm.	6.5 mm.	0.10 mm.
8.5 mm.	0.75 mm.	7.0 mm.	0.11 mm.
9.0 mm.	0.75 mm.	7.5 mm.	0.12 mm.

UNIT III

+2.50 D Single Cut Anterior Surface

L.D.	S.C.W.	O.Z.D.	C.T.
7.0 mm.	0.50 mm.	6.0 mm.	0.19 mm.
7.5 mm.	0.50 mm.	6.5 mm.	0.20 mm.
8.0 mm.	0.50 mm.	7.0 mm.	0.21 mm.
8.5 mm.	0.75 mm.	7.0 mm.	0.22 mm.
9.0 mm.	0.75 mm.	7.5 mm.	0.24 mm.

UNIT IV

+2.50 D Lenticular Cut Anterior Surface
(one set −6 D carrier and one set −9 D carrier)

L.D.	S.C.W.	O.Z.D.	Edge T.
7.5 mm.	0.75 mm.	6.0 mm.	0.13 mm.
8.0 mm.	0.75 mm.	6.5 mm.	0.13 mm.
8.5 mm.	0.75 mm.	7.0 mm.	0.13 mm.
9.0 mm.	0.75 mm.	7.5 mm.	0.13 mm.
9.5 mm.	1.00 mm.	7.5 mm.	0.13 mm.

UNIT V

−1.25 D Single Cut Anterior Surface

L.D.	S.C.W.	O.Z.D.	C.T.
7.5 mm.	0.50 mm.	6.5 mm.	0.16 mm.
8.0 mm	0.50 mm.	7.0 mm.	0.16 mm.
8.5 mm.	0.75 mm.	7.0 mm.	0.17 mm.
9.0 mm.	0.75 mm.	7.5 mm.	0.18 mm.
9.5 mm.	1.00 mm.	7.5 mm.	0.20 mm.
10.0 mm.	1.25 mm.	7.5 mm.	0.22 mm.

UNIT VI

−1.25 D Lenticular Cut Anterior Surface (−6 D carrier)

L.D.	S.C.W.	O.Z.D.	C.T.
7.5 mm.	0.75 mm.	6.0 mm.	0.12 mm.
8.0 mm.	0.75 mm.	6.5 mm.	0.12 mm.
8.5 mm.	0.75 mm.	7.0 mm.	0.13 mm.
9.0 mm.	0.75 mm.	7.5 mm.	0.13 mm.
9.5 mm.	1.00 mm.	7.5 mm.	0.13 mm.

UNIT VII

−6.00 D Single Cut Anterior Surface

L.D.	S.C.W.	O.Z.D.	C.T.
7.5 mm.	0.75 mm.	6.0 mm.	0.13 mm.
8.0 mm.	0.75 mm.	6.5 mm.	0.13 mm.
8.5 mm.	0.75 mm.	7.0 mm.	0.13 mm.
9.0 mm.	0.75 mm.	7.5 mm.	0.14 mm.
9.5 mm.	1.00 mm.	7.5 mm.	0.14 mm.

UNIT VIII

Aphakic +15 D Back Vertex Power
Single Cut Anterior Surface

L.D.	S.C.W.	O.Z.D.	Edge T.
7.5 mm.	0.50 mm.	6.5 mm.	0.12 mm.
8.0 mm.	0.50 mm.	7.0 mm.	0.12 mm.
8.5 mm.	0.50 mm.	7.5 mm.	0.12 mm.
9.0 mm.	0.75 mm.	7.5 mm.	0.12 mm.
9.5 mm.	0.75 mm.	8.0 mm.	0.12 mm.
10.0 mm.	1.00 mm.	8.0 mm.	0.12 mm.

UNIT IX

Aphakic +15 D Back Vertex Power
Lenticular Cut Anterior Surface (−8 D carrier)

L.D.	S.C.W.	O.Z.D.	Edge T.
8.0 mm.	0.75 mm.	6.5 mm.	0.12 mm.
8.5 mm.	0.75 mm.	7.0 mm.	0.12 mm.
9.0 mm.	0.75 mm.	7.5 mm.	0.12 mm.
9.5 mm.	0.75 mm.	8.0 mm.	0.12 mm.
10.0 mm.	1.00 mm.	8.0 mm.	0.12 mm.

UNIT X

Keratoconic −12 D
Lenticular Cut Anterior Surface
(plus carrier to 0.10 edge thickness) *

L.D.	S.C.W.	O.Z.D.	C.T.
7.5 mm.	1.00 mm.	5.5 mm.	0.08 mm.
8.0 mm.	1.00 mm.	6.0 mm.	0.08 mm.
8.5 mm.	1.00 mm.	6.5 mm.	0.08 mm.
9.0 mm.	1.25 mm.	6.5 mm.	0.08 mm.
9.5 mm.	1.25 mm.	7.0 mm.	0.08 mm.
10.0 mm.	1.25 mm.	7.5 mm.	0.08 mm.

* Base curve radii range from 6.10 to 7.40 in 0.10 mm. increments. Intermediate curve radius 2.0 mm. flatter than base curve radius. Peripheral curve radius 3.0 mm. flatter than base curve radius. Intermediate curve width is two-thirds of total secondary curve width. Blended lenses should be used.

UNIT XI

Prism Ballast Plano 1.5$^{\Delta}$

L.D.	S.C.W.	O.Z.D.	Apex T.
8.0 mm.	0.50 mm.	7.0 mm.	0.12 mm.
8.5 mm.	0.75 mm.	7.0 mm.	0.12 mm.
9.0 mm.	0.75 mm.	7.5 mm.	0.12 mm.
9.5 mm.	1.00 mm.	7.5 mm.	0.12 mm.

UNIT XII

Prism Ballast Plano 0.75$^{\Delta}$

L.D.	S.C.W.	O.Z.D.	Apex T.
8.0 mm.	0.50 mm.	7.0 mm.	0.12 mm.
8.5 mm.	0.75 mm.	7.0 mm.	0.12 mm.
9.0 mm.	0.75 mm.	7.5 mm.	0.12 mm.
9.5 mm.	1.00 mm.	7.0 mm.	0.12 mm.

REFERENCES

1. FILDERMAN, I. P., and WHITE, P. F.: Psychological, human relations, and practice management aspects of contact lens care—part one. J. Am. Optom. Assn., *36*(6):543–548, 1965.
2. HALE, J. R.: Emotional factors in fitting contact lenses. Optom. Weekly, *51*(45): 2349–2350, 1960.
3. WIENER, M. L.: A comparison of personality patterns of individuals requesting contact lenses and those rejecting them. Optom. Weekly, *55*(15):21–28, 1964.
4. BERK, R. L.: The psychological impact of contact lenses on children and youth. J. Am. Optom. Assn., *34*(15):1217–1222, 1963.
5. ORZACK, L. H.: The spread of contact lenses among college students: a sociological approach and research report. J. Am. Optom. Assn., *34*(8):628–633, 1963.
6. REMBA, M. J.: Doctor, can I wear contact lenses? Optom. Weekly, *55*(36):31–34, 1964.
7. COHEN, D. P.: Psychology and contact lenses. Optom. Weekly, *50*(44):2165–2166, 1959.
8. WESTHEIMER, G.: The visual world of the new contact lens wearer. J. Am. Optom. Assn., *34*(2):135–138, 1962.
9. WESTHEIMER, G.: Aberrations of contact lenses. Am. J. Optom. and Arch. Am. Acad. Optom., *38*(8):445–448, 1961.
10. SCHAPERO, M.: Physical considerations in contact lens fitting. Part I. Determinations from the case history. J. Am. Optom. Assn., *33*(3):215–218, 1961.
11. SARVER, M. D.: Record keeping and patient control procedures for the contact lens case. Encyclopedia Contact Lens Practice, *2*(11):7–23, chapter 5, 1961.
12. SARVER, M. D.: Prediction of residual astigmatism with contact lenses. Opt. J. and Rev. Optom., *100*(16):29–31, 1963.
13. SCHAPERO, M.: Physical considerations in contact lens fitting. Part III. Determinations from refraction, wearing. J. Am. Optom. Assn., *33*(5):351–353, 1961.
14. BRUCKER, D.: Tight lids and corneal edema. J. Am. Optom. Assn., *32*(8):625–626, 1961.
15. SCHAPERO, M.: Physical considerations in contact lens fitting. Part II. Determinations from the external exam. J. Am. Optom. Assn., *33*(4):300–304, 1961.
16. PHEIFFER, C. H.: Contact lenses and visual training complement each other. J. Am. Optom. Assn., *33*(8):578–582, 1962.

17. HAYNES, P. R.: Optometric examination in contact lens diagnosis. Encyclopedia Contact Lens Practice, *3*(15):1–36, chapter 2, 1962.
18. MARTIN, W. F.: Results of a research study on the vision of athletes. Optom. Weekly, *55*(29):23–27, 1964.
19. YARWOOD, R. A.: The use of contact lenses in all kinds of sports. J. Am. Optom. Assn., *31*(8):633–635, 1960.
20. STEWART, C. R.: Blending corneal lenses, Optom. Weekly, *54*(51):2359, 1963.
21. KORB, D. R., and FILDERMAN, I. P.: A new approach to contact lens ventilation. Optom. Weekly, *52*(49):2375–2380, 1961.
22. GORDON, S.: Some aspects of "venting" in corneal contact lenses. Encyclopedia Contact Lens Practice, *2*(11):6–34, chapter 6, 1961.
23. LEWISON, L., and HOLLANDER, H.: Report on new ultra-tiny vent-air grooved lens. Opt. J. and Rev. Optom., *93*(19):40, 1957.
24. MORRISON, R. J.: A new substance for contact lenses. Am. J. Optom., *39*(5): 252–256, 1962.
25. MORRISON, R. J.: Contact lens coating. Opt. J. and Rev. Optom., *100*(14):38–40, 1963.
26. BERMAN, M. R.: Some comments on the Erb method of contact lens wetting. Am. J. Optom. and Arch. Am. Acad. Optom., *40*(3):148–149, 1963.
27. GESSER, H. D., and FUNT, B. L.: A method of improving the wettability of contact lenses by free radical treatment. Am. J. Optom. and Arch. Am. Acad. Optom., *42*(5):321–324, 1965.
28. RENGSTROFF, R. H.: Corneal curvature and astigmatic changes subsequent to contact lens wear. J. Am. Optom. Assn., *36*(11):996–1000, 1965.
29. REMBA, M. J.: The effect of the eyelids on contact lens rotation—a detailed study. Contacto, *5*(4):123–132, 1961.
30. FILDERMAN, I. P.: The principles of the Bi-Ped contact lens. Southern J. Optom., *5*(5):5–9, 1963.
31. FILDERMAN, I. P., and WHITE, P. F.: Theoretical and clinical aspects of contact lens adherance and venting. Southern J. Optom., *6*(3):5–9 and 23–30, 1964.
32. POSTER, M. G.: Hydro-dynamics of corneal contact lenses. Am. J. Optom. and Arch. Am. Acad. Optom., *41*(7):422–425, 1964.
33. REMBA, M.: Maximum corneal exposure—a contact lens fitting philosophy. Optom. Weekly, *53*(7):285–289, 1962.
34. BRUCKER, D.: Theoretical considerations of gradually flattening peripheral curves and their modifications. Encyclopedia Contact Lens Practice, *2*(16):94–97, chapter 22, 1962.
35. MANDELL, R. B.: Linear clearance of contact lens peripheral curves. Am. J. Optom. and Arch. Am. Acad. Optom., *42*(12):742–747, 1965.
36. HOUSTON, R. J.: The function of the peripheral flange. Optom. Weekly, *52*(46): 2247–2253 and 2264–2265, 1961.
37. FILDERMAN, I. P.: Contact lens practice—a new perspective. Southern J. Optom., *6*(2):9–11 and 14–16, 1964.
38. FINGLES, H. M.: Factors governing adhesion from the mechanical standpoint. Opt. J. and Rev. Optom., *97*(18):39–42, 1960.
39. STEWART, C. R.: Corneal lens diameters and vertical positioning. J. Am. Optom. Assn., *34*(15):1223–1227, 1963.
40. BIER, N.: A study of the cornea in relation to contact lens practice. Am. J. Optom. and Arch. Am. Acad. Optom., *33*(6):291–304, 1956.
41. BIER, N.: The contour lens—a new form of corneal lens. J. Am. Optom. Assn., *28*(7):394–397, 1957.
42. MOSS, H. I.: An approach to prescribing corneal type contact lenses. Am. J. Optom. and Arch. Am. Acad. Optom., *35*(5):262–268, 1958.

43. MOSS, H. I.: The contour principle of contact lens fitting. J. Am. Optom. Assn., *29*(9):579–581, 1958.
44. MOSS, H. I.: A clinical experimental study of corneal contours in fitting contact lenses. Am. J. Optom. and Arch. Am. Acad. Optom., *36*(6):313–317, 1959.
45. WESLEY, N. K., and JESSEN, G. N.: The Sphercon lens—a new development. Optom. Weekly, *47*(39):1740–1741, 1956.
46. ISEN, A. A.: Two complementary techniques for fitting small corneal lenses. Optom. Weekly, *54*(51):2355–2358, 1963.
47. JESSEN, G. N.: New bifocal technique results in more comfortable single vision lenses. Contacto, *5*(7):237–243, 1961.
48. MORRISON, R.: Small–thin contact lens use. Optom. Weekly, *54*(19):853–855, 1963.
49. BAYSHORE, C. A.: Report on 276 patients fitted with micro-corneal lenses, apical clearance and central ventilation. Am. J. Optom. and Arch. Am. Acad. Optom., *39*(10):552–553, 1962.
50. BAYSHORE, C. A.: Report on 600 cases of micro-corneal lenses fitted with apical clearance. Am. J. Optom. and Arch. Am. Acad. Optom., *40*(6):351–353, 1963.
51. ISEN, A. A.: Two complementary techniques for fitting small corneal lenses. Optom. Weekly, *54*(52):2387–2389, 1963.
52. FILDERMAN, I. P.: Principles of the contact lens Pupilens. Optom. Weekly, *53*(46):2269–2273, 1962.
53. FILDERMAN, I. P.: Principles of the contact lens Pupilens. Optom. Weekly, *53*(49):2389–2396, 1962.
54. FILDERMAN, I. P.: Contact lens designs related to lower lid bearing. Optom. Weekly, *55*(24):27–33, 1964.
55. FILDERMAN, I. P.: Contact lens practice—a new perspective. Southern J. Optom., *7*(2):7–10 and 29–32, 1965.
56. HAYNES, P. R.: Custom fitting procedures for prescribing corneal contact lenses. J. Am. Optom. Assn., *35*(3):187–214, 1964.
57. BIER, N.: The fallacy of the ophthalmometer. Brit. J. Phys. Opt., *21*(4):224–233, 1964.
58. CHIQUIAR-ARIAS, M.: Contact lens base curve determination—by central or peripheral keratometry. Optom. Weekly, *56*(48):35–38, 1965.
59. CHIQUIAR-ARIAS, M.: Are we measuring the true apex of the cornea with the keratometer? Contacto, *4*(6):195–198, 1960.
60. GORDON, S.: Contact lens hydration: a study of the wetting-drying cycle. Optom. Weekly, *56*(14):55–62, 1965.
61. MORRISON, R. J., KAUFMAN, K. J., and CERULLI, E.: Base curve–changes of polymethylmethacrylate contact lenses. Am. J. Optom. and Arch. Am. Acad. Optom., *42*(1):17–20, 1965.
62. OSTRICH, A. D., and PAILET, E.: Hydration of contact lenses. Optom. Weekly, *51*(27):1408–1409, 1960.
63. HAYNES, P. R.: Comments on design and specification of diagnostic lenses. Encyclopedia Contact Lens Practice, *3*(14):19–40, chapter 4, 1962.
64. GATES, H., and EWELL, D.: Frequency distribution of base curves and dioptric powers. Encyclopedia Contact Lens Practice, *1*(5):8–9, chapter 30, 1960.
65. ISEN, A. A.: Effective trial contact lens procedure. Encyclopedia Contact Lens Practice, *1*(4):14–16, recent developments section, 1960.
66. HAYNES, P. R., BRUNGARDT, T. F., and POLLOCK, E. D.: Use of fluorescein in the fitting of contact lenses. Encyclopedia Contact Lens Practice, *1*(4):3–46, chapter 10, 1960.
67. BRUNGARDT, T. F.: Fluorescein patterns: they are accurate and they can be mastered. J. Am. Optom. Assn., *32*(12):973–974, 1961.

68. LESTER, R. W.: Fluorescein and contact lenses. Contacto, *2*(4):91–95, 1958.
69. BRONSTEIN, L.: Accuracy of fluorescein for determining corneal curvature. Contacto, *3*(6):170–171, 1959.
70. ELMSTROM, G. P.: A note on contact lens staining by strip fluorescein. Am. J. Optom. and Arch. Am. Acad. Optom., *33*(11):614, 1956.
71. VODNOY, B. E.: Sterile fluorescein impregnated paper strips, a must in contact lens practice. J. Am. Optom. Assn., *36*(3):235–237, 1965.
72. ELLERBROCK, V. J.: The role of toric surfaces in contact lens practice. Am. J. Optom. and Arch. Am. Acad. Optom., *40*(8):439–446, 1963.
73. FILDERMAN, I. P.: Contact lens practice—a new perspective. Southern J. Optom., *6*(7):13–17 and 24–29, 1964.
74. KORB, D. R.: A preliminary report on toric contact lenses. Optom. Weekly, *51*(48):2501–2505, 1960.
75. HAYNES, P. R.: Corneal contact lenses with toric optical zones and spherical or toric peripheral zone. Part I. Theoretical considerations. Encyclopedia Contact Lens Practice, *2*(9):4–11, chapter 9, 1961.
76. HAYNES, P. R.: Corneal contact lenses with toric optical zones and spherical or toric peripheral zones. Part II. Induced residual astigmatism produced by a toric optical zone on a corneal lens. Encyclopedia Contact Lens Practice, *2*(9):12–15, chapter 9, 1961.
77. KORB, D. R.: Corneal contact lenses with toric optical zones and spherical or toric peripheral zones. Part III. Clinical considerations. Encyclopedia Contact Lens Practice, *2*(10):16–64, chapter 9, 1961.
78. REMBA, M. J.: The abc's of toric contact lens fitting. Opt. J. and Rev. Optom., *99*(24):25–30, 1962.
79. SCHAPERO, M.: The fitting of highly toric corneae with toric corneal contact lenses. Am. J. Optom. and Arch. Am. Acad. Optom., *30*(3):157–160, 1953.
80. BRUNGARDT, T. F.: The case against toric base curve contact lens construction. J. Am. Optom. Assn., *33*(11):830–832, 1962.
81. ELLERBROCK, V. J.: Quality control of toric contact lenses. Am. J. Optom. and Arch. Am. Acad. Optom., *40*(1):29–34, 1963.
82. HAYNES, P. R.: Corneal contact lenses with toric peripheral curves. Encyclopedia Contact Lens Practice, *1*(6):26–32, recent developments section, 1960.
83. KAPLAN, M. M.: Residual astigmia and the bitoric lens. Optom. Weekly, *54*(3): 99–105, 1963.
84. KAPLAN, M. M.: Residual astigmia and the pre-corneal fluid. Optom. Weekly, *53*(43):2138–2141, 1962.
85. KAPLAN, M. M.: Residual astigmia and the toric concavity. Optom. Weekly, *53*(26):1301–1305, 1962.
86. KAPLAN, M. M.: Residual astigmia and the toric concavity. Optom. Weekly, *53*(27):1339–1343, 1962.
87. SARVER, M. D.: A toric base corneal contact lens with spherical power effect. J. Am. Optom. Assn., *34*(14):1136–1137, 1963.
88. WEST, D. C.: Method for predicting cylinder when using toric base contact lenses. J. Am. Optom. Assn., *36*(3):231–234, 1965.
89. BAILEY, N. J.: Residual astigmatism with contact lenses. Part I. Incidence. Opt. J. and Rev. Optom., *98*(1):30–31, 1961.
90. BAILEY, N. J.: Residual astigmatism with contact lenses. Part II. Predictability. Opt. J. and Rev. Optom., *98*(2):40–45, 1961.
91. BAILEY, N. J.: Residual astigmatism with contact lenses. Part III. Possible sites. Opt. J. and Rev. Optom., *98*(3):31–32, 1961.
92. BAILEY, N. J.: Residual astigmatism with contact lenses. Part IV. Corrective techniques. Opt. J. and Rev. Optom., *98*(4):43–44, 1961.

93. CARTER, J. H.: Residual astigmatism of the human eye. Optom. Weekly, *54*(27):1271–1272, 1963.
94. FILDERMAN, I. P.: Contact lens practice—a new perspective. Southern J. Optom., *6*(8):11–17 and 32–33, 1964.
95. EWELL, D. G.: Meridional orientation of contact lenses. Contacto, *4*(9):415–423, 1960.
96. KORB, D. R.: Techniques to achieve centration with prism corneal contact lenses. Encyclopedia Contact Lens Practice, *4*(20):117–123, recent developments section, 1963.
97. KORB, D. R.: Recent developments in prism ballast lenses. Encyclopedia Contact Lens Practice, *3*(15):67–71, recent developments section, 1962.
98. KORB, D. R.: A survey of current fitting techniques for prism ballast corneal contact lenses. Encyclopedia Contact Lens Practice, *3*(17):88–97, recent developments section, 1962.
99. EWELL, D. G., GATES, H., and REMBA, M. J.: The prism ballast contact lens principle. Encyclopedia Contact Lens Practice, *2*(12):31–54, chapter 16, 1961.
100. HAYNES, P. R.: Elliptical, double truncated and oval contact lenses. Encyclopedia Contact Lens Practice, *2*(8):36–44, recent developments section, 1961.
101. EWELL, D. G.: Design and modification of a truncated edge. Encyclopedia Contact Lens Practice, *3*(15):81–84, chapter 22, 1962.
102. MOSS, H. L.: Semi-sclero-corneal flange lens for correcting residual astigmatism. J. Am. Optom. Assn., *31*(1):57–58, 1959.
103. HAYNES, P. R.: Concept of the limbal angle and the design of a semi-scleral-corneal contact lens. Encyclopedia Contact Lens Practice, *1*(5):18–25, recent developments section, 1960.
104. GOLDBERG, J. B.: A clinical procedure to determine the effective cylinder axis for prism ballast lenses. Encyclopedia Contact Lens Practice, *3*(15):55–62, chapter 16, 1962.
105. FILDERMAN, I. P.: Contact lens practice—a new perspective. Southern J. Optom., *6*(9):7–10, 1964.
106. WILLIAMS, C. E.: Contact lenses as subnormal vision aids. Contacto, *1*(4):69–78, 1957.
107. WILLIAMS, C. E.: The use of contact lenses in subnormal vision. Encyclopedia Contact Lens Practice, *3*(16):63–76, chapter 16, 1962.
108. HALL, K. C., and THOMPSON, K. E.: Some aspects of keratoconus. Contacto, *6*(7):207–211, 1962.
109. FILDERMAN, I. P.: Use of contact lens in case of monocular keratoglobus—a case report. Am. J. Optom. and Arch. Am. Acad. Optom., *27*(7):350–351, 1950.
110. FILDERMAN, I. P.: Contact lens practice—a new perspective. Southern J. Optom., *6*(5):9–13 and 35, 1964.
111. FILDERMAN, I. P., and ISEN, A. A.: The therapy of keratoconus. Opt. J. and Rev. Optom., *97*(5):33–35, 1960.
112. FILDERMAN, I. P., and ISEN, A. A.: A suggested therapy for cases of keratoconus. J. Am. Optom. Assn., *31*(8):623–626, 1960.
113. SARWAR, M.: Examination and assessment for surgery and for contact lenses. Brit. J. Phys. Opt., *21*(3):130–133, 1964.
114. ULLEN, R. L.: Keratoconus and contact lenses. Opt. J. and Rev. Optom., *98*(24):34–40, 1961.
115. WILLIAMS, C. E.: An interpretation of contact lens variables and a resultant keratoconus technique. J. Am. Optom. Assn., *31*(8):613–616, 1960.
116. ZEKMAN, T. N., and KRIMMER, B. M.: The treatment of conical cornea—introduction of a new multicurve fluidless corneal contact lens. Arch. Ophth., *54*(2):481–488, 1955.

117. FRANCESCHETTI, A.: Keratoconus, in *The Cornea World Congress,* King, J. H., and McTigue, J. W. (eds.). Washington, D. C., Butterworth, pp. 152–168, 1965.
118. FREEMAN, E.: Pinhole contact lenses. Am. J. Optom., *29*(7):347–352, 1952.
119. FILDERMAN, I. P.: The telecon lens for the partially sighted. Am. J. Optom. and Arch. Am. Acad. Optom., *36*(3):135–136, 1959.
120. FILDERMAN, I. P.: Telecon lens system, a modified Galilean telescope. Contacto, *3*(4):94–96, 1959.
121. FILDERMAN, I. P.: Clinical procedure for adapting the telecon lens. J. Am. Optom. Assn., *30*(8):561–562, 1959.
122. FILDERMAN, I. P.: Spectacle lens—contact lens system. Southern J. Optom., *4*(6):5–7, 10 and 30, 1962.
123. FILDERMAN, I. P.: The spectacle lens—contact lens system. Brit. J. Phys. Opt., *21*(4):195–196, 1964.
124. ISEN, A. A.: Feinbloom miniscope contact lens. Encyclopedia Contact Lens Practice, *3*(13):53–55, 1961.
125. JESSEN, G. N.: Re-evaluation of scleral contact lens fitting. Contacto, *7*(8):5–8, 1963.
126. LUDLAM, W. M.: Clinical experience with the contact lens telescope. Am. J. Optom. and Arch. Am. Acad. Optom., *37*(7):363–372, 1960.
127. ABEL, P.: The aphakic patient in traffic. Optom. Weekly, *54*(35):1647, 1963.
128. WELSH, R. C.: Experimental simulation of aphakia. Brit. J. Ophth., *49*(2):84–86, 1965.
129. COWAN, A.: Monocular aphakia. Arch. Ophth., *50*(1):16–18, 1953.
130. ROSENBLOOM, A. A.: The correction of unilateral aphakia with corneal contact lenses. Am. J. Optom. and Arch. Am. Acad. Optom., *30*(10):536–542, 1953.
131. GOAR, E. L.: The management of monocular cataracts. Arch. Ophth., *54*(1): 73–76, 1955.
132. OGLE, K. N., BURIAN, H. M., and BANNON, R. E.: On the correction of unilateral aphakia with contact lenses. Arch. Ophth., *59*(5):639–652, 1958.
133. DYER, J. A., and OGLE, K. N.: Correction of unilateral aphakia with contact lenses. Am. J. Ophth., *50*(1):11–17, 1960.
134. SPAETH, P. G., and O'NEILL, P. M.: Functional results with contact lenses in unilateral congenital cataracts, high myopia, and traumatic cataracts. Am. J. Ophth., *49*(3):548–554, 1960.
135. WELSH, R. C.: The roving ring scotoma: with its jack-in-the-box phenomenon of strong-plus (aphakic) spectacle lenses. Am. J. Ophth., *51*(6):1277–1281, 1961.
136. BALDWIN, W. R.: Cataract surgical procedures and contact lenses. J. Am. Optom. Assn., *33*(8):583–584, 1962.
137. THOMAS, R. L.: When to fit the contact lens after cataract surgery. Contacto, *1*(4):64–67, 1957.
138. WELSH, R. C.: Contact lenses for aphakics. Arch. Ophth., *64*(2):251–253, 1960.
139. ISEN, A. A.: Fitting contact lenses on aphakic patients. Encyclopedia Contact Lens Practice, *1*(5):3–12, chapter 16, 1960.
140. ALPEREN, S. E.: Contact lens fitting for aphakia. J. Am. Optom. Assn., *31*(8): 617–620, 1960.
141. NEILL, J. C.: Contact lenses and aphakia. Am. J. Optom. and Arch. Am. Acad. Optom., *39*(4):169–187, 1962.
142. ULLEN, R. L.: Fitting corneal lenses to aphakics—advantages and problems. Opt. J. and Rev. Optom., *100*(4):37–40 and 46, 1963.
143. BAILEY, N. J.: Special contact lenses and their application. Part I. Bifocal design. Opt. J. and Rev. Optom., *96*(24):41–50, 1959.

144. FILDERMAN, I. P.: Contact lens practice—a new perspective. Southern J. Optom., *6*(4):10–15, 1964.
145. HAYNES, P. R.: The fitting of bifocal contact lenses. Encyclopedia Contact Lens Practice, *2*(7):1–42, chapter 31, 1960.
146. EWELL, D. G.: Bifocal contact lenses. Contacto, *5*(4):147–153, 1961.
147. BALDWIN, W.: The application of bifocal contact lenses to thirty presbyopes. Optom. Weekly, *55*(26):23–27, 1964.
148. GENEVAY, N. C., Jr.: Paraseg K inside segment bifocal contact lens. Optom. Weekly, *52*(11):515–516, 1961.
149. GENEVAY, N. C., Jr.: Paraseg K inside segment bifocal contact lens. Encyclopedia Contact Lens Practice, *2*(11):49–51, recent developments section, 1961.
150. GREEN, M.: Preliminary report on a new bifocal contact lens. Contacto, *5*(3): 83–89, 1961.
151. BREGER, J. L.: Contact lenses for the presbyope. Optom. Weekly, *55*(22):22–24, 1964.
152. HAYNES, P. R.: The McKay Taylor additive bifocal—a new experimental bifocal contact lens system. Encyclopedia Contact Lens Practice, *3*(18):102–105, recent developments section, 1962.
153. AKIYAMA, K.: Study of contact lenses for presbyopia. Contacto, *4*(5):149–152, 1960.
154. AKIYAMA, K.: The general study of rectangular bifocal contact lenses. Contacto, *4*(10):461–467, 1960.
155. AKIYAMA, K.: Rectangular bifocal contact lenses—clinical application. Contacto, *5*(11):349–353, 1961.
156. WESLEY, N. K., and JESSEN, G. N.: The Sphercon bifocal contact lens. Optom. Weekly, *49*(13):583–585, 1958.
157. DE CARLE, J.: De Carle bifocal contact lens. Contacto, *3*(1):5–9, 1959.
158. DE CARLE, J.: Further developments of bifocal contact lenses. Contacto, *4*(6): 185–193, 1960.
159. COLLINS, I. W.: Preliminary report: a bifocal lens. J. Am. Optom. Assn., *29*(7): 453–454, 1958.
160. MOSS, H. I.: The bi-profile corneal lens. Optom. Weekly, *54*(18):801–805, 1963.
161. ARNER, R. S.: A fitting procedure for the Moss-Arner bifocal contact lens. Am. J. Optom. and Arch. Am. Acad. Optom., *42*(8):464–472, 1965.
162. MOSS, H. I.: The Moss-Arner bifocal contact lens. J. Am. Optom. Assn., *37*(3): 252–253, 1966.
163. ST. PALLEY, S. L.: The "Polivision" multifocal lens—theory and design. Opt. J. and Rev. Optom., *96*(7):40–42, 1959.
164. SOEHNGES, W. P.: Multifocal micro pupil lens. Contacto, *6*(6):156–159 and 170–171, 1962.
165. BAILEY, N. J.: Special contact lenses and their application. Part I. A brief resume of pinhole contact lenses. Opt. J. and Rev. Optom., *97*(1):32–33, 1960.
166. ARNER, R. S.: A simplified design for the Moss bifocal contact lens. Am. J. Optom. and Arch. Am. Acad. Optom., *40*(10):629–635, 1963.
167. BAILEY, N. J.: Inspection of a contact lens with a stereomicroscope. Optom. Weekly, *50*(47):2317–2319, 1959.
168. BAILEY, N. J.: The examination and verification of a contact lens. J. Am. Optom. Assn., *30*(8):557–560, 1959.
169. HAYNES, P. R.: Quality control and inspection of contact lenses. Encyclopedia Contact Lens Practice, *1*(6):1–64, chapter 23, 1960.
170. HUANG, D. T.: Technique of contact lens inspection. Optom. Weekly, *52*(10): 459–464, 1961.

171. BAILEY, N. J.: The refractive power of a contact lens. Optom. Weekly, *51*(21): 1071–1074, 1960.
172. SARVER, M. D.: Verification of contact lens power. J. Am. Optom. Assn., *34*(16): 1304–1306, 1963.
173. KORB, D. R.: Recent developments in edge contours and edge thickness with specific reference to measurement with an edge thickness gauge. Encyclopedia Contact Lens Practice, *3*(16):77–87, recent developments section, 1962.
174. FIELD, K. K.: Lensometer contact lens inspection. Opt. J. and Rev. Optom., *99*(2):41–44, 1962.
175. LANGSEN, A. L.: Contact lens lensometer inspection. Optom. Weekly, *52*(19): 923–924, 1961.
176. WILHELM, A. C., and WILHELM, R. F.: Lensometer technique for contact lens inspection. Optom. Weekly, *52*(42):2120–2121, 1961.
177. TAJIRI, A.: Impression technique to determine edge contour of contact lenses. Contacto, *4*(9):391–397, 1960.
178. SARVER, M. D., and KERR, K.: A radius of curvature measuring device for contact lenses. Am. J. Optom. and Arch. Am. Acad. Optom., *41*(8):481–489, 1964.
179. WEST, D. C.: A preliminary report on a comparative study of two methods for evaluating the contact lens ocular zone radius. J. Am. Optom. Assn., *35*(12):1065–1066, 1964.
180. BREZEL, D.: An instrument for measuring the base curve of contact lenses. J. Am. Optom. Assn., *31*(5):379–380, 1959.
181. LAYCOCK, D.: A microlens measuring aid. Am. J. Optom. and Arch. Am. Acad. Optom., *34*(10):538–539, 1957.
182. BRUNGARDT, T.: A fast, accurate, and practical measurement of the secondary curve radius. J. Am. Optom. Assn., *34*(2):131–134, 1962.
183. BAYSHORE, C. A.: Secondary radius measurements and toric fitting. J. Am. Optom. Assn., *36*(3):224–226, 1965.
184. HAYNES, P. R.: Modification of contact lenses. Encyclopedia Contact Lens Practice, *1*(2):3–76, chapter 22, 1960.
185. HAYNES, P. R.: Comments on the fabrication of peripheral curves. Encyclopedia Contact Lens Practice, *2*(8):77–80, chapter 22, 1961.
186. ISEN, A. A.: *Supplementary Instruction Bulletin I, Contac-nique Unit.* Buffalo, N. Y., Frontier Contact Lens Co., 1959.
187. ISEN, A. A.: *Instructions for Contac-nique No. 2, New Edging System.* Buffalo, N. Y., Frontier Contact Lens Co., 1961.
188. CEPERO, G.: Conical and concentrical polishing. Contacto, *3*(2):28–34, 1959.
189. SOPER, J. W., and GIRARD, L. J.: Modification of the semi-finished corneal contact lens, in *Corneal Contact Lenses.* Saint Louis, C. V. Mosby Co., pp. 169–197, 1964.
190. MARANO, J. A.: Office procedure for adding plus and minus power to contact lenses. Optom. Weekly, *52*(36):1735–1737, 1961.
191. BAGNELL, B. L.: Initial insertion of lenses on the new patient. Contacto, *5*(11): 367–373, 1961.
192. FAGEDES, H. E.: Insertion, removal, and recentering of corneal contact lenses. Optom. Weekly, *52*(24):1199–1205, 1961.
193. PARTIN, R.: A clinical procedure for contact lens assistants. Opt. J. and Rev. Optom., *100*(3):27–30, 1963.
194. RICHARDSON, E.: Instruction of patients in their care of their contact lenses. Optom. Weekly, *56*(22):26–27, 1965.
195. PLAYER, H. S.: Instruction and training of the contact lens patient. J. Am. Optom. Assn., *35*(4):344–353, 1965.

196. BRUCKER, D., and MALIN, A. H.: How to prepare contact lenses for use on the eye. Am. J. Optom. and Arch. Am. Acad. Optom., *38*(5):265–268, 1961.
197. VODNOY, B. E.: Contact lens cleanliness and proper patient control—a grave responsibility. Optom. Weekly, *56*(27):23–26, 1965.
198. HALL, N. C., and KREZANOSKI, J. Z.: Microbiological aspects of contact lens wear. Encyclopedia Contact Lens Practice, *4*(20):27–31, chapter 30, 1963.
199. FILDERMAN, I. P.: The pharmacist and the contact lens patient. Opt. J. and Rev. Optom., *101*(11):28–29, 1964.
200. SZEKELEY, I. J., and KREZANOSKI, J. Z.: Hygienic contact lens care and patient comfort. Am. J. Optom. and Arch. Am. Acad. Optom., *37*(11):572–579, 1960.
201. CLIFTON, C. E., and HALL, N. C.: Re-sterilizing activity of certain contact lens solutions. Contacto, *3*(10):301–302, 1959.
202. HAMMER, M. E., and WATKINS, C. E.: The formulation and evalution of contact lens solutions. Contacto, *6*(4):95–98, 1962.
203. JIMISON, R. E.: Compatibility of contact lens solutions. Opt. J. and Rev. Optom., *102*(11):46–52, 1965.
204. RANKIN, B. F.: Contact lens solutions—a pharmacist's approach. Optom. Weekly, *52*(21):1019–1024, 1961.
205. RANKIN, B. F.: Suggested considerations for contact lens solutions. Contacto, *6*(5):137–139, 1962.
206. RANKIN, B. F.: An important consideration for contact lens solutions. Contacto, *6*(3):69–74, 1962.
207. RICHARDS, J. P.: Antibacterial properties of contact lens wetting and storage solutions. Brit. J. Phys. Opt., *21*(3):147–156, 1964.
208. SZEKELY, I. J.: Contact lens solutions. Optom. Weekly, *51*(33):1734–1735, 1960.
209. SZEKELY, I. J.: The eye, the contact lens, and the contact lens solution. Contacto, *6*(12):347–354 and 362, 1962.
210. SZEKELY, I. J., HIND, H. W., and KREZANOSKI, J. Z.: Accessory contact lens solutions. Encyclopedia Contact Lens Practice, *4*(20):13–26, 1963.
211. SZEKELY, I. J., KREZANOSKI, J. Z., and HIND, H. W.: Hygienic storage and handling of contact lenses. Encyclopedia Contact Lens Practice, *4*(22):43–50, chapter 30, 1963.
212. SZEKELY, I. J., and RIEGELMAN, S.: Corneal lens storage: a critical appraisal. Brit. J. Phys. Opt., *21*(4):239–249, 1964.
213. HIND, H. W., and SZEKELY, I. J.: Wetting and hydration of contact lenses. Contacto, *3*(3):65–68, 1959.
214. HIND, H. W., SZEKELY, I. J., and KREZANOSKI, J. Z.: Contact lens wetting and comfort. Encyclopedia Contact Lens Practice, *4*(21):32–42, chapter 30, 1963.
215. KREZANOSKI, J. Z.: What is wetting? Contacto, *7*(4):20–22, 1963.
216. SZEKELY, I. J., and HIND, H. W.: Treated polyvinyl alcohol for contact lens solution. United States patent 3,183,152, 1965.
217. ALLEN, H. F.: To wet or not to wet. Arch. Ophth., *67*(2):119–120, 1963.
218. KAPETANSKY, F. M., SUIE, T., GRACY, A. D., and BITONTE, J. L.: Contact lens bacteriology. Am. J. Ophth., *57*(2):255–258, 1964.
219. OBEAR, M. F., and WINTER, F. C.: Contact lens storage. Am. J. Ophth., *57*(3):441–443, 1964.
220. BAILEY, N. J.: Contact lenses must be kept wet. J. Am. Optom. Assn., *31*(12):985, 1960.
221. BAILEY, N. J.: Contact lens storage: a bacteriological study. Am. J. Optom. and Arch. Am. Acad. Optom., *43*(4):244–248, 1966.
222. HALL, N. C., and KREZANOSKI, J. Z.: Antimicrobial synergism in a contact lens soaking solution. New Eng. J. Optom., *14*(9):229–233, 1963.

223. BETTMAN, J. W.: Contact lens storage, wet or dry? Am. J. Ophth., *56*(1):77–84, 1963.
224. DABEZIES, O. H.: Storage of contact lenses. Am. J. Ophth., *59*(4):684–696, 1965.
225. SHPRITZ, M. H.: Problems associated with cleaning and hydration of contact lenses. Optom. Weekly, *52*(20):973–975, 1961.
226. HIND, H. W., and SZEKELY, I. J.: Scleral contact lens solutions. Encyclopedia Contact Lens Practice, *3*(17):5–11, chapter 30, 1962.
227. KOETTING, R. A., and MUELLER, R. C.: A routine for examination of contact lens patients. Am. J. Optom. and Arch. Am. Acad. Optom., *38*(4):211–220, 1961.
228. HAYNES, P. R.: The physical and physiological basis of edge reflections and marginal confusion with clinical comments on their correction. Encyclopedia Contact Lens Practice, *1*(5):6–12, chapter 25, 1960.
229. FARNUM, F. E.: Causes and correction of light dispersion. Contacto, *3*(10):298–300, 1959.
230. BLACK, C. J.: Corneal staining. Contacto, *1*(1):3–6, 1957.
231. ACKERLY, E.: Effects of contact lenses on the cornea. Contacto, *3*(6):145–152, 1959.
232. DICK, R. B.: The incidence and classification of corneal lesions in beginning contact lens wearers. J. Am. Optom. Assn., *33*(3):219–221, 1961.
233. MISAGE, R. J.: Changes in corneal curvature with contact lens wear. J. Am. Optom. Assn., *33*(8):590–592, 1962.
234. DIXON, J. M., and LAWACZECK, E.: Corneal dimples and bubbles under corneal contact lenses. Am. J. Ophth., *54*(5):827–831, 1962.
235. DIXON, J. M.: Ocular changes due to contact lenses. Am. J. Ophth., *58*(3):424–441, 1964.
236. KEMMETMULLER, H.: Medical effects on the eye from wearing contact lenses. Contacto, *8*(3):40–49, 1964.
237. MORRISON, R. J., KAUFMAN, K. J., and CERULLI, E.: Effect of contact lenses on the cornea after various periods of wear. Am. J. Optom. and Arch. Am. Acad. Optom., *41*(11):688–690, 1964.
238. PRATT-JOHNSON, J., and WARNER, D.: Corneal curvature changes. Am. J. Ophth., *60*(5):852–855, 1965.
239. RENGSTROFF, R. H.: The Fort Dix report—a longitudinal study of the effects of contact lenses. Am. J. Optom. and Arch. Am. Acad. Optom., *42*(3):153–163, 1965.
240. KORB, D. R.: Corneal transparency with emphasis on the phenomenon of central circular clouding. Encyclopedia Contact Lens Practice, *4*(20):106–115, recent developments section, 1963.
241. BRONSTEIN, L.: Symptomatology of corneal type lenses. Contacto, *1*(2):31–35, 1957.
242. POSTER, M.: Symptomatology as related to the structural nature of a contact lens. Contacto, *4*(10):477–479, 1960.
243. FIRESTONE, L. E.: Contact lens problems and practical corrective techniques. Contacto, *5*(6):207–216, 1961.
244. DE LAMATER, F.: Mucus control in contact lens practice. Optom. Weekly, *53*(47):2315–2316, 1962.
245. STEWART, C. R.: Blinking and corneal lenses. J. Am. Optom. Assn., *37*(3):243–247, 1966.
246. GROSVENOR, T. P.: The relationship between contact lenses and visual training. J. Am. Optom. Assn., *32*(8):621–624, 1961.

247. ROSENWASSER, H.: Contact lenses: diagnosis and adjustment of lid sensitivity problems. Opt. J. and Rev. Optom., *97*(4):62–64, 1960.
248. DICKINSON, F.: Heat, sunglare, and dust are factors in contact lens fitting in South Africa. Am. J. Optom. and Arch. Am. Acad. Optom., *37*(4):201–209, 1960.
249. FILDERMAN, I. P., and WHITE, P. F.: Psychological, human relations and practice management aspects of contact lens care. Part II. J. Am. Optom. Assn., *36*(7):637–643, 1965.
250. MOSS, H. I.: The practical aspects of contact lens practice. J. Am. Optom. Assn., *27*(9):510–513, 1956.
251. MOSS, H. L.: Contact lens records, forms, and routine. J. Am. Optom. Assn., *30*(8):563–566, 1959.
252. ABRAMS, B. S.: Contact lenses and office management. Optom. Weekly, *51*(2): 67–70, 1960.
253. MASTEN, G. W.: Practice management in contact lens practice. J. Am. Optom. Assn., *31*(8):630–632, 1960.
254. SILBERT, M.: Problems of patient management and control with contact lenses. Optom. Weekly, *52*(26):1287–1291, 1961.
255. ELMSTROM, G. P.: Contact lens practice management. Contacto, *5*(1):27–28, 1961.
256. SCHWARTZ, A.: Corneal contact lens insurance, Lowell Glatt (ed.). Opt. J. and Rev. Optom., *95*(17):31–33, 1958.
257. ELMSTROM, G. P.: Trends in contact lens insurance. Optom. Weekly, *51*(26): 1350–1351, 1960.
258. GLATT, L. D.: Contact lens insurance—an objective view. Opt. J. and Rev. Optom., *98*(12):39–45, 1961.
259. BAILEY, N. J.: Possible factors in the control of myopia with contact lenses. Contacto, *2*(5):114–117, 1958.
260. ELMSTROM, G. P., and KOHN, H.: *Synopsis of the Legal Aspects of Contact Lens Practice for Optometrists.* Minneapolis, Minn., Burgess Publishing Co., 1964.
261. ELMSTROM, G. P.: The legal aspects of contact lens practice. J. Am. Optom. Assn., *35*(9):775–777, 1964.
262. ULLEN, R. L.: Legal implications in fitting contact lenses. J. Am. Optom. Assn., *33*(4):288–291, 1961.
263. BRAFF, S. M.: Scleral lenses in contact lens practice. Am. J. Optom. and Arch. Am. Acad. Optom., *39*(4):195–202, 1962.
264. BRAFF, S. M.: History of scleral contact lenses. Encyclopedia Contact Lens Practice, *3*(17):3–10, chapter 34, 1962.
265. BRAFF, S. M.: The design and development of scleral contact lenses. J. Am. Optom. Assn., *36*(3):217–223, 1965.
266. McKELLEN, G. D.: The fitting of the transcurve lens. Encyclopedia Contact Lens Practice, *4*(19):23–32, chapter 40, 1962.
267. BRAFF, S. M.: The wide angle contact lens. Encyclopedia Contact Lens Practice, *4*(22):53–58, chapter 40, 1963.
268. FORKNALL, A. J.: Some notes on haptic lenses. Brit. J. Phys. Opt., *16*(2):96–115, 1959.
269. FORKNALL, A. J., and McKELLEN, G. D.: Long tolerances with haptic lenses. Encyclopedia Contact Lens Practice, *4*(19):1–22, chapter 40, 1962.
270. BRAFF, S. M.: Eye impressions without anesthesia. Encyclopedia Contact Lens Practice, *4*(19):45–46, chapter 40, 1962.
271. RIDLEY, F. K.: Scleral contact lenses. Arch. Ophth., *70*(6):740–745, 1963.
272. JENKIN, L.: Fitting haptic lenses by impression technique. Brit. J. Phys. Opt., *21*(3):163–168, 1964.

273. FLETCHER, R. J.: The haptic contact lens prescription. J. Am. Optom. Assn., *36*(3):227–230, 1965.
274. STONE, J.: Checking preformed contact lenses. Brit. J. Phys. Opt., *21*(4):264–286, 1964.
275. SALVATORI, P. L.: Modifications to scleral lenses. Encyclopedia Contact Lens Practice, *4*(19):47–52, chapter 40, 1962.
276. NIERENBERG, B. L.: Some applications of contact lens prostheses. Opt. J. and Rev. Optom., *91*(20):37–41, 1954.
277. HALL, K. C.: A special contact lens for complete ptosis. J. Am. Optom. Assn., *30*(2):121–123, 1958.
278. KOETTING, R. A.: The ocular prosthesis in optometric practice. Optom. Weekly, *56*(45):26–28, 1965.
279. NEILL, J. C.: The cosmetic contact lens—a case report. Am. J. Optom. and Arch. Am. Acad. Optom., *27*(7):329–332, 1950.
280. BIER, N.: Contact lenses and ocular disfigurement. Optom. Weekly, *47*(45):2016–2017, 1956.
281. SALVATORI, P. L.: Cosmetic contact lenses. Contacto, *1*(4):79–80, 1957.
282. POLICOFF, W. W.: Cosmetic contact lenses. Contacto, *6*(3):65–67, 1962.
283. BALL, G. V.: Characteristics of tinted contact lenses. Brit. J. Phys. Opt., *21*(4): 219–223, 1964.
284. KLEYHAUER, A. D.: Tinted contact lenses: equivalent light absorption of spectacle lenses. J. Am. Optom. Assn., *35*(6):487–488, 1964.
285. RICHARDS, O. W., and GROLMAN, B.: Avoid tinted contact lenses when driving at night. J. Am. Optom. Assn., *34*(1):53–55, 1962.
286. MAZOW, B.: Slit-lamp biomicroscopy in contact lens fitting. J. Am. Optom. Assn., *29*(7):447–449, 1958.
287. LESTER, R. W.: The use of the biomicroscope in contact lens fitting. Optom. Weekly, *50*(46):2261–2270, 1959.
288. GOODLAW, E. I.: Bio-microscope in contact lens work. Contacto, *3*(4):81–92, 1959.
289. NEILL, J. C.: Slit lamp diagnosis and procedures in contact lens practice. Am. J. Optom. and Arch. Am. Acad. Optom., *37*(6):273–294, 1960.
290. HAYNES, P. R.: Tracer systems for evaluating the flow and drainage of precorneal fluid in the retrolens space. Encyclopedia Contact Lens Practice, *2*(11): 45–48, recent developments section, 1961.
291. KORB, D. R.: Recent developments in the observation of the cornea-lens relationship. Encyclopedia Contact Lens Practice, *3*(18):98–101, recent developments section, 1962.
292. HAYNES, P. R.: Techniques for evaluating the attack of the upper eyelid on a contact lens. Encyclopedia Contact Lens Practice, *3*(15):72–74, recent developments section, 1962.
293. RUBIN, L.: A modification for radius charts used with the keratometer. Contacto, *6*(1):25, 1962.
294. ISEN, A. A.: Methods that help achieve accurate ophthalmometry. J. Am. Optom. Assn., *30*(10):723–724, 1959.
295. SHICK, C. R.: A simple mire modification to improve keratometer efficiency. J. Am. Optom. Assn., *34*(5):388–390, 1962.
296. SMITH, J. H.: A technique to improve the accuracy of ophthalmometer readings. J. Am. Optom. Assn., *34*(16):1312, 1963.
297. RUBIN, L.: Extending the range of the ophthalmometer and keratometer. Opt. J. and Rev. Optom., *98*(8):41–42, 1961.
298. GIRARD, L. J., SOPER, J. W., and SAMPSON, W. G.: *Corneal Contact Lenses.* Saint Louis, C. V. Mosby Co., 1964.

299. FILDERMAN, I. P., and White, P. F.: Contact lens optics—applied clinical aspects. Southern J. Optom., *7*(4):10–13, 16, and 28–31, 1965.

300. FILDERMAN, I. P., and WHITE, P. F.: Contact lens optics—applied clinical aspects. Southern J. Optom., *7*(5):12–17 and 26, 1965.

301. FILDERMAN, I. P., and WHITE, P. F.: Contact lens optics—applied clinical aspects. Southern J. Optom., *7*(6):13–17, 1965.

302. FILDERMAN, I. P., and WHITE, P. F.: Contact lens optics—applied clinical aspects. Southern J. Optom., *7*(7):7–11 and 18–19, 1965.

303. HAYNES, P. R.: Optics of contact lenses—introduction. Encyclopedia Contact Lens Practice, *1*(1):2–6, chapter 14, 1959.

304. SARVER, M. D.: Fluid lens power effect with contact lenses. Am. J. Optom. and Arch. Am. Acad. Optom., *39*(8):434–437, 1962.

305. SARVER, M. D.: Calculation of the optical specifications of contact lenses. Am. J. Optom. and Arch. Am. Acad. Optom., *40*(1):20–28, 1963.

306. BRAFF, S. M.: Power determination for contact lenses. Encyclopedia Contact Lens Practice, *2*(9):27–29, chapter 32, 1961.

307. MANDELL, R. B.: A simplified method to calculate front surface radius of contact lenses. Am. J. Optom. and Arch. Am. Acad. Optom., *41*(2):102–105, 1964.

308. ARNER, R. S., and BRAFF, S. M.: A simplified computation of the curve of a contact lens. *35*(9):773–774, 1964.

309. SCHAPERO, M.: Optics of contact lenses—bitoric corneal lenses. Encyclopedia Contact Lens Practice, *3*(17):7–19, chapter 14, 1962.

310. KOETTING, J. F.: Optical considerations in fitting toroidal back surface lenses; and the management of residual astigmatism. Contacto, *9*(1):14–22 and 27, 1965.

311. BOEDER, P.: Power and magnification properties of contact lenses. Arch. Ophth., *19*(1):54–67, 1938.

312. ALPERN, M.: Further comment on accommodation and convergence with contact lenses. Am. J. Optom. and Arch. Am. Acad. Optom., *27*(5):238–241, 1950.

313. TOCHER, R.: Astigmatism due to the tilt of a contact lens. Am. J. Optom. and Arch. Am. Acad. Optom., *39*(1):3–16, 1962.

314. SARVER, M. D.: The effect of contact lens tilt upon residual astigmatism. Am. J. Optom. and Arch. Am. Acad. Optom., *40*(12):730–744, 1963.

315. LUDLAM, W. M., and WITTENBERG, S.: Measurements of the ocular dioptric elements utilizing photographic methods. Part II. Cornea—theoretical considerations. Am. J. Optom. and Arch. Am. Acad. Optom., *43*(4):249–267, 1966.

316. MANDELL, R. B.: Keratopography. Encyclopedia Contact Lens Practice, *3*(18): 12–51, chapter 7, 1962.

317. KNOLL, H. A.: Corneal contours in the general population as revealed by the photokeratoscope. Am. J. Optom. and Arch. Am. Acad. Optom., *38*(7):389–397, 1961.

318. REYNOLDS, A. E.: Corneal topography as found by photo-electronic keratoscopy. Contacto, *3*(8):229–233, 1959.

319. RZYMKOWSKY, J.: Stereophotographic and stereophotogrametric reproduction of the cornea and sclera of the living eye. Am. J. Optom. and Arch. Am. Acad. Optom., *31*(8):416–422, 1954.

320. BONNETT, R., and COCHET, P.: New method of topographical ophthalmometry—its theoretical and clinical application. Am. J. Optom. and Arch. Am. Acad. Optom., *39*(5):227–251, 1962.

321. KAYES, J., and HELMBERG, A.: The fine structure of Bowman's layer and the basement membrane of the corneal epithelium. Am. J. Ophth., *50*(5-part 2): 1013–1021, 1960.

322. KRAUSE, A. C.: Biochemistry of the eye. Arch. Ophth., *15*(3):522–543, 1936.

323. ADLER, F. H.: *Physiology of the Eye—Clinical Application,* 3d Ed. St. Louis, C. V. Mosby Co., pp. 48–52, 1959.
324. HEALD, K., and LANGHAM, M. E.: Permeability of the cornea and the blood–aqueous barrier to oxygen. Brit. J. Ophth., *40*(12):705–720, 1956.
325. LAST, R. J.: *Wolff's Anatomy of the Eye and Orbit,* 5th Ed. Philadelphia, W. B. Saunders Co., p. 34, 1961.
326. WEEKERS, R.: Biochemistry of the normal and abnormal cornea. Ophthalmologica, *100:*136–149, 1940.
327. KOHRA, T.: On the metabolism of the cornea. Acta Societatis Ophthalmologicae Japonicae, *40:*1595, 1936.
328. HERRMANN, H., and MOSES, S. G.: Content and state of glutathione in the tissues of the eye, J. Biolog. Chem., *158:*33–45, 1945.
329. LEINFELDER, P. J.: Aerobic glycolysis of corneal tissue. Trans. Am. Ophth. Soc., *46:*412–422, 1948.
330. LAST, R. J.: *Wolff's Anatomy of the Eye and Orbit,* 5th Ed. Philadelphia, W. B. Saunders Co., 1961.
331. ADLER, F. H.: *Physiology of the Eye—Clinical Application,* 3d Ed. St. Louis, C. V. Mosby Co., p. 66, 1959.
332. CASPERSON, T., and ENGSTROM, A.: The transparency of corneal tissues. Nordisk Medicin, *30:*1279, 1946.
333. MAURICE, D. M.: The structure and transparency of the cornea. J. Phys., *136*(2): 263–286, 1957.
334. VAN WALBECK, K., and HEUMANN, H.: Studies of corneal transparency under various experimental conditions. Arch. Ophth., *46*(5):482–487, 1951.
335. KRAUSE, A. C.: The chemical constitution of the cornea. Am. J. Ophth., *15*(5): 422–424, 1932.
336. ADLER, F. H.: *Physiology of the Eye—Clinical Application,* 3d Ed. St. Louis, C. V. Mosby Co., p. 47, 1959.
337. ADLER, F. H.: *Physiology of the Eye—Clinical Application,* 3d Ed. St. Louis, C. V. Mosby Co., p. 45, 1959.
338. BERLINER, M. L.: *Biomicroscopy of the Eye,* Vol. 1, Rev. Ed. New York, Paul B. Hoeber, Inc., p. 393, 1949.
339. THOMAS, C. I.: *The Cornea.* Springfield, Ill., Charles C. Thomas, p. 118, 1955.
340. ADLER, F. H: *Physiology of the Eye—Clinical Application,* 3d Ed. St. Louis, C. V. Mosby Co., p. 83, 1959.
341. HAMANO, H.: Topical and systemic influences of wearing contact lenses. Contacto, *4*(2):41–48, 1960.
342. ADLER, F. H.: *Physiology of the Eye—Clinical Application,* 3d Ed. St. Louis, C. V. Mosby Co., p. 79, 1959.
343. LEBENSOHN, J. E.: The nature of photophobia. Arch. Ophth., *12*(3):380–390, 1934.
344. LAST, R. J.: *Wolff's Anatomy of the Eye and Orbit,* 5th Ed. Philadelphia, W. B. Saunders Co., pp. 33–41, 1961.
345. VOTOCKOVA, J., OBENBERGER, J., and PRAUS, R.: Study of the biochemical activity of the cornea in longer time intervals after elimination of the precorneal vascular plexus (in Czech). Ceskoslovenska Ophthalmol., *16:*316–328, 1960. (Abstract Ophthalmic Literature, *14:*269, 1960.)
346. POTTS, A. M., COHEN, B., and GOODMAN, D.: Corneal water transport as measured with tritiated water. Am. J. Ophth., *47*(1-part 2):419–426, 1959.
347. MAURICE, D. M.: The movement of fluorescein and water in the cornea. Am. J. Ophth., *49*(5-part 1):1011–1016, 1960.
348. ADLER, F. H.: *Physiology of the Eye—Clinical Application,* 3d Ed. St. Louis, C. V. Mosby Co., p. 48, 1959.

349. ADLER, F. H.: *Physiology of the Eye—Clinical Application,* 3d Ed. St. Louis, C. V. Mosby Co., p. 51, 1959.
350. SIMPSON, G. V.: Corneal edema. Trans. Am. Ophth. Soc., *47*:692–737, 1949.
351. ADLER, F. H.: *Physiology of the Eye—Clinical Application,* 3d Ed. St. Louis, C. V. Mosby Co., p. 52, 1959.
352. POTTS, A. M., GOODMAN, D., and JOHNSON, L. V.: The nutritional supply of corneal regions in experimental animals. Part III. Further studies on the corneal transport of inorganic ions. Am. J. Ophth., *38*(1-part 2):174–181, 1954.
353. COGAN, D. G., and KINSEY, V. E.: Physiologic studies on the cornea. Science, *95*:607–608, 1942.
354. SWAN, K. C., and WHITE, N. G.: Corneal permeability. Part I. Factors affecting penetration of drugs into the cornea. Am. J. Ophth., *25*(9):1043–1058, 1942.
355. COGAN, D. G., HIRSCH, E. O., and KINSEY, V. E.: The cornea. Part VI. Permeability characteristics of the excised cornea. Arch. Ophth., *31*(5):408–412, 1944.
356. COGAN, D. G.: Applied anatomy and physiology of the cornea. Trans. Am. Acad. Ophth. and Otolaryng., *55*:329–359, 1951.
357. MARIN-AMAT, M.: Les variations physiologiques de la courbure de la cornée pendant la vie; leur importance et transcendance dans la refraction oculaire. Bulletin de la Société Belge d'Ophthalmol., No. 113:251–293, 1956.
358. THOMAS, C. I.: *The Cornea.* Springfield, Ill., Charles C. Thomas, p. 134, 1955.
359. AURELL, G., and HOLMGREN, H.: On the metachromatic staining of the corneal tissue and some observations on its transparency. Acta Ophthalmol., *31*(1): 1–27, 1953.
360. COGAN, D. G., and KINSEY, V. E.: The cornea. Part I. Transfer of water and sodium chloride by osmosis, and diffusion through the excised cornea. Arch. Ophth., *27*(3):466–476, 1942; Part II. Transfer of water and sodium chloride by hydrostatic pressure through the excised cornea. Arch. Ophth., *27*(4):696–704, 1942.
361. CHRISTENSEN, L.: Cornea and sclera; annual review. Arch. Ophth., *59*(2): 280–301, 1958. See p. 281.
362. BOCK, R. H., and MAUMENEE, A. E.: Corneal fluid metabolism; experiments and observations. Arch. Ophth., *50*(3):282–285, 1953.
363. HARRIS, J. E.: The physiologic control of corneal hydration. Am. J. Ophth., *44*(5-part 2):262–280, 1957.
364. DUKE-ELDER, S., and PERKINS, E. S. (eds.): *The Transparency of the Cornea; a Symposium.* Springfield, Ill., Charles C. Thomas, 1960.
365. MAURICE, D. M.: The structure and transparency of the cornea. J. Phys., *136*(2): 263–286, 1957.
366. AURELL, G., and HOLMGREN, H.: Metachromatic substance in cornea, with special reference to question of transparency. Nordisk Medicin, *30*:1277, 1946.
367. SMELSER, G. K., and OZANICS, V.: Importance of atmospheric oxygen for maintenance of the optical properties of the human cornea. Science, *115*:140, 1952.
368. ACKERLY, E.: Clinical physiology of the eye with contact lenses. Internat. Ophth. Clinics, *1*(2):311–325, 1961.
369. FRIEDENWALD, J. S., and BUSCHKE, W.: Mitotic and wound-healing activities of the corneal epithelium. Arch. Ophth., *32*(5):410–413, 1944.
370. FRIEDENWALD, J. S., and BUSCHKE, W.: The influence of some experimental variables on the epithelial movements in the healing of corneal wounds. J. Cellular and Comp. Phys., *23*:95–107, 1944.
371. THOMAS, C. I.: *The Cornea.* Springfield, Ill., Charles C. Thomas, p. 160, 1955.
372. BERLINER, M. L.: *Biomicroscopy of the Eye,* Vol. 1, Rev. Ed. New York, Paul B. Hoeber, p. 401, 1949.

373. COGAN, D. G.: Vascularization of the cornea. Trans. Am. Ophth. Soc., *46*:457–471, 1948.
374. GRAYSON, M., and BOLING, R.: Clinical application of contact lenses, in *Contact Lens Management,* Morgan Raiford (ed.). Boston, Little, Brown and Co., pp. 31–40, 1962.
375. HALE, J. R.: Contact lens application in four cases of congenital nystagmus. Optom. Weekly, *53*(37):1799–1803, 1962.
376. KENNEDY, J. R.: Contact lenses in complicated glaucoma. Am. J. Optom. and Arch. Am. Acad. Optom., *39*(7):369–373, 1962.
377. KOETTING, R. A.: The influence of oral contraceptives on contact lens wear. Am. J. Optom. and Arch. Am. Acad. Optom., *43*(4):268–274, 1966.
378. MARENCO, J. C., LIBERATORE, J. C., and VOSS, E. H.: Prognosis for adaptability to contact lenses. Contacto, *1*(3):51–58, 1957.
379. RAIFORD, M. B.: Examination for contact lenses, in *Contact Lens Management,* Morgan Raiford (ed.). Boston, Little, Brown and Co., pp. 41–54, 1962.
380. ROSENTHAL, J. W.: Clinical pathology in contact lenses, in *Contact Lens Management,* Morgan Raiford (ed.). Boston, Little, Brown and Co., pp. 221–236, 1962.
381. ROSENWASSER, H. M.: Effects of diuretics and tranquilizers on wearing contact lenses. Opt. J. and Rev. Optom., *100*(22):41–47, 1963.
382. Werner, D. L.: Lens difficulty in a patient with Bell's Palsy. Opt. J. and Rev. Optom., *99*(6):41–44, 1962.
383. WINKLER, C. H., and DIXON, J. M.: Bacteriology of the eye. Part III. A. Effect of contact lenses on the normal flora. B. Flora of the contact lens. Arch. Ophth., *72*(6):817–819, 1964.
384. *Parabolar Contact Lenses Fitting Manual.* West Hempstead, N. Y., Danker and Wohlk, 1962.
385. *Paraboloid Contact Lens Fitting Manual.* Raleigh, N. C., Paraboloid Contact Lens Laboratory, 1965.
386. FEINBLOOM, W.: Corneal contact lens having inner ellipsoidal surfaces. United States Patent 3,227,507, January 4, 1966.
387. ELLIOTT, D. O.: A preliminary report on use of gradient ellipsoidal curves related to fitting of contact lenses. Optom. Weekly, *55*(21):21–22, 1964.
388. NEEFE, C. W.: Corneal contact lens of wide fitting range with sine curve concave surface. United States Patent 3,187,338, June 1, 1965.
389. *Technique in the Fitting of Con-o-coid Corneal Contact Lenses.* Sarasota, Fla., Obrig Laboratories, 1967.
390. KAPLAN, M. M.: The aplanatic contact lens. Optom. Weekly, *58*(6):25–29, and *58*(7):42–45, 1967.
391. GONDIN, W. R., and SOHMER, B.: *Intermediate Algebra and Analytic Geometry Made Simple.* New York, Doubleday & Co., 1959.
392. GONDIN, W. R., and SOHMER, B.: *Advanced Algebra and Calculus Made Simple.* New York, Doubleday & Co., 1959.
393. GRANVILLE, W. A., SMITH, P. F., and LONGLEY, W. R.: *Elements of the Differential and Integral Calculus.* Boston, Ginn and Co., 1941.
394. VOLK, D.: Lens generating method. United States Patent 3,218,765, November 23, 1965.
395. VOLK, D.: Lens generating apparatus. United States Patent 3,267,617, August 23, 1966.
396. CHANDLER, C.: Personal communication, 1967.
397. SPEEN, G. B.: Optical apparatus for testing the accuracy of quadric surfaces. United States Patent 3,247,760, April 26, 1966.
398. EMSLEY, H. H.: *Aberrations of Thin Lenses—An Elementary Treatment for Technicians and Students.* London, Constable and Co., 1956.

399. ZOETHOUT, W. D.: *Physiological Optics,* 4th Ed., Chicago, The Professional Press, 1946.
400. DAVSON, H. (ed.): *The Eye,* New York, Academic Press, Vol. 4, 1962.
401. KAPLAN, M. M.: Personal communication, Mar. 1967.
402. KAPLAN, M. M.: A new theory of dynamic visual resolution and corneal accommodation. Optom. Weekly, *56*(37)–*56*(48), 1965.
403. ESTEVEZ, J. M. J., and RIDLEY, F.: Safety requirements for contact lenses—and their manipulation and use. Am. J. Ophth., *62*(1):132–139, 1966.
404. MEYERS, E. L.: The testing of and standards for plastics. *In Papers Presented at Second AOA Contact Lens Symposium,* St. Louis, American Optometric Association, 1966.
405. VAN ROGGEN, A.: Molecular structure and contact lenses. *In Papers Presented at Second AOA Contact Lens Symposium,* St. Louis, American Optometric Association, 1966.
406. CAPELLI, Q. A.: Water extractives from colored contact lenses—a report. Opt. J. and Rev. Optom., *103*(13):32–33, 1966.
407. CHALKLEY, T., SARNAT, L., and SHOCH, D.: Evaluation of "bacteriostatic" contact lenses, Am. J. Ophth., *61*(5-part I):866–869, 1966.
408. Ceskoslovenska Akademie Ved: A method of producing contact lenses. Great Britain Patent 990,207, Apr. 28, 1965.
409. Ceskoslovenska Akademie Ved: Contact lens. Great Britain Patent 1,004,424, Sept. 15, 1965.
410. WICHTERLE, O.: Process for producing shaped articles from three-dimensional hydrophilic high polymers. United States Patent 2,976,576, Mar. 28, 1961.
411. WICHTERLE, O.: A method of production of contact lenses. Commonwealth of Australia Patent 257,878, Nov. 1, 1962.
412. WICHTERLE, O.: Cross-linked hydrophilic polymers and articles made therefrom. United States Patent 3,220,960, Nov. 30, 1965.
413. WICHTERLE, O., and LIM, D.: Hydrophilic gels for biological use. Nature, *185*(4706): Jan. 9, 1960.
414. EWELL, D. G.: The current status of hydrophilic contact lens materials. Optom. Weekly, *56*(6):37–38, 1965.
415. JANACEK, J., and KOLARIK, J.: Structure and properties of hydrophilic polymers and their gels. III. Coll. Czech. Chem. Commun., 30, June 17, 1964.
416. BARES, J., and JANACEK, J.: Structure and properties of hydrophilic polymers and their gels. IV. Coll. Czech. Chem. Commun., June 17, 1964.
417. TAKAJASHI, G. H., GOLDSTICK, T. K., and FATT, I.: Physical properties of hydrophilic gel contact lenses. Brit. Med. Jour., p. 142, Jan. 1966.
418. TAKAJASHI, G. H., GOLDSTICK, T. K., and FATT, I.: Properties of hydrophilic lenses. The Optician, Feb. 11, 1966.
419. VON ROGGEN, A.: Molecular structure and contact lenses. Second AOA Contact Lens Symposium, St. Louis, Mo., 1966.
420. SEDLACEK, B.: A contribution to the study of optical properties of polymeric gels. Inst. of Mcrmclr. Chem., Prague, June 21, 1965.
421. KAPLAN, M. M.: Report of conference at the Inst. of Mcrmclr. Chem., Prague, to the Natl. Pat. Dev. Co., New York, Dec. 2–8, 1965.
422. GUMPELMAYER, T.: Stability of moulded micro-corneal lenses made from PMMA, in relation to water absorbtion of the material. Der Augenoptiker, *19*(11): 1964.
423. ISEN, A.: Course at the Am. Acad. of Optom., Chicago, Dec. 9, 1965.
424. ISEN, A.: Hydrophilic lenses. Paper presented in Buffalo, Apr. 17, 1966.
425. POLICOFF, W.: Hydrophilic lenses. Paper presented at the Am. Acad. of Optom., Chicago, Dec. 12, 1965.

426. MORRISON, R. J.: Hydrophilic contact lenses. Paper presented at the Am. Acad. of Optom., Chicago, Dec. 12, 1965.
427. KAPLAN, M. M.: Optical considerations of hydrophilic lenses. II. Hydration and dehydration. Optom. Weekly, *58*(21):25–29, 1967.
428. JANACEK, J., and KOLARIK, J.: Relaxation behavior of polymethacrylic acid esters swollen by low-molecular weight substances at temperatures below the glass transition point. Inst. of Mcrmlclr. Chem., Prague, Apr. 29, 1965.
429. HILL, R. M., and FATT, I.: How dependent is the cornea on the atmosphere? J. Am. Optom. Assn., *35*(10):873–876, 1964.
430. HILL, R. M., and FATT, I.: Oxygen deprivation of the cornea by contact lenses and lid closure. Am. J. Optom. and Arch. Am. Acad. Optom., *41*(11):678–687, 1964.
431. HILL, R. M., and VESPER, G.: Hydrophilic contact lenses. Precision Cosmet Digest, quoted by Policoff, W. in Ref. 425.
432. HILL, R. M., and FATT, I.: A contact lens from the cornea's point of view. Optom. Weekly, *56*(36):29–31, 1965.
433. JENKINS, L., and TYLER-JONES, R.: *Theory and Practice of Contact Lens Fitting.* London, The Hatton Press, 1964.
434. RYCROFT, B. W.: The new hydrophilic gel (soft) contact lens. Highlights of Ophth., *7*(4):252–253, 1964.
435. KELLY, T., BLACK, S., and BUTLER, D.: Preliminary report on corneal lenses in relation to myopia. Paper presented at the Cont. Lens Soc. Cong. held at Bath, Eng., May, 1964.
436. TURNER, R. A.: The appraisal of the problems of hydrophilic contact lenses. Aus. J. Optom., 41–46, Feb. 1965.
437. NEILL, J. C.: The gel lens. Paper presented at the Symp. of the Optom. Cntr. of N. Y., Apr. 1965.
438. Editorial: On hydrophilic lenses. Cont. Lens Soc. Conf., The Optician, *149*(3868): May 21, 1965.
439. NEILL, J. C.: An appraisal of "gel" contact lenses. The Optical World, July, 1965.
440. NEILL, J. C.: "Gel" contact lenses. Pa. Optom., July–Aug., 1965.
441. HART, R. S.: An interesting experience with hydrophilic contact lenses. The Optician, *150*(3886): Sept. 1965.
442. BLACKSTONE, D.: Hydrophilic gel lenses. The Optician, *150*(3889): Oct. 15, 1965.
443. GIRARD, L. J.: Interview to the press, reported by William Policoff, Ref. 425.
444. Editorial: Studies with hydrophilic lenses. The Optician, *150*(3892):453, Nov. 5, 1965.
445. BRAILSFORD, M. I.: Hydrophilic lenses. The Optician, *150*(3892):490, Nov. 12, 1965.
446. Editorial: Optometry round the world. Optom. Weekly, *56*(1): Dec. 23, 1965.
447. JENKINS, L.: Problems with hydrophilic contact lenses. Optom. Weekly, *56*(52): 113, Dec. 30, 1965.
448. BLACK, C.: Latest advances in contact lenses. Paper presented at the N. Y. Acad. of Med., Mar. 11, 1966.
449. MORRISON, R. J.: Hydrophilic contact lenses. J. Am. Optom. Assn., *37*(3):211–218, 1966.
450. MORRISON, R. J.: Preliminary report of hydrophilic gel contact lenses. First South African Intl. Cont. Lens Cong., Johannesburg, Sept. 6, 1965.
451. BLACKSTONE, M.: Hydrophilic lenses: some practical experiments. The Optician, *151*(3901):5, Jan. 1966.
452. SEDLACEK, J.: The correction of aphakia with hydrophilic contact lenses. OS. Oftal., *22*(1):76, 1966.

453. Editorial: Contact lenses get a softer touch. Business Week, p. 47, Apr. 30, 1966.
454. VESPER, G.: Refraction on the correction of aphakic persons with flexible corneal contact lenses, Surv. of Ophth., *11*(3):257–258, June, 1966.
455. FARNIK, L.: Czechoslovakia works on the new gel contact lenses. Mfg. Optician, pp. 161, 163, Aug. 1966.
456. NEILL, J. C.: The new gelatin contact lens and its clinical utility in contact lens practice. Southern J. Optom., *8*(5):15–17, 1966.
457. ULLEN, R.: Hydrophilic contact lenses—a critical analysis. Precision Cosmet Digest, Apr. 1965.
458. DREIFUS, M.: A new hydrogelic contact lens made from polyglycolmonomethacrylic acid. Der Augenoptiker, *19*(6): 1964.
459. KAPLAN, M. M.: Technical aspects of the hydrophilic lens. Paper presented at the third Ann. P. G. Seminar, Cnt. for Cont. Med. Ed., Ohio St. U. Med. Sch., Sept. 13, 1966.
460. KAPLAN, M. M.: Optical consideration of hydrogel contact lenses. Optom. Weekly, *57*(14):29–39, 1966.
461. KAPLAN, M. M.: Refractive keratoplasty—corneal bending. Am. J. Optom. and Arch. Am. Acad. Optom., in press.
462. Becker, W. E.: Corneal contact lens fabricated from transparent silicone rubber. United States Patent 3,228,741, Jan. 11, 1966.
463. BREGER, J. L.: Personal communication, November, 1966.
464. DAUDT, W. H.: Composition comprising a siloxane copolymer. United States Patent 3,036,985, May 29, 1962.
465. DOW CORNING CORP.: Contact Lenses. Great Britain Patent 927,202, May 29, 1963.
466. DOW CORNING CORP.: Improvements in or relating to the treating of silicone rubber. Great Britain Patent 1,038,855, August 10, 1966.
467. DOW CORNING CORP.: Blends of organosiloxane copolymers. Great Britain Patent 1,040,408, Aug. 24, 1966.
468. HILL, R. M.: Effects of a silicone rubber contact lens on corneal respiration, J. Am. Optom. Assn., *37*(12):1119–1121, 1966.
469. LAMOREAUX, H. F.: Transparent resinous organopolysiloxanes. United States Patent 3,197,432, July 27, 1965.
470. LAMOREAUX, H. F.: Optically clear organopolysiloxane resins. United States Patent 3,197,433, July 27, 1965.
471. MUELLER WELT CONTACT LENSES, INC.: Improvements in contact lenses and methods of making such lenses. Great Britain Patent 922,871, Apr. 3, 1963.
472. CRANDON, H. D.: Optical elements formed of resinous materials and process for making same. United States Patent 3,221,083, Nov. 30, 1965.
473. ERB, R. A.: Method for producing wettable surfaces on contact lenses by formulation of inorganic films. Office of Technical Services, School of Aviation Medicine, Report 61–42, Mar. 1961.
474. BLUE, H. D.: Method of producing permanent wettability on plastic contact lenses. J. Am. Optom. Assn., *37*(1):678–681, 1966.
475. GESSER, H. D., and FUNT, B. L.: A method of improving the wettability for contact lenses by free radical treatment. Am. J. Optom. and Arch. Am. Acad. Optom., *42*(5):321–324, 1965.
476. GUILBERT, J.: Contact lens fitting in France. J. Am. Optom. Assn., *34*(17):1403–1404, 1963.
477. KOETTING, R. A.: A corneal abrasive resistance test. Am. J. Optom. and Arch. Am. Acad. Optom., *42*(8):475–485, 1965.
478. ULLEN, R.: Predetermination of contact lens toleration—a preliminary study. Precision Cosmet Digest, *4*(2), 1963.

479. FARKAS, P., and KASSALOW, T. W.: Tear flow as a variable in the contact lens fitting procedure. Opt. J. and Rev. Optom., *98*(13):25, 1960.
480. ROSENWASSER, H. M.: A dermographic test to determine adaptation schedules for contact lenses. Opt. J. and Rev. Optom., *101*(7):28–29, 1964.
481. LUDLAM, W., and KAYE, M.: Optometry and the new metrology. Am. J. Optom. and Arch. Am. Acad. Optom., *43*(8):525–528, 1966.
482. MANDELL, R. B.: Corneal curvature measurements by the aid of moiré fringes. J. Am. Optom. Assn., *37*(3):219–220, 1966.
483. OSTER, G.: *The Science of Moiré Patterns.* Barrington, N. J., Edmund Scientific Co., 1965.
484. KOETTING, R. A.: Interpreting corneal contact lens base curve changes. Optom. Weekly, *57*(52):9–11, 1966.
485. *Toposcope Manual.* Norwalk, Conn., Optical Methods, Inc., 1966.

BIBLIOGRAPHY

In addition to the works cited, many other books and articles were consulted. They are listed in the following bibliography.

Abel, P.: Keratoconus and contact lenses. Optom. Weekly, *54*(30):1415–1416, 1963.

Abraham, S. V., and Shanedling, P. D.: The clinical status of contact lenses: results of a study by the questionnaire method. Am. J. Ophth., *33*(6):933–938, 1950.

Abrams, B. S.: Contact lenses in subnormal vision cases. Optom. Weekly, *45*(18):827–830, 1954.

Abrams, B. S.: Contact lenses in subnormal vision cases. Optom. Weekly, *45*(32):1383–1387, 1954.

Abrams, B. S.: A new concept of corneal lenses. Opt. J. and Rev. Optom., *91*(22):33–34, 1954.

Abrams, B. S.: New contact lens design—theory and description. Opt. J. and Rev. Optom., *94*(20):32–33, 1957.

Abrams, B. S., and Whitman, M.: An evaluation of Bier's contact lens application techniques. J. Am. Optom. Assn., *29*(7):455–456, 1958.

Abrams, B. S.: An O.D. reports on contact lens patents and litigation. J. Am. Optom. Assn., *31*(7):537–542, 1960.

Abrams, B. S.: The re-fitting of contact lenses. J. Am. Optom. Assn., *31*(10):901–904, 1960.

Abrams, B. S., and Bailey, N. J.: Children and contact lenses. Contacto, *4*(10):455–459, 1960.

Adler, F. H.: *Physiology of the Eye—Clinical Application,* 3d Ed. St. Louis, C. V. Mosby Co., 1959.

Agatston, H., Barnert, A. H., and Feldstein, M.: Corneal lenses in ophthalmic practice. Am. J. Ophth., *49*(2):277–286, 1960.

Alexander, F.: Spatial readjustments of aphakics. Optom. Weekly, *41*(39):1441–1442, 1950.

Allen, H. F.: The contact lens gap—delegation or default. Arch. Ophth., *65*(2):161–162, 1961.

Allen, M. J.: Case analysis and contact lenses. J. Am. Optom. Assn., *34*(3):211–212, 1962.

Alperen, S.: Contact lenses and automobile driving. J. Am. Optom. Assn., *32*(3):221–223, 1960.

Althisar, R.: Fabrication of toric back surfaces with Nissel toric generator. Encyclopedia Contact Lens Practice, *3*(17):4–5, 1962.

Anderson, A. L.: *Technique of Fitting Contact Lenses.* Minneapolis, Minn., McGill Lithograph Co., 1944.

Arbital, S.: A new micro lens fitting technique. Optom. Weekly, *47*(25):1128–1129, 1956.

Arbital, S.: Office contact lens modification. J. Am. Optom. Assn., *33*(2):131–134, 1961.

Arner, R. S.: The magic piece of plastic. Optom. Weekly, *54*(48):2235–2237, 1963.

Arner, R. S.: The invariants of corneal contact lens fitting. Optom. Weekly, *56*(30):13–18, 1965.

Arner, R. S., and Baublitz, F. U.: The use of the sagitta table in contact lens design and modification. Am. J. Optom. and Arch. Am. Acad. Optom., *41*(12):716–728, 1964.

Arruga, R.: Contact lenses in comparison with intraocular lenses. Contacto, *2*(1):17–20, 1958.

Baglien, J. W.: The use of toric corneal contact lenses. Optom. Weekly, *44*(4):129–130, 1953.

Baglien, J. W., and Middleton, R. V.: A telescopic device with corneal contact lenses. Optom. Weekly, *43*(2):39–41, 1952.

Bailey, N. J.: Photophobia and contact lenses. Contacto, *2*(3):79–81, 1958.

Bailey, N. J.: New contact lens developments. J. Am. Optom. Assn., *33*(8):573–577, 1962.

Baldwin, W. R.: Optometry's position in the contact lens field. Am. J. Optom. and Arch. Am. Acad. Optom., *40*(7):418–420, 1963.

Baldwin, W. R., and Shick, C. R.: *Corneal Contact Lenses: Fitting Procedures.* Philadelphia, Chilton Book Company, 1962.

Barksdale, C. B.: The attrition and control of myopia in some selected cases. Contacto, *4*(8):349–366, 1960.

Bayshore, C. A.: Exploration of the corneal curvature. Contacto, *3*(7):188–190, 1959.

Bayshore, C. A.: Apical clearance fitting of small ventilated contact lenses. Encyclopedia Contact Lens Practice, *3*(15):1–3, chapter 38, 1962.

Bayshore, C. A.: Bayshore technique of residual astigmatic correction. Encyclopedia Contact Lens Practice, *4*(24):65–66, chapter 9, 1963.

Bayshore, C. A.: A technique for fitting small minimal pressure contact lenses. Encyclopedia Contact Lens Practice, *4*(21):8–13, chapter 38, 1963.

Bayshore, C. A.: Fluid dynamics of the Bayshore technique. Encyclopedia Contact Lens Practice, *4*(24):15–20, chapter 38, 1963.

Bayshore, C. A.: The application, use and the value of aperture lenses. Optom. Weekly, *55*(47):18–19, 1964.

Bayshore, C. A.: Manufacturing considerations of the B-T lens. Optom. Weekly, *55*(17):21–22, 1964.

Bayshore, C. A.: Status of the Bayshore technique in contact lens fitting. Am. J. Optom. and Arch. Am. Acad. Optom., *41*(8):464–465, 1964.

Bayshore, C. A.: A new look at the patient in our reception room. Optom. Weekly, *56*(25):33–34, 1965.

Beacher, L. L.: *Contact Lens Technique,* 4th Ed. Newark, N. J., L. Lester Beacher, 1946.

Beacher, L. L.: Contact lenses: effectivity of refraction. Opt. J. and Rev. Optom., *93*(16):31–32, 1956.

Beacher, L. L.: Psychosis and neurosis encountered in contact lens fitting with case reports. Am. J. Optom. and Arch. Am. Acad. Optom., *35*(2):72–78, 1958.

Beacher, L. L.: Insertion technique for aphakics. Opt. J. and Rev. Optom., *96*(10): 38–39, 1959.

Beacher, L. L.: Possible complications in the wearing of contact lenses. Optom. Weekly, *52*(45):2197–2200, 1961.

Beacher, L. L.: Contact lenses—flatter or steeper than "k" reading. Opt. J. and Rev. Optom., *101*(12):35–36, 1964.

Beacher, L. L.: The problem of fainting when contact lenses are inserted. Optom. Weekly, *55*(51):9–10, 1964.

Beiman, J. A., and Blumenthal, D.: Personality study of contact lens patients, a preliminary report. Optom. Weekly, *51*(19):963–965, 1960.

Beiman, J. A.: Comparison of peripheral corneal measurement methods by means of graphic representation of compumatic findings. Contacto, *6*(9):269–283, 1962.

Beiman, J. A.: Fluorescent drilled dots for identifying contact lenses. Optom. Weekly, *57*(23):31–33, 1966.

Bennett, A. G.: *Optics of Contact Lenses,* 3d Ed. London, Eng., Association of Dispensing Opticians, 1963.

Bennett, A. G.: A new keratometer and its application to corneal topography. Brit. J. Phys. Opt., *21*(4):234–238, 1964.

Berliner, M. L.: *Biomicroscopy of the Eye,* Vol. I. New York, Paul B. Hoeber, 1949.

Bier, N.: Developments in contact lens practice. Am. J. Optom. and Arch. Am. Acad. Optom., *27*(4):200–207, 1950.

Bier, N.: *Contact Lens Routine and Practice,* 2d Ed. London, Eng., Butterworths Scientific Publications, 1957.

Bier, N.: Contact lenses. Contacto, *2*(1):4–16, 1958.

Bier, N.: Contact lenses. Contacto, *2*(2):44–51, 1958.

Bier, N.: Two new contact lens instruments. Optom. Weekly, *49*(43):2032–2033, 1958.

Bier, N.: *Correction of Subnormal Vision.* London, Eng., Butterworths, 1960.

Bier, N.: The contact lens projection spherometer. Optom. Weekly, *52*(15):730–731, 1961.

Bier, N.: Contact lens practice today. Optom. Weekly, *53*(15):685–691, 1962.

Bier, N.: An American notebook. Optom. Weekly, *57*(20):39–44, 1966.

Birnbaum, J.: A case history on the use of contact lenses in correcting keratoconus. Opt. J. and Rev. Optom., *90*(23):30–32, 1953.

Blair, W. A.: Photo electronic keratoscopy testing. Contacto, *4*(7):217–227, 1960.

Blair, W. A.: Equivalent values in peripheral keratometer measurements. Contacto, *5*(7):249–250, 1961.

Boring, E., Langfeld, H., and Weld, H.: *Introduction to Psychology.* New York, John Wiley and Sons, 1946.

Borish, I. M.: *Clinical Refraction,* 2d Ed. Chicago, Professional Press, 1954.

Boyts, W.: An optometrist patient reports on lenses. Opt. J. and Rev. Optom., *94*(12): 42, 1957.

Braff, S.: The use of corneal contact lenses in high hyperopia. Am. J. Optom. and Arch. Am. Acad. Optom., *28*(7):369–371, 1951.

Braff, S.: Contact lenses as an occupational requirement—a case report. Am. J. Optom. and Arch. Am. Acad. Optom., *29*(6):318–319, 1952.

Braff, S.: Some reflections on contact lens progress. Optom. Weekly, *55*(38):25–27, 1964.

Brawner, L. W., Jr., and Jessop, D. G.: A review of contact lens solutions. Contacto, *6*(2):49–51, 1962.

Brombach, T. A.: Contact lenses and visual fields. Contacto, *5*(8):265–277, 1961.

Bronstein, L.: Non-critical power effect. Contacto, *3*(2):44–45, 1959.

Bronstein, L.: Vistacon. Contacto, *4*(4):125–128, 1960.

Bronstein, L.: Experiments in keratometry. Contacto, *6*(10):298–301, 1961.

Brown, D. V. L.: Traumatic fracture of plastic contact lenses. Arch. Ophth., *72*(3): 319–322, 1964.

Brown, W.: Minimum standards of contact lens practice. Optom. Weekly, *56*(36): 57–60, 1965.

Brucker, D.: Prisms and contact lenses. Optom. Weekly, *52*(29):1428–1429, 1961.

Brucker, D.: The refitting of contact lenses. Optom. Weekly, *55*(19):35–36, 1964.

Brucker, D., and Carter, D. B.: Corneal metabolism and contact lenses. Encyclopedia Contact Lens Practice, *2*(8):42–50, chapter 8, 1961.

Brungardt, T. F.: Study of corneal contour measurements. Am. J. Optom. and Arch. Am. Acad. Optom., *39*(11):596–602, 1962.

Brungardt, T. F.: The hi-riding contact lens. Optom. Weekly, *54*(30):1409–1414, 1963.

Brungardt, T. F.: Sagittal height of the cornea. Am. J. Optom. and Arch. Am. Acad. Optom., *42*(9):525–533, 1965.

Bryan, W. E.: Corrections of strabismus with contact lenses. J. Am. Optom. Assn., *31*(8):621–622, 1960.

Cappelli, Q. A.: Determining final powers of bitoric lenses. Brit. J. Phys. Opt., *21*(4): 256–263, 1964.

Carlson, A. G.: Sleep and the corneal-type contact lens. Optom. Weekly, *50*(4):159–161, 1959.

Carlson, J.: Contact lenses—basic factors in checking the progression of myopia. Opt. J. and Rev. Optom., *95*(19):37–42, 1958.

Cepero, G.: The angled peripheral curve lens. Contacto, *5*(2):51–56, 1961.

Cepero, G.: An ophthalmologist looks at corneal transparency. Contacto, *6*(8):228–229, 1962.

Chang, T. C.: Psychological aspects of contact lens fitting. Contacto, *5*(7):251–256, 1961.

Chayet, J.: Cycloplegics, skiascopy and refraction procedure in contact lens fitting. Contacto, *7*(3):3–4, 1963.

Chiquiar-Arias, M.: Refractive orthoptic techniques and contact lens fitting. Contacto, *3*(2):37–43, 1959.

Chiquiar-Arias, M.: A predetermined wearability contact lens fitting technique. Contacto, *4*(9):403–413, 1960.

Chiquiar-Arias, M.: Can we measure the true apex of the cornea with directed keratometry? Contacto, *5*(6):201–204, 1961.

Chiquiar-Arias, V.: Two unusual cases for study in contact lens fitting. Optom. Weekly, *53*(41):2023–2026, 1962.

Chiquiar-Arias, V.: The C.A. dynamic fluoroscopic technique. Contacto, *7*(4):3–17 and 22, 1963.

Chiquiar-Arias, V.: Reshaping the cornea in keratoconus. Contacto, *8*(1):6–10, 1964.

Chiquiar-Arias, V., Liberatore, J. C., Voss, E. H., and Chiquiar-Arias, M.: A new technique in fitting contact lenses in keratoconus. Contacto, *3*(12):393–415, 1959.

Cinefro, J.: The importance of thickness in contact lens fitting. Contacto, *5*(3):101–107, 1961.

Clark, J. E.: Power measurement of toroidal lenses. Contacto, *7*(5):5–6 and 10, 1963.

Cline, H.: The science of keratometry—I. Opt. J. and Rev. Optom., *94*(16):29–31, 1957.

Cline, H.: The science of keratometry—II. Opt. J. and Rev. Optom., *94*(17):36–37, 1957.

Cline, H.: The science of keratometry—III. Opt. J. and Rev. Optom., *94*(18):35–36, 1957.

Cline, H.: The science of keratometry—IV. Opt. J. and Rev. Optom., *94*(19):40–42, 1957.

Cline, H.: The science of keratometry—V. Opt. J. and Rev. Optom., *94*(20):31 and 47, 1957.

Clunes, R. B.: Prescribing the proper diameter of corneal contact lenses. J. Am. Optom. Assn., *30*(8):567–568, 1959.

Conlon, J. R., Jr.: Use of a trial set in patient screening. Contacto, *3*(7):203–204, 1959.

Covington, W., and Gordon, S.: Peripheral design considerations in prescribing plus-powered contact lenses. Optom. Weekly, *53*(40):1971–1974, 1962.

Creighton, C. P.: A computational form for contact lens thickness. Optom. Weekly, *55*(44):34–36, 1964.

Creighton, C. P.: *Contact Lenses Fabrication Tables.* Tonawanda, N. Y., John R. Creighton, 1964.

Cronin, J. A.: Increasing the demand for contact lenses. Opt. J. and Rev. Optom., *87*(24):46 and 54, 1950.

Cutler, H.: Fitting contact lenses with identical twins. Contacto, *4*(4):131–134, 1960.

Davis, H. E.: Techniques in the fitting of bifocal contact lenses. Contacto, *3*(3):70–71, 1959.

Davis, H. E.: Why the small contact lens? Brit. J. Phys. Opt., *21*(4):215–218, 1964.

Dick, R. B.: A case report on contact lenses in constant use for a 3-month period. Am. J. Optom. and Arch. Am. Acad. Optom., *35*(5):248–250, 1958.

Dick, R. B.: Incidence of corneal insult in contact lens wearers—a preliminary report. J. Am. Optom. Assn., *32*(8):632–634, 1961.

Dickins, R., and Fletcher, R.: Contact lens measurements: a comparison of several devices. Brit. J. Phys. Opt., *21*(2):107–115, 1964.

Dickinson, F.: Refractive diagnosis aided by contact lens techniques. Am. J. Optom. and Arch. Am. Acad. Optom., *30*(4):210–215, 1953.

Dickinson, F.: The "verification system" in corneal lens fitting. Encyclopedia Contact Lens Practice, *2*(9):4–8, chapter 35, 1961.

Dickinson, F.: The history of the International Society of Contact Lens Specialists. Contacto, *6*(6):152–153, 1962.

Dickinson, F.: The role of the keratometer—a survey of fifty cases. Contacto, *6*(6): 160–161 and 168–169, 1962.

Dickinson, F.: On the impact of interprofessional relations on contact lens practice in Great Britain. Contacto, *6*(8):220–224, 1962.

Dickinson, F.: Adaptation of corneal lens design for swimming. Contacto, *8*(1):4–5 and 23, 1964.

Dickinson, F., and Hall, K. G. C.: *An Introduction to the Prescribing and Fitting of Contact Lenses.* London, Eng., Hammond, Hammond and Co., 1946.

Dine, L. A.: Contact lens photography. Am. J. Optom., *39*(10):548–551, 1962.

Dowaliby, M.: Eyewear for the contact lens patient. Optom. Weekly, *52*(42):2054–2056, 1961.

Dowaliby, M.: An optometrist learns to wear contact lenses. Optom. Weekly, *54*(14): 611–613, 1963.

Duke-Elder, S.: *Parsons' Diseases of the Eye,* 13th Ed. New York, Macmillan Co., 1959.

Dupont, I. P.: A case in point. Contacto, *3*(6):172–173, 1959.

Dzik, D.: From the world of the blind to the world of the sighted. Contacto, *4*(6): 201–203, 1960.

Ellerbrock, V. J.: Variables in corneal topography. Am. J. Optom. and Arch. Am. Acad. Optom., *38*(10):556–563, 1961.

Elliott, D. O.: Minimum standards for contact lenses. Optom. Weekly, *46*(15):605–606, 1955.

Elliott, D. O.: Drafting the requirements for a minimum clearance corneal contact lens. Am. J. Optom., *33*(11):602–603, 1956.

Elliott, D. O.: A preliminary report on use of gradient ellipsoidal curves related to fitting of contact lenses. Optom. Weekly, *55*(21):21–22, 1964.

Ellison, L. B.: A case in point—protection afforded by corneal contact lenses. Contacto, *4*(3):101–102, 1960.

Elmstrom, G. P.: Corneal contact lenses in police work. J. Am. Optom. Assn., *25*(10): 136–138, 1953.

Elmstrom, G. P.: Contact lens standards. Contacto, *6*(11):332–334, 1962.

Elmstrom, G. P.: *Optometric Practice Management.* Philadelphia, Chilton Book Company, 1963.

Elmstrom, G. P., and Kohn, H.: *Synopsis of the Legal Aspects of Contact Lens Practice for Optometrists.* Minneapolis, Minn., Burgess Publishing Co., 1964.

Embrey, L. O.: Satisfied contact lens patient. Contacto, *3*(5):133–135, 1959.

Englemann, O. R.: Dynascopy as an aid in contact lens fitting. Contacto, *3*(8):239–241, 1959.

Enoch, J. M., and McGraw, J. L.: Contact lenses: some aspects of visual acuity and photophobia. Am. J. Optom. and Arch. Am. Acad. Optom., *31*(1):12–28, 1954.

Enoch, J. M., and McGraw, J. L.: Contact lenses: some aspects of visual acuity and photophobia. Am. J. Optom. and Arch. Am. Acad. Optom., *31*(2):78–87, 1954.

Erb, R. A.: Method for producing wettable surfaces on contact lenses by formulation of inorganic films. Office of Technical Services, School of Aviation Medicine Report 61–42, Mar. 1961.

Erickson, C. E.: *Slit Lamp Procedures in Fitting Contact Lenses.* Bothell, Wash., Olympic Litho, 1964.

Erlanger, J.: Observations on contact lens practice, Am. J. Optom. and Arch. Am. Acad. Optom., *32*(1):41–44, 1955.

Eure, S. B.: A case in point—training subnormal vision with contact lenses. Contacto, *4*(5):173–177, 1960.

Eure, S. B., and Taylor, W. L.: Observations on an attempt to eliminate nystagmus in an albino patient. Optom. Weekly, *56*(23):23–28, 1965.

Evershed-Martin, L.: Patient—first and last. Contacto, *2*(2):61–63, 1958.

Evershed-Martin, L.: The search for a common factor in successful contact lens prescribing. Brit. J. Phys. Opt., *21*(4):200–202, 1964.

Fagedes, H. E.: Three emergencies in contact lens practice. Optom. Weekly, *54*(46): 2148–2150, 1963.

Fagedes, H. E.: Elements of a semiannual contact lens progress study. J. Am. Optom. Assn., *35*(12):1054–1060, 1964.

Fagedes, H. E.: Instructions for contact lens patients. Optom. Weekly, *57*(12):19–21, 1966.

Farkas, P., and Kassalow, T. W.: Regression of the successful contact lens patient. Opt. J. and Rev. Optom., *99*(17):19–20, 1962.

Farkas, P., and Kassalow, T. W.: Spherical or specialty contact lenses—which to try first? Opt. J. and Rev. Optom., *101*(3):30–31, 1964.

Farkas, P., and Kassalow, T. W.: A guide to refitting the unsuccessful contact lens patient. J. Am. Optom. Assn., *36*(3):214–216, 1965.

Farkas, P., and Kassalow, T. W.: Contact lenses and the keratoconus patient. J. Am. Optom. Assn., *37*(3):254–255, 1966.

Farnum, F. E.: Subsequent keratometer readings as a guide for lens adjustment. Contacto, *2*(4):103–104, 1958.

Farnum, F. E.: Refinements in contact lens adjustments to increase wearing time. Am. J. Optom. and Arch. Am. Acad. Optom., *36*(7):382–384, 1959.

Farnum, F. E.: The ophthalmometer in corneal contact lens practice. J. Am. Optom. Assn., *30*(8):569, 1959.

Fehr, R.: Uses of contact lenses in radiation research. Contacto, *3*(10):307–309, 1959.

Feinberg, R.: A new technique in vision testing for contact lens specialists. Optom. Weekly, *50*(32):1599, 1959.

Feinbloom, W.: The gyroscope contact lens and corneal diopter plot. Opt. J. and Rev. Optom., *93*(9):25–27 and 65, 1956.

Filderman, I. P.: Contact lens practice—a new perspective. Southern J. Optom., *5*(6): 7–11, 1963.

Filderman, I. P.: Contact lens practice—a new perspective. Southern J. Optom., *5*(7): 11–12, 1963.

Filderman, I. P.: Contact lens practice—a new perspective. Southern J. Optom., *5*(8): 9–16, 1963.

Filderman, I. P.: Contact lens practice—a new perspective. Southern J. Optom., *5*(10): 11–13, 20, 23, 26, 29, and 44–45, 1963.

Filderman, I. P.: Contact lens practice—a new perspective. Southern J. Optom., *6*(1): 7–10 and 25–26, 1964.

Filderman, I. P.: The relationship of contact lenses to corneal physiology. Am. J. Optom., *41*(1):17–36, 1964.

Finklestein, I.: The biophysics of corneal scatter and diffraction of light induced by contact lenses. Am. J. Optom., *29*(4):185–208, 1952.

Finklestein, I.: The biophysics of corneal scatter and diffraction of light induced by contact lenses. Am. J. Optom., *29*(5):231–258, 1952.

Firestone, L. E.: The value of a good contact lens case. Optom. Weekly, *50*(5):222, 1959.

Fisher, E.: Clinical observations on the fitting of micro-lenses. Am. J. Optom. and Arch. Am. Acad. Optom., *32*(6):289–294, 1955.

Fitzgerald, J. R., Kapustiak, W., and McCarty, J. L.: Contact lens corneal ulcer. Am. J. Ophth., *54*(2):307–308, 1962.

Fletcher, R.: A study of the total light flux admitted to the interior of the eye through contact lenses. Brit. J. Phys. Opt., *21*(3):134–146, 1964.

Fonda, G.: *Management of the Patient With Subnormal Vision.* Saint Louis, C. V. Mosby Co., 1965.

Fontana, F. D.: Case in point—corneal scarring and contact lenses. Contacto, *4*(8): 377–381, 1960.

Fontana, F. D.: Remolding and therapy of the cornea through the use of contact lenses. Optom. Weekly, *53*(21):991–993, 1962.

Freeman, M. H.: The measurement of contact lens curvatures. Am. J. Optom. and Arch. Am. Acad. Optom., *42*(11):693–701, 1965.

Friedberg, M.: Contact lens apertures and toric curve designs. J. Am. Optom. Assn., *32*(8):642–644, 1961.

Fryer, D., Henry, E., and Sparks, C.: *General Psychology,* 4th Ed. New York, Barnes and Noble, 1954.

Gabe, M.: A new preformed scleral lens. Optom. Weekly, *56*(15):23–26, 1965.

Gale, J.: Dynoscopy in contact lens fitting. Optom. Weekly, *49*(29):1364–1365, 1958.

Gamboney, E.: Use of trial lenses in contact lens fitting. Contacto, *5*(2):63–65, 1961.

Gamboney, E.: The partial control of motion of contact lenses by the use of prism ballast and toric base curve lenses. Contacto, *7*(3):5–8, and 16, 1963.

Gardner, S. A.: Case history—a contact lens in phthisis bulbi. Optom. Weekly, *47*(31): 1361, 1956.

Geldbart, R. G.: Contact lenses—as a service. Optom. Weekly, *49*(5):188, 1958.

Genevay, N. C., Jr.: A new inside segment bifocal contact lens. Contacto, *5*(2):59–60, 1961.

Gettes, B. C., and Ravdin, E. M.: Monocular aphakia and exotropia corrected by contact lenses. Am. J. Ophth., *32*(6-part I):850–851, 1949.

Giraldi, O. T.: Dresser drawer wearing. Contacto, *4*(3):93–94, 1960.

Giraldi, O. T.: Fitting contact lenses for all-day wear. Optom. Weekly, *51*(21):1075, 1960.

Giraldi, O. T.: Fluorescein refracting room. Contacto, *7*(2):5, 1963.

Girard, L. J. (ed.): *Corneal Contact Lenses.* Saint Louis, C. V. Mosby Co., 1964.

Girard, L. J., Camp, R. N., Lamb, V. R., Richardson, C. R., and Soper, J. W.: Iris corneal lens. Am. J. Ophth., *52*(2):264–265, 1961.

Girard, L. J., Soper, J. W., and Camp, R. N.: The contact lens problem. Am. J. Ophth., *52*(5-part I):706–710, 1961.

Girard, L. J., Friedman, B., Moore, C. D., Blav, R. I., Brinkhorst, C. B., and Gobin, M. H.: Intraocular implants and contact lenses. Arch. Ophth., *68*(6):762–775, 1962.

Girard, L. J., and Soper, J. W.: Flush-fitting scleral contact lenses. Am. J. Ophth., *61*(5-part II):1109–1123, 1966.

Glatt, L.: Cosmetic use of a corneal lens—case report. Opt. J. and Rev. Optom., *97*(23): 24–26, 1960.

Glazer, W. H.: A successful contact lens experiment. Opt. J. and Rev. Optom., *96*(8): 46, 1959.

Glazer, W. H.: A discussion of prisms. Opt. J. and Rev. Optom., *98*(10):39, 1961.

Goar, E. L., Krieger, A. A., Kronfeld, P. C., Masters, R. J., and Thorpe, H. E.: *Slit Lamp Biomicroscopy.* Omaha, Neb., Douglas Printing Co., 1961.

Goldberg, J. B.: Comparison of fluidless contact lenses. Optom. Weekly, *43*(14):585–588, 1953.

Goldberg, J. B.: Fitting the cornea and determining the lens size. Opt. J. and Rev. Optom., *96*(20):40–42, 1959.

Goldberg, J. B.: Corneal contact lenses: initial and final values. Optom. Weekly, *51*(3):121–125, 1960.

Goldberg, J. B.: Bifocal contact lens procedure. Contacto, *5*(6):218–225, 1961.

Goldberg, J. B.: The influence of physiologic factors in contact lens design. Optom. Weekly, *52*(37):1785–1790, 1961.

Goldberg, J. B.: The influence of physiologic factors in contact lens design. Optom. Weekly, *52*(38):1843–1846, 1961.

Goldberg, J. B.: Lens evaluation inadequacies. Contacto, *5*(11):357–358, 1961.

Goldberg, J. B.: Some notes on contact lenses with mention of corneal epithelium turnover. Am. J. Optom. and Arch. Am. Acad. Optom., *38*(2):87–94, 1961.

Goldberg, J. B.: Clinical application of toric base curve contact lenses. Optom. Weekly, *53*(39):1911–1915, 1962.

Goldberg, J. B.: The fallacy of the ophthalmometer in contact lens practice. J. Am. Optom. Assn., *33*(8):593–594, 1962.

Goldberg, J. B.: Transition zone between optic diameter and bevel. Contacto, *6*(3): 79–80, 1962.

Goldberg, J. B.: A commentary on fitting small size corneal contact lenses. J. Am. Optom. Assn., *35*(3):215–220, 1964.

Goldberg, J. B.: The correction of residual astigmatism with circular design prism ballast contact lenses. Optom. Weekly, *55*(41):27–30, 1964.

Goldberg, J. B.: The correction of residual astigmatism with corneal contact lenses. Brit. J. Phys. Opt., *21*(3):169–174, 1964.

Golden, D.: Observations on fluidless contact lenses. Opt. J. and Rev. Optom., *87*(23): 44–46, 1950.

Golden, D.: A new development in contact lenses. Opt. J. and Rev. Optom., *89*(3):32–33, 1952.

Golden, D.: Correction of keratoconus and high astigmatism with contact lenses. Opt. J. and Rev. Optom., *90*(18):35–36, 1953.

Golden, D.: The Airflo-non-pressure lens—theory and description. Opt. J. and Rev. Optom., *94*(21):47 and 52, 1957.

Goodlaw, E. I.: Use of slit lamp biomicroscopy in the fitting of contact lenses. Encyclopedia Contact Lens Practice, *3*(13):5–48, chapter 11, 1961.

Goodlaw, E. I.: Avoiding the hazards and pitfalls in prescribing and fitting contact lenses. Optom. Weekly, *53*(29):1431–1437, 1962.

Goodlaw, E. I.: Avoiding the hazards and pitfalls in prescribing and fitting contact lenses. Optom. Weekly, *53*(30):1481–1484, 1962.

Goodlaw, E. I.: Use of slit lamp biomicroscopy in the fitting of contact lenses, Encyclopedia Contact Lens Practice, *4*(22):49–66, chapter 11, 1963.

Goodman, R. A.: Danger of corneal pressure in fitting contact lenses. Opt. J. and Rev. Optom., *94*(7):37–40, 1957.

Gordon, S.: The correction of residual astigmatism through toric inside contact lenses. Optom. Weekly, *52*(4):186–192, 1961.

Gordon, S.: An evaluation of small, thin contact lenses. Optom. Weekly, *55*(5):21–25, 1964.

Gordon, S., and Maslinger, B.: Minimized lens "settling." Opt. J. and Rev. Optom., *97*(16):39–40, 1960.

Graham, R.: Corneal lenses—a supplementary report. Am. J. Optom. and Arch. Am. Acad. Optom., *29*(3):137–141, 1952.

Graham, R.: Photophobia and contact lenses. Contacto, *3*(10):315–317, 1959.

Grant, A. H.: SCAL: skindiver's contact air lens. Opt. J. and Rev. Optom., *100*(21): 22–25, 1963.

Grant, A. H.: This is scal—skin diver's contact air lens. Optom. Weekly, *55*(22):17–19, 1964.

Grant, A. H.: One-hand technique of contact lens insertion. Optom. Weekly, *56*(9): 19, 1965.

Grant, A. H.: The Grant hyperbola. J. Am. Optom. Assn., *37*(6):550–552, 1966.

Greene, L. M.: History of contact lenses in England from medical standpoint. Contacto, *7*(7):5–11, 1963.

Greene, L. M.: Ocular physiological factors influencing a contact lens practice. Contacto, *7*(8):10–16, 1963.

Groppi, J. J.: A study of trends in contact lens adjustment. Contacto, *4*(9):398–399, 1960.

Groppi, J. J., and Mandel, A. M.: Corneal curvature changes after fitting contact lenses. Contacto, *2*(3):72–73, 1958.

Gross, R.: General considerations in contact lens laboratory. Optom. Weekly, *51*(25): 1301–1303, 1960.

Grosvenor, T. P.: Clinical use of the keratometer in evaluating the corneal contour. Am. J. Optom. and Arch. Am. Acad. Optom. *38*(5):237–246, 1961.

Grosvenor, T. P.: *Contact Lens Theory and Practice.* Chicago, Professional Press, 1963.

Grosvenor, T. P.: Contact lens fitting in New Zealand and Australia. Am. J. Optom. and Arch. Am. Acad. Optom., *42*(6):351–358, 1965.

Grosvenor, T. P.: Physiological factors in contact lens wearing. Optom. Weekly, *57*(13): 13–19, 1966.

Guilbert, J.: Contact lens fitting in France. J. Am. Optom. Assn., *34*(17):1403–1405, 1963.

Gyorffy, I.: Contact lens fitting in Hungary. Contacto, *3*(10):289–297, 1959.

Gyorffy, I.: Sports and contact lenses—observation of 400 cases. Contacto, *4*(11):495–499, 1960.

Gyorffy, I.: The history of the moulded all-plastic lens. Brit. J. Phys. Opt., *21*(4):291–292, 1964.

Haines, H. F.: Monocular anterior corneal staphyloma corrected with contact lens with resultant binocular fusion—a case report. Am. J. Optom. and Arch. Am. Acad. Optom., *27*(3):137–139, 1950.

Hale, J. R.: Preliminary microlens report. Optom. Weekly, *46*(20):437–438, 1955.

Hale, J. R.: Management of teenage contact lens patients. Optom. Weekly, *56*(49):21–25, 1965.

Hall, K. C.: Experiences in fitting microlenses. Contacto, *2*(2):57–60, 1958.

Hall, K. C.: A visit to the first contact lens department in Soviet Russia. Contacto, *4*(11):509–520, 1960.

Hall, K. C.: A comprehensive study of keratoconus. Optom. Weekly, *55*(48):19–23, 1964.

Hall, K. C.: A comprehensive study of keratoconus. Optom. Weekly, *55*(49):17–24, 1964.

Hall, K. C.: A comprehensive study of keratoconus. Optom. Weekly, *55*(50):31–34, 1964.

Hall, K. C.: A comprehensive study of keratoconus. Optom. Weekly, *55*(51):11–15, 1964.

Haluschak, M.: There is no ideal contact lens patient. Optom. Weekly, *54*(11):480–481, 1963.

Hamano, H.: Topical and systemic influences of wearing contact lenses. Contacto, *4*(2):41–48, 1960.

Hamano, H., Yasuhara, M., and Moromoto, S.: Effects of wind and humidity on the wearing of contact lenses. Contacto, *6*(10):293–297, 1962.

Hamilton, C. B.: An investigation of corneal profiles. Contacto, *7*(3):9–16, 1963.

Hamm, H. A.: Plastics used in contact lenses. Contacto, *6*(2):43–45, 1962.

Handal, J. P.: Some considerations concerning corneal topography and the determination of contact lens base curves. Contacto, *7*(6):8–15 and 31–32, 1963.

Harris, H. S.: The corneal lens. Am. J. Optom. and Arch. Am. Acad. Optom., *27*(2):64–87, 1950.

Hart, R.: Nineteen diopters of corneal astigmatism corrected with contact lens. Opt. J. and Rev. Optom., *94*(13):42, 1957.

Hartstein, J.: Newer corneal types of contact lenses. Am. J. Ophth., *45*(5):919–920, 1958.

Haynes, P. R.: Aperture venting techniques in corneal contact lenses. Encyclopedia Contact Lens Practice, *1*(4):9–13, recent developments section, 1960.

Haynes, P. R.: Comments on factors which must be considered in the fitting of contact lenses. J. Am. Optom. Assn., *32*(4):299–302, 1960.

Haynes, P. R.: Comments on lens designs and fitting techniques of corneal contact lenses. Encyclopedia Contact Lens Practice, *1*(3):8–41, chapter 8, 1960.

Haynes, P. R.: Fitting of contact lenses on patients manifesting keratoconus. Encyclopedia Contact Lens Practice, *1*(5):13–30, chapter 16, 1960.

Haynes, P. R.: Exact theory for the calculation of peripheral thickness values in corneal contact lenses with multiple peripheral curves. Encyclopedia Contact Lens Practice, *2*(12):6–18, chapter 4, 1961.

Haynes, P. R.: Custom fitting procedures for prescribing corneal contact lenses. Part I. Encyclopedia Contact Lens Practice, *4*(23):77–136, chapter 8, 1963.

Haynes, P. R.: Custom fitting procedures for prescribing corneal contact lenses. Part II. Encyclopedia Contact Lens Practice, *4*(24):137–189, chapter 8, 1963.

Haynes, P. R., and McEachern, C.: Keratometer readings for keratoconus. Contacto, *2*(1):35–38, 1958.

Hebbard, F. W.: Contact lenses in civil aviation: current status. J. Am. Optom. Assn., *34*(8):618–622, 1963.

Henao, H. R.: Contact lenses in keratoplasty. Contacto, *3*(8):235–237, 1959.

Hersh, D.: Modern contact lenses for keratoconus. Optom. Weekly, *49*(31):1397–1398, 1958.

Hersh, D.: Bifocal contact lenses in migraine induced aniseikonic effect, and hyperphoria. Optom. Weekly, *50*(12):555–559, 1959.

Hersh, D.: Effect of corneal planning—a case report. Opt. J. and Rev. Optom., *97*(12): 37–39, 1960.

Hersh, D.: Use of eccentrically ground secondary curve in relief of "fine" contact lens symptoms. Optom. Weekly, *51*(8):377–379, 1960.

Hersh, D.: A study of contact lens nomenclature. Opt. J. and Rev. Optom., *98*(9): 29–31 and 45, 1961.

Hersh, D.: Tinted contact lenses—a new lens coloring concept. Optom. Weekly, *56*(42): 37–39, 1965.

Hier, J.: Where we stand on contact lens fitting in 1960. Am. J. Optom. and Arch. Am. Acad. Optom., *37*(12):642–648, 1960.

Hill, R. M.: Oxygen uptake of the cornea following contact lens removal. J. Am. Optom. Assn., *36*(10):913–915, 1965.

Hill, R. M.: The Corneal Biophysics Laboratory, School of Optometry, The Ohio State University. J. Am. Optom. Assn., *37*(3):221–223, 1966.

Hill, R. M.: Relative effects of static reservoir volumes on corneal respiration. Am. J. Optom. and Arch. Am. Acad. Optom., *43*(2):88–95, 1966.

Hill, R. M.: Respiratory profiles of the corneal epithelium. Part I. Control profiles and effects of the non-aperture lens. Am. J. Optom. and Arch. Am. Acad. Optom., *43*(4):233–237, 1966.

Hill, R. M., and Fatt, I.: Oxygen deprivation of the cornea by contact lenses and lid closure. Am. J. Optom. and Arch. Am. Acad. Optom., *41*(11):678–687, 1964.

Hill, R. M., and Fatt, I.: Oxygen measurements under a contact lens. Am. J. Optom. and Arch. Am. Acad. Optom., *41*(6):382–387, 1964.

Hill, R. M., and Fatt, I.: A contact lens from the cornea's point of view. Optom. Weekly, *56*(36):29–31, 1965.

Hill, R. M., and Leighton, A. J.: Physiological time courses associated with contact lenses. Temperature. Part I. Animal time courses with scleral lenses. Am. J. Optom. and Arch. Am. Acad. Optom., *40*(8):427–438, 1963.

Hill, R. M., and Leighton, A. J.: Physiological time courses associated with contact lenses—temperature. Part II. Animal time courses with corneal lenses. Am. J. Optom. and Arch. Am. Acad. Optom., *41*(1):3–9, 1964.

Hill, R. M., and Leighton, A. J.: Temperature changes of human cornea and tears under a contact lens. Part I. The relaxed open eye, and the natural and forced closed eye conditions. Am. J. Optom., *42*(1):9–16, 1965.

Hill, R. M., and Leighton, A. J.: Temperature changes of human cornea and tears under a contact lens. Part II. Effects of intermediate lid apertures and gaze. Am. J. Optom. and Arch. Am. Acad. Optom., *42*(2):71–77, 1965.

Hill, R. M., and Leighton, A. J.: Temperature changes of human cornea and tears under contact lenses. Part III. Ocular sensation. Am. J. Optom. and Arch. Am. Acad. Optom., *42*(10):584–588, 1965.

Hirsch, M.: Is the fitting of contact lenses an optometric specialty? Am. J. Optom. and Arch. Am. Acad. Optom., *36*(5):248–251, 1959.

Hirsch, M.: Instrumentation as a reflection of a new trend in contact lens fitting. Am. J. Optom. and Arch. Am. Acad. Optom., *37*(4):210–212, 1960.

Hirsch, M.: Contact lenses do not belong in the market place. Am. J. Optom. and Arch. Am. Acad. Optom., *38*(6):349–350, 1961.

Hodd, F. A. B.: Changes in corneal shape induced by the use of alignment fitted corneal lenses. Contacto, *9*(3):18–24, 1965.

Hofstetter, H. W.: A keratoscopic survey of 13,395 eyes. Am. J. Optom. and Arch. Am. Acad. Optom., *36*(1):3–11, 1959.

Hopps, H. C.: *Principles of Pathology*. New York, Appleton-Century-Crofts, 1959.

Huang, D. T.: An aphakic case fitted with aperture contact lenses. Contacto, *7*(2): 17–19, 1963.

Huang, D. T., and Reilly, J. M.: A modification technique of a contact lens toric secondary curve. Optom. Weekly, *56*(43):23–24, 1965.

Hughes, R. E.: Residual astigmatism correction. Contacto, *4*(8):369–375, 1960.

Hummel, D.: Present status of contact lens practice. Am. J. Optom. and Arch. Am. Acad. Optom., *35*(6):327–331, 1958.

Iacono, G. D.: Psychological considerations in contact lens practice. Contacto, *4*(6): 205–209, 1960.

Iacono, G. D.: A positive approach to contact lens practice. Contacto, *5*(8):279–280, 1961.

Isen, A. A.: The relationship of edge thickness to center thickness of a contact lens. Optom. Weekly, *50*(53):2581–2582, 1959.

Isen, A. A.: A rationale for fitting contact lenses. Optom. Weekly, *51*(6):269–273, 1960.

Isen, A. A.: The fabrication or modification of toric peripheral curves. Encyclopedia Contact Lens Practice, *3*(16):92–93, chapter 22, 1962.

Jackson, W. R.: Medic alert offers contact lens public service. J. Am. Optom. Assn., *33*(8):595–596, 1962.

Jackson, W. R.: Urge your contact lens patients to join the medic-alert foundation. Optom. Weekly, *56*(23):29–30, 1965.

Jaeckle, C. E.: Contact lenses and the physician. Opt. J. and Rev. Optom., *98*(7):33–36, 1962.

Jenkin, L.: Contact lens fitting in Great Britain. Optom. Weekly, *41*(21):767, 1950.

Jenkin, L.: Contact lens fitting in Great Britain. Contacto, *2*(4):97–101, 1958.

Jenkin, L., and Tyler-Jones, R.: *Theory and Practice of Contact Lens Fitting.* London, Eng., Hatton Press Ltd., 1964.

Jessen, G. N.: The long term effects on the cornea and the visual system with contact lenses. Contacto, *5*(4):137–145, 1961.

Jessen, G. N.: Bifocal contact lenses—a survey. Contacto, *6*(2):53–56, 1962.

Jessen, G. N.: Contact lenses and visual training. Contacto, *6*(5):121–126 and 134–135, 1962.

Jessen, G. N.: Orthofocus techniques. Contacto, *6*(7):200–204, 1962.

Jessen, G. N.: World wide summary of contact lens techniques. Am. J. Optom. and Arch. Am. Acad. Optom., *39*(12):680–682, 1962.

Jessen, G. N.: Contact lenses as a therapeutic device. Am. J. Optom. and Arch. Am. Acad. Optom., *41*(7):429–435, 1964.

Jessen, G. N.: Baseball and contact lenses. Am. J. Optom. and Arch. Am. Acad. Optom., *43*(5):320–324, 1966.

Jessen, G. N., and Wesley, N. K.: A new development in multi-focal contact lenses. Contacto, *9*(3):11–14, 1965.

Jessop, D. G.: Plotting corneal topography. Contacto, *5*(2):69–74, 1961.

Jessop, D. G.: Tear layer reduction factor. Contacto, *5*(5):189–191, 1961.

Jessop, D. G.: Peripheral keratometric findings. Contacto, *6*(1):19–23, 1962.

Jessop, D. G.: Peripheral corneal readings—corneal isopters. Contacto, *7*(2):7–16, 1963.

Jessop, D. G.: Para-central readings and apical clearance fitting. Contacto, *9*(1):10–13, 1965.

Johnson, R. A.: A group survey of contact lens office procedures. Optom. Weekly, *56*(4):21–25, 1965.

Kabakoff, B. J.: Contact lens management of the geriatric aphakic. Opt. J. and Rev. Optom., *100*(9):35–38, 1963.

Kapetansky, F. M., Suie, T., and Bitonte, J. L.: Bacteriological studies. Contacto, *9*(1): 6–9, 1965.

Kelly, T. S.-B., and Butler, D.: Preliminary report on corneal lenses in relation to myopia. Brit. J. Phys. Opt., *21*(3):175–186, 1964.

Kemmetmuller, H.: The fluid lens as a most important aid in fitting corneal lenses. Contacto, *5*(4):115–119, 1961.

Kemmetmuller, H.: Corneal lenses and keratoconus. Contacto, *6*(7):188–193, 1962.

Kennedy, J. R.: Developments in the contact lens field—future direction. Opt. J. and Rev. Optom., *96*(15):42, 1959.

Kennedy, J. R.: Contact lens procedure in exophthalmos. J. Am. Optom. Assn., *31*(8): 627–629, 1960.

Kennedy, J. R.: Safe contact lens follow-up care. Optom. Weekly, *55*(25):23–25, 1964.

Kershner, L. W.: Current concepts in corneal lens fitting. Opt. J. and Rev. Optom., *98*(21):27–30, 1961.

Kershner, L. W.: Refitting problem cases with smaller corneal lenses. Opt. J. and Rev. Optom., *101*(13):28–30, 1964.

Kienast, E. J.: Contact lens inspection. Optom. Weekly, *51*(26):1347–1349, 1960.

Kimura, S. J.: Fluorescein paper: a simple means of insuring the use of sterile fluorescein. Am. J. Ophth., *344*(3):446–447, 1951.

King, J. H., Jr., and McTigue, J. W. (eds): *The Cornea World Congress*. Washington, D. C., Butterworths, 1965.

Kinsey, V. E.: An explanation of the corneal haze and halos produced by contact lenses. Am. J. Ophth., *35*(5-part I):691–695, 1952.

Kleyhauer, A.: A lens edge treatment for office application. Contacto, *4*(5):167–169, 1960.

Knoll, H. A.: Photokeratoscopy and corneal contours. Encyclopedia Contact Lens Practice, *2*(9):6–11, chapter 7, 1961.

Koetting, R. A.: Minimizing problems resulting from changes in contact lens radius. Optom. Weekly, *54*(43):1999–2002, 1963.

Koetting, R. A.: Ten second fluorescein pattern photography. Am. J. Optom. and Arch. Am. Acad. Optom., *40*(11):684–693, 1963.

Koetting, R. A.: Mucous formation in cases of aphakia. Opt. J. and Rev. Optom., *101*(19):29–30, 1964.

Koetting, R. A.: Special considerations in the fitting of contact lenses in aphakia. Am. J. Optom. and Arch. Am. Acad. Optom., *41*(4):248–260, 1964.

Koetting, R. A.: Advantages of contact lenses fitted early in aphakia. J. Am. Optom. Assn., *37*(3):239–242, 1966.

Kokoski, C. S., and Schwartz, S. M.: A study of the effects of various soaking solutions on the wettability of plastic lens surfaces. Contacto, *7*(5):15–21, 1963.

Konyama, K.: Contact lens treatment in amblyopia. Contacto, *4*(1):17–21, 1960.

Korb, D. R.: Application of multiple microholes. J. Am. Optom. Assn., *32*(11):891–892, 1961.

Korb, D. R.: A preliminary report on continuing performance of toric inner surface contact lenses. Contacto, *5*(10):317–323, 1961.

Korb, D. R.: Recent advances in corneal lens fenestration. Encyclopedia Contact Lens Practice, *3*(14):58–66, recent developments section, 1962.

Kraus, D. E., and Zabner, L. E.: The hand slit lamp and Touhy corneal lenses. Optom. Weekly, *45*(39):1565, 1954.

Lake, L. H.: Contact lenses in the treatment of infantile and juvenile aphakia. Brit. J. Phys. Opt., *21*(4):287–290, 1964.

Lansche, R. K., and Lee, R. C.: Acute complications from present day corneal contact lenses. Arch. Ophth., *64*(2):275–285, 1960.

Last, R. J.: *Wolff's Anatomy of the Eye and Orbit,* 5th Ed. Philadelphia, W. B. Saunders Co., 1961.

Lee, S. K.: New way to visual happiness. Contacto, *2*(5):135–136, 1958.

Leigh, E. R.: Optical properties of contact lenses. Am. J. Ophth., *59*(5):909–913, 1965.

Lester, R. W.: Contact lens checking in the office. Contacto, *1*(3):44, 1957.

Lester, R. W.: The full circle of contact lens care. J. Am. Optom. Assn., *29*(7):442–444, 1958.

Lester, R. W.: New contact lens form. Contacto, *3*(5):117–124, 1959.

Lester, R. W.: The use of the biomicroscope in contact lens fitting. Am. J. Optom. and Arch. Am. Acad. Optom., *40*(6):309–331, 1963.

Levenson, D.: Keratoconus. Contacto, *3*(7):181–186, 1959.

Levey, E. M.: A case history of two years continuous wearing of contact lenses, followed by six months of non-continuous wearing. Am. J. Optom. and Arch. Am. Acad. Optom., *41*(12):703–715, 1964.

Levey, E. M.: The sports wearer of contact lenses—a new approach. Brit. J. Phys. Opt., *21*(4):197–199, 1964.

Levey, E. M.: The sports wearer of contact lenses, a new approach. Am. J. Optom. and Arch. Am. Acad. Optom., *42*(1):21–23, 1965.

Levy, O. R.: Artificial eye fitting. Optom. Weekly, *43*(42):1688–1689, 1952.

Lewis, E. L.: Protective corneal lens for prolonged procedures, Am. J. Ophth., *45*(6): 922, 1958.

Lewison, L.: A chart of contact lens fitting procedure. Opt. J. and Rev. Optom., *93*(24): 52, 1956.

Long, W.: Basic principles in fitting the fluidless contact lens. Optom. Weekly, *43*(10): 359–362, 1952.

Loring, J. H.: Visual acuity in 5 selected contact lens cases not correctable to standard acuity. Optom. Weekly, *49*(43):2031–2032, 1958.

Lutes, H. R.: The importance of the storage case for contact lenses. Optom. Weekly, *56*(35):33–34, 1965.

Magatani, H.: Limitless wearing of contact lenses without interruption. Contacto, *4*(3):81–87, 1960.

Magatani, H.: Optical and biological problems of refraction and contact lenses. Contacto, *6*(1):5–13, 1962.

Malin, A. H.: A method of fitting contact lenses and correcting aphakia. Am. J. Optom. and Arch. Am. Acad. Optom., *35*(11):580–589, 1958.

Manas, L.: Using a functional "K" factor in contact lens fitting. Optom. Weekly, *52*(4):170–175, 1961.

Mandel, A. M.: Keratoconus and contact lenses. Contacto, *3*(4):101–104, 1959.

Mandel, A. M.: Mucus and contact lenses. Contacto, *4*(5):159–164, 1960.

Mandelbaum, J.: Corneal vascularization following use of contact lenses. Arch. Ophth., *71*(5):633–635, 1964.

Mandell, R. B.: The calculation of contact lens edge thickness. Optom. Weekly, *55*(3): 19–21, 1959.

Mandell, R. B.: Profile methods of measuring corneal curvature. J. Am. Optom. Assn., *32*(8):627–631, 1961.

Mandell, R. B.: Methods to measure the peripheral corneal curvature—part one: photokeratoscopy. J. Am. Optom. Assn., *33*(2):137–139, 1961.

Mandell, R. B.: Methods to measure the peripheral corneal curvature—part two: geometric construction and "computers." J. Am. Optom. Assn., *33*(8):585–589, 1962.

Mandell, R. B.: Methods to measure the peripheral corneal curvature—part three: ophthalmometry. J. Am. Optom. Assn., *33*(12):889–892, 1962.

Mandell, R. B.: Reflection point ophthalmometry. Am. J. Optom. and Arch. Am. Acad. Optom., *39*(10):513–537, 1962.

Mandell, R. B.: Corneal areas utilized in ophthalmometry. Am. J. Optom. and Arch. Am. Acad. Optom., *41*(3):150–153, 1964.

Mandell, R. B.: *Contact Lens Practice: Basic and Advanced.* Springfield, Ill., Charles C. Thomas, 1965.

Mandell, R. B.: Keratometry and contact lens practice. Optom. Weekly, *56*(18):69–75, 1965.

Mandell, R. B.: Corneal curvature measurements by the aid of moiré fringes. J. Am. Optom. Assn., *37*(3):219–220, 1966.

Manwiller, R. S.: Twelve consecutive case reports from the contact lens clinic of the Pennsylvania State College of Optometry. Am. J. Optom. and Arch. Am. Acad. Optom., *27*(10):477–483, 1950.

Marano, J. A.: A computer for contact lens cylinder axis. Contacto, *4*(11):503–506, 1960.

Marano, J. A.: Front surface cylindrical contact lenses. Optom. Weekly, *53*(37):1803–1804, 1962.

Marriott, P. J., and Woodward, E. G.: A method of measuring the corneal clearance of a haptic lens. Brit. J. Phys. Opt., *21*(2):61–83, 1964.

Martin, W. F.: A research study on athletes' vision. Contacto, *7*(1):5–9 and 22, 1963.

Martin, W. F., and Jensen, R. D.: Size and peripheral curve factors in contact lens fitting. Contacto, *4*(5):155–158, 1960.

Mast, A. R.: Derivation of the radius of the anterior curve of contact lenses accounting for the presence and refraction of the lachrymal fluid and thickness. Optom. Weekly, *55*(19):19–25, 1964.

May, C. H.: Comparative study of visual performance before and after contact lenses. Contacto, *4*(2):51–53, 1960.

May, C. H.: Corneal profile by photographic means. Contacto, *7*(4):18–19, 1963.

May, C. H.: New method of measuring peripheral curves. Contacto, *7*(7):15–21, 1963.

May, M. C.: Investigation of corneal curvature. Contacto, *1*(1):7–9, 1957.

Mazow, B.: Pupilens—a preliminary report. Contacto, *2*(5):128–131, 1958.

Mazow, B.: *Synopsis of Corneal Contact Lens Fitting for Optometrists.* Minneapolis, Minn., Burgess Publishing Co., 1962.

McCaslin, M. F.: Effects of invisible lens aberrations: a clinical experiment. Arch. Ophth., *62*(3):434–437, 1959.

McCormack, H. G.: The relative value of factors that influence lens centering. Contacto, *6*(11):325–332, 1962.

McCormack, H. G.: The computergraph. Contacto, *9*(1):23–27, 1965.

Middleton, J. M.: Use of contact lenses by a three-year-old partial albinotic with high myopia. Eye, Ear, Nose, and Throat Monthly, *38*(7):565–568, and 574, 1959.

Miller, B.: Can progressive myopia be prevented by corneal lenses? Contacto, *6*(7):196–199, 1962.

Miller, D.: Basic physiology involved in fitting corneal lenses. Opt. J. and Rev. Optom., *94*(17):40–45, 1957.

Miller, D.: Physical forces applied to a corneal contact lens. Arch. Ophth., *70*(6):823–829, 1963.

Mizutani, Y.: Selected problems and solutions in contact lens fitting. Contacto, *4*(10):439–452, 1960.

Monoplex Eye Fitting Manual. Southbridge, Mass., American Optical Co., 1950.

Moore, L.: Sub-normal vision and contact lenses. Contacto, *3*(7):192–201, 1959.

Moore, L.: The contact lens for subnormal visual acuity. Brit. J. Phys. Opt., *21*(4):203–204, 1964.

Morris, F. M.: Contact lenses in aviation and space. J. Am. Optom. Assn., *34*(8):623–627, 1963.

Morris, F. M.: Contact lenses for flying personnel—a clinical investigation. Contacto, *8*(1):12–15 and 23–25, 1964.

Morrison, R. J.: Contact lenses and the progression of myopia. Optom. Weekly, *48*(34):1487–1488, 1956.

Morrison, R. J.: Contact lenses and the progression of myopia. J. Am. Optom. Assn., *28*(12):711–713, 1957.

Morrison, R. J.: Contact lenses: a review of their many uses. J. Am. Optom. Assn., *29*(7):445–446, 1958.

Morrison, R. J.: Observations on contact lenses and progression of myopia. Contacto, *2*(1):20–25, 1958.

Morrison, R. J.: Keratoconus, aphakia, and contact lenses. J. Am. Optom. Assn., *32*(4): 311–313, 1960.

Morrison, R. J.: Routine care of the contact lens patient. Optom. Weekly, *51*(38): 1971–1974, 1960.

Morrison, R. J.: The use of contact lenses in adolescent myopia. Am. J. Optom. and Arch. Am. Acad. Optom., *37*(3):165–168, 1960.

Morrison, R. J.: Some observations on bifocal contact lenses. Opt. J. and Rev. Optom., *98*(7):32–35, 1961.

Morrison, R. J.: After-care of the contact lens patient. Brit. J. Phys. Opt., *21*(4):209–214, 1964.

Morrison, R. J., and Mallinger, B.: Keratoconus. Encyclopedia Contact Lens Practice, *2*(12):3–10, chapter 18, 1961.

Morrison, R. J., Kaufman, K. J., and Cerulli, E.: Oblique bitorics—a method to calculate and/or check prescriptions as indicated on the lensometer. J. Am. Optom. Assn., *36*(12):1068–1069, 1965.

Morse, W., and Wingo, G. M.: *Psychology and Teaching.* Chicago, Scott Foresman and Co., 1962.

Moss, H. I: Micro-lens prescribing. Opt. J. and Rev. Optom., *94*(3):36–40, 1957.

Moss, H. I.: The contour principle in corneal contact lens prescribing for keratoconus. J. Am. Optom. Assn., *30*(8):570–572, 1959.

Moss, H. I.: The scleral contact lens and its values in today's practice. Am. J. Optom. and Arch. Am. Acad. Optom., *36*(11):591–594, 1959.

Moss, H. I.: The contour principle. Encyclopedia Contact Lens Practice, *2*(8):51–67, chapter 8, 1961.

Moss, H. I.: Bifocal contact lenses—a review. Am. J. Optom. and Arch. Am. Acad. Optom., *39*(12):653–668, 1962.

Moss, H. I.: Confusion resulting from "on k" in corneal lens prescribing. Am. J. Optom. and Arch. Am. Acad. Optom., *39*(5):264–268, 1962.

Moss, H. I.: The haptic contact lens and its value in today's practice. Encyclopedia Contact Lens Practice, *3*(17):4–7, chapter 38, 1962.

Moss, H. I.: A review of small corneal lenses and the lens-cornea relationship. Am. J. Optom. and Arch. Am. Acad. Optom., *41*(10):609–615, 1964.

Moss, H. I.: Corneal contact lenses and myopia. Optom. Weekly, *57*(12):22–23, 1966.

Moss, H. I., and Brungardt, T. F.: *Fluorescein Studies, Corneal Contact Lenses.* Topeka, Kan., Duffens Contact Lens Co., 1963.

Moss, H. I., and Moss, H. L.: The complete contact lens practice. Optom. Weekly, *47*(35):1524–1525, 1956.

Mosse, P.: Underwater contact lenses. Brit. J. Phys. Opt., *21*(4):250–255, 1964.

Mueller-Welt, A.: Trial case fittings. Contacto, *1*(2):28–30, 1957.

Murrell, S. C., and Henderson, J. P.: Contact lenses, salts and intraocular tension. Contacto, *2*(6):145–1457, 1958.

Muth, C. R.: Nystagmus fitted with toric base curve lenses. Contacto, *5*(6):229–230, 1961.

Nagel, C., and Monical, J. B.: The design and development of a contact lens for underwater seeing. Am. J. Optom. and Arch. Am. Acad. Optom., *31*(9):468–472, 1954.

Neefe, C. W.: An approach to the design of a better convex edge contour for contact lenses. Contacto, *3*(9):273–275, 1959.

Neill, J. C.: Contact lens fitting in the United States. Am. J. Optom. and Arch. Am. Acad. Optom., *28*(12):616–623, 1951.

Neill, J. C.: Graduate education for contact lens fitting. Am. J. Optom. and Arch. Am. Acad. Optom., *33*(8):432–436, 1956.

Neill, J. C.: Contact lenses and the older patient, in *Vision of the Aging Patient,* Hirsch, M. J., and Wick, R. E. (eds.). Philadelphia, Chilton Book Company, pp. 257–263, 1960.

Neill, J. C.: A contact lens practitioner looks at corneal transparency. Contacto, *6*(8): 225–227, 1962.

Neill, J. C.: Contact lenses for young people, in *Vision of Children,* Hirsch, M. J., and Wick, R. E. (eds.). Philadelphia, Chilton Book Company, pp. 361–370, 1963.

Neill, J. C., and Hanna, J. J.: Study of the effect of various media on the radii of micro corneal contact lenses. Contacto, *7*(9):10–13, 1963.

Neitzel, D. J.: Evaluation of contact lens variables. Contacto, *3*(6):154–155, 1959.

Nevyast, J.: A biochemist looks at corneal transparency. Contacto, *6*(8):235–237, 1962.

Newman, B. Y.: Enthusiasm—the key to success with contact lens patients. Optom. Weekly, *55*(47):15–17, 1964.

Nierenberg, B. L.: Applied psychology and the contact lens patient. Opt. J. and Rev. Optom., *91*(1):29–32 and 50, 1954.

Nissel, G.: The second world survey. Contacto, *7*(8):20–26, 1963.

Nolan, J. A.: Progress of myopia and contact lenses. Contacto, *8*(1):25–26, 1964.

Norm, M. S.: Vital staining in practice using a mixed stain and alcian blue. Brit. J. Phys. Opt., *21*(4):293–298, 1964.

Norris, G.: A contact lens removal technique. Opt. J. and Rev. Optom., *98*(23):19, 1961.

Nupuf, J.: Subjective responses to queries on changes in visual acuity while wearing contact lenses. J. Am. Optom. Assn., *34*(4):297–306, 1962.

Obrig, T. E.: *Contact Lenses.* Philadelphia, Chilton Book Company, 1942.

Obrig, T. E., and Salvatori, P. L.: *Contact Lenses,* 3d Ed. New York, Obrig Laboratories, 1957.

Paige, N. A.: The power of positive suggestion in fitting contact lenses. Optom. Weekly, *55*(27):15–16, 1964.

Panter, I.: Legal aspects of fitting contact lenses. Contacto, *2*(1):27–31, 1958.

Pascal, J. I.: *Studies in Visual Optics.* St. Louis, C. V. Mosby Co., 1952.

Passmore, C.: Abrasions from corneal contact lenses. Contacto, *4*(11):489–491, 1960.

Pheiffer, C. H.: The contact lens characteristics for an optimal fit. J. Am. Optom. Assn., *32*(6):451–452, 1961.

Player, H. S.: An investigation on the use of contact lenses in sports. J. Am. Optom. Assn., *30*(1):33–36, 1958.

Player, H. S.: The contact lens field—a time for re-evaluation. Optom. Weekly, *52*(4): 167–169, 1961.

Poksay, R. A.: The personal diary of a new contact lens patient. Optom. Weekly, *50*(32):1554, 1959.

Pollock, E. D.: Basic principles and variables of the corneal type lens. Opt. J. and Rev. Optom., *92*(15):29–36, 1955.

Pollock, E. D.: Observations on the fitting of the micro-lens. Opt. J. and Rev. Optom., *93*(6):39–41 and 47, 1956.

Pollock, E. D.: Adjustments on corneal type lenses. J. Am. Optom. Assn., *29*(7):450–452, 1958.

Pollock, E. D.: Contact lenses and your practice. Contacto, *2*(3):75–77, 1958.

Pollock, E. D.: Changes in fluorescein patterns. Contacto, *3*(5):113–115, 1959.

Prior, J. A., and Silberstein, J. S.: *Physical Diagnosis—The History and Examination of the Patient.* St. Louis, C. V. Mosby Co., 1959.

Racusen, F. R., Corral, E., and McGee, T. F.: An exploratory investigation of factors associated with success or failure in contact lens wearing. Am. J. Optom. and Arch. Am. Acad. Optom., *41*(4):232–240, 1964.

Raiford, M. B. (ed.): *Contact Lens Management*. Boston, Little, Brown and Co., 1962.

Rengstroff, R. H.: Contact lens application and myopia research in the Army. Optom. Weekly, *56*(10):34–35, 1965.

Reynolds, A. E.: A practical fitting process for scleral contact lenses. Contacto, *1*(3): 45–48, 1957.

Reynolds, A. E.: Fitting a bifocal contact lens. Contacto, *2*(2):64–66, 1958.

Reynolds, A. E.: Anatomical and topographical considerations in contact lens fitting. Contacto, *4*(12):550–558, 1960.

Reynolds, A. E., and Kratt, H. J.: The photo-electronic keratoscope. Contacto, *3*(3): 53–59, 1959.

Richards, O. W.: Tinted contact lenses: a handicap for night driving. J. Am. Optom. Assn., *35*(6):494, 1964.

Richardson, E. F.: Importance of making contact lens adjustments in the office. Optom. Weekly, *57*(12):24, 1966.

Rochte, A. R.: A case in point—case record of a patient with retrolental fibroplasia fitted with a contact lens. Contacto, *4*(7):237–242, 1960.

Rosen, D. M.: Causes of contact lens wearing failure. Optom. Weekly, *54*(40):1877–1878, 1963.

Rosenbloom, A. A.: Contact lens research needs—a bold look ahead. Part I. Optom. Weekly, *52*(42):2107–2111, 1961.

Rosenbloom, A. A.: Contact lens research needs—a bold look ahead. Part II. Optom. Weekly, *52*(44):2149–2153, 1961.

Rosenwasser, H. M.: A case in point—the fitting of toric peripheral curve contact lenses. Contacto, *4*(2):59–61, 1960.

Rosenwasser, H. M.: Physiological considerations of corneal turgescence. Opt. J. and Rev. Optom., *97*(17):39–41, 1960.

Rottmann, J. H.: Corneal astigmatism and corneal lenses. Optom. Weekly, *53*(18): 839–841, 1962.

Rubin, L.: A device for measuring peripheral radii. Opt. J. and Rev. Optom., *99*(5): 44–46, 1962.

Rubinstein, D. M.: Contact lenses—a re-evaluation. Opt. J. and Rev. Optom., *89*(6): 36 and 74, 1952.

Rusnak, E. F.: Relationship of size and central thickness. Contacto, *3*(5):126–128, 1959.

Rybachok, O. G.: An anatomist looks at corneal transparency. Contacto, *6*(8):232–234, 1962.

Rycroft, B. W. (ed.): *Corneal Grafts*. St. Louis, C. V. Mosby Co., 1955.

Saks, S. J.: Fluctuations in refractive state in adapting, and long term contact lens wearers. J. Am. Optom. Assn., *37*(3):229–238, 1966.

Saliba, N.: Considerations in fitting contact lenses. Opt. J. and Rev. Optom., *87*(5): 37, 1950.

Saliba, N.: The decline of contact lenses. Opt. J. and Rev. Optom., *88*(4):54, 1951.

Saliba, N.: A case of keratoconus fitted with micro-lenses. Opt. J. and Rev. Optom., *94*(24):54, 1957.

Salvatori, P. L.: *A Scientific Method of Fitting Contact Lenses*. New York, Philip L. Salvatori, 1947.

Sarver, M. D.: Verification of contact lens power. Encyclopedia Contact Lens Practice, *4*(24):45–49, chapter 32, 1963.

Sarwar, M.: Contact lenses and corneal opacities. Am. J. Ophth., *34*(12):1747–1749, 1951.

Sarwar, M.: Medical uses of contact lenses. Brit. J. Phys. Opt., *8*(2):108–111, 1951.

Sato, T., and Magatani, H.: New approach to curvature calculation. Contacto, *2*(5): 120–127, 1958.

Sato, T., and Saito, N.: Contact lenses for babies and children. Contacto, *3*(12):419–424, 1959.

Schapero, M.: A corneal contact lens record form. Opt. J. and Rev. Optom., *89*(5):30–31, 1952.

Schapero, M.: New contact lens record form. Contacto, *3*(6):167–168, 1959.

Schapero, M.: A survey of current fitting techniques for corneal contact lenses. Am. J. Optom. and Arch. Am. Acad. Optom., *37*(10):533–546, 1960.

Schecter, L.: Some rules of thumb for bifocal contact lenses. Optom. Weekly, *50*(21): 1007–1108, 1959.

Schwartz, A., Glatt, L. (ed.): The human factor in contact lens insurance. Opt. J. and Rev. Optom., *96*(19):32–33, 1959.

Schwartz, A., and Pincus, A. R.: Legal aspects of insurance. Opt. J. and Rev. Optom., *96*(3):33–35, 1959.

Schwartz, A., and Glatt, L.: Contact lenses for children and adolescents—a survey. J. Am. Optom. Assn., *32*(2):143–146, 1960.

Scott, D., and Sirkis, A.: Increasing the wearing time of contact lenses. Optom. Weekly, *41*(35):1288–1289, 1950.

Sellers, F. J. E.: Corneal fit criteria—part 1. Contacto, *6*(9):257–259, 1962.

Sellers, F. J. E.: Bifocal contact lenses for all? Contacto, *7*(6):27–29, 1963.

Sellers, F. J. E.: Fenestrations first—not last. Contacto, *8*(2):17–18 and 23–30, 1964.

Sheiman, J.: Some pointers on fitting toric base contact lenses. Opt. J. and Rev. Optom., *99*(1):21–22, 1962.

Shlaifer, A.: Physiological aspects of corneal transparency. Contacto, *6*(8):238–241, 1962.

Shnider, H. A.: Diabetes mellitus and contact lenses. J. Am. Optom. Assn., *36*(8): 706–710, 1965.

Silberstein, I. W.: Contact lenses in industry. Am. J. Optom. and Arch. Am. Acad. Optom., *39*(3):111–129, 1962.

Silbert, M.: Minimum lid sensation as a contact lens fitting factor. Opt. J. and Rev. Optom., *92*(18):56–58, 1955.

Silbert, M.: Fitting a corneal lens for comfort following iridectomy. Opt. J. and Rev. Optom., *95*(4):41–44, 1958.

Silbert, M.: Contact lenses—case reports. Opt. J. and Rev. Optom., *97*(6):38, 1960.

Silbert, M.: How to get along with your contact lens laboratory. Opt. J. and Rev. Optom., *98*(9):33–36, 1961.

Silbert, M.: Comments on myopia control by contact lenses. Optom. Weekly, *53*(20): 961–963, 1962.

Silbert, M.: Cornea-limbus-scleral lens. Opt. J. and Rev. Optom., *99*(9):35–36, 1962.

Silbert, M.: Contact lens edges—contour and thickness. Contacto, *9*(1):28–33, 1965.

Silverstein, S. W.: Silvent contact lens design. Opt. J. and Rev. Optom., *90*(6):50–51, 1953.

Silverstein, S. W.: Case report of aniridia in a seven-year-old patient. Opt. J. and Rev. Optom., *91*(23):32–34, 1954.

Simmons, B. J.: You can sleep with contact lenses. Optom. Weekly, *49*(23):1062, 1958.

Simmons, E. F.: Contact lenses—helpful procedures. Opt. J. and Rev. Optom., *99*(4): 44, 1962.

Simpson, W.: Environmental factors involved in wearing contact lenses. Optom. Weekly, *46*(50):2067, 1955.

Skeffington, A. M.: Contact lenses in functional optometric application. Optom. Weekly, *50*(36):1743–1747, 1959.

Sloan, D. P.: A report on continuous contact lens wearing. Contacto, *4*(4):117–122, 1960.

Sloan, D. P.: A further report on continuous contact lens wearing. Contacto, *5*(1): 13–18, 1961.

Sloan, D. P.: A further report on continuous contact lens wearing. Contacto, *8*(1): 16–19, 1964.

Smelser, G. K.: Relation of factors involved in maintenance of optical properties of cornea to contact lens wear. Arch. Ophth., *47*(3):328–343, 1952.

Smelser, G. K., and Chen, D. K.: Physiological changes in the cornea induced by contact lenses. Arch. Ophth., *53*(5):676–679, 1955.

Smith, W.: Orthoptics in the adaptive procedure of contact lens cases. Opt. J. and Rev. Optom., *97*(9):37–38, 1960.

Smither, M.: Case in point. Contacto, *4*(1):25–26, 1960.

Soehnges, W. P.: Measuring corneal reflection for osmotic changes. Optom. Weekly, *48*(52):2427–2428, 1957.

Soehnges, W. P.: Comparative temperature measurements in the use of contact lenses. Contacto, *2*(3):86, 1958.

Soehnges, W. P.: Measurement of light reflection of the cornea to show osmotic changes. Contacto, *2*(2):53–56, 1958.

Soper, J. W., Sampson, W. G., and Girard, L. J.: Corneal topography, keratometry and contact lenses. Arch. Ophth., *67*(6):753–760, 1960.

Southall, J. P. C.: *Mirrors, Prisms, and Lenses—A Text-book of Geometrical Optics*, 3d Ed. New York, Dover Publications, 1964.

Sparer, J. P. (ed.): *Personality, Stress and Tuberculosis*. New York, International Universities Press, 1956.

Sperling, A.: *Psychology Made Simple*. Garden City, N. Y., Doubleday and Co., 1957.

Spring, T. F.: Aphakia and contact lenses. Contacto, *5*(1):5–8, 1961.

Spring, T. F.: Contact lenses and corneal effects. Contacto, *5*(5):185–186, 1961.

Steele, E.: Contact lens clinics of the London refractive hospitals. Am. J. Optom. and Arch. Am. Acad. Optom., *28*(11):560–563, 1951.

Steele, E.: The future of contact lenses. Opt. J. and Rev. Optom., *88*(6):35–36 and 40, 1951.

Steele, E.: Observation in the fitting of corneal contact lenses. Am. J. Optom. and Arch. Am. Acad. Optom., *36*(4):194–199, 1959.

Steele, E.: The control of eccentrically locating corneal contact lenses. Brit. J. Phys. Opt., *21*(4):205–208, 1964.

Steele, E.: The control of high riding corneal contact lenses. Contacto, *9*(3):6–8, 1965.

Stephens, W. B.: Contact lenses at body temperature. Am. J. Optom. and Arch. Am. Acad. Optom., *38*(6):358, 1961.

Stern, J.: An analysis of power changes on contact lenses. Part I. Adding minus. Opt. J. and Rev. Optom., *102*(3):27–31 and 34, 1965.

Stern, J.: An analysis of power changes on contact lenses. Part II. Effect on eye; lens verification, precorneal tear layer. Opt. J. and Rev. Optom., *102*(4):35–38, 1965.

Stern, J.: An analysis of power changes on contact lenses. Part III. Adding plus: suggested method for power changes. Opt. J. and Rev. Optom., *102*(5):48–49, 1965.

Strughold, H.: The sensitivity of cornea and conjunctiva of the human eye and use of contact lenses. Am. J. Optom. and Arch. Am. Acad. Optom., *30*(12):625–630, 1953.

Sullivan, J. C.: Office-centered contact lens adjustments. Optom. Weekly, *51*(8):379–380, 1960.

Swanson, W. L.: Results of edge contouring of contact lenses. Optom. Weekly, *51*(43): 2255–2257, 1960.

Taher, Z.: A modified method for curvature width measurement in corneal lenses. Contacto, *8*(2):11, 1964.

Tajiri, A.: Sclerals or corneals. J. Am. Optom. Assn., *36*(3):245–246, 1965.

Tajiri, A.: Dimple contact lenses. Am. J. Optom. and Arch. Am. Acad. Optom., *42*(4): 248–249, 1965.

Tarbis, R.: Your first contact lens patient. Contacto, *2*(3):83–85, 1958.

Tarbis, R.: Clinical observations on 33 contact lens patients. Contacto, *3*(10):311–313, 1959.

Thomas, C. I.: *The Cornea.* Springfield, Ill., Charles C. Thomas, 1955.

Thomas, P. F.: Basic concepts of corneal correction. J. Am. Optom. Assn., *32*(1):40–44, 1960.

Thomas, P. F., and Williams, O. A.: Notes on fitting contact micro-lenses. Am. J. Optom. and Arch. Am. Acad. Optom., *35*(7):373–375, 1958.

Thurmond, R. H.: Heterophoric patient. Contacto, *3*(6):164–165, 1959.

Toline, E., Baylor, E. R., and Shaw, E.: Contact lenses fitted to the eyes of fish. Am. J. Optom. and Arch. Am. Acad. Optom., *40*(4):140–142, 1963.

Tomlinson, K.: Contact lens practice: the early years. Brit. J. Phys. Opt., *21*(3):157–162, 1964.

Tortolero, J.: Corneal tissue changes following corneal contact lens wear. Contacto, *5*(5):161–173, 1961.

Tortolero, J.: Glaucoma and contact lenses. Contacto, *8*(2):6–10 and 31, 1964.

Tortolero, J., Wesley, N. K., and Bronstein, L.: *Fluorescein Staining—Characteristics of Corneal Insult.* Chicago, Plastic Contact Lens Co., 1959.

Tower, P.: Contact lenses for correction of myopia complicated by lesions of retina and choroid. Arch. Ophth., *38*(4):521–528, 1947.

Ullen, R. L.: Early visual development with implications for contact lens practice. Optom. Weekly, *51*(33):1719–1724, 1960.

Ullen, R. L.: Early visual development with implications for contact lens practice. Optom. Weekly, *51*(34):1765–1770, 1960.

Ullen, R. L.: A contact lens fitting procedure. Optom. Weekly, *53*(45):2225–2229, 1962.

Ullen, R. L.: Front versus back vertex power readings on contact lenses. J. Am. Optom. Assn., *34*(4):307–309, 1962.

Ullen, R. L.: Physiological factors involved in the fitting of contact lenses. Optom. Weekly, *53*(17):793–796, 1962.

Ullen, R. L.: A rationale on contact lens edge construction and inspection. Encyclopedia Contact Lens Practice, *3*(16):85–91, chapter 22, 1962.

Ullen, R. L.: Appearance of epithelial edema in fitting corneal lenses. Opt. J. and Rev. Optom., *100*(18):31–34, 1963.

Van Such, J. E.: Reducing lid tension with spectacles in fitting contact lenses to patients with keratoconus. Contacto, *4*(5):165, 1960.

Vanysek, J., and Altman, J.: Non-corrective uses of contact lenses. Contacto, *3*(8):213–218, 1959.

Vaughn, B. T.: Adjustments to minimize spectacle blur. Contacto, *2*(6):153–154, 1958.

Vaughn, D., Cook, R., and Asbury, T.: *General Ophthalmology,* 3d Ed. Los Altos, Calif., Lange Medical Publications, 1962.

Vics, I. I.: A report on 10 cases fitted with the Feinbloom self-centering corneal contact lens. Am. J. Optom. and Arch. Am. Acad. Optom., *28*(3):147–153, 1951.

Vics, I. I.: Hypnosis as a modality in contact lens fitting. Opt. J. and Rev. Optom., *97*(21):29–33, 1960.

Vodnoy, B. E.: The use of prism ballast contact lenses with triple truncation in hyperphoria. Optom. Weekly, *54*(45):2087–2088, 1963.

Vodnoy, B. E.: Some principles for corneal contact lens practice. Am. J. Optom. and Arch. Am. Acad. Optom., *42*(10):619–625, 1965.

Vogel, L. R.: A method of contact lens fitting. Optom. Weekly, *53*(12):533–535, 1962.

Voss, E. H., and Liberatore, J. C.: Fitting the apex of keratoconus. Contacto, *6*(7):212–214, 1962.

Voss, E. H., and Liberatore, J. C.: Psychological considerations and hypnosis in contact lens fitting. Contacto, *6*(6):164–167 and 172–173, 1962.

Wachs, H.: Clinical use of slit lamp in refining the fit of contact lenses. Contacto, *4*(3):89–92, 1960.

Waggoner, H. W.: Ocular prosthetics. J. Am. Optom. Assn., *37*(1):30–39, 1966.

Wakita, S.: Some factors for the determination of the size of contact lenses. Contacto, *6*(2):37–40, 1962.

Walton, J.: Education in contact lens practice. Brit. J. Phys. Opt., *21*(3):123–129, 1964.

Warren, E. F.: The fitting of contact lenses in optometric practice. J. Am. Optom. Assn., *27*(3):161–162, 1955.

Warren, E. F.: The fitting of contact lenses in optometric practice—Kruckenberg's spindle, Staehli's line, or k.p.'s? J. Am. Optom. Assn., *27*(4):227–228, 1955.

Warren, E. F.: Tropias and contact lenses. J. Am Optom. Assn., *29*(2):113–114, 1957.

Warren, E. F.: Detection of keratoconus. Contacto, *2*(1):32–34, 1958.

Warren, G. T., and Warren, E. F.: Reducing the angle of error and divergence. Opt. J. and Rev. Optom., *91*(16):33–36, 1954.

Warren, G. T., and Warren, E. F.: Contact lenses—patient handling and motivation. Opt. J. and Rev. Optom., *92*(8):38–39, 1955.

Wasserman, M. A.: The miniscule nt process in contact lenses. Optom. Weekly, *52*(19): 934–935, 1961.

Watkins, C. E.: The formulation and evaluation of contact lens cleaning solutions. Contacto, *6*(4):97–100, 1962.

Watkins, J. R.: Scllentecorel by the four "c" method. Contacto, *8*(1):27–38, 1964.

Watkins, J. R.: Corneal topography and contact lens relationships. J. Am. Optom. Assn., *37*(3):224–228, 1966.

Weber, J. M.: The use of contact illumination for improved contact lens management. J. Am. Optom. Assn., *35*(8):669–674, 1964.

Wechsler, S.: A study of magnification as applied to contact lenses. Contacto, *1*(2): 23–27, 1957.

Wechsler, S.: A study of magnification as applied to contact lenses. Contacto, *1*(3):49–50, 1957.

Weinstein, H. I.: FDA authority and responsibility for contact lenses. Opt. J. and Rev. Optom., *102*(23):24–26, 1965.

Weiss, H.: Contact lenses as a means for correction of astigmatism. Optom. Weekly, *52*(31):1511–1516, 1961.

Weiss, N. J.: Basic principles in contact lenses fitting. Am. J. Optom. and Arch. Am. Acad. Optom., *35*(12):613–628, 1958.

Weiss, S. G.: Some preliminary observations on the Touhy corneal lens. Am. J. Optom. and Arch. Am. Acad. Optom., *27*(8):404–406, 1950.

Weisser, S. D.: A specialized adjustment procedure with spinning tool. Opt. J. and Rev. Optom., *98*(6):39–40, 1961.

Weisser, S. D.: Contact lens inspection. Opt. J. and Rev. Optom., *100*(5):47, 1963.

Welsh, R. C.: Corneal contact lens trial sets for postoperative cataract patients. Arch. Ophth., *65*(3):427–432, 1961.

Welsh, R. C., Fall, E. E., and Ahorner, F.: Hand neutralization of aphakic-range contact lenses. Arch. Ophth., *73*(5):621–622, 1965.

Welt, A. M.: The Mueller Welt fluidless contact lens. Optom. Weekly, *41*(23):831–834, 1950.

Wesley, N. K.: Contact lenses as a diagnostic instrument. Optom. Weekly, *45*(41): 1647–1648, 1954.

Wesley, N. K.: The Wiesbaden scleral glass blown lens. Optom. Weekly, *48*(44):2071–2072, 1957.

Wesley, N. K.: Residual astigmatism. Contacto, *3*(9):269–271, 1959.

Wesley, N. K.: Factors affecting adhesion of contact lenses to the cornea. Contacto, *4*(3):97–99, 1960.

Wesley, N. K.: A new contact lens for toroidal eyes. Opt. J. and Rev. Optom., *97*(20): 39–43, 1960.

Wesley, N. K.: Telecon lens—a case history. Contacto, *4*(1):7–15, 1960.

Wesley, N. K.: Inside toric curve contact lens fitting. Contacto, *5*(1):31–45, 1961.

Wesley, N. K.: Impact of contact lenses on a national basis. Am. J. Optom. and Arch. Am. Acad. Optom., *39*(5):269–274, 1962.

Wesley, N. K.: More facts about toric base curve lenses. Contacto, *6*(1):25–30, 1962.

Wesley, N. K.: Corneal contour and contact lenses. Am. J. Optom. and Arch. Am. Acad. Optom., *40*(3):150–155, 1963.

Wesley, N. K.: Non-index bifocal. Contacto, *8*(1):22–23, 1964.

Wesley, N. K., and Jessen, G. N.: The fluidless contact lens. Optom. Weekly, *42*(32): 1265–1266, 1951.

Wesley, N. K., and Jessen, G. N.: Symptoms and corrections in fitting contact lenses. Optom. Weekly, *42*(44):1713–1717, 1951.

Wesley, N. K., and Jessen, G. N.: *Contact Lens Practice.* Chicago, Professional Press, 1953.

Wesley, N. K., and Jessen, G. N.: Orthoptics and contact lenses. Contacto, *2*(6):149–150, 1958.

Wesley, N. K., and Jessen, G. N.: *Basic Sphercon Contact Lens Fitting Manual,* 8th Ed. Chicago, Plastic Contact Lens Co., 1959.

Westsmith, R. A.: Patients' acceptance of corneal microlenses—a study based on a questionnaire survey, Am. J. Ophth., *46*(6):869–872, 1958.

Westsmith, R. A.: Uses of a monocular contact lens. Am. J. Ophth., *46*(1-part I):81, 1958.

Wilhelm, W. D.: A case in point—use of bitoric contact lenses. Contacto, *5*(5):175–176, 1961.

Williams, O. A.: Notes on psychological fitting in contact lens practice. Am. J. Optom. and Arch. Am. Acad. Optom., *37*(11):588–591, 1960.

Williams, O. A.: Principles associated with peripheral curvature in corneal lens design. Encyclopedia Contact Lens Practice, *2*(12):68–75, chapter 8, 1961.

Woo Kong, B.: A new mounting method for optically measuring contact lens surfaces. Optom. Weekly, *50*(16):760–761, 1959.

Woolf, D.: Social and psychological impact of contact lenses on children and youth. J. Am. Optom. Assn., *34*(14):1138–1143, 1963.

Woolf, H. D.: The Woolf slit lamp inspection adapter for contact lenses. Optom. Weekly, *52*(23):1165, 1961.

Worst, J. G. F.: A new method for fixing diagnostic contact lenses. Am. J. Ophth., *48*(6):849–850, 1959.

Wray, A.: Relationship between contact lenses and aniseikonia—a case report. Optom. Weekly, *53*(22):1031–1034, 1962.

Yonenaga, N. T.: Importance of tear flow in relation to contact lenses. Contacto, *5*(9): 293–298, 1961.

Yonenaga, N. T.: Lacrimal characteristics in contact lens fitting. Contacto, *6*(4):103–105, 1961.

York, M. A., Jr.: *Laboratory Manual for Contact Lenses.* Memphis, Tenn., Southern College of Optometry, 1964.

Zabner, L.: The economics of contact lens fitting. Opt. J. and Rev. Optom., *90*(2):32–33, 1953.

Zabner, L.: Some basic concepts of contact lenses. Optom. Weekly, *46*(6):217–219, 1955.

Index

C

G

H

S

U

V

W

X, Y, Z

THE AUTHORS

Drs. Irving P. Filderman and Paul F. White are well known in the ophthalmic field as practitioners, educators, and authors of many articles.

Dr. Filderman graduated from Southern College of Optometry in 1939 and holds a Masters Degree in Education from Memphis State University. In 1946, as Professor of Optometry, he taught the first contact lens and subnormal vision courses introduced at Southern College of Optometry, and was affiliated with the college until 1952. Dr. Filderman is a Fellow of the American Academy of Optometry and a Diplomate of its Contact Lens and Subnormal Vision Section. His contact lens and subnormal vision lens inventions are recognized and patented in countries throughout the world. In addition to continued research, Dr. Filderman maintains a private practice in Memphis, Tennessee.

Dr. White graduated from The Massachusetts College of Optometry in 1961, and has done postgraduate work at several colleges and universities. Along with his extensive research and writing about contact lenses and subnormal vision aids, Dr. White maintains a private practice. He is Assistant Professor and Chief of the Contact Lens Department of The Massachusetts College of Optometry, Boston, Massachusetts. Dr. White is also Director of the Contact Lens Section of The Massachusetts Optometric Clinic, in Boston.